Targeted Radionuclide Tumor Therapy

Torgny Stigbrand • Jörgen Carlsson
Gregory P. Adams
Editors

Targeted Radionuclide Tumor Therapy

Biological Aspects

Springer

Editors
Torgny Stigbrand
University of Umea
Department of Immunology
Umea, Sweden

Gregory P. Adams
Fox Chase Cancer Center
Department of Medical Oncology
Philadelphia, USA

Jörgen Carlsson
Uppsala University
Rudbeck Laboratory
Uppsala, Sweden

ISBN 978-90-481-7956-5 e-ISBN 978-1-4020-8696-0

Printed on acid-free paper

9 8 7 6 5 4 3 2 1

springer.com

Preface

The last three decades have provided opportunities to explore the potential of treating malignant diseases with antibodies or other targeting molecules labelled with nuclides. While considerable advances have been reported, there is still a significant amount of work left to accomplish before our ambitions can be achieved.

It now seems timely to review the accomplishments achieved to date and to clarify the challenges that remain. The choice of radionuclide, the conjugation procedure employed, and the selection of suitable targets were early issues that were faced by our field that still persist, however we can now tackle these obstacles with significantly better insight. The expanding array of new targeting molecules (recombinant antibodies, peptides and agents based upon alternate scaffolds) may increase the therapeutic efficacy or even modify the radiation sensitivity of the targeted tumor cell. The title of this book "Targeted Radionuclide Tumour Therapy – Biological Aspects" was selected to reinforce the concept that a major focus of this volume was devoted to understanding the biological effects of targeting and radiation. These important issues have not previously been the primary focus in this context. Furthermore, our rapidly expanding knowledge of different types of cell death and the increasingly likely existence of cancer stem cells suggests to us that even more efficient approaches in targeting might be possible in the future.

The development of targeted therapy is a true multidisciplinary enterprise involving physician scientists from the fields of nuclear medicine, radiation therapy, diagnostic radiology, surgery, gynaecology, pathology and medical oncology/haematology. It also involves many preclinical scientists working with experimental animal models, immunochemistry, recombinant antibody technologies, radiochemistry, radiation physics (dosimetry) and basic cell biology including the study of cell signalling pathways and the mechanisms of cellular death.

Certainly several challenges remain in bringing targeted therapy into mainstream of treatment modalities, but in many of the chapters significant improvements in targeting efficiency are observed and may indicate future efficacy and acceptance, maybe not as a single treatment modality, but in combination with other strategies.

It is the ambition of the editors to enable, with this volume, deeper insights in the process of improving targeted therapy for this diverse group of scientists. Clearly, some of the obstacles to gaining wider clinical acceptance might partly be related to this necessity of multidisciplinary collaborations. A number of disciplines, many of them mentioned above, have to both collaborate and coordinate with each other in order to control the chain of judgement necessary for the treatment of each patient. All these requirements may not always be available or easy to accomplish. This is a management paradigm shift, which usually would take some time. However, we hope that the chapters in this book will convince you, the reader, that a critical mass of knowledge regarding how to effectively use targeted radionuclide therapy has been accumulated. We believe, and hope that you will agree, that the time now has come when targeted therapy can soon be added to standard oncology treatment regimens.

As editors we would also like to express our sincere gratitude to all the authors that contributed to this book.

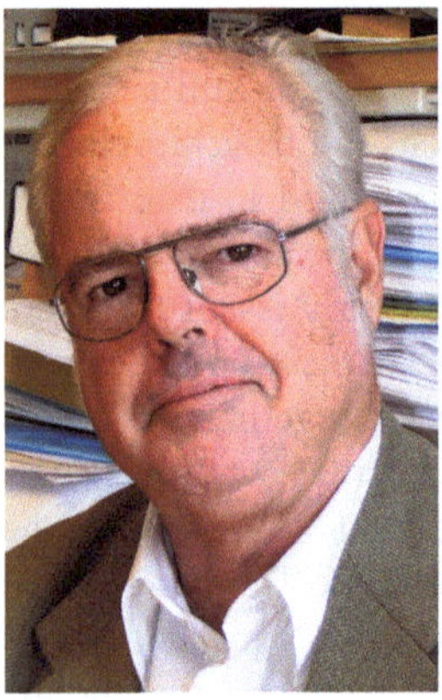

Torgny Stigbrand

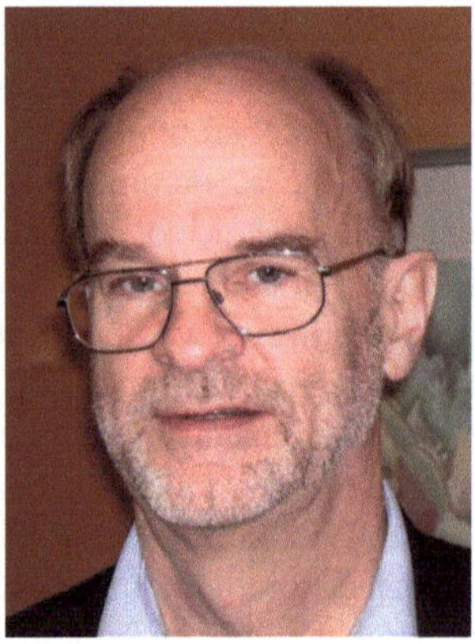

Jörgen Carlsson

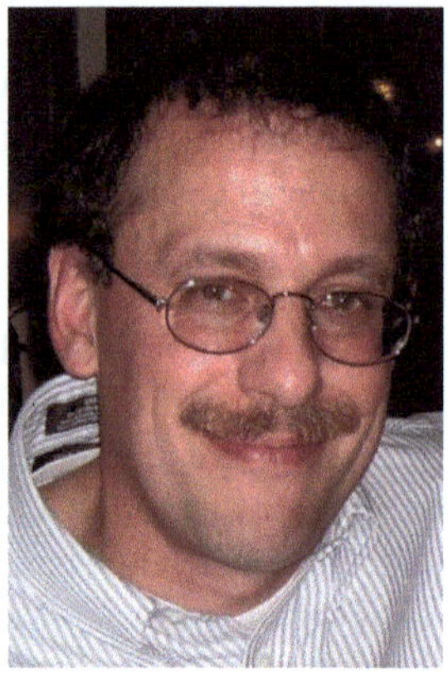

Gregory Adams

Contents

Contributors

Adams, Gregory P., Ph.D.
Department of Medical Oncology, Fox Chase Cancer Center, 333 Cottman Ave, Philadelphia, PA 19111, USA

Bruland, Øyvind S., M.D., Ph.D.
Faculty of Medicine, University of Oslo and Department of Oncology, The Norwegian Radium Hospital, N-0310 Oslo, Norway

Carlsson, Jörgen, Ph.D.
Department of Oncology, Radiology and Clinical Immunology, Rudbeck Laboratory, Uppsala University, SE-751 85, Uppsala, Sweden

Collis, Spencer J., Ph.D.
DNA Damage Response Laboratory, Cancer Research UK, Clare Hall Laboratories, Blanche Lane, South Mimms, EN6 3LD, UK

Jostein, Dahle, Ph.D.
Department of Radiation Biology, The Norwegian Radium Hospital, N-0310 Oslo, Norway

De Jong, Marion, Ph.D.
Department of Nuclear Medicine, Erasmus MC, Room V-218,'s Gravendijkwal 230, 3015 CE Rotterdam, The Netherlands

de Visser, Monique, Ph.D., Department of Nuclear Medicine, Erasmus MC,'s Gravendijkwal 230, 3015 CE Rotterdam, The Netherlands

Ekerljung, Lina, Ph.D.-student
Department of Oncology, Radiology and Clinical Immunology, Rudbeck Laboratory, Uppsala University, SE-751 85, Uppsala, Sweden

Eriksson, David, Ph.D.
Department of Immunology, Clinical Microbiology, University of Umeå, SE-901 85, Umeå, Sweden

Gedda, Lars, Ph.D.
Department of Oncology, Radiology and Clinical Immunology, Rudbeck Laboratory, Uppsala University, SE-751 85, Uppsala, Sweden

Johansson, Lennart, Ph.D.
Department of Radiation Physics, University of Umeå, SE-901 85, Umeå, Sweden

Joiner, Michael C., Ph.D.
Department of Radiation Oncology, Wayne State University, Gershenson Radiation Oncology Center, 4100 John R, Detroit, MI 48201–2013, USA

Krenning, Eric P., M.D., Ph.D.
Department of Nuclear Medicine, Erasmus MC, Rotterdam, The Netherlands

Krueger, Sarah A., Ph.D.
Department of Radiation Oncology, William Beaumont Hospital, 3811 W. Thirteen Mile Rd, 105-RI, Royal Oak, MI 48073–0213, USA

Kwekkeboom, Dik J., M.D.
Department of Nuclear Medicine, Erasmus MC,'s Gravendijkwal 230, 3015 CE Rotterdam, The Netherlands

Larsen, Roy H., Ph.D.
Department of Radiation Biology, The Norwegian Radium Hospital, N-0310 Oslo, Norway

Lee, Sze-Ting, Ph.D.-student
Department of Nuclear Medicine and Centre for PET; Department of Medicine, University of Melbourne; and Ludwig Institute for Cancer Research, Austin Hospital, Heidelberg, Victoria, 3084, Australia

Lennartsson, Johan, Ph.D.
Ludwig Institute for Cancer Research, Uppsala University, Box 595, SE-751 24, Uppsala, Sweden

Lundqvist, Hans, Ph.D.
Department of Oncology, Radiology and Clinical Immunology, Rudbeck Laboratory, Uppsala University, SE-751 85, Uppsala, Sweden

Marples, Brian, Ph.D.
Department of Radiation Oncology, William Beaumont Hospital, 3811 W. Thirteen Mile Rd, 105-RI, Royal Oak, MI 48073–0213, USA

Frejd, Fredrik Y., Ph.D.
Affibody AB, Voltavägen 13 Box 20137, SE-161 02 Bromma, Sweden

Olsen, Dag Rune, Ph.D.
Department of Radiation Biology, The Norwegian Radium Hospital, N-0310 Oslo, Norway

Prise, Kevin M., Ph.D.
Professor of Radiation Biology, Centre for Cancer Research and Cell Biology, Queen's University Belfast, 97 Lisburn Rd, Belfast, BT9 7BL, UK

Riklund, Katrine, M.D., Ph.D.
Department of Diagnostic Radiology, University of Umeå, SE-901 85, Umeå, Sweden

Scott, Andrew M., M.D., Ph.D.
Department of Nuclear Medicine and Centre for PET; Department of Medicine, University of Melbourne; and Ludwig Institute for Cancer Research, Austin Hospital, Heidelberg, Victoria, 3084, Australia

Sgouros, George, Ph.D.
The Russel H. Morgan Department of Radiology and Radiological Science Johns Hopkins University, School of Medicine, Baltimore, Maryland, USA

Stenerlöw, Bo, Ph.D.
Department of Oncology, Radiology and Clinical Immunology, Rudbeck Laboratory, Uppsala University, SE-751 85, Uppsala, Sweden

Stigbrand, Torgny, M.D., Ph.D.
Department of Immunology, Clinical Microbiology, University of Umeå, SE-90185, Umeå, Sweden

Tolmachev, Vladimir, Ph.D.
Department of Oncology, Radiology and Clinical Immunology, Rudbeck Laboratory, Uppsala University, SE-751 85, Uppsala, Sweden

Valkema, Roelf, M.D.
Department of Nuclear Medicine, Erasmus MC,'s Gravendijkwal 230, 3015 CE Rotterdam, The Netherlands

Verwijnen, Suzanne M., Ph.D.
Department of Nuclear Medicine, Erasmus MC,'s Gravendijkwal 230, 3015 CE Rotterdam, The Netherlands

Chapter 1
Introduction to Radionuclide Therapy

Jörgen Carlsson[1], Torgny Stigbrand[2], and Gregory P. Adams[3]

Summary This introductory chapter is written for those who are new to the field and desire a short overview of the present status of clinical and preclinical radionuclide therapy. In particular, this chapter provides an overview of the radiophysical concepts and key aspects of dosimetry and treatment planning that are beyond the scope of this book's focus on biological aspects of radionuclide therapy. Finally, a discussion on the choice of radionuclides and the availability of radiopharmaceuticals is provided.

The Editors View

The editors consider radionuclide therapy, to a large extent, as a potentially powerful method to eradicate disseminated tumor cells and small metastases. In contrast, bulky tumors and large metastases will likely have to be treated with surgery, external radiation therapy or chemotherapy before the remaining tumor cells might be reasonably treated with radionuclide therapy. The promising therapeutic results for hematological tumors [1], see also chapter 20, provide a reasonable expectation that radionuclide therapy will ultimately be effective for the treatment of disseminated cells from solid tumors.

Significant advances have recently been made in the characterization of new molecular target structures (chapters 2, 3, 7, 11, 18 and 20) and Fig. 1.1 schematically illustrates this. Furthermore, there is an increased knowledge in the pharmacokinetics, cellular processing and principles for modification of the radionuclide uptake for different types of targeting agents (chapters 4–8, 10, 11, 18 and 20).

[1]Unit of Biomedical Radiation Sciences, Department of Oncology, Radiology and Clinical Immunology, Rudbeck Laboratory, Uppsala University, SE-751 85, Uppsala, Sweden

[2]Department of Immunology, Clinical Microbiology, University of Umeå, SE-90185, Umeå, Sweden

[3]Department of Medical Oncology, Fox Chase Cancer Center, Philadelphia, PA 19111, USA

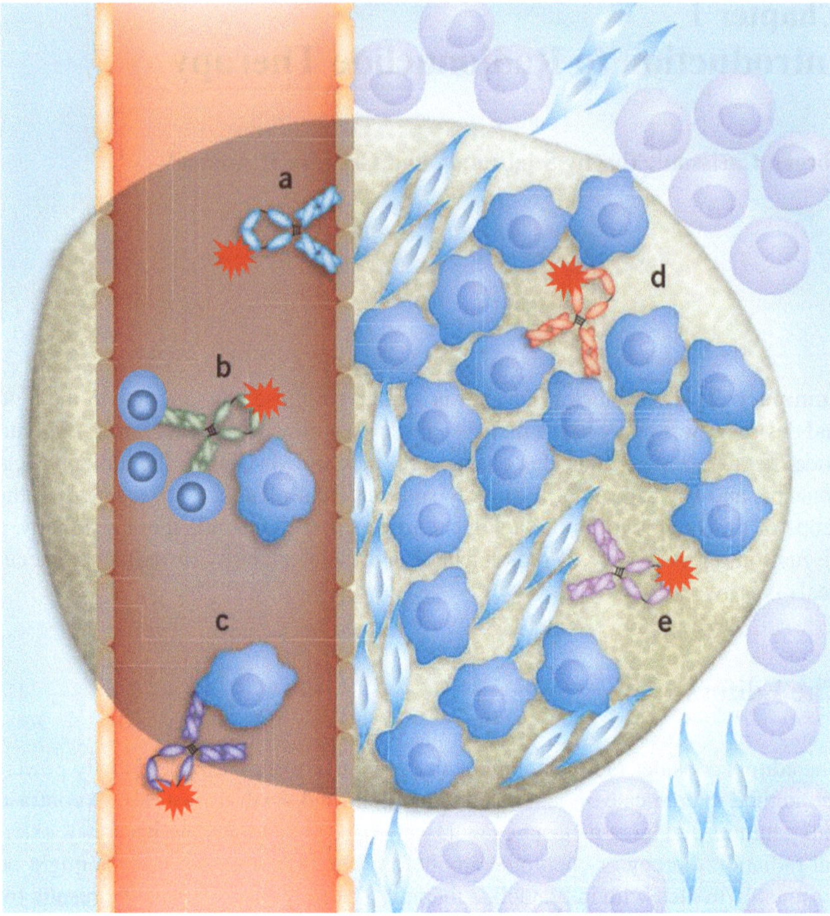

Fig. 1.1 Schematic drawing of potential targets for radionuclide therapy in a primary tumor or metastasis area. The radionuclide labelled targeting agents (e.g. monoclonal antibodies) can be used to target cancer-associated blood vessels (a), lymphoma or leukemia cell associated targets (e.g. CD20) in the blood flow (b), growth factor or other receptors on disseminated cells from a solid tumour (c) or on such cells that already have formed metastases (d). Also stroma cells and matrix components in the tumor area can be targets (e). The red stars indicate radioactive nuclides on the antibodies (Modified from [2]. With permission from the Nature Publishing Group)

There is also improved understanding of the factors of importance for the choice of appropriate radionuclides with respect to their decay properties and the therapeutic applications (chapters 7–11 and 20). Taken together, this suggests to the editors that this field is on the verge of experiencing major clinical advances.

However, we still need additional knowledge about the effects of low dose-rate (<1 Gy/h) radiation (chapter 16), programmed cell death (e.g. apoptosis) (chapter 12), cell cycle disturbances (chapter 14), bystander effects (chapter 17) and hyper radiosensitivity (chapter 19) for various tumor cell types and for critical normal tissues exposed to targeted radionuclide therapy. Our knowledge in the area of tolerance doses for normal tissues when the radiation is delivered at low dose-rate is also very limited.

The disparate effects resulting from applying different qualities of radiation, e.g. low- versus high-LET, is also an interesting aspect that deserves further investigation (chapters 9–11). Furthermore, new concepts, such as the assumed existence of cancer stem cells (chapter 15) and possibilities to enhance the effects of targeted radionuclide therapy using various agents, such as chemotherapy agents and tyrosine kinase inhibitors (chapter 18), must be considered to better exploit the rapidly emerging knowledge of basic tumor biology. A striking example of that is the possibility for "double action" (chapter 13) or "autosensitization" (chapter 18) in which the targeting agent not only delivers therapeutically active radionuclides to tumor associated antigens and receptors, but also, simultaneously radiosensitizes the targeted tumor cells by triggering an intracellular signaling cascade (e.g. one that blocks radiation induced DNA-repair).

This book examines the topics mentioned above. This is important because in order for the field of radionuclide therapy to mature from one associated with palliation to one capable of curing patients with advanced malignancies it will be necessary to consider the basic biological factors that are believed to determine the outcome of radionuclide therapy.

Disseminated Tumor Cells and Radionuclide Therapy

As mentioned above, surgery and external radiation therapy are the major treatment modalities used for primary tumors and large metastases. Chemotherapy is used for disseminated disease and may be curative in cases of lymphomas, testicular tumors and tumors in the pediatric group or in solid tumors when used in combination with other modalities. However, in the vast majority of cases, there is no curative treatment available for the quantitatively large groups of patients with disseminated adenocarcinomas (e.g. breast, prostate, colorectal, lung and ovarian tumors) and squamous cell carcinomas (e.g. lung, esophagus and head-neck tumors). For most of these patients, a palliative effect and/or prolonged survival can at best be achieved with chemotherapy. This is also true for malignant gliomas and various other types of disseminated tumors, e.g. malignant melanomas and neuroendocrine tumors. Other, or complementary, treatment modalities seem therefore to be necessary to achieve considerable improvements in the treatment of the common types of disseminated malignant diseases, e.g. immunotherapy, anti-angiogenesis therapy, gene therapy or radionuclide therapy or possibly combinations of these (Fig. 1.2).

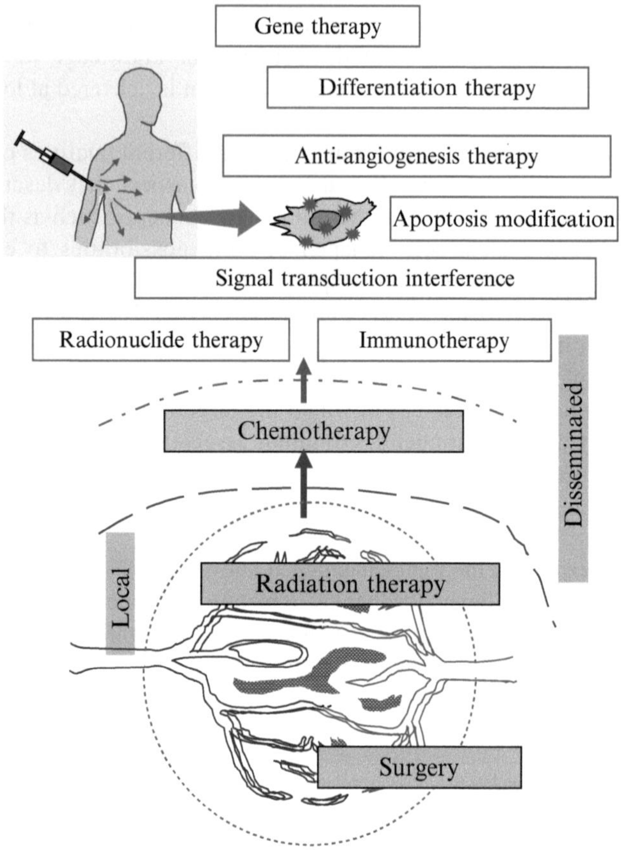

Fig. 1.2 Schematic illustration of strategies for tumor therapy. Surgery and external radiation therapy form the basis when locally growing tumor masses are treated. Chemotherapy in various forms is applied when there is tumor cell dissemination (symbolically shown above the dashed line). New therapy approaches (indicated with red frames above the dash-dotted line) will be tried when chemotherapy is not effective in its present forms. The new approaches are based on e.g. signal transduction interference with kinase inhibitors or modification of apoptotic processes. Some general and "biology-based" concepts are immunotherapy, differentiation therapy, anti-angiogenesis therapy and gene therapy. Radionuclide therapy is based on the same effect mechanism as external radiation therapy, namely induction of severe DNA-damage, and is therefore a form of radiotherapy. However, radionuclide therapy is placed among the new forms of "biology-based" therapies because it is dependent to a large extent on antigen and receptor expression and the biological factors regulating that (Modified from [45]. With permission from Elsevier Science Ltd.)

Present Status of Radionuclide Therapy

Chapter 20 in this book provides an in depth overview of the present status of clinical radionuclide therapy and we can also recommend recent reviews on the subject [2–6]. Although radionuclide therapy has been available for many years, few methods are routinely used on a large scale. The exceptions are ^{131}I iodide, which has been used for a long time for therapy of thyroid cancer [5, 7, 8] and ^{32}P-orthophosphate for therapy of polycythemia and thrombocythemia [9, 10]. However, recently major successes have been achieved with the targeted radionuclide therapy of lymphomas (reviewed in chapter 20). Radiolabeled anti-CD20 antibodies Bexxar (^{131}I) and Zevalin (^{90}Y) provide significant improvement of response rate in comparison to use of the non-radiolabeled corresponding antibodies [1, 11], suggesting to us that this approach may soon experience more widespread use.

Other examples of recent successes with radiopharmaceuticals include ^{131}I or ^{125}I labeled MIBG (meta-iodobenzylguanidine) for treatment of pheochromocytoma and neuroblastoma [12–14] and the promising attempts to use ^{177}Lu labeled somatostatin analogues for treatment of neuroendocrine tumors [15–17] (see also chapter 7). Palliative treatments of skeletal metastases are routinely performed using radioactive calcium or phosphate analogues or other substances [18–20] and new approaches applying high-LET radiation have also been attempted as described in chapters 9 and 10.

In cases when the absorbed radiation dose to bone marrow stem cells is estimated to be too high, it has been necessary to prepare for stem cell transplantation prior to radionuclide therapy or combined chemo- and radionuclide therapy. This has, for example, been the case when large amounts of β-emitting radionuclides have been given for treatments of lymphomas and has been associated with favorable outcomes when stem cell transplantation was used in combination with high-dose chemotherapy and systemic radiotherapy [21, 22].

However, more research is necessary concerning advantages and disadvantages of stem cell transplantation in combination with radionuclide therapy. Actually, the need for stem cell transplantation will probably be much lower, or even eliminated, when short range α- and ß-emitters can be delivered with targeting agents that give a higher degree of specificity for tumor cell uptake.

Clinical Versus Preclinical Results

During the past two decades significant amounts of clinical and preclinical research have been devoted to targeted radionuclide therapy using radiolabeled monoclonal antibodies and receptor binding agents specific for CD antigens, somatostatin receptors, EGFR-family receptors and a range of other tumor-associated targets. Furthermore, various forms of antibody fragments, peptides and other molecules have also been employed (chapters 2–7 and 20). Only a few clinical studies have demonstrated a significant number of complete remissions. Thus, the potential for long-term cure has been limited. The best clinical results so far have been achieved for the treatment of lymphomas [1, 11].

However, there is enormous potential for improved clinical outcomes using radionuclide therapy [4]. Preclinical research has demonstrated the potential for cure of both primary and disseminated tumors [23–28] (see also references in chapter 18) and such studies have enabled a selection of appropriate radionuclides and stimulated the development of a variety of new compounds. However the problem of a limited knowledge concerning the way to successfully transfer preclinical successes to the clinical setting remains.

Choice of Radionuclides

While it may not be oblivious to individuals not actively involved in the field of nuclear medicine, the choice of radionuclide is a very important consideration. Several types of radionuclides are suitable for therapy and these are well reviewed in chapter 8. The three major groups are β-particle emitting radionuclides (e.g. ^{67}Cu, ^{90}Y, ^{131}I, ^{177}Lu, ^{186}Re and ^{188}Re), Auger electron cascades (e.g. ^{111}In and ^{125}I) and α-particle emitting radionuclides (e.g. ^{211}At, ^{212}Bi, ^{213}Bi, ^{225}Ac and ^{227}Th). High-energy β-particles, such as ^{90}Y and ^{188}Re, are not efficient for killing single disseminated cells or small metastases, since only a small fraction of the electron energy will be deposited in such small targets. Most of the energy will instead travel beyond the tumor target to be absorbed in surrounding, often healthy, tissues. High-energy β particles might on the other hand be important for treatment in cases of non-uniform radioactivity distribution in large tumor areas. Irradiation from the targeted cells will then enable a more uniform dose-distribution and potentially elicit therapeutic effects on non-targeted tumor cells [29, 30]. In addition, it might be advantageous to use radionuclide cocktails to minimize the impact of heterogeneity [31].

Radionuclides emitting low energy β-particles such as ^{67}Cu, ^{131}I and ^{177}Lu and α particles (chapter 8) (or short-range electrons [32]) are options for treatment of small tumor deposits or even single disseminated tumor cells. However, a comparatively large amount of radionuclides per cell is needed when low energy β-particles (or low energy electrons) are used, thereby requiring a well-developed targeting process. By using α-particle emitting nuclides, or suitable Auger-electron emitters if nuclear localization is possible (chapter 11), fewer radionuclides per cell are needed. Recently, principles for local α-particle cascades were described whereby two or more α particles are emitted almost instantaneously and are therefore likely to contribute to the radiation dose in the vicinity of the site of the original decay (chapters 9 and 10).

The physical half-life of the radionuclides should preferably be in the same order of magnitude as the biological half-life of the radionuclide or the radionuclide conjugate. An overly long physical half-life increases the amount of radionuclides that must be delivered to the tumor cells to achieve therapeutic levels of decays before excretion. An extremely short physical half-life may not allow sufficient time for the tumor-targeting process to take place, resulting in the majority of the radioactive decays occurring in the vicinity of healthy, and often sensitive, tissues. It seems reasonable to assume that the most suitable physical half-lives range from a few hours up to a few days when targeting of disseminated cells is desired. Longer physical half-lives (up to one or a few weeks) might be needed to achieve significant uptake in solid tumor masses.

Dosimetry and Treatment Planning

The radiophysical and technical aspects of targeted radionuclide therapy are important subjects but are not the focus of this book. Imaging techniques are briefly mentioned in a few chapters and dosimetry is not at all discussed. These subjects are instead covered by review articles [33] and other books [34–40]. However, as these are important considerations in radionuclide therapy a short overview of key aspects of dosimetry and treatment planning is provided below.

Tissue and organ level. Radionuclides associated with radiopharmaceuticals of therapeutic interest are taken up and excreted in a variety of ways in tumor cells and normal tissues. There is a continuous redistribution of radionuclides in the body and they are typically ultimately eliminated from the body, primarily by renal and faecal excretion. It is, of course, important to visualize and quantify the varying distributions.

The dosimetry used today is mainly based on conventional planar scintigraphy. It is highly desirable to improve the methods for quantification of radionuclide uptake in normal tissues and tumor areas and to use more quantitative methods. This can be achieved through the use of photon or positron emitting radionuclides suitable for SPECT [41] or PET [42, 43] imaging (SPECT = Single Photon Emission Computed Tomography, PET = Positron Emission Tomography), thereby making reliable dosimetry and radionuclide treatment planning possible. The PET technique is especially well suited for this.

For treatment planning, radionuclides intended for imaging should be used prior to radionuclide therapy. However, these radionuclides can also be used during therapy in order to allow calculations or corrections of achieved radiation doses. Suitable radionuclides for SPECT include ^{99m}Tc, ^{111}In and ^{123}I. ^{111}In and ^{123}I can also be used as SPECT-tracers in planning for therapy with radiometals and radiohalogens, respectively. Suitable radionuclides for PET include ^{18}F, ^{64}Cu, ^{68}Ga, ^{76}Br, ^{86}Y, ^{110}In and ^{124}I. The metals ^{64}Cu, ^{68}Ga, ^{86}Y and ^{110}In and the halogens ^{76}Br and ^{124}I can be used as PET-tracers in planning for therapy with radiometals and radiohalogens, respectively. There are also radionuclides, such as ^{177}Lu, that simultaneously deliver both therapeutically-relevant radiation doses through the emitted β-particles and photons capable of being monitored in a gamma camera.

The mean absorbed dose to normal tissues, primary tumors and large metastases can be estimated in this manner with reasonably high levels of accuracy and the results can be verified and supplemented, at least in experimental studies, using activity measurements taken on excised tissue samples. However, the dose to single disseminated tumor cells can only be roughly estimated. There is also a need for improved dosimetry, especially for determining the dose to bone marrow, which is often a critical dose-limiting organ in radionuclide therapy. The strategy with targeted radionuclide therapy will be, as it is for external radiotherapy, to exploit the full tolerance radiation dose of critical normal tissues and thereby to maximize the amount given to the tumor cells.

The mean absorbed dose to large solid tumor masses and to critical normal tissues can be estimated reasonably well using the MIRD-formulation (MIRD = Medical Internal Radiation Dose) [34, 38, 44] using data from SPECT or PET studies. The amount of radionuclides excreted from the body can also be estimated by measurements of urine, faeces and, in some cases, by analyses of the remaining radioactivity in the body. Individual treatment planning should be routinely performed before radionuclide therapy to minimize the risk for under- or overdosing. However, it is necessary to consider that the kinetics of a radiopharmaceutical drug may in some cases be changed from the administration of a small test activity for treatment planning to the administration of larger amounts suitable for therapy.

It is possible that the absorbed dose to the tumor cells, in many cases, has been too low due to unfavorable pharmacokinetics of the therapeutic agent. Actually, the absorbed doses necessary for successful radionuclide therapy are not well known, nor are the tolerance doses for normal tissues. Studies regarding radiobiological effects have mainly been performed using external radiation generally with dose rates of about 1–2 Gy/min or more. In contrast, radionuclide therapy yields low dose rates, most often below 1 Gy/h (see chapter 16), making the use of external radiation derived absorbed dose values and tolerances questionable in these applications.

Cellular level. The radiation dose to single disseminated tumor cells can possibly only be estimated if representative samples of such cells are isolated from the body, e.g. by purification from the blood or by careful analysis of such cells from biopsies. Reasonable estimates of variations in dose at the cellular level can probably be achieved through computer calculations when the average amount of bound radionuclide is known. Knowledge of the subcellular radionuclide distribution will likely also be critical, especially for radionuclides emitting short-range particles.

For high-LET (LET = Linear Energy Transfer) particles, such as Auger electrons and α particles, microdosimetric concepts must be considered. Identical macroscopic radiation doses calculated with MIRD formalism can give quite different biological effects depending on the subcellular localization of the radionuclides.

Availability of Radiopharmaceuticals

An additional consideration that must be addressed is the potential reluctance of the pharmaceutical industry to produce radiopharmaceuticals. This is in part due to limited shelf life resulting from the physical half-life of the radionuclides and to complications associated with radiolysis during storage. It is our belief that these concerns may be solved in the future if the pharmaceutical industry focuses on producing non-radioactive substances designed for simple and effective radioactive labeling at the local hospital.

The substances could have a chelate coupled to them (chapter 8), as is presently the case for the somatostatin analogue octreoscan (chapter 7) and certain antibody preparations (chapter 4). This would allow them to be labeled with readily available metal radionuclides such as ^{177}Lu or ^{90}Y, different isotopes of indium or rhenium and potentially with short-lived α emitters such as ^{213}Bi. They could also be prefabricated to allow for halogen labeling with isotopes of iodine and the α-emitter ^{211}At, although such labelings would require a more complex procedure (see chapter 8).

The radionuclides could be produced locally at the nuclear medicine department with applied generators or accelerators or they could be bought from companies specializing in radionuclide production. It is important to note that the availability of radiopharmaceuticals will not be a severe problem if radionuclide therapy proves to be routinely effective in the clinical setting. Actually, radionuclide therapy might not be more complicated than chemotherapy combined with external radiotherapy provided that the non-radioactive substances prepared for radiolabeling are commercially available and that the radionuclides are available at the hospital [45].

References

1. Witzig TE (2006) Radioimmunotherapy for B-cell non-Hodgkin lymphoma. Best Pract Res Clin Haematol 19(4):655–68. Review.
2. Adams GP, Weiner LM (2005) Monoclonal antibody therapy of cancer. Nat Biotechnol 23(9):1147–57. Review.
3. Goldenberg DM, Sharkey RM (2006) Advances in cancer therapy with radiolabeled monoclonal antibodies. Q J Nucl Med Mol Imaging 50(4):248–64. Review.
4. DeNardo SJ, DeNardo GL (2006) Targeted radionuclide therapy for solid tumors: an overview. Int J Radiat Oncol Biol Phys 66(2 Suppl):S89–95. Review.
5. Oyen WJ, Bodei L, Giammarile F, Maecke HR, Tennvall J, Luster M, Brans B (2007) Targeted therapy in nuclear medicine–current status and future prospects. Ann Oncol 18(11):1782–92. Review.
6. Boerman OC, Koppe MJ, Postema EJ, Corstens FH, Oyen WJ (2007) Radionuclide therapy of cancer with radiolabeled antibodies. Anticancer Agents Med Chem 7(3):335–43. Review.
7. Pacini F, Schlumberger M, Harmer C, Berg GG, Cohen O, Duntas L, Jamar F, Jarzab B, Limbert E, Lind P, Reiners C, Sanchez Franco F, Smit J, Wiersinga W (2005) Post-surgical use of radioiodine ^{131}I in patients with papillary and follicular thyroid cancer and the issue of remnant ablation: a consensus report. Eur J Endocrinol 153:651–9.
8. Woodrum DT, Gauger PG (2005) Role of ^{131}I in the treatment of well differentiated thyroid cancer. J Surg Oncol 89:114–21.
9. Berlin NI (2000) Treatment of the myeloproliferative disorders with 32P. Eur J Haematol 65(1):1–7. Review.
10. Berlin NI (2002) Polycythemia vera: diagnosis and treatment 2002. Expert Rev Anticancer Ther 2(3):330–6. Review.
11. Davis TA, Kaminski MS, Leonard JP, Hsu FJ, Wilkinson M, Zelenetz A, Wahl RL, Kroll S, Coleman M, Goris M, Levy R, Knox SJ (2004) The radioisotope contributes significantly to the activity of radioimmunotherapy. Clin Cancer Res 10:7792–7798.
12. Chrisoulidou A, Kaltsas G, Ilias I, Grossman AB (2007) The diagnosis and management of malignant phaeochromocytoma and paraganglioma. Endocr Relat Cancer 14(3):569–85. Review.
13. Howman-Giles R, Shaw PJ, Uren RF, Chung DK (2007) Neuroblastoma and other neuroendocrine tumors. Semin Nucl Med 37(4):286–302. Review.

14. Scholz T, Eisenhofer G, Pacak K, Dralle H, Lehnert H (2007) Clinical review: current treatment of malignant pheochromocytoma. J Clin Endocrinol Metab 92(4):1217–25. Review.
15. Kwekkeboom DJ, Mueller-Brand J, Paganelli G, Anthony LB, Pauwels S, Kvols LK, O'dorisio TM, Valkema R, Bodei L, Chinol M, Maecke HR, Krenning EP (2005) Overview of results of peptide receptor radionuclide therapy with 3 radiolabeled somatostatin analogs. J Nucl Med 46(Suppl 1):62S–66S.
16. Forrer F, Valkema R, Kwekkeboom DJ, de Jong M, Krenning EP (2007) Peptide receptor radionuclide therapy. Best Pract Res Clin Endocrinol Metab 21:111–29.
17. Van Essen M, Krenning EP, De Jong M, Valkema R, Kwekkeboom DJ (2007) Peptide Receptor Radionuclide Therapy with radiolabelled somatostatin analogues in patients with somatostatin receptor positive tumours. Acta Oncol 46(6):723–34. Review.
18. Finlay IG, Mason MD, Shelley M (2005) Radioisotopes for the palliation of metastatic bone cancer: a systematic review. Lancet Oncol 6:392–400.
19. Bauman G, Charette M, Reid R, Sathya J (2005) Radiopharmaceuticals for the palliation of painful bone metastasis-a systemic review. Radiother Oncol 75:258–270.
20. Lawrentschuk N, Davis ID, Bolton DM, Scott AM (2007) Diagnostic and therapeutic use of radioisotopes for bony disease in prostate cancer: current practice. Int J Urol 14:89–95.
21. Press OW, Eary JF, Gooley T, Gopal AK, Liu S, Rajendran JG, Maloney DG, Petersdorf S, Bush SA, Durack LD, Martin PJ, Fisher DR, Wood B, Borrow JW, Porter B, Smith JP, Matthews DC, Appelbaum FR, Bernstein ID (2000) A phase I/II trial of iodine-131 tositumomab (anti-CD20), etoposide, cyclophosphamide, and autologous stem cell transplantation for relapsed B-cell lymphomas. Blood 96:2934–42.
22. Molina A, Krishnan A, Fung H, Flinn IW, Inwards D, Winter JN, Nademanee A (2007) Use of radioimmunotherapy in stem cell transplantation and posttransplantation: focus on yttrium 90 ibritumomab tiuxetan. Curr Stem Cell Res Ther 2(3):239–48. Review.
23. Buchsbaum DJ (2000) Experimental radioimmunotherapy. Semin Radiat Oncol 10(2):156–67.
24. Behr TM, Blumenthal RD, Memtsoudis S, et al. (2000) Cure of metastatic human colonic cancer in mice with radiolabeled monoclonal antibody fragments. Clin Cancer Res 6(12):4900–7.
25. Barendswaard EC, Humm JL, O'Donoghue JA, et al. (2001) Relative therapeutic efficacy of (125)I- and (131)I-labeled monoclonal antibody A33 in a human colon cancer xenograft. J Nucl Med 42(8):1251–6.
26. de Jong M, Breeman WAP, Bernard BF, et al. (2001) [^{177}Lu-DOTA^{0}, Tyr^{3}]octreotate for somatostatin receptor-targeted radionuclide therapy. Int J Cancer 92:628–33.
27. Kassis AI, Adelstein SJ (2005) Radiobiologic principles in radionuclide therapy. J Nucl Med 46(Suppl 1):4S–12S. Review.
28. Murray D, McEwan AJ (2007) Radiobiology of systemic radiation therapy. Cancer Biother Radiopharm 22(1):1–23. Review.
29. O'Donoghue JA, Bardies M, Wheldon TE (1995) Relationships between tumor size and curability for uniformly targeted therapy with beta-emitting radionuclides. J Nucl Med 36(10):1902–09.
30. Hartman T, Lundqvist H, Westlin JE, Carlsson J (2000) Radiation doses to the cell nucleus in single cells and cells in micrometastases in targeted therapy with 131I labelled ligands or antibodies. Int J Radiat Oncol Biol Phys 46(4):1025–1036.
31. de Jong M, Breeman WA, Valkema R, Bernard BF, Krenning EP (2005) Combination radionuclide therapy using 177Lu- and 90Y-labeled somatostatin analogs. J Nucl Med 46(Suppl 1):13S–7S.
32. Bernhardt P, Forssell-Aronsson E, Jacobsson L, Skarnemark G (2001) Low-energy electron emitters for targeted radiotherapy of small tumours. Acta Oncol 40(5):602–8.
33. Wessels BW, Syh JH, Meredith RF (2006) Overview of dosimetry for Systemic Targeted Radionuclide Therapy (STaRT). Int J Radiat Oncol Biol Phys 66(2 Suppl):S39–45. Review.
34. Ell PJ, Gambhir S (2004) Nuclear Medicine in Clinical Diagnosis and Treatment. Elsevier Health Sciences, Edinburgh, UK (ISBN: 9780443073120).

35. Ramer K, Alavi A (2005) Nuclear Medicine Technology. Springer, New York (ISBN: 3540253742).
36. Schiepers C (2005) Diagnostic Nuclear Medicine. Springer, Germany (ISBN: 9783540423096).
37. Zaidi H (2005) Quantitative Analysis in Nuclear Medicine Imaging. Springer, New York (ISBN: 9780387238548).
38. Saha GB (2006) Physics and Radiobiology of Nuclear Medicine. Springer, New York (ISBN: 9780387307541).
39. Christian PE, Waterstram-Rich K (2007) Nuclear Medicine and Pet/Ct Technology and Techniques. Elsevier Health Sciences, St. Louis, MO (ISBN: 9780323043953).
40. Morton KA, Nance RW, Clark PB, Christensen CR, O'Malley JP, Blodgett TM, Waxman AD, Stevens JS, Drosten R, Chinn CA (2007) Nuclear Medicine. W.B. Saunders, Edinburgh, UK (ISBN: 9781416033394).
41. Evans ES, Hahn CA, Kocak Z, Zhou SM, Marks LB (2007) The role of functional imaging in the diagnosis and management of late normal tissue injury. Semin Radiat Oncol 17(2):72–80. Review.
42. Saleem A, Charnley N, Price P (2006) Clinical molecular imaging with positron emission tomography. Eur J Cancer 42(12):1720–7. Review.
43. Brans B, Bodei L, Giammarile F, Linden O, Luster M, Oyen WJ, Tennvall J (2007) Clinical radionuclide therapy dosimetry: the quest for the "Holy Gray". Eur J Nucl Med Mol Imaging 34(5):772–86. Review.
44. Thomas SR (2007) From the SNM MIRD committee. J Nucl Med 48(2):33N–34N.
45. Carlsson J, Forssell AE, Hietala SO, Stigbrand T, Tennvall J (2003) Tumour therapy with radionuclides; assessment of progress and problems. Radiother Oncol 66(2):107–17.

Chapter 2
Therapeutically Used Targeted Antigens in Radioimmunotherapy

Torgny Stigbrand[1], David Eriksson[1], Katrine Riklund[2], and Lennart Johansson[3]

Summary Many antigens have been tested as targets for radioimmunotherapy with intact antibodies. Some of the early used targets have been found to be of decreasing interest due to low expression, extensive shedding or other reasons. Others have been found more useful due to their accessibility, amount available in the tumours, or the biological properties of the target antigen. In this chapter some of the most used antigens and their characteristics are presented.

Introduction

An increasing number of promising antigens on malignant cells for monitoring malignant diseases have recently been reviewed [1]. Several of the seventy markers in that review have also been investigated for putative use in radioimmunotherapy, and this chapter will focus on some of them.

The ideal antigen for targeting should be readily accessible, expressed mainly within the targeted tissue, if possible, and should be present in substantial amounts. In the early history of targeting experiments, many of the antigens referred to as "tumour markers" were employed and even secreted products were used for targeting. Several of these early secreted targets have turned obsolete today and have disappeared or are used in very limited extent (HCG, α-fetoprotein) and instead new aspects on the nature of the target have come into focus. Some of the major antigens in use will be presented here.

The amount available and accessibility of the antigen in combination of biological properties affect the outcome of targeting. The selectivity in tissue expression is also of importance. Some antigens may be regarded as disease specific for certain malignancies, while others are expressed in different type of tumours. Such ubiquitously

[1]Department of Immunology, University of Umeå, SE-90185, Umeå, Sweden

[2]Departments of Clinical Microbiology, Diagnostic Radiology, University of Umeå, SE-90185, Umeå, Sweden

[3]Department of Radiation Physics, University of Umeå, SE-90185, Umeå, Sweden

T. Stigbrand et al. (eds.) *Targeted Radionuclide Tumor Therapy*,

expressed targets may have advantages at clinical radioimmunotherapy in a wider perspective. Several of the most used antigens today are expressed in several tumour tissues as for example, CEA, TAG-72, HER2/neu, EGFR and VEGF. CEA is expressed in colorectal, gastric, pancreatic, non-small cell lung and breast carcinomas. TAG-72 is similarly expressed in colorectal, gastric, pancreatic, ovarian, endometrial, breast, non-small cell lung cancer and prostate carcinomas. The expression of EGFR and HER2 is described in detail in chapter 3 but shortly described also below. In order to minimize hematopoietic toxicity at radioimmunotherapy, it is a significant advantage if the tissue expression is limited to the diseased tissue.

One aspect, today more in focus than earlier, is the metabolic behaviour of the targeted antigen. Some antigens, possible to target, may reside on the plasma membranes of the malignant cells, but also extracellularly located target molecules within the tumour tissue may be considered, if they are present in significant amounts, e.g. in the tumour stroma or tumour vasculature.

Many useful membrane antigens exert their biological role by recycling between the plasma membrane of the host cell and the interior of the same cell, providing a mechanism for internalization of antibodies by the targeted malignant cell. At the same time, however, the antibody will be exposed to the intracellular degradation machinery, including proteolytic cleavages of the labelled compound, with possibilities to separate the nuclide from its carrier. This causes a consecutive and continuous transport out of the cell of the nuclide as a low molecular weight compound, which will be subjected to urinary excretion.

Improved cellular retention can be achieved by the use radioactive metals (e.g. ^{90}Y or ^{177}Lu) which, after degradation of the targeting agent, bind to intracellular structures or by the use of residualizing reagents during coupling of radioactive halogens (e.g. ^{131}I or ^{211}At) to the targeting agent, see chapter 8 for more details.

Some of the antigens widely used are released or even secreted from the tumours and this causes appearance of circulating intact or degraded products of these antigens within the vasculature, which may interfere with the efficiency in the targeting by consuming the labelled antibodies with subsequent degradation within the reticuloendothelial system. Both CEA and TAG-72 appear in blood in soluble form in low amounts, and will compromise binding to the tumour, while for example CD20 is an excellent target because it is neither shed, nor internalized and furthermore expressed by almost all B-cell tumours. The properties of this antigen may be one of the important reasons for the positive outcome when treating different types of lymphomas.

Some of the most used antigens are presented below.

CEA

When the concept of oncofoetal antigens was introduced, following the discovery of CEA by Gold and Freeman [2], CEA was soon to be the very first antigen to be used both as a tumour marker and as target for intervention in the treatment of malignant diseases [3, 4].

The human CEA family has been fully characterized and comprises 29 genes, out of which 18 are expressed [5]. The CEA subgroup members are cell membrane associated and presents a complex expression pattern in normal and cancerous epithelial tissues. The form used as target is a heavily glycosylated single polypeptide chain of 180kDa. CEA is an important tumour marker for colorectal cancer, but is expressed in many other tumours and regarded as a pancarcinoma marker.

Today CEA not only has become one of the most extensively used tumour markers, but also, due to its pronounced expression in many carcinomas, a widely used target antigen for radioimmunotherapy. Several interesting reports have been presented during the last years with this antigen and one trend is to use tailored constructs with several binding sites towards the antigen and the nuclides. Sharkey et al. generated a multivalent, bispecific antibody against CEA with a tenfold increase in uptake in a preclinical test with human colon xenografts and could reach tumour to non-tumour ratios up to 100 [6].

Similarly a streptavidin-conjugate of the chimeric antiCEAantibody T84.66 was also found to reach high ratios with an extremely rapid clearance from the blood and other organs [7]. This ^{90}Y-labelled antibody has also been tested on patients with uptake and radiation delivery to smaller nodal lesions [8].

An interesting new concept, the "dock-and-lock" approach to generate trivalent, bispecific antibodies against CEA was recently presented, with two binding sites for CEA and one for the nuclide. This construct displayed high specific targeting to pancreatic and colon cancer xenografts [9, 10]. A number of pretargeting reports furthermore support the usefulness of CEA as a target and improved localization has been reported, and provide experimental evidence for clinical application of radioimmunotherapy [11–15].

TAG-72

TAG-72 was initially identified 1985 as the target antigen of an antibody B72.3 raised against a membrane-enriched fraction of a metastatic breast carcinoma [16]. TAG-72 is a high molecular weight glycoprotein complex (240–400kDa), which is also expressed on 80% of colorectal carcinomas, with very limited expression in normal tissues [17]. It should today also be regarded as a pancarcinoma antigen. A second generation of antibodies towards this antigen has been generated, CC49 being one of them [18, 19]. The TAG-72 antigen contains several carbohydrate epitopes and this CC49 antibody reacts with the sialyl-Tn and sialyl-T epitopes of the antigen. Since multiple epitopes can be present on a single target antigen, this may contribute to improved efficiency both when the antigen is the target or in monitoring assays.

The initial use of this antigen in radioimmunotherapy was limited, with sporadic positive effects and the murine antibody was highly immunogenic [20–23]. During the last years several reports have been presented, confirming TAG-72 over-expression in several tumour types [24]. Recombinant antibodies against TAG-72 have demonstrated excellent pharmacokinetics and biodistribution targeting this antigen [25–28]. Furthermore, the heterogenous expression of some antigens in ovarian tumours have been compensated for by using several radiolabeled antibodies at the same time, one of them against TAG-72, a procedure which improved the targeting efficiency [29].

HER2/neu (c-erbB-2)

HER2 is a glycosylated protein with a molecular weight of 185 kDa. It has no known natural ligand. Instead it is activated via heterodimerization to other receptors in the EGFR-family. Activation leads to down-stream signalling to a large extent controlling cell proliferation and apoptosis (chapter 3).

HER2 is expressed, to a limited extent, in the epithelia of lung, bladder, pancreas and prostate. The ectodomain of this protein can, at least in experimental systems, be proteolytically cleaved off from the intact receptor and released in soluble form [30]. However, this seems not to occur, or at least only occur at a low level, in clinical cases since a constant strong tumour cell membrane associated overexpression of HER2 has been reported in an overwhelming number of cases (chapter 3).

Cell membrane associated HER2 overexpression has been studied mainly in breast cancer but has been observed also in several other malignancies such as prostate, ovarian and lung carcinomas [31–34]. HER2 is a potentially interesting target for radionuclide therapy, especially breast cancers that have primary or induced resistance to Herceptin treatment. Chapter 3 gives more detailed discussions about HER2 and other members of the EGFR-family as targets for radionuclide therapy.

EGFR

The epidermal growth factor receptor, EGFR, is a transmembrane glycoprotein that is activated by the binding of EGF, TGF-α and a few other ligands to the extracellular part of the receptor. Following activation, intracellular kinases are phosphorylated resulting in down-stream signalling controlling proliferation, differentiation, apoptosis and migration (chapter 3).

Elevated levels of the receptor (and often also of the ligands) have been observed in numerous cancer types, especially in various forms of squamous cell carcinomas, e.g. head & neck and non-small cell lung cancers, but a reasonably high expression has also been reported for adenocarcinomas such as breast, ovarian and colorectal cancers [35]. There are several recent reviews written on the expression of EGFR in various tumours and that is summarized in chapter 3 of this volume. EGFR expression has been studied as a potential target for intracavitary anti-EGFR radionuclide therapy of gliomas [36]. Genomic rearrangements can cause expression of modified receptors, which also can be considered for radioimmunotherapeutic trials [37].

A33

The A33 antigen has been extensively investigated. It is a transmembrane antigen which has lower molecular weight than e.g. EGFR and HER2, since the molecular weight for A33 is only 43 kDa. It belongs to the Ig superfamily and is expressed in normal gastrointestinal epithelia as well as in carcinomas of colon and rectum, where it is homogenously expressed in 95% of the tumours [38, 39]. Recently the antigen has been used for several radioimmunotherapeutic trials with excellent targeting, but only a few patients demonstrated stable disease while the others presented progressive disease [40–42].

MUC-1

MUC-1 belongs to the mucin family of proteins and is overexpressed in more than 90% of breast and other glandular epithelial cancers in a hypoglycosylated form. The core peptides of the extracellular domain are exposed, which is the structure employed for targeting [43]. Highly conserved repeats of 20 amino acids, VNTR, vary between 20 and 125 in the protein, depending on the allele. Each tandem repeat contains five potential glycosylation sites, which constitute the structure exploited for therapy. These core peptides in the repeats are masked in normal cells, but become exposed in tumour cells [43].

The major part of antibodies raised against this antigen reacts with carbohydrate epitopes within these repeats, as investigated in an ISOBM workshop with 56 monoclonal antibodies to this antigen [44]. In one report Nicholson et al. [45] were able to demonstrate that MUC-1 targeted radioimmunotherapy can be working. It was shown that out of 21 patients, with ovarian cancer with no remaining macroscopic disease after cytoreductive surgery, 16 were still alive ten years after radioimmunotherapy, which was significantly better than the median survival of less than four years in a control group.

VEGF

The vascular endothelial growth factor (VEGF) occupies a unique position in this context, since it is not expressed on the tumour cells, but was initially identified as a tumour-derived and excreted factor capable of increasing vascular permeability [46, 47]. In the embryo, VEGF and its isoforms are critical for normal vessel development and these peptide hormones can exert apoptotic, mitogenic and permeability-increasing activities specific for the vascular endothelium. A number of different isoforms of VEGF exist due to different splicing of a single gene with eight exons [48]. A family of peptides closely related to VEGF (VEGF-B – VEGF-E) are also known to stimulate angiogenesis.

VEGF and related factors have been demonstrated to increase in serum levels in various cancers and have been suggested to be used to monitor disease progress and response to treatment [49]. High levels have also been correlated to advanced stages or with a worse prognosis in tumours of the bladder, brain, breast, colon, lung, ovary, renal cell carcinoma, squamous cell carcinoma of the neck and neuroblastoma [50–58]. Recently in a preclinical investigation an ^{131}I-labeled antibody against VEGF was reported to cause growth retardation [59].

CD20

CD20 occupies a unique role in radioimmunotargeting by being widely used for the treatment of different lymphomas. It was initially discovered already 1981 by Nadler et al. [60]. It is a 33–36-kDa transmembrane phosphoprotein involved in the activation, proliferation and differentiation of B-lymphocytes [61]. The predicted amino acid sequence of the CD20 suggests four transmembrane-spanning regions with both the N- and C-terminals located intracellularly in the cytoplasm, which may contribute to the restricted mobility.

Activation of CD20 by binding of antibodies directed towards the extracellular domain of CD20 leads to tyrosine kinase pathway activation and modulation of cell cycle progression via interaction with src-related kinases. Binding of unlabeled humanized antibodies to this antigen can cause cell death via complement-dependant cellular cytotoxicity or antibody-dependant cellular cytotoxicity. Several investigators have documented variations in the surface intensity of the antigen of malignant B-cells in lymphoproliferative diseases, an observation which might affect the efficiency in therapeutic outcome [62].

The introduction of radioimmunotherapy and also the naked antibodies for haematological diseases has revolutionized the field of cancer treatment in the last decade. For recent reviews – see [63, 64] and chapter 20. Many positive reports on the efficiency of such treatments have been presented [65–67].

The Cytokeratins

The cytokeratins occupy a unique position within the group of antigens that can be targeted. These intermediate filaments are abundantly expressed intracellularily in all epithelial tissues in certain combinations. When released into the circulation they can be used as powerful tumour markers for several malignant diseases. Their unique repetitive structures, with comparatively low solubility, enable the cytokeratins to remain in place, within the tumour following cytotoxic therapy, and can by such mechanisms increase their level of antigen significantly by external radiotherapy or other cytotoxic drugs. (See also chapter 4) [68–70].

Conclusions

The targets for radioimmunotherapy and their impact on treatment results differ significantly, and the favourable properties of the well exposed CD20 partially contributes to the positive outcome when treating lymphomas, compared to solid tumours.

One of the reasons why the efficiency has so far been low at treating solid tumours might be that there is often too low amounts of specific target antigens. Exceptions might be targeting of EGFR and HER2 where we expect promising results when large scale clinical trials with strongly receptor expressing tumours start.

However, searching new antigens is still a needed activity. Release of antigens already within the tumour might be another possibility to increase targeting efficiency. External beam radiation, causing partial necrosis within the tumour, may cause significant exposure of intermediate filaments, which due to low solubility might remain within the tumour site and could be used as targets.

Acknowledgements Financial support from the Swedish Cancer Society, the County of Västerbotten and the Medical Faculty at Umeå University for research related to the content of this chapter is acknowledged.

References

1. Voorzanger-Rousselot N, Garnero P: Biochemical markers in oncology. Part I: Molecular basis. Part II: Clinical uses. Cancer Treat Rev 2007; 33:230–283.
2. Gold P, Freedman SO: Specific carcinoembryonic antigens of the human digestive system. J Exp Med 1965; 122:467–481.
3. Mach JP, Carrel S, Merenda C, Sordat B, Cerottini JC: In vivo localisation of radiolabelled antibodies to carcinoembryonic antigen in human colon carcinoma grafted into nude mice. Nature 1974; 248:704–706.
4. Goldenberg DM, DeLand F, Kim E, Bennett S, Primus FJ, van Nagell JR, Jr., Estes N, DeSimone P, Rayburn P: Use of radiolabeled antibodies to carcinoembryonic antigen for the detection and localization of diverse cancers by external photoscanning. N Engl J Med 1978; 298:1384–1386.
5. Hammarstrom S: The carcinoembryonic antigen (cea) family: Structures, suggested functions and expression in normal and malignant tissues. Semin Cancer Biol 1999; 9:67–81.
6. Sharkey RM, Cardillo TM, Rossi EA, Chang CH, Karacay H, McBride WJ, Hansen HJ, Horak ID, Goldenberg DM: Signal amplification in molecular imaging by pretargeting a multivalent, bispecific antibody. Nat Med 2005; 11:1250–1255.
7. Jia F, Shelton TD, Lewis MR: Preparation, characterization, and biological evaluation of a streptavidin-chimeric t84.66 conjugate for antibody pretargeting. Cancer Biother Radiopharm 2007; 22:654–664.
8. Wong JY, Chu DZ, Williams LE, Liu A, Zhan J, Yamauchi DM, Wilczynski S, Wu AM, Yazaki PJ, Shively JE, Leong L, Raubitschek AA: A phase I trial of (90)y-dota-anti-cea chimeric t84.66 (ct84.66) radioimmunotherapy in patients with metastatic cea-producing malignancies. Cancer Biother Radiopharm 2006; 21:88–100.

9. Goldenberg DM, Rossi EA, Sharkey RM, McBride WJ, Chang CH: Multifunctional antibodies by the dock-and-lock method for improved cancer imaging and therapy by pretargeting. J Nucl Med 2008; 49:158–163.
10. Sharkey RM, Karacay H, Vallabhajosula S, McBride WJ, Rossi EA, Chang CH, Goldsmith SJ, Goldenberg DM: Metastatic human colonic carcinoma: Molecular imaging with pretargeted spect and pet in a mouse model. Radiology 2008; 246:497–507.
11. Kraeber-Bodere F, Rousseau C, Bodet-Milin C, Ferrer L, Faivre-Chauvet A, Campion L, Vuillez JP, Devillers A, Chang CH, Goldenberg DM, Chatal JF, Barbet J: Targeting, toxicity, and efficacy of 2-step, pretargeted radioimmunotherapy using a chimeric bispecific antibody and 131i-labeled bivalent hapten in a phase I optimization clinical trial. J Nucl Med 2006; 47:247–255.
12. Lankester KJ, Maxwell RJ, Pedley RB, Dearling JL, Qureshi UA, El-Emir E, Hill SA, Tozer GM: Combretastatin a-4-phosphate effectively increases tumor retention of the therapeutic antibody, 131i-a5b7, even at doses that are sub-optimal for vascular shut-down. Int J Oncol 2007; 30:453–460.
13. Chatal JF, Campion L, Kraeber-Bodere F, Bardet S, Vuillez JP, Charbonnel B, Rohmer V, Chang CH, Sharkey RM, Goldenberg DM, Barbet J: Survival improvement in patients with medullary thyroid carcinoma who undergo pretargeted anti-carcinoembryonic-antigen radioimmunotherapy: A collaborative study with the french endocrine tumor group. J Clin Oncol 2006; 24:1705–1711.
14. Karacay H, Brard PY, Sharkey RM, Chang CH, Rossi EA, McBride WJ, Ragland DR, Horak ID, Goldenberg DM: Therapeutic advantage of pretargeted radioimmunotherapy using a recombinant bispecific antibody in a human colon cancer xenograft. Clin Cancer Res 2005; 11:7879–7885.
15. Li GP, Zhang H, Zhu CM, Zhang J, Jiang XF: Avidin-biotin system pretargeting radioimmunoimaging and radioimmunotherapy and its application in mouse model of human colon carcinoma. World J Gastroenterol 2005; 11:6288–6294.
16. Johnson VG, Schlom J, Paterson AJ, Bennett J, Magnani JL, Colcher D: Analysis of a human tumor-associated glycoprotein (tag-72) identified by monoclonal antibody b72.3. Cancer Res 1986; 46:850–857.
17. Thor A, Ohuchi N, Szpak CA, Johnston WW, Schlom J: Distribution of oncofetal antigen tumor-associated glycoprotein-72 defined by monoclonal antibody b72.3. Cancer Res 1986; 46:3118–3124.
18. Batra SK, Jain M, Wittel UA, Chauhan SC, Colcher D: Pharmacokinetics and biodistribution of genetically engineered antibodies. Curr Opin Biotechnol 2002; 13:603–608.
19. Meredith RF, Bueschen AJ, Khazaeli MB, Plott WE, Grizzle WE, Wheeler RH, Schlom J, Russell CD, Liu T, LoBuglio AF: Treatment of metastatic prostate carcinoma with radiolabeled antibody cc49. J Nucl Med 1994; 35:1017–1022.
20. Divgi CR, Scott AM, Dantis L, Capitelli P, Siler K, Hilton S, Finn RD, Kemeny N, Kelsen D, Kostakoglu L, et al.: Phase I radioimmunotherapy trial with iodine-131-cc49 in metastatic colon carcinoma. J Nucl Med 1995; 36:586–592.
21. Meredith RF, Khazaeli MB, Liu T, Plott G, Wheeler RH, Russell C, Colcher D, Schlom J, Shochat D, LoBuglio AF: Dose fractionation of radiolabeled antibodies in patients with metastatic colon cancer. J Nucl Med 1992; 33:1648–1653.
22. Meredith RF, Khazaeli MB, Plott WE, Grizzle WE, Liu T, Schlom J, Russell CD, Wheeler RH, LoBuglio AF: Phase II study of dual 131i-labeled monoclonal antibody therapy with interferon in patients with metastatic colorectal cancer. Clin Cancer Res 1996; 2:1811–1818.
23. Murray JL, Macey DJ, Kasi LP, Rieger P, Cunningham J, Bhadkamkar V, Zhang HZ, Schlom J, Rosenblum MG, Podoloff DA: Phase II radioimmunotherapy trial with 131i-cc49 in colorectal cancer. Cancer 1994; 73:1057–1066.
24. Ponnusamy MP, Venkatraman G, Singh AP, Chauhan SC, Johansson SL, Jain M, Smith L, Davis JS, Remmenga SW, Batra SK: Expression of tag-72 in ovarian cancer and its correlation with tumor stage and patient prognosis. Cancer Lett 2007; 251:247–257.

25. Chauhan SC, Jain M, Moore ED, Wittel UA, Li J, Gwilt PR, Colcher D, Batra SK: Pharmacokinetics and biodistribution of 177lu-labeled multivalent single-chain fv construct of the pancarcinoma monoclonal antibody cc49. Eur J Nucl Med Mol Imaging 2005; 32:264–273.
26. Goel A, Colcher D, Baranowska-Kortylewicz J, Augustine S, Booth BJ, Pavlinkova G, Batra SK: Genetically engineered tetravalent single-chain fv of the pancarcinoma monoclonal antibody cc49: Improved biodistribution and potential for therapeutic application. Cancer Res 2000; 60:6964–6971.
27. Kashmiri SV, Shu L, Padlan EA, Milenic DE, Schlom J, Hand PH: Generation, characterization, and in vivo studies of humanized anticarcinoma antibody cc49. Hybridoma 1995; 14:461–473.
28. Larson SM, El-Shirbiny AM, Divgi CR, Sgouros G, Finn RD, Tschmelitsch J, Picon A, Whitlow M, Schlom J, Zhang J, Cohen AM: Single chain antigen binding protein (sfv cc49): First human studies in colorectal carcinoma metastatic to liver. Cancer 1997; 80:2458–2468.
29. Chauhan SC, Vinayek N, Maher DM, Bell MC, Dunham KA, Koch MD, Lio Y, Jaggi M: Combined staining of tag-72, muc1, and ca125 improves labeling sensitivity in ovarian cancer: Antigens for multi-targeted antibody-guided therapy. J Histochem Cytochem 2007; 55:867–875.
30. Langton BC, Crenshaw MC, Chao LA, Stuart SG, Akita RW, Jackson JE: An antigen immunologically related to the external domain of gp185 is shed from nude mouse tumors overexpressing the c-erbb-2 (her-2/neu) oncogene. Cancer Res 1991; 51:2593–2598.
31. Han H, Landreneau RJ, Santucci TS, Tung MY, Macherey RS, Shackney SE, Sturgis CD, Raab SS, Silverman JF: Prognostic value of immunohistochemical expressions of p53, her-2/neu, and bcl-2 in stage I non-small-cell lung cancer. Hum Pathol 2002; 33:105–110.
32. Ross JS, Fletcher JA: The her-2/neu oncogene in breast cancer: Prognostic factor, predictive factor, and target for therapy. Oncologist 1998; 3:237–252.
33. Calvo BF, Levine AM, Marcos M, Collins QF, Iacocca MV, Caskey LS, Gregory CW, Lin Y, Whang YE, Earp HS, Mohler JL: Human epidermal receptor-2 expression in prostate cancer. Clin Cancer Res 2003; 9:1087–1097.
34. Hogdall EV, Christensen L, Kjaer SK, Blaakaer J, Bock JE, Glud E, Norgaard-Pedersen B, Hogdall CK: Distribution of her-2 overexpression in ovarian carcinoma tissue and its prognostic value in patients with ovarian carcinoma: From the Danish malova ovarian cancer study. Cancer 2003; 98:66–73.
35. Salomon DS, Brandt R, Ciardiello F, Normanno N: Epidermal growth factor-related peptides and their receptors in human malignancies. Crit Rev Oncol Hematol 1995; 19:183–232.
36. Carlsson J, Ren ZP, Wester K, Sundberg AL, Heldin NE, Hesselager G, Persson M, Gedda L, Tolmachev V, Lundqvist H, Blomquist E, Nister M: Planning for intracavitary anti-egfr radionuclide therapy of gliomas. Literature review and data on egfr expression. J Neurooncol 2006; 77:33–45.
37. Ohman L, Gedda L, Hesselager G, Larsson R, Nister M, Stigbrand T, Wester K, Carlsson J: A new antibody recognizing the viii mutation of human epidermal growth factor receptor. Tumour Biol 2002; 23:61–69.
38. Ritter G, Cohen LS, Nice EC, Catimel B, Burgess AW, Moritz RL, Ji H, Heath JK, White SJ, Welt S, Old LJ, Simpson RJ: Characterization of posttranslational modifications of human a33 antigen, a novel palmitoylated surface glycoprotein of human gastrointestinal epithelium. Biochem Biophys Res Commun 1997; 236:682–686.
39. Heath JK, White SJ, Johnstone CN, Catimel B, Simpson RJ, Moritz RL, Tu GF, Ji H, Whitehead RH, Groenen LC, Scott AM, Ritter G, Cohen L, Welt S, Old LJ, Nice EC, Burgess AW: The human a33 antigen is a transmembrane glycoprotein and a novel member of the immunoglobulin superfamily. Proc Natl Acad Sci USA 1997; 94:469–474.
40. Almqvist Y, Steffen AC, Tolmachev V, Divgi CR, Sundin A: In vitro and in vivo characterization of 177lu-hua33: A radioimmunoconjugate against colorectal cancer. Nucl Med Biol 2006; 33:991–998.

41. Sakamoto J, Oriuchi N, Mochiki E, Asao T, Scott AM, Hoffman EW, Jungbluth AA, Matsui T, Lee FT, Papenfuss A, Kuwano H, Takahashi T, Endo K, Old LJ: A phase I radioimmunolocalization trial of humanized monoclonal antibody hua33 in patients with gastric carcinoma. Cancer Sci 2006; 97:1248–1254.
42. Chong G, Lee FT, Hopkins W, Tebbutt N, Cebon JS, Mountain AJ, Chappell B, Papenfuss A, Schleyer P, Paul U, Murphy R, Wirth V, Smyth FE, Potasz N, Poon A, Davis ID, Saunder T, O'Keefe GJ, Burgess AW, Hoffman EW, Old LJ, Scott AM: Phase I trial of 131i-hua33 in patients with advanced colorectal carcinoma. Clin Cancer Res 2005; 11:4818–4826.
43. Singh R, Bandyopadhyay D: Muc1: A target molecule for cancer therapy. Cancer Biol Ther 2007; 6:481–486.
44. Price MR, Rye PD, Petrakou E, Murray A, Brady K, Imai S, Haga S, Kiyozuka Y, Schol D, Meulenbroek MF, Snijdewint FG, von Mensdorff-Pouilly S, Verstraeten RA, Kenemans P, Blockzjil A, Nilsson K, Nilsson O, Reddish M, Suresh MR, Koganty RR, Fortier S, Baronic L, Berg A, Longenecker MB, Hilgers J, et al.: Summary report on the isobm td-4 workshop: Analysis of 56 monoclonal antibodies against the mucl mucin. San Diego, California, November 17–23, 1996. Tumour Biol 1998; 19(Suppl 1):1–20.
45. Nicholson S, Gooden CS, Hird V, Maraveyas A, Mason P, Lambert HE, Meares CF, Epenetos AA: Radioimmunotherapy after chemotherapy compared to chemotherapy alone in the treatment of advanced ovarian cancer: A matched analysis. Oncol Rep 1998; 5:223–226.
46. Senger DR, Galli SJ, Dvorak AM, Perruzzi CA, Harvey VS, Dvorak HF: Tumor cells secrete a vascular permeability factor that promotes accumulation of ascites fluid. Science 1983; 219:983–985.
47. Leung DW, Cachianes G, Kuang WJ, Goeddel DV, Ferrara N: Vascular endothelial growth factor is a secreted angiogenic mitogen. Science 1989; 246:1306–1309.
48. Tischer E, Mitchell R, Hartman T, Silva M, Gospodarowicz D, Fiddes JC, Abraham JA: The human gene for vascular endothelial growth factor. Multiple protein forms are encoded through alternative exon splicing. J Biol Chem 1991; 266:11947–11954.
49. Kuroi K, Toi M: Circulating angiogenesis regulators in cancer patients. Int J Biol Markers 2001; 16:5–26.
50. Crew JP, O'Brien T, Bradburn M, Fuggle S, Bicknell R, Cranston D, Harris AL: Vascular endothelial growth factor is a predictor of relapse and stage progression in superficial bladder cancer. Cancer Res 1997; 57:5281–5285.
51. Vaquero J, Zurita M, Morales C, Cincu R, Oya S: Expression of vascular permeability factor in glioblastoma specimens: Correlation with tumor vascular endothelial surface and peritumoral edema. J Neurooncol 2000; 49:49–55.
52. Linderholm B, Lindh B, Tavelin B, Grankvist K, Henriksson R: P53 and vascular-endothelial-growth-factor (vegf) expression predicts outcome in 833 patients with primary breast carcinoma. Int J Cancer 2000; 89:51–62.
53. Tokunaga T, Oshika Y, Abe Y, Ozeki Y, Sadahiro S, Kijima H, Tsuchida T, Yamazaki H, Ueyama Y, Tamaoki N, Nakamura M: Vascular endothelial growth factor (vegf) mrna isoform expression pattern is correlated with liver metastasis and poor prognosis in colon cancer. Br J Cancer 1998; 77:998–1002.
54. Fontanini G, Faviana P, Lucchi M, Boldrini L, Mussi A, Camacci T, Mariani MA, Angeletti CA, Basolo F, Pingitore R: A high vascular count and overexpression of vascular endothelial growth factor are associated with unfavourable prognosis in operated small cell lung carcinoma. Br J Cancer 2002; 86:558–563.
55. Fujimoto J, Sakaguchi H, Aoki I, Khatun S, Tamaya T: Clinical implications of expression of vascular endothelial growth factor in metastatic lesions of ovarian cancers. Br J Cancer 2001; 85:313–316.
56. Jacobsen J, Rasmuson T, Grankvist K, Ljungberg B: Vascular endothelial growth factor as prognostic factor in renal cell carcinoma. J Urol 2000; 163:343–347.
57. Sauter ER, Nesbit M, Watson JC, Klein-Szanto A, Litwin S, Herlyn M: Vascular endothelial growth factor is a marker of tumor invasion and metastasis in squamous cell carcinomas of the head and neck. Clin Cancer Res 1999; 5:775–782.

58. Eggert A, Ikegaki N, Kwiatkowski J, Zhao H, Brodeur GM, Himelstein BP: High-level expression of angiogenic factors is associated with advanced tumor stage in human neuroblastomas. Clin Cancer Res 2000; 6:1900–1908.
59. Chen J, Wu H, Han D, Xie C: Using anti-vegf mcab and magnetic nanoparticles as double-targeting vector for the radioimmunotherapy of liver cancer. Cancer Lett 2006; 231:169–175.
60. Nadler LM, Ritz J, Hardy R, Pesando JM, Schlossman SF, Stashenko P: A unique cell surface antigen identifying lymphoid malignancies of b cell origin. J Clin Invest 1981; 67:134–140.
61. Manshouri T, Do KA, Wang X, Giles FJ, O'Brien SM, Saffer H, Thomas D, Jilani I, Kantarjian HM, Keating MJ, Albitar M: Circulating cd20 is detectable in the plasma of patients with chronic lymphocytic leukemia and is of prognostic significance. Blood 2003; 101:2507–2513.
62. Keating M, O'Brien S: High-dose rituximab therapy in chronic lymphocytic leukemia. Semin Oncol 2000; 27:86–90.
63. Emmanouilides C: Radioimmunotherapy for non-hodgkin lymphoma: Historical perspective and current status. J Clin Exp Hematop 2007; 47:43–60.
64. Emmanouilides C: Current treatment options in follicular lymphoma: Science and bias. Leuk Lymphoma 2007:1–12.
65. Green DJ, Pagel JM, Pantelias A, Hedin N, Lin Y, Wilbur DS, Gopal A, Hamlin DK, Press OW: Pretargeted radioimmunotherapy for b-cell lymphomas. Clin Cancer Res 2007; 13:5598s–5603s.
66. Pagel JM, Hedin N, Subbiah K, Meyer D, Mallet R, Axworthy D, Theodore LJ, Wilbur DS, Matthews DC, Press OW: Comparison of anti-cd20 and anti-cd45 antibodies for conventional and pretargeted radioimmunotherapy of b-cell lymphomas. Blood 2003; 101:2340–2348.
67. Witzig TE: Radioimmunotherapy for b-cell non-hodgkin lymphoma. Best Pract Res Clin Haematol 2006; 19:655–668.
68. Johansson A, Sandstrom P, Ullen A, Behravan G, Erlandsson A, Levi M, Sundstrom B, Stigbrand T: Epitope specificity of the monoclonal anticytokeratin antibody ts1. Cancer Res 1999; 59:48–51.
69. Ullen A, Sandstrom P, Ahlstrom KR, Sundstrom B, Nilsson B, Arlestig L, Stigbrand T: Use of anticytokeratin monoclonal antiidiotypic antibodies to improve tumor/nontumor ratio in experimental radioimmunolocalization. Cancer Res 1995; 55:S5868–S5873.
70. Eriksson D, Joniani HM, Sheikholvaezin A, Lofroth PO, Johansson L, Ahlstrom KR, Stigbrand T: Combined low dose radio- and radioimmunotherapy of experimental hela hep 2 tumours. Eur J Nucl Med Mol Imaging 2003; 30:895–906.

Chapter 3
EGFR-Family Expression and Implications for Targeted Radionuclide Therapy

Jörgen Carlsson

Abbreviations EGFR, Epidermal growth factor receptor; HER, Human epidermal growth factor receptor

Summary High expression in the primary tumor of receptors in the EGFR-family is most often also accompanied by a similar high expression in corresponding metastases. This makes these receptors interesting as putative targets for targeted radionuclide therapy of metastases and disseminated tumor cells. The expression of all four family members, EGFR, HER2, HER3 and HER4 is reviewed in this chapter. Studies on breast, urinary bladder, colorectal, prostate, head and neck, esophageal and glioma tumors are described and possible strategies for targeted radionuclide therapy are discussed. Quantification of receptor expression and the possible influence of genomic stability on the expression are also discussed.

Introduction

It is well known that there is no successful curative treatment for the quantitatively large groups of adenocarcinoma patients with disseminated tumor cells and distant metastases (e.g. breast, prostate, colorectal, lung and ovarian tumors). The situation is equally difficult considering disseminated squamous cell carcinomas (e.g. lung, esophagus and head-neck tumors). In most of these cases, a palliative effect and prolonged survival can at best be achieved with chemotherapy. This is also true for various other types of disseminated tumors, e.g. malignant melanomas, neuroendocrine tumors and urinary bladder tumors as well as for locally, intra-CNS, spread malignant gliomas. In order for receptor targeted radionuclide therapy to be an efficient complement or alternative to chemotherapy, it is necessary that the

Unit of Biomedical Radiation Sciences, Department of Oncology, Radiology and Clinical Immunology, Rudbeck Laboratory, Uppsala University, SE-751 85, Uppsala, Sweden

T. Stigbrand et al. (eds.) *Targeted Radionuclide Tumor Therapy*,

disseminated tumor cells and metastases express the target structure to a similar extent as the corresponding primary tumors.

When the target for radionuclide therapy is a growth factor receptor within the epidermal growth factor receptor, EGFR, family, there are several reports in the literature that high expression in the primary tumor, most often is accompanied by high expression in the metastases. The reason for this is probably that the tumor cells are dependent on the growth stimulation from the growth factor-growth factor receptor interactions. If tumor cells, e.g. due to genomic instability, lose the growth factor receptor expression they might also lose their growth advantage and be overgrown by tumor cells with high receptor expression.

Examples of important growth factor receptor families are the EGFR, InsulinR, PDGFR, VEGFR and FGFR families [1]. These are of protein tyrosine kinase, PTK, type. Most of these receptors and their ligands can be aberrantly expressed in various cancers [2] and this gives possibilities for design of new forms of therapy. Various receptors have already been targets in preclinical and clinical tests with radionuclide therapy as exemplified in several reviews [3–8].

The content of this chapter focus on the expression of native receptors in the epidermal growth factor receptor, EGFR, family. Tumors expressing mutated EGFR-family receptors are rather sensitive to tyrosine kinase inhibitors, while most tumors expressing an excess of native EGFR-family receptors seem to be less sensitive. However, EGFR-family targeted radionuclide therapy is mainly targeting the native receptors and the effect of radiation is not, when the dose is high, dependent on whether the targeting agent interferes with intracellular signaling cascades. The killing capacity of ionizing radiation is of course well known and treatment induced resistance has, to the author's knowledge, not been reported. Thus, targeted radionuclide therapy can be complementary, or even superior, to the application of tyrosine kinase inhibitors. There are actually increasing numbers of not yet exploited possibilities to use EGFR-family receptors as targets in radionuclide therapy, as will be indicated in this chapter. If such an approach is successful, then more patients can be treated with a curative intention instead of palliation.

The EGFR-Family and Cancer

The expression of receptors in tumors and their corresponding metastases is available for the epidermal growth factor receptor, EGFR, family members, i.e. EGFR (ErbB-1/HER1), HER2 (ErbB-2), HER3 (ErbB-3), and HER4 (ErbB-4). They present an extracellular ligand binding domain, a hydrophobic transmembrane domain and an intracellular domain with protein-tyrosine kinase activity. However, HER3 has no intrinsic tyrosine kinase activity. EGF and five other ligands bind to EGFR and neuregulins (NRG:s) are the ligands for HER3 and HER4. HER2 has, so far, no known ligand [9, 10].

The receptors are usually active in a dimeric form via homo- or heterodimerisation after ligand mediated stimulation. The interactions between different receptor pairs represent mechanisms for signal diversification and they initiate intracellular signaling via various phosphorylation steps. Since HER2 has no known ligand and HER3 has no intrinsic tyrosine kinase activity, the signal transduction of HER2 and HER3 is mediated via heterodimerisation with each other or other receptors in the family. Since there are four known members within this receptor family, and several ligands, multiple possibilities of hetero- and homodimers mediating signals to control proliferation, apoptosis, migration and differentiation exist [9, 10]. Overexpression of EGFR and HER2 has often been associated with malignant transformation. Therapeutic targeting has actually becoming a clinical reality for tumors expressing high levels of EGFR and HER2 [9–14]. Immunohistochemical stainings of EGFR and HER2 have demonstrated pronounced membranous staining. Furthermore, EGFR and HER2 have been reported to be expressed in high levels in both tumors and metastases. Both EGFR and HER2 can be considered good targets for radionuclide based tumor therapy.

The expression of EGFR in normal tissues has been documented many years back [15, 16]. The distribution of HER2 in normal tissues differs from that of EGFR with much lower expression [17, 18]. Distributions of EGFR and HER2 in various tissues can be found at the human protein atlas (http://www.proteinatlas.org). HER2 is expressed to a lesser extent than EGFR in liver and in various epithelial tissues. HER2 is weakly expressed on hepatocytes and in the bile ducts, where the expression of EGFR is significant. EGFR is also expressed more than HER2 in the digestive tract, skin, and reproductive organs. Thus, HER2 is of interest as a specific tumor target for systemic therapy with radionuclide labeled targeting agents, since the uptake in most normal tissues is expected to be limited. An exception from applicability seems to be if the extracellular domain of HER2 is, to a large extent, cleaved by proteases as has in a few cases been reported. EGFR is less attractive as tumor target when the targeting agents has to be given systemically. EGFR is attractive mainly when the tumor uptake is higher than in most normal tissues and preferentially when local delivery of the targeting agent can be made.

It remains to be determined whether HER3 and HER4 receptors are suitable for radionuclide targeted therapy. One problem seems to be that HER3 and HER4, immunohistochemically, IHC, often seems to be cytoplasmic [19–22]. This staining pattern is not understood and it can not be excluded that, in spite of the cytoplasmic staining, there is also a fraction of these receptors in the cellular membrane. Most data is available for HER3 and it has been reported that there is mainly cytoplasmic staining of HER3 in esophageal, ovarian, lung, and breast cancer [23–25], while both cytoplasmic and significant membrane staining of HER3 has been reported for colorectal carcinomas [26]. HER3 can be overexpressed in many types of malignancies [27].

A number of human tissues and some human mammary carcinoma cell lines have HER4 transcripts [19] but the role of HER4 in cancer is not clear [20, 28, 29]. It has actually been reported for breast cancer, that high expression of HER4 correlates with increased survival time [30–32].

For the future, it is probably of importance to study coexpression of the receptors in tumor samples since it has been suggested that various forms of coexpression may be associated with the malignant phenotype [9, 10]. Targeting against e.g. EGFR-HER2 or HER2-HER3 dimers might increase the tumor specificity and give possibilities to decrease the radionuclide uptake in normal tissues. The potential disadvantage is that it might be too few of the dominating forms of dimers to allow for dimer-receptor specific delivery of therapeutical amounts of radionuclides. However, for imaging it might be enough. More research is needed to evaluate this.

There is of course a general interest, for diagnostics, imaging and therapy, to study targeting of receptors in the EGFR-family. Metastases are sometimes obvious or detectable with available diagnostic tools such as computed tomography or magnetic resonance tomography, but can also be confirmed microscopically following surgery. However, it is likely that technologies within nuclear medicine present higher sensitivity in detecting small tumor cell clusters. Even more important might be to analyze whether they present high receptor expression or not. This will facilitate the decision regarding treatment modality. If the metastases display strong receptor expression, the possibility for targeted radionuclide therapy could open up. Imaging of receptor expression to follow therapeutic efficacy is also of interest.

Studies comparing the expression of EGFR-family members in primary tumors and corresponding metastases are given below for some tumor types. Breast cancer and HER2 expression are dealt with first because more information is available. Thereafter, EGFR-family receptor expression in primary tumors and corresponding metastases of urinary bladder, colorectal, prostate, head and neck and esophageal tumors are described. The EGFR expression in gliomas is also discussed. EGFR is furthermore an interesting target for therapy of non-small cell lung cancer, but this is not discussed in this review.

Breast Cancer

There is a need for new therapy modalities to improve the survival for patients with disseminated breast cancer. An often employed approach is to target the antibody trastuzumab (Herceptin™) to the HER2 receptor, when it is overexpressed [14, 33–35]. HER2 is overexpressed in 25–30% of all breast cancers and in a higher percentage in the more malignant subgroup that form lymph node or distant metastases [14] and has been reported to be even higher than 50% when only breast cancer patients with x-ray verified bone metastases are considered [36].

It has been shown that a fraction of patients with high expression of HER2 does not respond to trastuzumab treatment whether the antibody is given alone or in combination with chemotherapy. The reason for resistance to trastuzumab will not be discussed in detail here, but several ideas have been brought forward [37, 38] such as compensatory increased signaling via the IGF-I receptor [39] and reduced action of the PI3K inhibitor PTEN [40]. Another obvious explanation to trastuzumab resistance might be heterogeneity in the expression of HER2 between primary and metastatic tumor cells. It has earlier been feared that overexpression of HER2 may sometimes be lost in metastases, but as seen from the results in Table 3.1 this is not the case.

The success of radionuclide therapy in breast cancer is only dependent on the expression of HER2 and not if the receptor function can be blocked or not. Thus, it seems as breast cancer patients not responding to trastuzumab treatment, in spite of strong HER2 expression, instead could be treated with HER2 targeted radionuclide therapy. The aim of published meta analyses by Carlsson et al. [36] and Regitnig et al. [41] was to further add to the body of data on HER2 expression in breast cancer metastases and review previously published studies. A summary of the immunohistochemical, IHC, studies mentioned in these articles, including also results from a more recent publication, is given in Table 3.1.

Examples on FISH determinations of the HER2 gene amplification (the erbB-2 gene) in primary breast cancer tumors and the corresponding metastases are shown in Table 3.2. It is obvious that the expression of HER2 in metastases, as measured with IHC and FISH, is generally similar in both local and distant metastases, as in the corresponding primary breast tumors. Furthermore, it has been found by Schindlbeck et al. [42] that HER2 expression was as high in isolated breast cancer tumor cells in the bone marrow as in primary breast cancer tumors. The results in the publication by Hanna et al. [43] indicated that intratumoral heterogeneity of HER2 expression can exist but probably is rare. An example of HER2 staining in a primary breast cancer and the corresponding lymph node metastasis, is shown in Fig. 3.1.

Table 3.1 Examples from the literature on HER2 expression, measured with immunohistochemistry (IHC), in primary breast tumors and corresponding metastases

Report	Percentage IHC overexpression primary tumors	Percentage IHC overexpression in metastases	Comments
Masood and Bui [166]	32% (n = 56)	32% (n = 56)	2+ or 3+, HercepTest
Shimizu et al. [167]	38% (n = 21)	38% (n = 21)	+/– scale, not HercepTest
Simon et al. [168]	24.8% (n = 125)	21.6% (n = 125)	2+ or 3+ HercepTest and /or positive FISH
Tanner et al. [169]	28% (n = 46)	28% (n = 46)	0–3+ scale, not HercepTest
Gancberg et al. [170]	29% (n = 100)	27% (n = 100)[a]	2+ or 3+, HercepTest
Vincent-S et al. [171]	25% (n = 44)	20.5% (n = 44)[b]	+/– scale, not HercepTest
Tsutsui et al. [172]	25% (n = 76)	25% (n = 76)	0, +, + + scale, not HercepTest
Sekido et al. [173]	27% (n = 44)	23% (n = 44)[c]	2+ or 3+, HercepTest
Carlsson et al. [36]	55% (n = 47)	55% (n = 47)[d]	2+ or 3+, HercepTest
Zidan et al. [174]	24% (n = 58)	35% (n = 58)[a]	2+ or 3+, HercepTest

[a]Mainly distant metastases.

[b]Liver and lung metastases.

[c]Metastatic and recurrent tumors.

[d]Only patients that had x-ray verified bone metastases were included. Lymph node metastases were analyzed in all cases except in the studies by Gancberg et al. [170], Vincent-Salomon et al. [171] and Zidan et al. [174] where distant metastases were analyzed.

Table 3.2 Examples of results from HER2 gene amplification analyses of primary breast cancers and corresponding metastases

Xu et al. [175]: "HER2 gene amplification was consistent in multifocal metastases"
Gancberg et al. [170]: "Similar HER2 gene amplification between primary and metastatic samples"
Bozzetti et al. [176]: "Similar HER2 gene amplification between primary and metastatic samples"
Regitnig et al. [41]: "Similar HER2 gene amplification between primary tumor and lymph node metastases"
Regitnig et al. [41]: "Increased HER2 gene amplification in distant metastases in relation to primary tumors"
Gong et al. [177]: "Similar HER2 gene amplification between primary and metastatic samples"
Gong et al. [177]: "Similar HER2 gene amplification between locoregional and distant metastases"
López-Guerrero et al. [178]: "Recurrent breast cancers have a higher fraction of HER2 amplification than the primary tumors"
Tapia et al. [179]: "The HER2 status remains highly conserved as breast cancers metastasize"
Vincent-Salomon et al. [180]: "The HER2 status remained rather stable between bone metastases and the primary tumor"
Palmieri et al. [181]: "Brain breast cancer metastases have a higher fraction of HER2 amplification than the primary tumors"

The results given by Regitnig et al. [41], Gancberg et al. [170], Gong et al. [177] and Palmieri et al. [181], were also supported by results with immunohistochemistry (HercepTest).

The expression in breast cancer of all four EGFR-family receptors has been evaluated in a few cases and it was demonstrated that all four receptors can be expressed [30–32, 44]. HER3 was expressed at least as frequent as HER2, while the frequency of EGFR expression was similar to the expression of HER2. HER4 was somewhat less expressed than HER2 and the expression of HER4 was reported to be associated with good survival prognosis, while expression of EGFR, HER2 and HER3 was associated with bad prognosis. It should also be noted that the intensity level of EGFR expression in breast cancer seems generally lower than for HER2. This is most clearly demonstrated in an old but well performed quantitative estimation of EGFR and HER2 expression where it was demonstrated that HER2 is overexpressed in most cases, while EGFR is underexpressed when related to normal breast tissue [45].

As indicated earlier in this chapter, HER3 seems not to be a suitable target for radionuclide therapy, at least not as a single target, since there are indications from several pathological investigations on various tumors, that HER3 staining is mainly cytoplasmic, while the cell membrane bound fraction of HER3 is difficult to see. This is also supported by the IHC images presented at the human protein atlas (http://www.proteinatlas.org/). The same cytoplasmic pattern is also seen for HER4 staining. This is an obvious controversy since molecular biology studies report on HER3 and HER4 as cell membrane associated receptors expressing a transmembrane region. It cannot be excluded that HER3 and HER4 are, to a large extent, associated with intracellular membranes. Furthermore, it cannot be excluded that

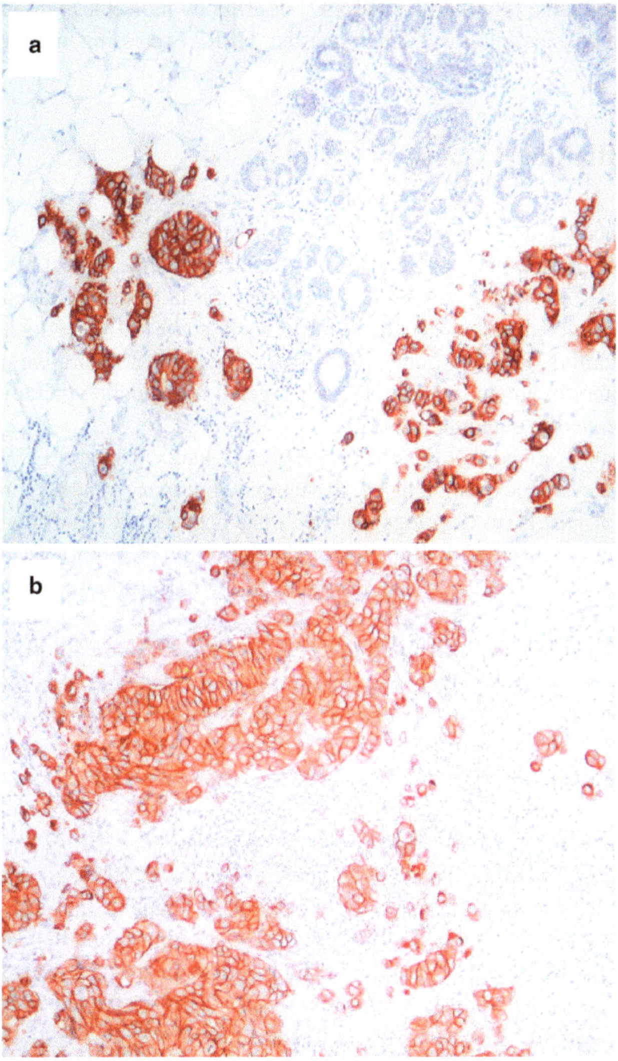

Fig. 3.1 Typical red-brown IHC HER2-stainings of sections from a primary breast cancer (A) and the corresponding lymph node metastasis (B). Note the homogeneous membrane staining of virtually all tumor cells (From [36]. With permission from the Nature Publishing Group)

preforms of HER3 and HER4 in the cytoplasm are stained. However, if HER3 and HER4 are externally exposed in the cellmembrane, they might be there for only a short time due to a possible rapid internalization. The latter could also contribute to the main staining of the cytoplasm.

To summarize, the stability in the HER2 expression is encouraging for efforts to try therapy of disseminated breast cancer with radionuclide labeled HER2 binders such as trastuzumab [46], pertuzumab [47] or affibody molecules [48]. This is especially urgent considering trastuzumab resistant HER2 expressing breast cancers.

Urinary Bladder Cancer

The incidence of urinary bladder cancer is increasing and there is a need for improved diagnostic methods and therapy. Metastases appear most often in lymph nodes, but also in lung, liver and skeleton. Surgery and external radiation therapy are treatment modalities for localized tumors while chemotherapy is used for disseminated tumors. However, chemotherapy is generally not curative and other or complementary treatment modalities, e.g. targeted radionuclide therapy, are necessary to improve the outcome [49–52].

It has been assumed that the epidermal growth factor receptor, EGFR, could be a target for systemic treatment of disseminated urinary bladder tumors. High expression of EGFR (in the range 40–98%) has been found [53–56] and has been related to tumor stage and malignancy grade. Bue et al. [53] reported that EGFR is expressed to a similar level in metastases as in the corresponding primary urinary bladder tumors (65.0% and 70.0%, respectively). Rotterud et al. [55] also reported similar EGFR frequencies in metastases as in the corresponding primary tumors (36.0% and 39.2%, respectively). Expression of EGFR has also been found in small cell carcinomas of the urinary bladder [57]. However, EGFR receptors are also distributed among various normal tissues [15, 16] so it has been assumed that HER2, with a lower expression in normal tissues, is a better target for systemic therapy of urinary bladder cancers.

Thus, a possible urinary bladder tumor associated target is HER2 and the expression frequency has been reported to be in the range 35–98% [49, 54–56, 58–60]. In a study on a limited number of urinary bladder cancer patients (n = 21) it was found that HER2 was overexpressed in 81% of the primary tumors and in 67% of the corresponding metastases and that all HER2 positive metastases were from HER2 positive primary tumors [54]. A tendency towards a lower degree of expression in more distant metastases was also seen and the need for further studies on a larger material was stressed, since the number of samples were too few in this study. Another study (n = 39) concluded that overexpression of HER2 in the primary tumor consistently predicts overexpression in distant or regional metastasis but also that a few HER2 negative primary tumors demonstrated HER2 overexpression in their corresponding metastasis [61].

In a more recent study, the HER2 expression was analyzed in a larger patient material (n = 90) to find a possible difference in receptor expression between primary tumors and metastases at different locations. It was found that there were high HER2 levels in 79% of the primary tumors and 62% in the corresponding metastases. Furthermore, there was a tendency towards a lower fraction of HER2 positive metastases with increasing “distance” from HER2 positive primary tumors. In ten studied sentinel node metastases, coming from HER2 positive primary tumors, all except one were HER2 positive. Considering all regional metastases coming from HER2 positive primary tumors, 28 out of 33 were HER2 positive while for distant metastases the corresponding values were 18 out of 31 [49]. Thus, there seems to be nearly similar HER2 expression in the metastases as in the corresponding primary urinary bladder cancers [49, 54, 55, 61].

The frequency of HER2 positive primary tumors, 79%, in the study by Gårdmark et al. [49], was higher than in many other studies on urinary bladder cancers (e.g. see [54] and references therein). One explanation for the higher value is that only patients with histologically verified metastatic tumor growth and only tumors of high grade were included. A poor correlation between erbB-2 gene amplification and HER2 overexpression has been reported for urinary bladder tumors [58, 59], which is in contrast to the findings for breast cancer. Histological sections from primary urinary bladder tumors and corresponding metastases, stained for HER2, are shown in Fig. 3.2.

The expression of HER3 has been reported to be 99% [56] and 47.0% [55] in primary metastasizing urinary bladder cancers. It has also been reported that HER3 is expressed to nearly the same level in metastases as in the corresponding primary tumors (39.2% and 47.0%, respectively) [55]. It is uncertain if the intensity of the expression in the cell membrane is enough to target HER3 receptors for radionuclide therapy. The expression of HER4 has been reported to be 63% [56] and 41.2% [55] in primary metastasizing urinary bladder cancers. Rotterud et al. [55] also reported that HER4 is expressed to the same level in metastases as in the corresponding primary tumors (40.0% and 41.2%, respectively). It is uncertain, also in the case of HER4, if the intensity of the cell membrane associated expression is enough to target these receptors for radionuclide therapy.

It seems as patients with positive expression of receptors in the EGFR-family in their primary urinary bladder tumors, also express the same receptors in their metastases. Thus, EGFR-family targeted radionuclide therapy, especially targeting HER2, might be an alternative or complement to other therapy modalities for

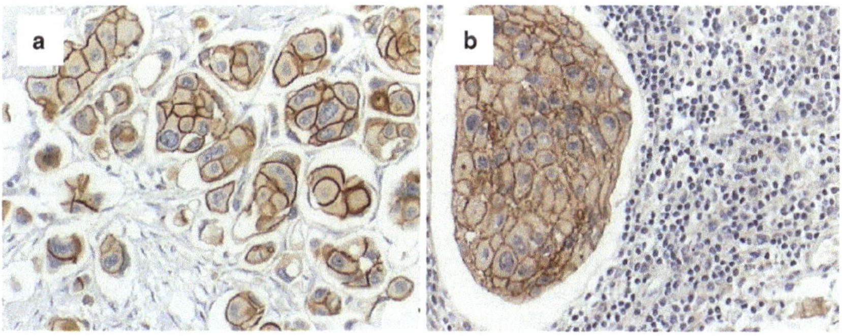

Fig. 3.2 Typical brown IHC HER2-stainings of sections from a primary urinary bladder cancer (A) and the corresponding lymph node metastasis (B). Note the homogeneous membrane staining of virtually all tumor cells (From [54]. With permission from Taylor & Francis Publishing)

urinary bladder cancers. The possibility of targeting more than one receptor at the time (e.g. EGFR and HER2 or HER2 and HER3) is also worth to consider.

Colorectal Cancer

In recent reviews on therapy of colorectal cancer it has been stated that EGFR is often overexpressed in primary colorectal cancers and that overexpression is associated with short time survival of the patients [62, 63]. There is a wide span between reported levels of EGFR-expression in the primary colorectal tumors and individual studies have reported EGFR expression in 20–95% of the studied cases ([64–70], and references given in Table 3.3). EGFR positive cells have also been detected in peripheral blood from colon cancer patients [71, 72]. No expression of the mutated EGFRvIII receptor has so far been found in colorectal cancers [70]. There are several studies analyzing EGFR expression in colorectal primary tumors and corresponding metastases (see Table 3.3). There is obviously a rather good agreement between the reported frequencies of expression in the primary tumors and the metastases, irrespective of lymph node or liver metastases are considered.

HER2 has also been reported to be overexpressed in primary colorectal cancers. The determinations vary within the wide range of 3–82% [64, 65, 67, 73–78]. In the report by Knosel et al. [76] there is also a summary of 10 previously published, during 1994–2001, investigations including 1,007 patients, on HER2 expression in primary colorectal cancers. More than half of the investigated cases were HER2 positive. HER2 expression has also been associated with poor survival and dissemination [76]. HER2 expression in metastases has been less studied and has so far been reported to be in the range 36–54% [75, 76, 79].

Thus, HER2 is rather often expressed in colorectal cancers and the frequency is probably about half of all cases. Furthermore, the general impression from the studies is that even if the obtained frequency numbers often can be rather high, the intensity of expression and the frequency of positive cells within each colorectal tumor are

Table 3.3 Examples of EGFR expression, measured with immunohistochemistry (IHC), in primary colorectal carcinomas and corresponding metastases

Report	Primary tumor	Li-metastases	Ln-metastases	Comment
Saeki et al. [79]	51.1% (n = 45)	NA	61.5% (n = 13)	SN
DeJong et al. [182]	30% (n = 33)	13% (n = 45)	NA	SN
Goldstein et al. [183]	20–33% (n = 102)	39.7% (n = 45)	32.9% (n = 97)	0–3+ scale
Scartozzi et al. [184]	53% (n = 53)	46% (n = 39)	NA	≥1% of cells
Italiano et al. [185]	80% (n = 45)	81.2% (n = 79)	NA	≥1% of cells
Bralet et al. [186]	95% (n = 40)	79% (n = 64)	88% (n = 27)	≥1% of cells
Shia et al. [187]	85% (n = 123)	79% (n = 24)[a]	NA	0–3+ scale
Scartozzi et al. [188]	52% (n = 98)	48% (n = 84)	NA	1+ to 3+ scale

Li = Liver, Ln = Lymph node, NA = Not analyzed, SN = Scoring method not known

[a]Only six liver metastases, the rest lung metastases.

generally lower than for breast cancers. Thus, it seems as colorectal cancer might not be as suitable for HER2 radionuclide targeting as breast cancers. However, more research on this is necessary. The reported large variations in both EGFR and HER2 expression are probably due to both different patient inclusion criteria and methodological differences (especially regarding IHC, e.g. applying different retrieval methods) between laboratories.

HER3 has previously been reported to be expressed in 36–89% of colorectal cancers [65, 67, 80–82]. A recent study on 106 patient cases by Kountourakis et al. [26] reported that HER3 membrane and cytoplasmic staining was seen in 17.0% and 28.3% of the cases, respectively. Examples of HER3 stainings in colorectal cancers are shown in Fig. 3.3.

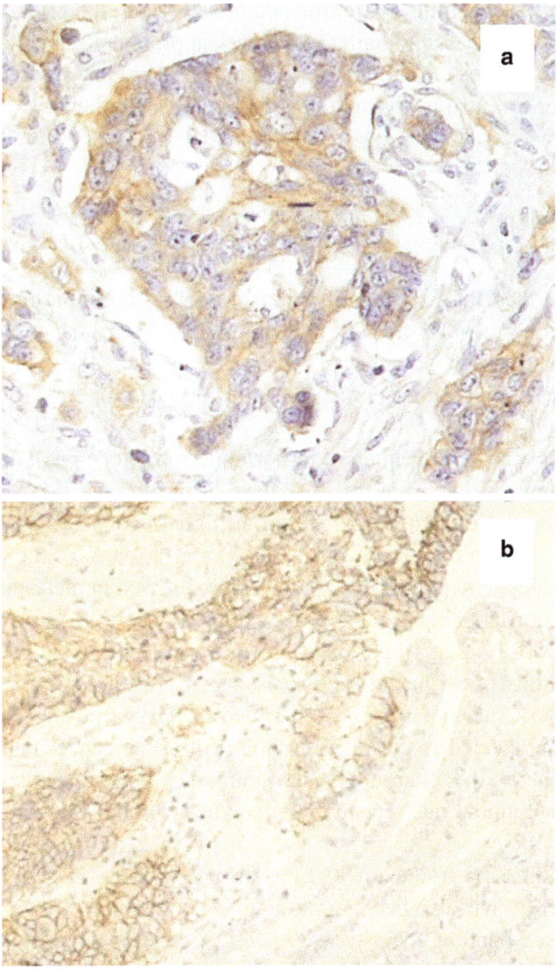

Fig. 3.3 Immunohistochemical HER3-stainings (brown) of sections from primary colorectal cancers. The stainings were weak membranous and cytoplasmic in (A) and mainly weak membranous in (B) (From [26]. With kind permission)

HER4 has previously been reported to be expressed in 22% of colorectal cancers [67]. The recent study on 106 patient cases by Kountourakis et al. [26] reported that HER4 membrane and cytoplasmic staining was seen in 18.9% and 30.2% of the cases, respectively.

It seems as EGFR and HER2 expression is rather frequent in colorectal cancers. However, there seems to be low amounts of both types of receptors per cell. This indicates that there might be necessary with “double targeting”, i.e. radiolabeled targeting agents can be given as a cocktail with binders to both EGFR and HER2. According to the results by Kountourakis et al. [26], HER3 and HER4 might also be considered. Bifunctional antibodies or affibody molecules, with capacity to bind with one arm to e.g. EGFR and with the other to e.g. HER2 is also a possible approach. However, the concept of double receptor targeting has to be analyzed further and tried in preclinical experiments. If successful, the principle can then be tried for radionuclide based imaging in patients, applying radionuclides suitable for gamma- or PET cameras. If the tumor specificity and uptake is good then there can be considerations of also using radionuclides suitable for therapy.

Prostate Cancer

It has been reported that EGFR is more expressed in hormone refractory than in hormone sensitive prostate cancers [83–85] and that blocking of EGFR possibly can decrease the invasive potential of prostate cancer cells [86, 87]. The frequency of EGFR expression in primary prostate cancer has been reported to be in the range 40–45% [88, 89].

The HER2 expression frequency in hormone refractory prostate cancer is not settled and values in the range 20–70% have been reported [88–90]. In addition, HER2 has been reported to be expressed at high frequencies in prostate cancer metastases and has, in one study, been found in up to 90% of the analyzed cases [91]. Myers et al. [92] reported that HER2 was expressed in metastases to a similar level as in the corresponding primary prostate tumors. There are also studies reporting low frequencies of HER2 expression in prostate cancers [93] and there is one study actually reporting almost no HER2 expression in prostate cancers and the corresponding lymph node metastases [94]. However, HER2 positive prostate cancer cells have been detected in peripheral blood of prostate cancer patients [95]. The situation regarding HER2 targeting with antibodies without radioactivity of hormone refractory tumors has recently been studied without, so far, positive results [96, 97].

A HER3 expression frequency of 21% has been reported [88] in primary prostate cancers. HER3 has also been reported to be expressed in both primary prostate cancers and corresponding metastases [92, 98]. A secreted isoform of HER3, called MDA-BF-1, has been reported to be expressed in metastatic prostate cancer [99]. HER4 expression in prostate cancer has, in one recent study, been reported to be 29% [88].

Thus, prostate cancers seem to have capacity to express all EGFR-family receptors, especially EGFR and HER2. Solit and Rosen [100] have summarized the situation regarding the use of tyrosine kinase inhibitors blocking HER2 and EGFR in hormone refractory prostate cancers and concluded that there seemed to be no response. Thus, in those cases with significant levels of receptors expressed, but with tumor cells resistant to tyrosine kinase inhibitors, targeted radionuclide therapy can be an interesting alternative. However, in parallel to colorectal carcinomas, the EGFR and HER2 receptors seem not to be highly expressed neither in frequency of patients nor per tumor cell [97, 100–106]. This indicates that there is, as for colorectal carcinomas, a possible need for"double targeting", i.e. radiolabeled targeting agents might be given as a cocktail with binders to both EGFR and HER2 (and possibly also HER3). Bifunctional antibodies or affibody molecules, with capacity to bind two different receptors, is probably a possible approach for imaging and radionuclide therapy of disseminated prostate cancers. More research is needed regarding this.

Esophageal Tumors

The expression of epidermal growth factor receptor, EGFR, has been studied in primary esophageal cancers, and overexpression is common [22, 23, 107–110] and is also associated with poor prognosis [111, 112]. The reported EGFR expression frequencies were, in most of these reports, within the range 50–80%. The EGFR targeted drugs that are now commercially available, including small-molecule tyrosine kinase inhibitors (e.g. Iressa and Tarceva), as well as the antibody cetuximab (Erbitux) have, with the exception of Iressa, not yet been tried for therapy of esophageal cancers. Iressa has been used as second-line treatment of advanced esophageal cancer patients in one clinical trial showing limited success [113]. Kinase domain EGFR mutations have been found in esophageal tumors [114] but so far not exploited for therapy.

The frequency of HER2 expression in esophageal carcinoma has been reported to vary in the wide range of 0–65% [22, 110, 115–118]. High HER2 expression has actually only been found in 2–10% of the studied patients [22, 107, 115, 118]. However, two studies have reported HER2 overexpression in more than half of the patients [23, 119]. Thus, there is an obvious controversy regarding HER2 expression in esophageal carcinoma. There might be many reasons for the observed differences, including patient selection, methodology of the IHC procedures, scoring and the definition of overexpression.

HER3 expression can be found in normal squamous epithelium of esophagus [120], but so far, the literature on HER3 expression in esophageal carcinoma is limited. In a study by Wei et al. [22], HER3 staining was restricted to the cytoplasm, exhibiting diffuse and/or granular cytoplasmic staining (Fig. 3.4E) and HER3 expression was observed in about half of the primary tumors. Positive HER3 staining has previously been reported in about 64% of primary esophageal

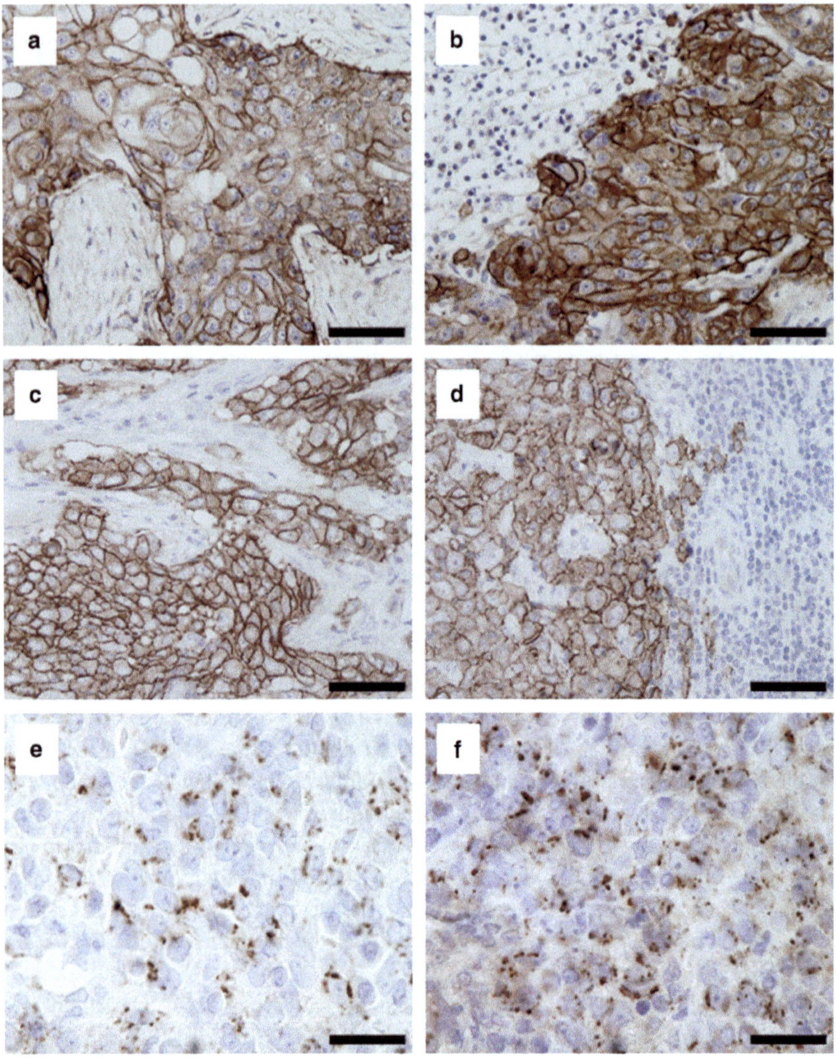

Fig. 3.4 Comparisons of the immunohistochemical brown receptor stainings of primary esophageal squamous cell cancers (A, C and E) and corresponding metastases (B, D and F) from three patients. (A and B): EGFR-stainings. (C and D): HER2 stainings. (E and F): HER3 stainings. The bars in A–D correspond to 50 μm and the bars in E and F correspond to 20 μm (From [22]. With permission from International Journal of Oncology)

cancers [23]. The author has not seen reports on the expression of HER4 in esophageal tumors.

At least one investigation has been carried out to characterize possible differences in the EGFR, HER2 and HER3 expression between the primary esophageal tumors and metastases. The expression was investigated immunohistochemically in both lymph node metastases and corresponding primary tumors (n = 51) [22]. The major part of the cases were squamous cell carcinomas, ESCC (n = 40). EGFR overexpression was found in 67.5% of both the ESCC primary tumors and the corresponding lymph node metastases. HER2 overexpression was found only in three of all the primary ESCC tumors and only two of the lymph node metastases. The HER3 staining was mainly cytoplasmic and granular and was observed in about half of the cases, both for primary tumors and the corresponding lymph node metastases. Examples of EGFR, HER2 and HER3 stainings in the studied squamous esophagus carcinomas and corresponding metastases are shown in Fig. 3.4.

Regarding other previous comparisons between primary tumors and metastases the author has found only one more report [121] which reported that 88% of the metastatic lymph nodes (n = 46) were EGFR positive. In the cases with EGFR expression in the primary tumors, 94.3% of the lymph node metastases were EGFR positive.

The conclusion is that EGFR expression is stable when comparing the lymph node metastases with the primary esophageal cancer [22, 121]. Actually, it seems that EGFR expression in the primary tumors can predict EGFR-positive lymph node metastases with a reasonably high probability. Thus, the stability in EGFR expression is encouraging for efforts to develop radionuclide based EGFR targeting strategies.

There are, to the knowledge of the authors, only three studies in the literature concerning the stability of HER2 expression between primary esophageal tumors and the corresponding lymph node metastases [22, 116, 118]. In the study by Mimura et al. [116] only three cases with HER2 expression were found out of 66 primary tumors. HER2 overexpression was preserved in the metastatic lymph nodes in all three cases. In the studies by Wei et al. [22] and Reichelt et al. [118] there was also a low HER2 expression frequency and a reasonably good agreement between the HER2 expression in the primary tumors and the corresponding metastases. Thus, the frequency of HER2 overexpression in esophageal cancer seems to be low, which suggests a limited role of this receptor as a target for treatment. For the few patients with strong HER2 membrane staining in the primary tumor, the same HER2 expression in the lymph node metastases is expected, which might be of interest for HER2 targeted therapy in those few cases. However, EGFR seems to be the major target candidate for radionuclide therapy of esophageal tumors.

Head and Neck Squamous Carcinomas

Squamous cell carcinomas of the head and neck region, HNSCC, spread locally in the near epithelium and later they form lymph node metastases [122]. Treatment with surgery and external radiotherapy of patients with HNSCC is difficult since the normal epithelium near the primary tumor might be invaded with single tumor cells and small islands of microscopic tumors. Chemotherapy is included when dissemination is suspected, but with limited positive results. The search for prognostic markers to predict clinical behavior and metastatic potential of a tumor has made some progress but there is a need for new forms of diagnostics and treatment. One such approach is receptor mediated tumor targeting using radiolabeled antibodies or ligands [3, 21].

The EGFR biology in HNSCC has been reviewed recently [122] and overexpression of EGFR is common [21, 123–129]. The reported overexpression frequencies are most often in the range 30–50% and in some cases even up to 80–90%. Thus, EGFR is a potential target for radionuclide therapy.

Expression of HER2 has been reported in HNSCC although at low frequencies, 0–30%, and also, in most cases, with lower intensity in the staining than for EGFR [21, 124, 127, 128, 130–133]. Thus, HER2 seems to be a less interesting target than EGFR for radionuclide therapy of HNSCC.

HER3 has been shown to be overexpressed in 20–70% of the studied HNSCC cases and associated with malignant progression [21, 122, 124, 134, 135]. The HER3 staining has been reported to by mainly cytoplasmic [21]. HER3 can also be expressed in the normal surface squamous epithelium of the tongue, oropharynx and esophagus [120]. There are reports on coexpression of HER3 with other EGFR-family members in HNSCC [124, 136, 137]. HER4 is expressed in 25–60% of the studied HNSCC cases [21, 122, 124]. The HER4 staining intensity has been reported to be low and mainly cytoplasmic [21]. The role of HER4 in HNSCC tumor development is not clear.

In the study by Ekberg et al. [21], the expression of all four EGFR-family receptors in HNSCC of the oral cavity and base of the tongue was compared with their corresponding metastases and normal epithelium in a limited number of patients (n = 19). It was found that EGFR had a similar and high expression in both primary tumors and the corresponding metastases, while the expression in normal epithelium was lower in most cases. Thus, EGFR seemed generally stable when comparing primary tumors with the corresponding metastases. HER2 was not expressed to the same extent and intensity as EGFR [21]. However, when HER2 was expressed, it was in most cases expressed to the same extent and intensity in the metastases as in the primary tumors. HER3 and HER4 were expressed to about the same level in the primary HNSCC as in the metastases. No overexpression of HER3 and HER4 in the tumors was seen as compared to normal epithelium. Examples of EGFR, HER2, HER3 and HER4 stainings in HNSCC of the oral cavity are shown Fig. 3.5. Examples of stainings in normal oral epithelium are shown Fig. 3.6.

Since the EGFR-family receptors form heterodimers and seem to be coexpressed in HNSCC [122, 124, 135–137] further work is needed on this. It is possible that a better specificity can be achieved if a targeting agent is directed against a heterodimer structure characteristic of the HNSCC tumor cells. Whether that will give low normal tissue uptake and at the same time enough amount of radiolabeled targeting agents in the tumor cells to allow for therapy is unclear.

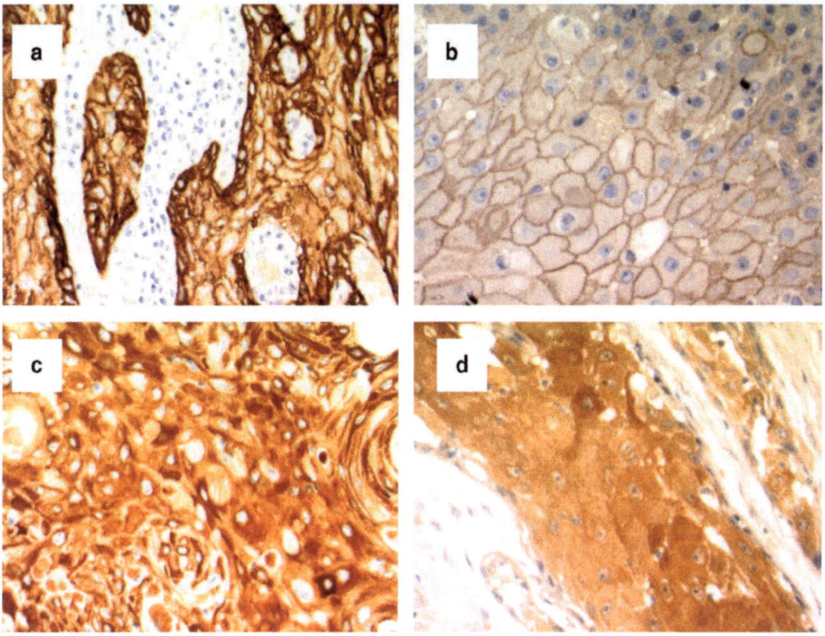

Fig. 3.5 Examples of immunostaining in of head and neck squamous carcinomas, HNSCC, of the oral cavity. EGFR (A), HER2 (B), HER3 (C) and HER4 (D) (From [21]. With permission from International Journal of Oncology)

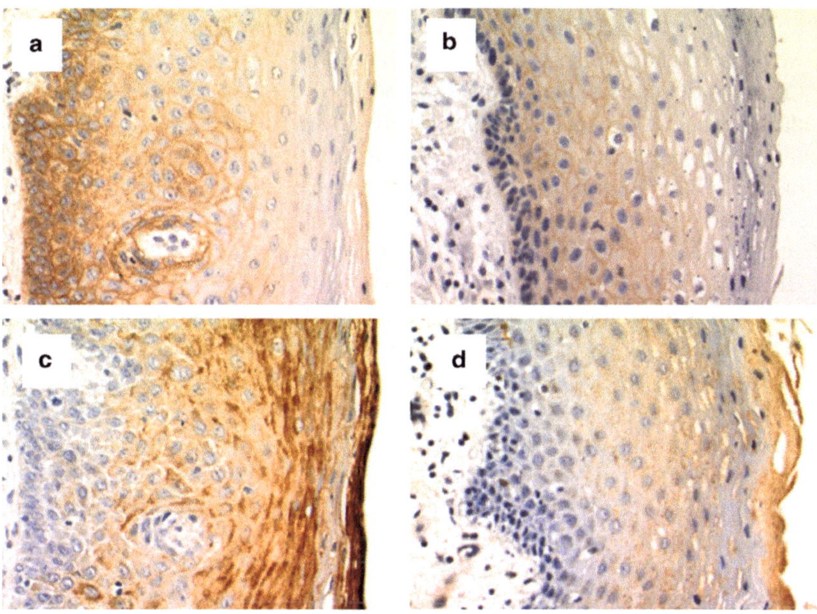

Fig. 3.6 Examples of immunostainings of normal oral epithelium for EGFR (A), HER2 (B), HER3 (C) and HER4 (D) (From [21]. With permission from International Journal of Oncology)

Gliomas

It is known that gliomas do not generate metastases outside CNS. Thus, comparisons of receptor expression between the primary tumor and metastases cannot be made. Instead, the relation between the primary tumor and the locally migrating glioma cells within CNS is discussed regarding the expression of EGFR.

The most common brain tumors in adults, and also the most aggressive, are the glioblastomas, GBM. The GBM cells display good migration potential and appear to invade normal brain tissue along the white matter tracts, around nerve cells and along perivascular spaces. GBMs are so far considered incurable [138]. One usually distinguishes between primary GBMs and secondary GBMs [139]. Secondary GBMs arise in somewhat younger patients with a previous lower-grade astrocytoma [140] and these tumors seldom express EGFGR, while primary GBMs most often have overexpression of EGFR [139, 141]. EGFR overexpression in the primary GBMs correlates with decreased survival [139, 142]. It has been indicated that EGFR overexpression is most pronounced at the tumor cell invading edges [143]. At least half of all analyzed GBM patients have overexpression of EGFR in their tumors [141, 142, 144].

Patients with GBM are often treated with surgery to remove the bulky part of the tumor and the cavity margin is then irradiated [145]. Despite this, recurrence occurs in almost all patients and the median survival time is less than 1.5 years [145–147]. Chemotherapy is often given with a palliative intention. Temozolomide in combination with radiotherapy has recently been shown to increase median survival time with some months and to increase the two years survival from 8% to 26% [148]. However, several other chemotherapeutics have proved not to be efficient [138].

Intracavitary radionuclide therapy has since long been claimed to be a promising modality for postoperative treatment of GBM, since the migrating tumor cells might thereby be reached and killed [149]. The subject has been reviewed when the extracellular matrix component tenascin was targeted with radiolabeled antibodies. The survival time after such intracavitary radionuclide therapy was prolonged, when compared to other forms of GBM therapy, but no cure was achieved [150].

HER2 has been reported to be only expressed in 10–15% of the studied GBM patients and is also related to poor survival [151, 152]. The author has not found reports on the frequency of HER3 and HER4 expression in GBMs.

Thus, it is possible that targeting of the epidermal growth factor receptor, EGFR, via intracavitary injections of radiolabeled EGFR-binding agents can improve both the possibility to image the tumor extension and to carry out therapy. However, targeting EGFR with radiolabeled anti-EGFR antibodies via intravenous or intra-arterial injections has previously been reported but has, so far, not given satisfactory treatment results [153–156].

A review on EGFR as a possible target for radionuclide based intracavitary therapy of GBM:s has recently been published [157]. It was concluded that the therapeutical efforts made so far using antibodies have given limited effects, probably due to low radiation doses to the migrating tumor cells. The low radiation doses might be due to limited penetration of the antibodies. The possibility to target

EGFR with lower molecular weight substances, e.g. radiolabeled ligands or affibody molecules, was recommended.

However, there seems to be a lack of knowledge on the degree of intratumoral variation of EGFR expression in GBM. In the limited study by Carlsson et al. [157], the EGFR expression seemed rather homogeneous over large areas in the clinical samples (n = 16). Examples of EGFR stainings in GBM are shown in Fig. 3.7. It was discussed that loss of EGFR expression might not be the critical factor for successful intracavitary radionuclide therapy. Instead, it is likely that the penetration property of the targeting agent is critical. It was indicated that low molecular weight targeting agents might be preferable to antibodies due to better penetration properties. However, studies on penetration are necessary to verify, since there might be a "cavity wound" barrier, which might make it difficult also for low molecular weight substances to penetrate. Transport in the extracellular spaces, i.e. in the cerebrospinal fluid and in the extracellular matrix, might also be a problem.

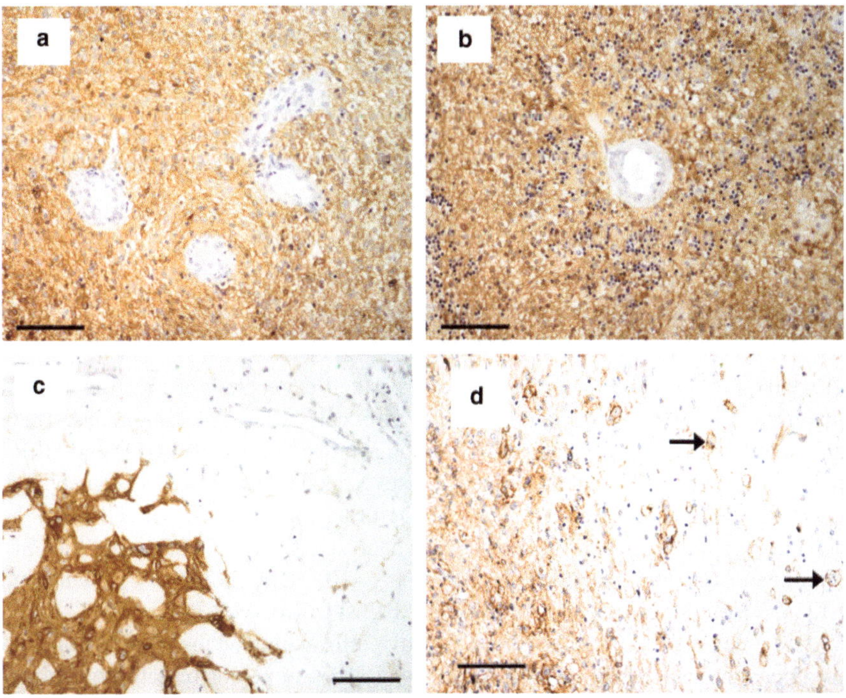

Fig. 3.7 Examples of EGFR expression in GBM tumors. Strong membranous and homogeneous EGFR staining in large tumor areas with, at least three, EGFR-negative blood vessels are shown in (A). A similar strong membranous and homogeneous EGFR staining is shown in (B), but in this case with infiltrating lymphocytes (and only one big blood vessel). (C) Shows strong and homogeneous EGFR staining of tumor cells infiltrating, from the lower left part, a loose "scar-like" area containing non-tumor cells. E shows homogeneous but weak EGFR staining of tumor cells in the tumor front infiltrating the normal brain tissue (to the right). Two examples of spread tumor cells in D are indicated with arrows. The bars correspond in all figures to 100 μm (From [157]. With permission from International Journal of Neurooncology)

The mutated EGFRvIII receptor has also been suggested as a target in glioma treatment [158, 159]. However, this mutated receptor is less represented than the wild type EGFR in GBM:s. An interesting observation from the results of IHC on the glioma samples, as studied by Ohman et al. [160], was that the staining of EGFRvIII to a large extent seemed cytoplasmic. Published results have shown that the expression of EGFRvIII is, in addition, also cell membrane associated [158]. EGFRvIII is known to be in the constitutively signaling (ligand independent) and when positioned in the cellular membrane it can not be excluded that also signaling for internalization takes place constitutively. If so, the EGFRvIII will only shortly visit the cellular membrane and then be internalized [160].

The observed homogeneity of EGFR expression was surprising considering the genomic instability and heterogeneity that characterize GBM:s. However, overexpression of EGFR is, at least in primary GBMs, one of the steps in the development of malignancy, and tumor cells that lose or down regulate EGFR will probably be outgrown in an expanding tumor cell population.

The general conclusion is that intracavitary radionuclide GBM therapy has proven to prolong survival but not to be curative when the extracellular matrix component tenascin has been the target. EGFR is an interesting target for intracavitary GBM radionuclide therapy that, in cases with high and homogeneous EGFR expression, might improve current therapeutical results. Further investigations on EGFR expression in distantly migrating glioma cells as well as further studies on the homogeneity in EGFR expression are necessary.

Quantification of Receptor Expression

Quantification of the number of receptors per cell is generally difficult in clinical material. The most reliable data is instead from cell cultures measurements. There are actually several published reports on the average number of EGFR and HER2 per cultured tumor cell. In most of these cases Scatchard analysis has been applied. One example is that there seems to be in the order of 10^6 EGFR per cell when the squamous carcinoma cells A431 have been analyzed ([161] and references therein). Another example is that there seems to be $\approx 10^6$ HER2 receptors per cultured SKOV-3 (ovarian cancer) and per SKBR3 (breast cancer) cell.

It is much more difficult to get quantitative information on the number of receptors per tumor cell from patient samples (biopsies or tumor resection material). Analysis of the number of receptors per cell can not, at least to the knowledge of the author, be made from tissue sections. Furthermore, it is well known that immunohistochemical stainings are not quantitative even if it is obvious that a weak staining corresponds to a low receptor expression and a strong staining should correspond to high expression. However, indirect comparisons can be made. For example, SKOV-3 cells have been grown as transplanted tumors and these cells have about 10^6 HER2 per cell when analyzed *in vitro*. The tumors were then fixed, embedded in paraffin, sectioned and stained for HER2 in the same way as tissue preparations from patients normally are processed [162]. It could be seen that these tumors gave a similar strong HER2 staining as HER2 positive breast cancer tumors from patients [36] scored as 2+/3+ using the established HercepTest® criteria. Since the same staining techniques were applied for both the transplanted tumors and the patient samples, and the stainings were carried out at the same laboratory, it is reasonable to assume that also the patient tumors had about 10^6 receptors per cell. Actually, it is often said, informally, among pathologists that the 3+ score in the HercepTest® criteria correspond to about that number of HER2 receptors.

However, the author has also, with a rubber policeman, scraped EGFR and HER2 positive cultured tumor cells with about 10^6 receptors per cell, from culture dishes and centrifuged them to a pellet and then processed them as if they were biopsy preparations from patients. In these cases the immunohistochemical stainings had presented a somewhat weaker staining than clinical material from gliomas and urinary bladder cancers (EGFR) and breast cancers (HER2) indicating the possibility that the tumor cells in the clinical samples had even more than 10^6 receptors per cell (not published data). This is reported here only to emphasize the uncertainty of receptor quantification in patient samples. It is necessary to establish methods for quantitative and representative evaluation of especially EGFR and HER2 expression in patient tumors. Such information is desired to allow for better prediction of the suitability of receptor targeted radionuclide therapy for individual patients, i.e. to allow for "personalized medicine".

An attempt has been made to quantify the EGFR expression in patient samples of head and neck squamous cell carcinoma (HNSCC) using a radioimmunoassay. The assay using ^{125}I-cetuximab was first validated and then applied to quantify expression of EGFR, in patient samples. Results were compared to immunohistochemical stainings. The assay provided sensitive quantitative values generally in agreement with the expected qualitative immunohistochemistry (IHC) results [163]. It was concluded that the radioimmunoassay is simple, reliable, and can be performed on a small amount (50 mg) of tissue. This assay could be a useful tool in the growing field of personalized cancer therapy, and can at least be used as a complement to IHC.

Genomic Instability as a Threat to Targeted Radionuclide Therapy

The stability in EGFR and HER2 expression, as reported above, seems surprising in the light of the genomic instability that characterize most malignant tumors. Tumors are formed via multistep carcinogenesis involving defect onco-, suppressor-, cell cycle- and apoptosis regulating genes [2, 164, 165]. EGFR and HER2 overexpression can be regarded as overexpression of oncogene products and the often related gene amplification as an oncogene amplification. It is likely that EGFR and HER2 overexpression is, at least for many tumors, one of the steps in the multistep process towards malignancy and that loss or a decrease in expression of these receptors therefore might decrease the growth potential of the tumors. Tumor cells that lose or downregulate EGFR or HER2 will then be outgrown in an expanding tumor cell population [3]. They can possibly also be directed towards apoptosis since it has been indicated that changes in HER2 expression can, at least in combination with therapy, modify the route to apoptosis [9, 10].

The arguments given above about the lack of influence of genomic instability on EGFR and HER2 expression are of obvious interest when targeted radionuclide therapy is considered. It is expected that an efficient therapy, based on targeting of the receptors, would tend to induce survival selection for cells with low or no expression. However, as discussed above, such cells might have a decreased growth potential and, during therapy they can even be triggered to apoptosis. Thus, it is likely that EGFR and HER2 are suitable targets for radionuclide targeted therapy also if treatment induced selection is considered [3, 36].

Discussion

It seems as the expression of EGFR and HER2 often is similar in metastases as in the corresponding primary tumor, at least in most of the tumor types discussed above. EGFR targeting drugs are clinically available, including small-molecule tyrosine kinase inhibitors (e.g. Iressa and Tarceva), as well as the chimeric monoclonal antibody cetuximab (Erbitux) and the humanized antibody trastuzumab (Herceptin). However, these agents seem generally to stop tumor growth temporarily and the tumors unfortunately continue to grow if delivery of these drugs is interrupted. Some of these drugs also enhance the effect of chemotherapy. However, both EGFR and HER2 are, in these cases, probably better candidates for targeted radionuclide therapy of disseminated tumor cells and metastasis and such therapy relies on several years of experience to kill cells with ionizing radiation.

It actually seems as target expression is not a major problem, rather, it is likely that the design of suitable targeting agents with low uptake in critical normal tissues, and suitable biodistribution and pharmacokinetics, is the major challenge for the future. However, there is good hope for a good development of that, as is described in several chapters in this book. New knowledge is continuously emerging related to receptor targeting. Pharmacokinetics and cellular processing of different types of targeting agents increases and the research dealing with molecular design of new targeting agents is rapidly expanding. The development of peptides and small proteins with specificity against tumor cells is one strategy. The area of antibody engineering is also rapidly developing and various forms of antibody fragments are developed such as minimal recognizing units, single chain fragments, scFv, and dimeric scFv. Liposomes containing toxic substances and conjugated with targeting agents might be of special interest for killing of disseminated tumor cells that remain in the systemic circulation. Thus, there are several possibilities for new and complementary strategies when targeting of disseminated growth factor expressing tumors are considered. It should also be noted that resistance induction has so far not been associated with radiation treatment in spite of more than 100 years of experience of radiation therapy of tumors.

Furthermore, it seems that tumors expressing mutated EGFR-family receptors (especially in the case of EGFR) are rather sensitive to tyrosine kinase inhibitors while the majority of tumors expressing native EGFR-family receptors are not. Planned radionuclide therapy is mainly considering targeting of native receptors, which open up for such therapy of large groups of patients. Thus, targeted radionuclide therapy can be a complement, or even a better alternative, to application of tyrosine kinase inhibitors. There are increasing numbers of not exploited possibilities to use EGFR-family receptors as targets in radionuclide therapy, as discussed in this chapter. One example is the potential possibility to target more than one receptor at the time, e.g. EGFR together with HER2, as suggested for urinary bladder, colorectal and prostate cancers ("double targeting").

Conclusion

Growth factor receptors of the EGFR-family are suitable targets for radionuclide therapy since they, when highly expressed, appear in a similar extent in both in the primary tumor and the corresponding disseminated tumor cells and metastases. HER2 is the obvious candidate for radionuclide therapy of trastuzumab resistant HER2 expressing disseminated breast cancers. EGFR and HER2 are together ("double targeting") potential candidates for radionuclide therapy of disseminated bladder, colorectal and prostate cancers. EGFR is the major candidate for radionuclide therapy of disseminated head and neck and esophageal squamous carcinomas and for intracavitary radionuclide therapy of gliomas.

Progress and problems when applying tumor therapy with radionuclides has been reviewed recently [3–8]. It was concluded that targeted radionuclide therapy with radiolabeled anti-CD20 antibodies is an accepted modality for treatment of chemotherapy resistant lymphoma, and for neuroendocrine tumors using somatostatin analogues. However, treatment of most other tumors so far has been unsuccessful. The promising therapeutic results for lymphomas give hope that targeted radionuclide therapy will be successful also for treatment of disseminated cells and metastases from solid tumors. The availability of suitable growth factor receptors indicates that this will be the case. Such radionuclide therapy has the potential to switch palliative to curative treatment.

Acknowledgements Financial support from the Swedish Cancer Society, grant 0980-B06-19XBC, and Vinnova, grant 2004-02159, for research related to the content of this article is acknowledged. Thanks also to the journals that allowed the author to reproduce, and in some cases slightly modify, figures from previously published articles (see figure texts for details).

References

1. McGill MA, McGlade CJ (2004) Cellular signaling. In: The Basic Science of Oncology (editors: Tannock IF, Hill RP, Bristow RC and Harrington L). McGraw-Hill Medical Publishing Division, New York (ISBN-13: 978-0-07-138774-3), Chapter 8, pp142–166
2. Pecorino L (2005) Molecular Biology of Cancer. Mechanisms, Targets and Therapeutics. Oxford University Press, Oxford (ISBN 0-19-926472-4)
3. Carlsson J, Forssell AE, Hietala SO, Stigbrand T, Tennvall J (2003) Tumour therapy with radionuclides: assessment of progress and problems. Radiother Oncol 66: 107–17
4. Adams GP, Weiner LM (2005) Monoclonal antibody therapy of cancer. Nat Biotechnol 23(9): 1147–57. Review
5. DeNardo SJ, DeNardo GL (2006) Targeted radionuclide therapy for solid tumors: an overview. Int J Radiat Oncol Biol Phys 66(Suppl 2): S89–95. Review
6. Goldenberg DM, Sharkey RM (2006) Advances in cancer therapy with radiolabeled monoclonal antibodies. Q J Nucl Med Mol Imaging 50(4): 248–64. Review
7. Witzig TE (2006) Radioimmunotherapy for B-cell non-Hodgkin lymphoma. Best Pract Res Clin Haematol 19(4): 655–68. Review
8. Wong JY (2006) Systemic targeted radionuclide therapy: potential new areas. Int J Radiat Oncol Biol Phys 66(Suppl 2): S74–82. Review
9. Citri A, Yarden Y (2006) EGF-ERBB signalling: towards the systems level. Nat Rev Mol Cell Biol 7(7): 505–16
10. Bublil EM, Yarden Y (2007) The EGF receptor family: spearheading a merger of signaling and therapeutics. Curr Opin Cell Biol 19(2): 124–34. Review
11. Hynes NE, Lane HA (2005) ERBB receptors and cancer: the complexity of targeted inhibitors. Nat Rev Cancer 5(5): 341–54.
12. Scaltriti M, Baselga J (2006) The epidermal growth factor receptor pathway: a model for targeted therapy. Clin Cancer Res 12(18): 5268–72. Review
13. Mendelsohn J, Baselga J (2006) Epidermal growth factor receptor targeting in cancer. Semin Oncol 33: 369–85
14. Baselga J, Perez EA, Pienkowski T, Bell R (2006) Adjuvant trastuzumab: a milestone in the treatment of HER-2-positive early breast cancer. Oncologist 11(Suppl 1): 4–12. Review
15. Gusterson B, Cowley G, Smith JA, Ozanne B (1984) Cellular localisation of human epidermal growth factor receptor. Cell Biol Int Rep 8: 649–58
16. Damjanov I, Mildner B, Knowles BB (1986) Immunohistochemical localization of the epidermal growth factor receptor in normal human tissues. Lab Invest 55: 588–92
17. Natali PG, Nicotra MR, Bigotti A, Venturo I, Slamon DJ, Fendly BM, Ullrich A (1990) Expression of the p185 encoded by HER2 oncogene in normal and transformed human tissues. Int J Cancer 45: 457–61
18. Press MF, Cordon-Cardo C, Slamon DJ (1990) Expression of the HER-2/neu proto-oncogene in normal human adult and fetal tissues. Oncogene 5: 953–62
19. Plowman GD, Culouscou JM, Whitney GS (1993) Ligand-specific activation of HER4/p180 erbB4, a fourth member of the epidermal growth factor receptor family. Proc Natl Acad Sci USA 90(5): 1746–50
20. Srinivasan R, Gillett CE, Barnes DM, Gullick WJ (2000) Nuclear expression of the c-erbB 4/HER-4 growth factor receptor in invasive breast cancers. Cancer Res 60(6): 1483–7
21. Ekberg T, Nestor M, Engstrom M, Nordgren H, Wester K, Carlsson J, Anniko M (2005) Expression of EGFR, HER2, HER3, and HER4 in metastatic squamous cell carcinomas of the oral cavity and base of tongue. Int J Oncol 26(5): 1177–85
22. Wei Q, Chen L, Sheng L, Nordgren H, Wester K, Carlsson J (2007) EGFR, HER2 and HER3 expression in esophageal primary tumours and corresponding metastases. Int J Oncol 31: 493–9
23. Friess H, Fukuda A, Tang WH, Eichenberger A, Furlan N, Zimmermann A, Korc M, Buchler MW (1999) Concomitant analysis of the epidermal growth factor receptor family in esophageal

cancer: overexpression of epidermal growth factor receptor mRNA but not of c-erbB-2 and c erbB-3. World J Surg 23: 1010–8
24. Tanner B, Hasenclever D, Stern K, Schormann W, Bezler M, Hermes M, Brulport M, Bauer A, Schiffer IB, Gebhard S, Schmidt M, Steiner E, Sehouli J, Edelmann J, Lauter J, Lessig R, Krishnamurthi K, Ullrich A, Hengstler JG (2006) ErbB-3 predicts survival in ovarian cancer. J Clin Oncol 24: 4317–23
25. Leibl S, Bodo K, Gogg-Kammerer M, Hrzenjak A, Petru E, Winter R, Denk H, Moinfar F (2006) Ovarian granulosa cell tumors frequently express EGFR (Her-1), Her-3, and Her-4: an immunohistochemical study. Gynecol Oncol 101: 18–23
26. Kountourakis P, Pavlakis K, Psyrri A, Rontogianni D, Xiros N, Patsouris E, Pectasides D, Economopoulos T (2006) Prognostic significance of HER3 and HER4 protein expression in colorectal adenocarcinomas. BMC Cancer 6: 46
27. Gullick WJ (1996) The c-erbB3/HER3 receptor in human cancer. Cancer Surv 27: 339–49.
28. Srinivasan R, Poulsom R, Hurst HC, Gullick WJ (1998) Expression of the c-erbB-4/HER4 protein and mRNA in normal human fetal and adult tissues and in a survey of nine solid tumour types. J Pathol 185(3): 236–45
29. Gullick WJ (2003) c-erbB-4/HER4: friend or foe? J Pathol 200: 279–81
30. Pawlowski V, Revillion F, Hebbar M, Hornez L, Peyrat JP (2000) Prognostic value of the type I growth factor receptors in a large series of human primary breast cancers quantified with a real-time reverse transcription-polymerase chain reaction assay. Clin Cancer Res 6(11): 4217–25
31. Witton CJ, Reeves JR, Going JJ, Cooke TG, Bartlett JM (2003) Expression of the HER1-4 family of receptor tyrosine kinases in breast cancer. J Pathol 200(3): 290–7
32. Fuchs IB, Siemer I, Buhler H, Schmider A, Henrich W, Lichtenegger W, Schaller G, Kuemmel S (2006) Epidermal growth factor receptor changes during breast cancer metastasis. Anticancer Res 26(6B): 4397–401
33. Bartsch R, Wenzel C, Zielinski CC, Steger GG (2007) HER-2-positive breast cancer: hope beyond trastuzumab. BioDrugs 21(2): 69–77. Review
34. Moasser MM (2007) Targeting the function of the HER2 oncogene in human cancer therapeutics. Oncogene May 7 [Epub ahead of print]
35. Nahta R, Esteva FJ (2007) Trastuzumab: triumphs and tribulations. Oncogene 26(25): 3637–43
36. Carlsson J, Nordgren H, Sjostrom J, Wester K, Villman K, Bengtsson NO, Ostenstad B, Lundqvist H, Blomqvist C (2004) HER2 expression in breast cancer primary tumours and corresponding metastases. Original data and literature review. Br J Cancer 90: 2344–8
37. Lan KH, Lu CH, Yu D (2005) Mechanisms of trastuzumab resistance and their clinical implications. Ann N Y Acad Sci 1059: 70–5. Review
38. Nahta R, Yu D, Hung MC, Hortobagyi GN, Esteva FJ (2006) Mechanisms of disease: understanding resistance to HER2-targeted therapy in human breast cancer. Nat Clin Pract Oncol 3(5): 269–80. Review
39. Lu Y, Zi X, Pollak M (2004) Molecular mechanisms underlying IGF-I-induced attenuation of the growth-inhibitory activity of trastuzumab (Herceptin) on SKBR3 breast cancer cells. Int J Cancer 108: 334–41
40. Winter JL, Stackhouse BL, Russell GB, Kute TE (2007) Measurement of PTEN expression using tissue microarrays to determine a race-specific prognostic marker in breast cancer. Arch Pathol Lab Med 131(5): 767–72
41. Regitnig P, Schippinger W, Lindbauer M, Samonigg H, Lax SF (2004) Change of HER-2/neu status in a subset of distant metastases from breast carcinomas. J Pathol 203(4): 918–26
42. Schindlbeck C, Janni W, Shabani N, Rack B, Gerber B, Schmitt M, Harbeck N, Sommer H, Braun S, Friese K (2004) Comparative analysis between the HER2 status in primary breast cancer tissue and the detection of isolated tumor cells in the bone marrow. Breast Cancer Res Treat 87(1): 65–74
43. Hanna W, Nofech-Mozes S, Kahn HJ (2007) Intratumoral heterogeneity of HER2/neu in breast cancer – a rare event. Breast J 13(2): 122–9

44. Tovey SM, Witton CJ, Bartlett JM, Stanton PD, Reeves JR, Cooke TG (2004) Outcome and human epidermal growth factor receptor (HER)1-4 status in invasive breast carcinomas with proliferation indices evaluated by bromodeoxyuridine labelling. Breast Cancer Res 6(3): R246–51
45. Robertson KW, Reeves JR, Smith G, Keith WN, Ozanne BW, Cooke TG, Stanton PD (1996) Quantitative estimation of epidermal growth factor receptor and c-erbB-2 in human breast cancer. Cancer Res 56(16): 3823–30
46. Milenic DE, Garmestani K, Brady ED, Albert PS, Abdulla A, Flynn J, Brechbiel MW (2007) Potentiation of high-LET radiation by gemcitabine: targeting HER2 with trastuzumab to treat disseminated peritoneal disease. Clin Cancer Res 13(6): 1926–35
47. Persson M, Gedda L, Lundqvist H, Tolmachev V, Nordgren H, Malmstrom PU, Carlsson J (2007) [177Lu]pertuzumab: experimental therapy of HER-2-expressing xenografts. Cancer Res 67(1): 326–31
48. Tolmachev V, Orlova A, Pehrson R, Galli J, Baastrup B, Andersson K, Sandstrom M, Rosik D, Carlsson J, Lundqvist H, Wennborg A, Nilsson FY (2007) Radionuclide therapy of HER2 positive microxenografts using a 177Lu-labeled HER2-specific Affibody molecule. Cancer Res 67(6): 2773–82
49. Gardmark T, Wester K, De la Torre M, Carlsson J, Malmstrom PU (2005) Analysis of HER2 expression in primary urinary bladder carcinoma and corresponding metastases. BJU Int 95(7): 982–6
50. Alonzi R, Hoskin P (2005) Novel therapies in bladder cancer. Clin Oncol (R Coll Radiol) 17(7): 524–38. Review
51. Adam L, Kassouf W, Dinney CP (2005) Clinical applications for targeted therapy in bladder cancer. Urol Clin North Am 32(2): 239–46. Review
52. Baffa R, Letko J, McClung C, LeNoir J, Vecchione A, Gomella LG (2006) Molecular genetics of bladder cancer: targets for diagnosis and therapy. J Exp Clin Cancer Res 25(2): 145–60. Review
53. Bue P, Wester K, Sjostrom A, Holmberg A, Nilsson S, Carlsson J, Westlin JE, Busch C, Malmstrom PU (1998) Expression of epidermal growth factor receptor in urinary bladder cancer metastases. Int J Cancer 76: 189–93
54. Wester K, Sjostrom A, de la Torre M, Carlsson J, Malmstrom PU (2002) HER-2–a possible target for therapy of metastatic urinary bladder carcinoma. Acta Oncol 41: 282–8
55. Rotterud R, Nesland JM, Berner A, Fossa SD (2005) Expression of the epidermal growth factor receptor family in normal and malignant urothelium. BJU Int 95(9): 1344–50
56. Memon AA, Sorensen BS, Meldgaard P, Fokdal L, Thykjaer T, Nexo E (2006) The relation between survival and expression of HER1 and HER2 depends on the expression of HER3 and HER4: a study in bladder cancer patients. Br J Cancer 94: 1703–9
57. Wang X, Zhang S, MacLennan GT, Eble JN, Lopez-Beltran A, Yang XJ, Pan CX, Zhou H, Montironi R, Cheng L (2007) Epidermal growth factor receptor protein expression and gene amplification in small cell carcinoma of the urinary bladder. Clin Cancer Res 13(3): 953–7
58. Latif Z, Watters AD, Dunn I, Grigor K, Underwood MA, Bartlett JM (2004) HER2/neu gene amplification and protein overexpression in G3 pT2 transitional cell carcinoma of the bladder: a role for anti-HER2 therapy? Eur J Cancer 40(1): 56–63
59. Wulfing C, von Struensee D, Bierer S, Bogemann M, Hertle L, Eltze E (2005) Expression of Her2/neu in locally advanced bladder cancer: implication for a molecular targeted therapy Aktuelle Urol 36(5): 423–9
60. Hussain MH, MacVicar GR, Petrylak DP, Dunn RL, Vaishampayan U, Lara PN Jr, Chatta GS, Nanus DM, Glode LM, Trump DL, Chen H, Smith DC (2007) National Cancer Institute. Trastuzumab, paclitaxel, carboplatin, and gemcitabine in advanced human epidermal growth factor receptor-2/neu-positive urothelial carcinoma: results of a multicenter phase II National Cancer Institute trial. J Clin Oncol 25(16): 2218–24
61. Jimenez RE, Hussain M, Bianco FJ Jr, Vaishampayan U, Tabazcka P, Sakr WA, Pontes JE Wood DP Jr, Grignon DJ (2001) Her-2/neu overexpression in muscle-invasive urothelial carcinoma of the bladder: prognostic significance and comparative analysis in primary and metastatic tumors. Clin Cancer Res 7(8): 2440–7

62. Alekshun T, Garrett C. Targeted therapies in the treatment of colorectal cancers (2005) Cancer Control 12(2): 105–10. Review
63. Beaven AW, Goldberg RM (2006) Adjuvant therapy for colorectal cancer: yesterday, today, and tomorrow. Oncology (Williston Park) 20(5): 461–9. Review
64. Kluftinger AM, Robinson BW, Quenville NF, Finley RJ, Davis NL (1992) Correlation of epidermal growth factor receptor and c-erbB2 oncogene product to known prognostic indicators of colorectal cancer. Surg Oncol 1(1): 97–105
65. Porebska I, Harlozinska A, Bojarowski T (2000) Expression of the tyrosine kinase activity growth factor receptors (EGFR, ERB B2, ERB B3) in colorectal adenocarcinomas and adenomas. Tumour Biol 21(2): 105–15
66. Giralt J, de las Heras M, Cerezo L, Eraso A, Hermosilla E, Velez D, Lujan J, Espin E, Rosello J, Majo J, Benavente S, Armengol M, de Torres I (2005) Grupo Espanol de Investigacion Clinica en Oncologia Radioterapica (GICOR). The expression of epidermal growth factor receptor results in a worse prognosis for patients with rectal cancer treated with preoperative radiotherapy: a multicenter, retrospective analysis. Radiother Oncol 74(2): 101–8
67. Lee JC, Wang ST, Chow NH, Yang HB (2002) Investigation of the prognostic value of coexpressed erbB family members for the survival of colorectal cancer patients after curative surgery. Eur J Cancer 38(8): 1065–71
68. Resnick MB, Routhier J, Konkin T, Sabo E, Pricolo VE (2004) Epidermal growth factor receptor, c-MET, beta-catenin, and p53 expression as prognostic indicators in stage II colon cancer: a tissue microarray study. Clin Cancer Res 10(9): 3069–75
69. Giralt J, Eraso A, Armengol M, Rossello J, Majo J, Ares C, Espin E, Benavente S, de Torres I (2002) Epidermal growth factor receptor is a predictor of tumor response in locally advanced rectal cancer patients treated with preoperative radiotherapy. Int J Radiat Oncol Biol Phys 54(5): 1460–5
70. Azuma M, Danenberg KD, Iqbal S, El-Khoueiry A, Zhang W, Yang D, Koizumi W, Saigenji K, Danenberg PV, Lenz HJ (2006) Epidermal growth factor receptor and epidermal growth factor receptor variant III gene expression in metastatic colorectal cancer. Clin Colorectal Cancer 6(3): 214–8
71. De Luca A, Pignata S, Casamassimi A, D'Antonio A, Gridelli C, Rossi A, Cremona F, Parisi V, De Matteis A, Normanno N (2000) Detection of circulating tumor cells in carcinoma patients by a novel epidermal growth factor receptor reverse transcription-PCR assay. Clin Cancer Res 6(4): 1439–44
72. Clarke LE, Leitzel K, Smith J, Ali SM, Lipton A (2003) Epidermal growth factor receptor mRNA in peripheral blood of patients with pancreatic, lung, and colon carcinomas detected by RT-PCR. Int J Oncol 22(2): 425–30
73. Dursun A, Poyraz A, Suer O, Sezer C, Akyol G (2001) Expression of Bcl-2 and c-ErbB-2 in colorectal neoplasia. Pathol Oncol Res 7(1): 24–7
74. Koeppen HK, Wright BD, Burt AD, Quirke P, McNicol AM, Dybdal NO, Sliwkowski MX, Hillan KJ (2001) Overexpression of HER2/neu in solid tumours: an immunohistochemical survey. Histopathology 38(2): 96–104
75. McKay JA, Murray LJ, Curran S, Ross VG, Clark C, Murray GI, Cassidy J, McLeod HL (2002) Evaluation of the epidermal growth factor receptor (EGFR) in colorectal tumours and lymph node metastases. Eur J Cancer 38(17): 2258–64
76. Knosel T, Petersen S, Schwabe H, Schluns K, Stein U, Schlag PM, Dietel M, Petersen I (2002) Incidence of chromosomal imbalances in advanced colorectal carcinomas and their metastases. Virchows Arch 440(2): 187–94
77. Nathanson DR, Culliford AT 4th, Shia J, Chen B, D'Alessio M, Zeng ZS, Nash GM, Gerald W, Barany F, Paty PB (2003) HER 2/neu expression and gene amplification in colon cancer. Int J Cancer 105(6): 796–802
78. Uner A, Ebinc FA, Akyurek N, Unsal D, Mentes BB, Dursun A (2005) Vascular endothelial growth factor, c-erbB-2 and c-erbB-3 expression in colorectal adenoma and adenocarcinoma. Exp Oncol 27(3): 225–8

79. Saeki T, Salomon DS, Johnson GR, Gullick WJ, Mandai K, Yamagami K, Moriwaki S, Tanada M, Takashima S, Tahara E (1995) Association of epidermal growth factor-related peptides and type I receptor tyrosine kinase receptors with prognosis of human colorectal carcinomas. Jpn J Clin Oncol 25(6): 240–9
80. Ciardiello F, Kim N, Saeki T, Dono R, Persico MG, Plowman GD, Garrigues J, Radke S, Todaro GJ, Salomon DS (1991) Differential expression of epidermal growth factor-related proteins in human colorectal tumors. Proc Natl Acad Sci USA 88(17): 7792–6
81. Maurer CA, Friess H, Kretschmann B, Zimmermann A, Stauffer A, Baer HU, Korc M, Buchler MW (1998) Increased expression of erbB3 in colorectal cancer is associated with concomitant increase in the level of erbB2. Hum Pathol 29(8): 771–7
82. Kapitanovic S, Radosevic S, Slade N, Kapitanovic M, Andelinovic S, Ferencic Z, Tavassoli M, Spaventi S, Pavelic K, Spaventi R (2000) Expression of erbB-3 protein in colorectal adenocarcinoma: correlation with poor survival. J Cancer Res Clin Oncol 126(4): 205–11
83. Scher HI, Sarkis A, Reuter V, Cohen D, Netto G, Petrylak D, Lianes P, Fuks Z, Mendelsohn J, Cordon-Cardo C (1995) Changing pattern of expression of the epidermal growth factor receptor and transforming growth factor alpha in the progression of prostatic neoplasms. Clin Cancer Res 1(5): 545–50
84. Shah RB, Ghosh D, Elder JT (2006) Epidermal growth factor receptor (ErbB1) expression in prostate cancer progression: correlation with androgen independence. Prostate 66(13): 1437–44
85. Festuccia C, Gravina GL, Millimaggi D, Muzi P, Speca S, Ricevuto E, Vicentini C, Bologna M (2007) Uncoupling of the epidermal growth factor receptor from downstream signal transduction molecules guides the acquired resistance to gefitinib in prostate cancer cells. Oncol Rep 18(2): 503–11
86. Kim SJ, Uehara H, Karashima T, Shepherd DL, Killion JJ, Fidler IJ (2003) Blockade of epidermal growth factor receptor signaling in tumor cells and tumor-associated endothelial cells for therapy of androgen-independent human prostate cancer growing in the bone of nude mice. Clin Cancer Res 9(3): 1200–10
87. Festuccia C, Angelucci A, Gravina GL, Biordi L, Millimaggi D, Muzi P, Vicentini C, Bologna M (2005) Epidermal growth factor modulates prostate cancer cell invasiveness regulating urokinase-type plasminogen activator activity. EGF-receptor inhibition may prevent tumor cell dissemination. Thromb Haemost 93(5): 964–75
88. Hernes E, Fossa SD, Berner A, Otnes B, Nesland JM (2004) Expression of the epidermal growth factor receptor family in prostate carcinoma before and during androgen-independence. Br J Cancer 90(2): 449–54
89. Bartlett JM, Brawley D, Grigor K, Munro AF, Dunne B, Edwards J (2005) Type I receptor tyrosine kinases are associated with hormone escape in prostate cancer. J Pathol 205(4): 522–9
90. Morote J, de Torres I, Caceres C, Vallejo C, Schwartz S Jr, Reventos J (1999) Prognostic value of immunohistochemical expression of the c-erbB-2 oncoprotein in metastasic prostate cancer. Int J Cancer 84(4): 421–5
91. Carles J, Lloreta J, Salido M, Font A, Suarez M, Baena V, Nogue M, Domenech M, Fabregat X (2004) Her-2/neu expression in prostate cancer: a dynamic process? Clin Cancer Res 10(14): 4742–5
92. Myers RB, Srivastava S, Oelschlager DK, Grizzle WE (1994) Expression of p160erbB-3 and p185erbB-2 in prostatic intraepithelial neoplasia and prostatic adenocarcinoma. J Natl Cancer Inst 86(15): 1140–5
93. Reese DM, Small EJ, Magrane G, Waldman FM, Chew K, Sudilovsky D (2001) HER2 protein expression and gene amplification in androgen-independent prostate cancer. Am J Clin Pathol 116(2): 234–9
94. Liu HL, Gandour-Edwards R, Lara PN Jr, de Vere White R, LaSalle JM (2001) Detection of low level HER-2/neu gene amplification in prostate cancer by fluorescence in situ hybridization. Cancer J 7(5): 395–403
95. Ady N, Morat L, Fizazi K, Soria JC, Mathieu MC, Prapotnich D, Sabatier L, Chauveinc L (2004) Detection of HER-2/neu-positive circulating epithelial cells in prostate cancer patients. Br J Cancer 90(2): 443–8

96. Agus DB, Sweeney CJ, Morris MJ, Mendelson DS, McNeel DG, Ahmann FR, Wang J, Derynck MK, Ng K, Lyons B, Allison DE, Kattan MW, Scher HI (2007) Efficacy and safety of single-agent pertuzumab (rhuMAb 2C4), a human epidermal growth factor receptor dimerization inhibitor, in castration-resistant prostate cancer after progression from taxane-based therapy. J Clin Oncol 25(6): 675–81
97. de Bono JS, Bellmunt J, Attard G, Droz JP, Miller K, Flechon A, Sternberg C, Parker C, Zugmaier G, Hersberger-Gimenez V, Cockey L, Mason M, Graham J (2007) Open-label phase II study evaluating the efficacy and safety of two doses of pertuzumab in castrate chemotherapy naive patients with hormone-refractory prostate cancer. J Clin Oncol 25(3): 257–62
98. Yu Y, Chen W, Zhang Y, Hamburger AW, Pan H, Zhang Z (2007) Suppresion of salivary adenoid cystic carcinoma growth and metastases by ErbB3 binding protein Ebp1 gene transfer. Int J Cancer 120: 1909–13
99. Vakar-Lopez F, Cheng CJ, Kim J, Shi GG, Troncoso P, Tu SM, Yu-Lee LY, Lin SH (2004) Up-regulation of MDA-BF-1, a secreted isoform of ErbB3, in metastatic prostate cancer cells and activated osteoblasts in bone marrow. J Pathol 203(2): 688–95
100. Solit DB, Rosen N (2007) Targeting HER2 in prostate cancer: where to next? J Clin Oncol 25(3): 241–3
101. Schwartz S Jr, Caceres C, Morote J, De Torres I, Rodriguez-Vallejo JM, Gonzalez J, Reventos J (1999) Gains of the relative genomic content of erbB-1 and erbB-2 in prostate carcinoma and their association with metastasis. Int J Oncol 14(2): 367–71
102. Edwards J, Mukherjee R, Munro AF, Wells AC, Almushatat A, Bartlett JM (2004) HER2 and COX2 expression in human prostate cancer. Eur J Cancer 40(1): 50–5
103. Brys M, Stawinska M, Foksinski M, Barecki A, Zydek C, Miekos E, Krajewska WM (2004) Androgen receptor versus erbB-1 and erbB-2 expression in human prostate neoplasms. Oncol Rep 11(1): 219–24
104. Hegeman RB, Liu G, Wilding G, McNeel DG (2004) Newer therapies in advanced prostate cancer. Clin Prostate Cancer 3(3): 150–6. Review
105. Zellweger T, Ninck C, Bloch M, Mirlacher M, Koivisto PA, Helin HJ, Mihatsch MJ, Gasser TC, Bubendorf L (2005) Expression patterns of potential therapeutic targets in prostate cancer. Int J Cancer 113(4): 619–28
106. Edwards J, Traynor P, Munro AF, Pirret CF, Dunne B, Bartlett JM (2006) The role of HER1-HER4 and EGFRvIII in hormone-refractory prostate cancer. Clin Cancer Res 12(1): 123–30
107. Gibault L, Metges JP, Conan-Charlet V, Lozac'h P, Robaszkiewicz M, Bessaguet C, Lagarde N and Volant A (2005) Diffuse EGFR staining is associated with reduced overall survival in locally advanced oesophageal squamous cell cancer. Br J Cancer 93: 107–15
108. Hanawa M, Suzuki S, Dobashi Y, Yamane T, Kono K, Enomoto N, Ooi A (2006) EGFR protein overexpression and gene amplification in squamous cell carcinomas of the esophagus. Int J Cancer 118: 1173–80
109. Sunpaweravong P, Sunpaweravong S, Puttawibul P, Mitarnun W, Zeng C, Baron AE, Franklin W, Said S, Varella-Garcia M (2005) Epidermal growth factor receptor and cyclin D1 are independently amplified and overexpressed in esophageal squamous cell carcinoma. J Cancer Res Clin Oncol 131: 111–9
110. Langer R, Von Rahden BH, Nahrig J, Von Weyhern C, Reiter R, Feith M, Stein HJ, Siewert JR, Hofler H, Sarbia M (2006) Prognostic significance of expression patterns of c-erbB-2, p53, p16INK4A, p27KIP1, cyclin D1 and epidermal growth factor receptor in oesophageal adenocarcinoma: a tissue microarray study. J Clin Pathol 59(6): 631–4
111. Aloia TA, Harpole DH Jr, Reed CE, Allegra C, Moore MB, Herndon JE 2nd, D'Amico TA (2001) Tumor marker expression is predictive of survival in patients with esophageal cancer. Ann Thorac Surg 72: 859–66
112. Gibson MK, Abraham SC, Wu TT, Burtness B, Heitmiller RF, Heath E, Forastiere A (2003) Epidermal growth factor receptor, p53 mutation, and pathological response predict survival in patients with locally advanced esophageal cancer treated with preoperative chemoradiotherapy. Clin Cancer Res 9: 6461–8

113. Janmaat ML, Gallegos-Ruiz MI, Rodriguez JA, Meijer GA, Vervenne WL, Richel DJ, Van Groeningen C, Giaccone G (2006) Predictive factors for outcome in a phase II study of Gefitinib in second-line treatment of advanced esophageal cancer patients. J Clin Oncol 24: 1612–9
114. Kwak EL, Jankowski J, Thayer SP, Lauwers GY, Brannigan BW, Harris PL, Okimoto RA, Haserlat SM, Driscoll DR, Ferry D, Muir B, Settleman J, Fuchs CS, Kulke MH, Ryan DP, Clark JW, Sgroi DC, Haber DA, Bell DW (2006) Epidermal growth factor receptor kinase domain mutations in esophageal and pancreatic adenocarcinomas. Clin Cancer Res 12(14): 4283–7
115. Lam KY, Tin L, Ma L (1998) C-erbB-2 protein expression in oesophageal squamous epithelium from oesophageal squamous cell carcinomas, with special reference to histological grade of carcinoma and pre-invasive lesions. Eur J Surg Oncol 24: 431–5
116. Mimura K, Kono K, Hanawa M, Mitsui F, Sugai H, Miyagawa N, Ooi A, Fujii H (2005) Frequencies of HER-2/neu expression and gene amplification in patients with oesophageal squamous cell carcinoma. Br J Cancer 92: 1253–1260
117. Dreilich M, Wanders A, Brattstrom D, Bergstrom S, Hesselius P, Wagenius G, Bergqvist M (2006) HER-2 overexpression (3+) in patients with squamous cell esophageal carcinoma correlates with poorer survival. Dis Esophagus 19(4): 224–31
118. Reichelt U, Duesedau P, Tsourlakis MCh, Quaas A, Link BC, Schurr PG, Kaifi JT, Gros SJ, Yekebas EF, Marx A, Simon R, Izbicki JR, Sauter G (2007) Frequent homogeneous HER-2 amplification in primary and metastatic adenocarcinoma of the esophagus. Mod Pathol 20: 120–9
119. Akamatsu M, Matsumoto T, Oka K, Yamasaki S, Sonoue H, Kajiyama Y, Tsurumaru M, Sasai K (2003) c-erbB-2 oncoprotein expression related to chemoradioresistance in esophageal squamous cell carcinoma. Int J Radiat Oncol Biol Phys 57: 1323–7
120. Prigent SA, Lemoine NR, Hughes CM, Plowman GD, Selden C, Gullick WJ (1992) Expression of the c-erbB-3 protein in normal human adult and fetal tissues. Oncogene 7(7): 1273–8
121. Itakura Y, Sasano H, Shiga C, Furukawa Y, Shiga K, Mori S, Nagura H (1994) Epidermal growth factor receptor overexpression in esophageal carcinoma. An immunohistochemical study correlated with clinicopathologic findings and DNA amplification. Cancer 74: 795–804
122. Kalyankrishna S, Grandis JR (2006) Epidermal growth factor receptor biology in head and neck cancer. J Clin Oncol 24(17): 2666–72. Review
123. Rikimaru K, Tadokoro K, Yamamoto T, Enomoto S, Tsuchida N (1992) Gene amplification and overexpression of epidermal growth factor receptor in squamous cell carcinoma of the head and neck. Head Neck 14(1): 8–13
124. Xia W, Lau YK, Zhang HZ (1999) Combination of EGFR, HER-2/neu, and HER-3 is a stronger predictor for the outcome of oral squamous cell carcinoma than any individual family members. Clin Cancer Res 5(12): 4164–74
125. Santini J, Formento JL, Francoual M (1991) Characterization, quantification, and potential clinical value of the epidermal growth factor receptor in head and neck squamous cell carcinomas. Head Neck 13(2): 132–9
126. Albanell J, Codony-Servat J, Rojo F, Del Campo JM, Sauleda S, Anido J, Raspall G, Giralt J, Rosello J, Nicholson RI, Mendelsohn J, Baselga J (2001) Activated extracellular signal regulated kinases: association with epidermal growth factor receptor/transforming growth factor alpha expression in head and neck squamous carcinoma and inhibition by anti-epidermal growth factor receptor treatments. Cancer Res 61(17): 6500–10
127. Khademi B, Shirazi FM, Vasei M, Doroudchi M, Gandomi B, Modjtahedi H, Pezeshki AM, Ghaderi A (2002) The expression of p53, c-erbB-1 and c-erbB-2 molecules and their correlation with prognostic markers in patients with head and neck tumors. Cancer Lett 184(2): 223–30
128. Bei R, Budillon A, Masuelli L, Cereda V, Vitolo D, Di Gennaro E, Ripavecchia V, Palumbo C, Ionna F, Losito S, Modesti A, Kraus MH, Muraro R (2004) Frequent overexpression of

multiple ErbB receptors by head and neck squamous cell carcinoma contrasts with rare antibody immunity in patients. J Pathol 204(3): 317–25

129. Ongkeko WM, Altuna X, Weisman RA, Wang-Rodriguez J (2005) Expression of protein tyrosine kinases in head and neck squamous cell carcinomas. Am J Clin Pathol 124(1): 71–6
130. Craven JM, Pavelic ZP, Stambrook PJ (1992) Expression of c-erbB-2 gene in human head and neck carcinoma. Anticancer Res 12(6B): 2273–6
131. Giatromanolaki A, Koukourakis MI, Sivridis E, Fountzilas G (2000) c-erbB-2 oncoprotein is overexpressed in poorly vascularised squamous cell carcinomas of the head and neck, but is not associated with response to cytotoxic therapy or survival. Anticancer Res 20(2A): 997–1004.
132. Khan AJ, King BL, Smith BD, Smith GL, DiGiovanna MP, Carter D, Haffty BG (2002) Characterization of the HER-2/neu oncogene by immunohistochemical and fluorescence in situ hybridization analysis in oral and oropharyngeal squamous cell carcinoma. Clin Cancer Res 8(2): 540–8
133. Schartinger VH, Kacani L, Andrle J, Schwentner I, Wurm M, Obrist P, Oberaigner W, Sprinzl GM (2004) Pharmacodiagnostic value of the HER family in head and neck squamous cell carcinoma. ORL J Otorhinolaryngol Relat Spec 66(1): 21–6
134. Shintani S, Funayama T, Yoshihama Y, Alcalde RE, Matsumura T (1995) Prognostic significance of ERBB3 overexpression in oral squamous cell carcinoma. Cancer Lett 95(1–2): 79–83
135. O-charoenrat P, Rhys-Evans PH, Modjtahedi H, Eccles SA (2002) The role of c-erbB receptors and ligands in head and neck squamous cell carcinoma. Oral Oncol 38(7): 627–40. Review
136. Ibrahim SO, Vasstrand EN, Liavaag PG, Johannessen AC, Lillehaug JR (1997) Expression of c-erbB proto-oncogene family members in squamous cell carcinoma of the head and neck. Anticancer Res 17(6D): 4539–46
137. Bei R, Pompa G, Vitolo D (2001) Co-localization of multiple ErbB receptors in stratified epithelium of oral squamous cell carcinoma. J Pathol 195(3): 343–8
138. Giese A, Bjerkvig R, Berens ME, Westphal M (2003) Cost of migration: invasion of malignant gliomas and implications for treatment. J Clin Oncol 21: 1624–36
139. Rich JN, Bigner DD (2004) Development of novel targeted therapies in the treatment of malignant glioma. Nat Rev Drug Discov 3: 430–46
140. Benjamin R, Capparella J, Brown A (2003) Classification of glioblastoma multiforme in adults by molecular genetics. Cancer J 9: 82–90
141. Boskovitz A, Wikstrand CJ, Kuan CT, Zalutsky MR, Reardon DA, Bigner DD (2004) Monoclonal antibodies for brain tumour treatment. Expert Opin Biol Ther 4: 1453–71
142. Shinojima N, Tada K, Shiraishi S, Kamiryo T, Kochi M, Nakamura H, Makino K, Saya H, Hirano H, Kuratsu J, Oka K, Ishimaru Y, Ushio Y (2003) Prognostic value of epidermal growth factor receptor in patients with glioblastoma multiforme. Cancer Res 63: 6962–70
143. Okada Y, Hurwitz EE, Esposito JM, Brower MA, Nutt CL, Louis DN (2003) Selection pressures of TP53 mutation and microenvironmental location influence epidermal growth factor receptor gene amplification in human glioblastomas. Cancer Res 63: 413–6
144. Nicholas MK, Lukas RV, Jafri NF, Faoro L, Salgia R (2006) Epidermal growth factor receptor - mediated signal transduction in the development and therapy of gliomas. Clin Cancer Res 12(24): 7261–70. Review
145. Lang O, Liebermeister E, Liesegang J, Sautter-Bihl ML (1998) Radiotherapy of glioblastoma multiforme: feasibility of increased fraction size and shortened overall treatment. Strahlenther Onkol 174: 629–32
146. Barker FG 2nd, Chang SM, Gutin PH, Malec MK, McDermott MW, Prados MD, Wilson CB (1998) Survival and functional status after resection of recurrent glioblastoma multiforme. Neurosurgery 42: 709–20

147. Nieder C, Adam M, Molls M, Grosu AL (2006) Therapeutic options for recurrent high grade glioma in adult patients: recent advances. Crit Rev Oncol Hematol 60(3): 181–93. Review
148. Stupp R, Mason WP, van den Bent MJ, Weller M, Fisher B, Taphoorn MJ, Belanger K, Brandes AA, Marosi C, Bogdahn U (2005) Radiotherapy plus concomitant and adjuvant temozolomide for glioblastoma. N Engl J Med 352: 987–96
149. Blomquist E, Carlsson J (1991) Strategy for planned radiotherapy of malignant gliomas. Postoperative treatments with high dose proton irradiation and tumor seeking radionuclides. Int J Radiat Oncol Biol Phys 22: 259–63
150. Zalutsky MR (2004) Targeted radiotherapy of brain tumours. Br J Cancer 90: 1469–73
151. Koka V, Potti A, Forseen SE, Pervez H, Fraiman GN, Koch M, Levitt R (2003) Role of Her 2/neu overexpression and clinical determinants of early mortality in glioblastoma multiforme. Am J Clin Oncol 26(4): 332–5
152. Potti A, Forseen SE, Koka VK, Pervez H, Koch M, Fraiman G, Mehdi SA, Levitt R (2004) Determination of HER-2/neu overexpression and clinical predictors of survival in a cohort of 347 patients with primary malignant brain tumors. Cancer Invest 22(4): 537–44
153. Epenetos AA, Courtenay-Luck N, Pickering D, Hooker G, Durbin H, Lavender JP, McKenzie CG (1985) Antibody guided irradiation of brain glioma by arterial infusion of radioactive monoclonal antibody against epidermal growth factor receptor and blood group A antigen. Br Med J (Clin Res Ed) 290: 1463–6.
154. Kalofonos HP, Pawlikowska TR, Hemingway A, Courtenay-Luck N, Dhokia B, Snook D, Sivolapenko GB, Hooker GR, McKenzie CG, Lavender PJ (1989) Antibody guided diagnosis and therapy of brain gliomas using radiolabeled monoclonal antibodies against epidermal growth factor receptor and placental alkaline phosphatase. J Nucl Med 30: 1636–45
155. Brady LW, Miyamoto C, Woo DV, Rackover M, Emrich J, Bender H, Dadparvar S, Steplewski Z, Koprowski H, Black P (1992) Malignant astrocytomas treated with iodine-125 labeled monoclonal antibody 425 against epidermal growth factor receptor: a phase II trial. Int J Radiat Oncol Biol Phys 22: 225–30
156. Emrich JG, Brady LW, Quang TS, Class R, Miyamoto C, Black P, Rodeck U (2002) Radioiodinated (I-125) monoclonal antibody 425 in the treatment of high grade glioma patients: ten-year synopsis of a novel treatment. Am J Clin Oncol 25: 541–6.
157. Carlsson J, Ren ZP, Wester K, Sundberg AL, Heldin NE, Hesselager G, Persson M, Gedda L, Tolmachev V, Lundqvist H, Blomquist E, Nister M (2006) Planning for intracavitary anti-EGFR radionuclide therapy of gliomas. Literature review and data on EGFR expression. J Neurooncol 77(1): 33–45. Review
158. Wikstrand CJ, McLendon RE, Friedman AH, Bigner DD (1997) Cell surface localization and density of the tumor-associated variant of the epidermal growth factor receptor, EGFRvIII. Cancer Res 57: 4130–40
159. Kuan CT, Wikstrand CJ, Bigner DD (2001) EGF mutant receptor vIII as a molecular target in cancer therapy. Endocr Relat Cancer 8: 83–96
160. Ohman L, Gedda L, Larsson R, Stigbrand T, Wester K, Carlsson J (2002) A new antibody recognising the vIII mutation of human EGFR. Tumor Biol 23(2): 61–9
161. Nordberg E, Steffen AC, Persson M, Sundberg AL, Carlsson J, Glimelius B (2005) Cellular uptake of radioiodine delivered by trastuzumab can be modified by the addition of epidermal growth factor. Eur J Nucl Med Mol Imaging 32(7): 771–7
162. Steffen AC, Orlova A, Wikman M, Nilsson FY, Stahl S, Adams GP, Tolmachev V, Carlsson J (2006) Affibody-mediated tumour targeting of HER-2 expressing xenografts in mice. Eur J Nucl Med Mol Imaging 33(6): 631–8
163. Nestor M, Ekberg T, Dring J, van Dongen G, Wester K, Tolmachev V, Anniko M (2007) Quantification of CD44v6 and EGFR expression in head and neck squamous cell carcinoma using a single dose radioimmunoassay. Tumour Biol 28(5): 253–63
164. Bertram JS (2002) The molecular biology of cancer. Mol Aspects Med 21: 167–223
165. Onyango P (2002) Genomics and cancer. Curr Opin Oncol 14: 79–85
166. Masood S, Bui MM (2000) Assessment of Her-2/neu overexpression in primary breast cancers and their metastatic lesions: an immunohistochemical study. Ann Clin Lab Sci 30: 259–65

167. Shimizu C, Fukutomi T, Tsuda H, Akashi-Tanaka S, Watanabe T, Nanasawa T, Sugihara K (2000) C-erbB-2 protein overexpression and p53 immunoreaction in primary and recurrent breast cancer tissues. J Surg Oncol 73: 17–20
168. Simon R, Nocito A, Hubscher T, Bucher C, Torhorst J, Schraml P, Bubendorf L, Mihatsch MM, Moch H, Wilber K, Schotzau A, Kononen J, Sauter G (2001) Patterns of her-2/neu amplification and overexpression in primary and metastatic breast cancer. J Natl Cancer Inst 93: 1141–6
169. Tanner M, Jarvinen P, Isola J (2001) Amplification of HER-2/neu and topoisomerase IIalpha in primary and metastatic breast cancer. Cancer Res 61: 5345–8
170. Gancberg D, Di Leo A, Cardoso F, Rouas G, Pedrocchi M, Paesmans M, Verhest A, Bernard-Marty C, Piccart MJ, Larsimont D (2002) Comparison of HER-2 status between primary breast cancer and corresponding distant metastatic sites. Ann Oncol 13: 1036–43
171. Vincent-Salomon A, Jouve M, Genin P, Freneaux P, Sigal-Zafrani B, Caly M, Beuzeboc P, Pouillart P, Sastre-Garau X (2002) HER2 status in patients with breast carcinoma is not modified selectively by preoperative chemotherapy and is stable during the metastatic process. Cancer 94: 2169–73
172. Tsutsui S, Ohno S, Murakami S, Kataoka A, Kinoshita J, Hachitanda Y (2002) EGFR, c erbB2 and p53 protein in the primary lesions and paired metastatic regional lymph nodes in breast cancer. Eur J Surg Oncol 28: 383–7
173. Sekido Y, Umemura S, Takekoshi S, Suzuki Y, Tokuda Y, Tajima T, Osamura RY (2003) Heterogeneous gene alterations in primary breast cancer contribute to discordance between primary and asynchronous metastatic/recurrent sites: HER2 gene amplification and p53 mutation. Int J Oncol 22(6): 1225–32
174. Zidan J, Dashkovsky I, Stayerman C, Basher W, Cozacov C, Hadary A (2005) Comparison of HER-2 overexpression in primary breast cancer and metastatic sites and its effect on biological targeting therapy of metastatic disease. Br J Cancer 93(5): 552–6
175. Xu R, Perle MA, Inghirami G, Chan W, Delgado Y, Feiner H (2002) Amplification of Her 2/neu gene in Her-2/neu-overexpressing and -nonexpressing breast carcinomas and their synchronous benign, premalignant, and metastatic lesions detected by FISH in archival material. Mod Pathol 15: 116–24
176. Bozzetti C, Personeni N, Nizzoli R, Guazzi A, Flora M, Bassano C, Negri F, Martella E, Naldi N, Franciosi V, Cascinu S (2003) HER-2/neu amplification by fluorescence in situ hybridization in cytologic samples from distant metastatic sites of breast carcinoma. Cancer 99(5): 310–5
177. Gong Y, Booser DJ, Sneige N (2005) Comparison of HER-2 status determined by fluorescence in situ hybridization in primary and metastatic breast carcinoma. Cancer 103(9): 1763–9
178. Lopez-Guerrero JA, Llombart-Cussac A, Noguera R, Navarro S, Pellin A, Almenar S, Vazquez-Alvadalejo C, Llombart-Bosch A (2006) HER2 amplification in recurrent breast cancer following breast-conserving therapy correlates with distant metastasis and poor survival. Int J Cancer 118(7): 1743–9
179. Tapia C, Savic S, Wagner U, Schonegg R, Novotny H, Grilli B, Herzog M, Barascud AD, Zlobec I, Cathomas G, Terracciano L, Feichter G, Bubendorf L (2007) HER2 gene status in primary breast cancers and matched distant metastases. Breast Cancer Res 9(3): 1–8
180. Vincent-Salomon A, Pierga JY, Couturier J, d'Enghien CD, Nos C, Sigal-Zafrani B, Lae M, Freneaux P, Dieras V, Thiery JP, Sastre-Garau X (2007) HER2 status of bone marrow micrometastasis and their corresponding primary tumours in a pilot study of 27 cases: a possible tool for anti-HER2 therapy management? Br J Cancer 96(4): 654–9
181. Palmieri D, Bronder JL, Herring JM, Yoneda T, Weil RJ, Stark AM, Kurek R, Vega-Valle E, Feigenbaum L, Halverson D, Vortmeyer AO, Steinberg SM, Aldape K, Steeg PS (2007) Her-2 overexpression increases the metastatic outgrowth of breast cancer cells in the brain. Cancer Res 67(9): 4190–8
182. De Jong KP, Stellema R, Karrenbeld A, Koudstaal J, Gouw AS, Sluiter WJ, Peeters PM, Slooff MJ, De Vries EG (1998) Clinical relevance of transforming growth factor alpha,

epidermal growth factor receptor, p53, and Ki67 in colorectal liver metastases and corresponding primary tumors. Hepatology 28(4): 971–9

183. Goldstein NS, Armin M (2001) Epidermal growth factor receptor immunohistochemical reactivity in patients with American Joint Committee on Cancer Stage IV colon adenocarcinoma: implications for a standardized scoring system. Cancer 92(5): 1331–46
184. Scartozzi M, Bearzi I, Berardi R, Mandolesi A, Fabris G, Cascinu S (2004) Epidermal growth factor receptor (EGFR) status in primary colorectal tumors does not correlate with EGFR expression in related metastatic sites: implications for treatment with EGFR-targeted monoclonal antibodies. J Clin Oncol 22(23): 4772–8
185. Italiano A, Saint-Paul MC, Caroli-Bosc FX, Francois E, Bourgeon A, Benchimol D, Gugenheim J, Michiels JF (2005) Epidermal growth factor receptor (EGFR) status in primary colorectal tumors correlates with EGFR expression in related metastatic sites: biological and clinical implications. Ann Oncol 16(9): 1503–7
186. Bralet MP, Paule B, Adam R, Guettier C (2005) Loss of epidermal growth factor receptor expression in lymph node and liver metastases of colon carcinoma. J Clin Oncol 23(24): 5844–5
187. Shia J, Klimstra DS, Li AR, Qin J, Saltz L, Teruya-Feldstein J, Akram M, Chung KY, Yao D, Paty PB, Gerald W, Chen B (2005) Epidermal growth factor receptor expression and gene amplification in colorectal carcinoma: an immunohistochemical and chromogenic in situ hybridization study. Mod Pathol 18(10): 1350–6
188. Scartozzi M, Bearzi I, Berardi R, Mandolesi A, Fabris G, Cascinu S (2007) Epidermal growth factor receptor (EGFR) downstream signalling pathway in primary colorectal tumours and related metastatic sites: optimising EGFR-targeted treatment options. Br J Cancer 97(1): 92–7

Chapter 4
Targeting Tumours with Radiolabeled Antibodies

Torgny Stigbrand[1], David Eriksson[1], Katrine Riklund[2], and Lennart Johansson[3]

Summary The introduction of radiolabelled antibodies targeting the lymphocyte antigen CD20 in certain hematologic malignancies received positive attention and is now accepted as a treatment modality. Treating solid tumours with radiolabelled antibodies has, so far, not been met with the same appreciation and such therapy for the large groups of malignancies like colorectal, breast, prostate, ovarian, lung cancer and brain tumours still require improvements in order to gain acceptance. In this chapter limitations, possibilities and future directions to improve therapy with radiolabelled antibodies are discussed.

Introduction

The concept of "magic bullets", early launched by Paul Ehrlich, making use of the capacity in nature to generate an immense repertoire of immunoglobulins, was the start of a new era in cancer therapy. With the possibility to deliver drugs, toxins, enzymes or nuclides conjugated to antibodies to the diseased site and leave unaffected organs untouched, the selectivity in therapeutic interventions would increase dramatically and new therapeutic modalities could be envisioned. A number of reviews on the topic have recently been published [1–10]. In Table 4.1 are the major presently used targeting antibodies for malignant diseases presented.

The clear success of radiolabeled antibodies in the management of hematological malignancies was initiated by the introduction and commercial success of a few efficient antibodies targeting B-cell surface antigens, approved by the Food and Drug Administration (FDA) in United States. Thus, the dream of a "targeting therapy" was partially fulfilled with the introduction of Bexxar [11] and Zevalin [12], and this immediately generated a deeper interest for similar spectacular treatment modalities also for epithelial solid tumours.

[1]Department of Immunology, University of Umeå, SE-90185, Umeå, Sweden

[2]Department of Diagnostic Radiology, University of Umeå, SE-90185, Umeå, Sweden

[3]Department of Radiation Physics, University of Umeå, SE-90185, Umeå, Sweden

T. Stigbrand et al. (eds.) *Targeted Radionuclide Tumor Therapy*,

Table 4.1 Antibodies for detection or treatment of malignant diseases approved by FDA. (Data derived from [13, 14])

Generic name	Trade name	Type/target antigen	Treatment indication	Approval
Unconjugated				
Rituximab	Rituxan	Chi-Anti-CD20	B-cell lymphoma	1997
Trastuzumab	Herceptin	Hum-anti-HER2	Breast	1998
Alemtuzumab	CamPath	Hum anti-CD52	CLL	2001
Cetuximab	Erbitux	Chi-anti-	Colorectal Head/neck	2004 2006
Bevacizumab	Avastin	Chi-anti-VEGF	Colorectal	2006
Radioconjugates				
Satamomab pentedide	OncoScint[a]	^{111}In-mur-anti-TAG72	Colorectal Ovarian	1992
Nofetumomab merpentan	Verluma[a]	^{99m}Tc-mur-anti-EGP Fab	Small cell lung cancer	1996
Arcitumomab	CEA-Scan[a]	^{99m}Tc-mur-anti-CEA Fab	Colorectal	1996
Capromab pentedide	ProstaScint	^{111}In-mur-anti-PSMA	Prostate	1996
Ibritumomab tiuxetan	Zevalin	^{99m}Tc-mur-anti-CD20	B-cell lymphoma	2002
Tositumomab	Bexxar	^{131}I- mur-anti-CD20	B-cell lymphoma	2003
Drug conjugates				
Gemtuzumab ozogamicin	Mylotard	Hum-antiCD33	AML	2000

CLL = chronic lymphocytic leukaemia; AML = acute myelogenous leukaemia; Chi- = chimeric antibody; mur- = murine antibody; Hum- = human antibody
[a]No longer commercially available.

Looking back today at more than 50 years of trials and errors within the field of targeted therapy, the panorama of treatment outcomes should be looked upon as dichotomized. While many hematological malignancies are treated worldwide with significant success, the outcome when treating solid malignancies are modest irrespective of tumour type and organ of origin. This obvious difference is a challenge and one way to move forward with targeted therapy is to delineate and describe possible reasons for this dichotomy.

In this chapter the deviations in final outcome between these tumour groups will be discussed, and the parameters which would be of importance for further developing targeted therapy for solid tumours will be highlighted.

Hematological Malignancies

Lymphomas offer the advantage of expressing a number of hematopoietically related antigens on their plasma membranes, which are topologically easy to target and comparatively accessible for immunotherapy. The most abundant antigens used today include CD20 (B1), CD22 (LL2) and HLA-DR10β(Lym1) (antibodies within parenthesis) [15]. Two antibodies are widely used, Bexxar (a murine antibody conjugated with ^{131}I) and Zevalin (a murine antibody conjugated with ^{90}Y) and they both target CD20 with excellent clinical outcome. Between 20–40% complete remissions can be obtained and an overall response rate of 60–80% in patients with indolent lymphomas and related conditions [16]. Patients with significant bone marrow infiltration are however excluded in order not to cause potential haematological damage. It is generally concluded that these antibodies can provide clinically meaningful and durable responses even in patients where chemotherapy has failed [17].

The anti CD22 antibody, also initially a murine phenotype, was later humanized and was demonstrated to maintain significant positive effects in the clinic [18]. Furthermore, the antibodies targeting DR10β(Lym1) have been extensively studied by de Nardo and collaborators with demonstrated clinical effects on patients with non-Hodgkin lymphomas, when labelled with either ^{131}I or ^{67}Cu [19].

Solid Tumours

Colorectal cancer: Many efforts have been devoted to both image and treat malignancies of colorectal origin. The target antigens most abundantly used are Ep-CAM, A33, TAG-72 and CEA [20–22].

The most exploited antigen has been CEA with "better-than expected" outcome and observed switches from progressive disease to stable disease. Typically, as reviewed by Koppe et al. [10], reduction in circulating CEA can be observed together with decreases in symptoms and conversion to slower progression in fourteen different studies. The nature of the involved radionuclide also might affect the outcome [23–25]. Development of HAMA was observed in the major part of the studies in which murine antibodies were used. Some of the earlier used conjugates now have disappeared from the market.

The transmembrane glycoprotein A33 has been used with good targeting and 4 out of 15 patients presenting stable disease [26, 27]. On the contrary the murine CC49 antibody, both intact and in chimeric form, failed to produce significant clinical results against the same antigen [28, 29].

Breast cancer: Breast cancer has been studied intensively both from imaging and therapeutic point of view. Among the antigens employed are MUC1, CEA and L6. Also for this group of tumours, the benefits of radioimmunotherapy have been few compared to hematologic malignancies. The appearance of non-specific localization in tumour-negative nodes in breast cancer patients seems to be a property that weakens the clinical outcome, although up to 80% of the tumours have been possible to localize. In some investigations though, partial responses have been reached with up to 47% of the patients, despite failing earlier treatment [30–32]. Also antibodies against CEA have been tested and the derivative ^{131}I-NP was shown to present modest effects in 12 out of 35 patients with one partial remission, four minor responses and seven with stable disease [33, 34]. The L6 antigen, also present in substantial amounts in the breast epithelium, has been used for targeting both directly and as a part of combination strategies. Both positive and negative influences were reported on cure rate and toxicity [31, 35–37].

Prostate cancer: The most well known antibody for targeting prostate antigen is Capromad, directed against PSMA (prostate specific membrane antigen) and used as ^{111}In-labeled derivative for imaging of soft tissue metastases of prostate cancer ("Prostascint"). The antibody does not, however, localize to bone metastases due to the reactivity with a buried intracellular N-terminal target epitope. In therapeutic approaches no major responses have been observed [38, 39]. When extracellular epitopes of the PSMA antigen have been targeted, results have been slightly better with positive reports on hormone-refractive prostate cancer [41]. Also TAG-72 has been tested as target with negative results [40]. In combined experimental treatment investigations with radioimmunotherapy and chemotherapy, 67% cure rate has been reported, but neither RIT, nor chemotherapy alone could cure mice [42].

Ovarian cancer: Some initial positive reports on ovarian cancer, using an ^{90}Y labelled antibody against human milk fat globule (HMFG) to patients with minimal residual disease, have been reported [43], but the findings were not possible to repeat in an international, randomized multi-centre study. Several early experiments also demonstrated small, but not significant results [44–46]. In an evaluation of eight clinical radioimmunotherapy trials in ovarian cancer patients, the typical results were partial responses in less than 20% of the patients [10]. The positive outcome for ovarian cancer treatment thus seems to be elusive [47].

Lung cancer: Early attempts to identify advanced-stage disease, using a 99mTc-labelled anti SCLC (small cell lung cancer) antibody were partially positive and in 87% of the cases the extent of the disease was accurately determined [48, 49]. However 23% of the cases did present metastases later and this high false negative rate made this antibody less useful. In 2005, one report making use of an ^{90}Y-labelled anti SCLC antibody caused both toxic and immunological complications and no objective tumour responses [50].

Brain tumours: Gliomas have the capacity to rapidly infiltrate surrounding brain tissue and is the most common and lethal form of primary brain tumours. These tumours furthermore display significant resistance to chemotherapy and radiotherapy and are difficult to manage with cytoreductive surgery. Locoregional RIT treatment has been tried for these conditions [51]. One antigen expressed in many high grade gliomas is tenascin, which is an extracellular matrix glycoprotein, not abundantly expressed in normal glia cells. The murine antibody ^{131}I-81C6 against this alternatively spliced fibronectin-type molecule has shown promise in Phase 1 trials following intratumoral administration [52]. Some small clinical benefits have been observed also later with an average survival time increasing from 70 to 87 weeks, following intracavitary administration [53]. More recent investigations using locoregional application with ^{131}I-labeled antitenascin antibodies have been more encouraging [53, 54]. Also an anti-EGFR antibody has been used for intracavital administration and a relation between delivered dose and clinical outcome was observed [55]. A number of alternative three-step pretargeting reports have been presented with more obvious increases in survival time – increasing from 8 months (historical controls) to 34 months following treatment [56, 57]. The overall impression regarding brain tumours is that loco-regional therapy will generate more encouraging results, due to the high initial absorbed doses obtained.

Factors Affecting Therapeutic Outcome in Hematopoietic and Epithelial Tumours

The clinical success of radioimmunotherapy for solid tumours still seems to be a distant dream as judged from the comprehensive overview above. See also chapters 20 and 21 in this volume. Only small fractions of injected dose typically ends up in the tumour in patients and not more than 0.001–0.01% reach the tumour during a short period. In preclinical investigations however, much higher levels (5%) can be reached [58]. One of the reasons for this is that human tumour cell lines, often used in nude mice in preclinical experiments, are implanted in animals which do not express the targeted antigen at all anywhere, and this might cause unrealistic expectations when the model is transferred to clinical settings. For solid tumours very few complete remissions have been reported, although several minor, partial or mixed responses or stabilization of an earlier progressive disease have been reported. A delicate balance between myelotoxic side effects from the circulating large intact antibodies reaching the bone marrow and antibody accretion and residence time within the tumour has to be optimized, which was early recognized [59].

The limited success for radioimmunotherapy of solid tumours can be attributed to many factors. It should be remembered, though, that many of the clinical investigations evaluating radioimmunotherapy have been performed on heavily treated patients with advanced, mostly bulky, metastatic disease, which is a highly unfavourable setting for the application of radiolabeled antibodies. One of the major draw-backs, furthermore, may be the technology transfer when dealing with solid epithelial tumours in stead of lymphocytes, two cell types which display significant differences in behaviour when irradiated. Some of the differences will be delineated and discussed below.

Differences in Cell Death Mechanisms

One of the underlying reasons behind the refractoriness of solid tumours may be the way cell death is induced. As described elsewhere in this volume (chapters 12–14), a complex and interrelated system of activation pathways are in operation and related to irradiation induced death modalities. Radiation induced apoptosis has been considered to be one of the main cell death mechanisms following exposure to radiation [50]. In cells of lymphoid or myeloid origin, the early, rapid apoptosis, takes place only a few hours in the interphase [60] following irradiation exposure and does not require any cell division. Presently, however, the reasons for induction of different cell death types have been discussed and these considerations help to explain the absence of a simple link between apoptosis and clonogenicity and may give suggestions to how to overcome such restrictions [61].

Epithelial cells typically display a different type of death known as mitotic catastrophe, which takes place several days after the irradiation exposure, following mitosis. Finally this may induce a delayed type of apoptosis (see chapter 12). Direct comparisons between external radiation therapy and radioimmunotherapy have demonstrated, in preclinical studies, very disturbed morphological appearance of the targeted tumour tissue with appearance of giant cells, vacuolization and low growth potential and decrease in tumour volume, typical for induction of mitotic catastrophes with delayed type of apoptosis [62, 63].

The irradiation response in non-Hodgkin lymphoma patients usually occurs at very low absorbed doses, i.e. below 10 Gy [64–66]. An obvious dose-response relationship is likely, but not really proven. The antibodies used, however, do exert cytotoxic effects by themselves and can both contribute to increased sensitivity for irradiation and chemotherapy by activation of the cell. The antibodies can also, by joining forces with the complement system or by antibody dependent cell-mediated cytotoxicity eliminate the tumour cells. These mechanisms are not that easily observed with epithelial cells being targeted. These additional mechanisms may blur a direct linear relationship between doses and tumour growth inhibition. When naked antibodies against CD20 have been compared with identical radiolabeled antibodies, both do demonstrate significant effects, but the radiolabeled antibodies are more efficient [67–69]. Also antibodies targeting CD22 can induce measurable effects in naked form, which confirms that additional effects, besides irradiation contribute to the positive outcome [70–73]. It can thus be concluded that haematological malignancies can benefit to a higher degree on several independent killing mechanisms, compared to solid tumours, which should be kept in mind when the outcomes are compared.

One of the advantages with radioimmunotherapy, compared with chemotherapy, as demonstrated with hematologic malignancies is the much lower incidence of side-effects. Even if most of the clinical effects documented are based on single injections of radiolabeled antibodies, also multiple treatments given, present low toxicity with 50–60% objective response rates and long durations in treatment response [74–76]. It should however not be ruled out that several years have to pass before a complete evaluation of complications may be fully described. Both secondary cancers and myelodysplastic syndromes could be discussed, although the risks have been estimated to be very low [77].

Differences in Biological Properties of the Tumour Cells

The targeting of solid tumours is less efficient than targeting haematological malignancies. This depends partially also on several tumour-related factors. Solid tumours present a limited vascular supply, with anoxic regions at some distance from the vascular support. Furthermore, there is a heterogeneous uptake of antibody in the tumour, combined with increase in interstitial pressure and comparatively long transportation routes from the blood vessels [78]. This contributes to a hampered accumulation of antibodies in solid tumours compared to haematological malignancies.

Size of Targeting Molecules

Significant efforts have been devoted to generate derivatives, fragments or recombinant antibodies in order to affect targeting precision or clearing mechanisms (see also chapter 5 in this volume). The major part of all therapeutic approaches so far have been pursued with intact antibodies, which both display the inherent property of not being cleared fast and thus remain circulating for days during the targeting phase to the tumour. The major deterrent for using low molecular fragments, i.e. scFvs, diabodies or minibodies, with molecular weights below 50 kDa, is their extremely rapid clearance through the kidneys, which occur within hours [79–82]. This rapid clearance, however, certainly will cause a rapidly increasing tumour to non-tumour ratio, which is favourable from imaging point of view, but hampers both the residence time in the tumour and the absolute levels of targeting agents within the tumour. It seems today unlikely that any of these small, rapidly secreted, usually monovalent antibody construct will be able to efficiently jeopardize the future of a tumour cell, due to the transient, from the tumour disappearing antibody with its nuclide. Many attempts to generate recombinant antibodies, using a single scFv-fragment as starting point followed by creation of different types of multimers are partially hampered by low solubility properties of the constructs, despite tedious efforts, by site-directed-mutagenesis, to exchange amino acids known to be important for solubility both in vitro and during physiological conditions [80, 81]. It seems to be important to maintain antibody derivatives in divalent form (for affinity reasons) with molecular weights above 70 kDa in order to be above the threshold for renal excretion. The nature of the antigen may furthermore be crucial and the targeting efficiency can be very high if the antibodies may circulate for long periods without excretion due to small size. In preclinical investigations, using cytokeratin 8 as target, high amounts of activity could be visualized more than 30 days following administration of antibody, with absorbed doses of more than 10 Gy to the tumour [58, 83].

Another aspect that could negatively affect targeting with low molecular weight radionuclide-conjugates is reabsorption and uptake in the kidneys, where these compounds may exert toxic effects. By use of significant amounts of cationic amino acids, this uptake can however be partially avoided [84, 85]. In more recent investigations, targeting the somatostatin receptor, significant similar toxicities related to the kidney uptake has been documented [86–89]. Other compounds such as gelofusine and spirinolactone have been reported to confer a more rapid passage for these low molecular weight compounds through the kidney, lowering the toxic effects

[90–93]. Since all low molecular weight compounds have to pass through the kidney, any uptake in this organ should, if possible, be avoided.

Clearing of Redundant Antibody

A number of different mechanisms to clear redundant antibody has been brought forward in order to diminish irradiation effects on the bone marrow. For decades this has been one of the major factors that could improve efficiency, when improving treatment of solid tumours.

One of these techniques is the use of extracorporeal immuno-adsorption of antibodies remaining in the circulation. The technologies have not yet reached clinical acceptance, but from the very first attempts with extracorporeal circulation to selectively remove the labelled antibodies by passing plasma over antigen-coated agarose beads [94], the surgical intervention strategies have been modified and more simple to execute. It is possible to achieve a significant 95% reduction of circulating radioimmuno-conjugates, but only a reduction with 34% in the tumours [95, 96]. The authors conclude that this technology could contribute to reduce myelotoxicity with sustained concentration of immuno-conjugates in the tumours.

In a similar way the use of anti-idiotypic antibodies have been launched as aids for eliminating redundant antibodies. Cytokeratin 8 is an intermediate filament expressed intracellularly in many epithelial cells, and this antigen is deposited to a significant degree within experimental tumours due to low solubility. The detailed structure of the linear epitope, 26 amino acid long, has been revealed [97]. The immunoreactivity and epitope specificity of more than 30 monoclonal antibodies targeting this group of antigens have also been examined in a large collaborative investigation within ISOBM (International Society of Oncology and Biomarkers) [98]. The exquisite specificities of antidiotypic antibodies, intended for clearing of the idiotypes, are able to lower the levels of only the circulating radiolabeled antibodies within hours in preclinical investigations, and the levels of targeted antibodies can furthermore be titrated in vivo [99–102]. Extensive studies of the structural relation between idiotypic, anti-diotypic antibodies and their target antigen have been performed with modelling of the interaction surfaces [103–105]. The degradation of the complexes, following in vivo injection, occurs in the liver and the reticuloendothelial system with rapid excretion of the circulating nuclide in the urine. [101, 102]. These model systems indicate that it is technically possible to selectively eliminate one single injected radiolabeled antibody from the circulation within 24 hours, following administration of an anti-idiotypic antibody, and decrease total remaining activity in the body to 15–20%, still with 65% of the tumour activity in place [102]. This can be accomplished without any immunogenicity problems. These technologies, despite promising preclinical findings, have not however yet been established as useful modalities to reduce overload of targeting antibody in the clinic, but have not really been tested either. Figure 4.1 shows results from an experimental study using mice with transplanted tumors on their flanks. Reduced normal tissue uptake is seen after injection of an antiidiotypic antibody that, in the blood circulation bound the redundant primary radiolabelled antibody.

The introduction of different pretargeting techniques today seems to get consensus in terms of how to reach improvements in tumour to non-tumour ratios, in

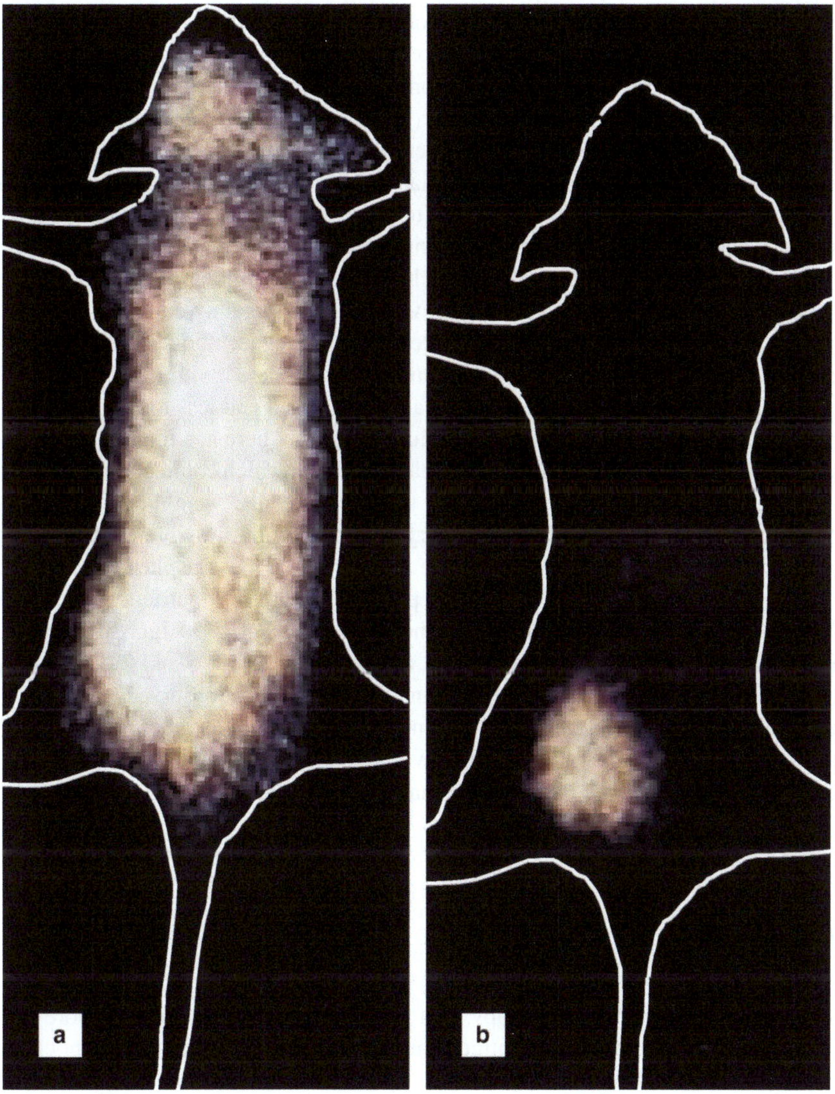

Fig. 4.1 (A) Scintigrafic evaluation of a mouse carrying a HeLa Hep2 tumour, 24 hours following i.p. injection of a ^{125}I-labeled mouse monoclonal anticytokeratin antibody TS1. Biodistribution of the antibody in the entire animal is seen. (B) The same animal, injected with half-equimolar amounts of an antiidiotypic anti TS1 antibody (αTS1). Scintigraphy performed 48 hours after injection of the antiidiotype. The tumour only can be visualized (Picture modified from [102])

combination with high accumulation within the tumours. A number of different approaches have been introduced, all striving to overcome the slow blood clearance of directly labelled antibodies by separating the targeting phase of the antibody from the delivery phase of the radionuclide [106, 107]. Following some early attempts with use of bispecific antibodies, Hnatowich et al. were the first to introduce the avidin (mammalian produced) and streptavidin (from bacteria) molecules and make use of their interaction with biotin, as a technology to separately gear the levels of nuclides and antibodies in vivo [108]. The typical "two-step" procedure includes three agents, one streptavidin conjugated scFv, a clearing agent and finally radiolabeled biotin [109–114]. Another approach is the "three-step" technique, employing biotinylated primary antibodies, which could be cleared or bridged with avidin or streptavidin, followed by radiolabeled biotin [115]. The streptavidin multivalency for biotin enables its binding to the complex. The monovalency of the scFvs, when used, and the immunogenicity of streptavidin might negatively affect the targeting efficiency. Several approaches using bispecific antibodies have also been presented, with even up to four scFvs within the targeting construct [111].

It is reasonable to conclude that different pretargeting techniques offer the highest efficiency in targeting yield today, and when compared with directly labelled antibodies, both larger absorbed doses can be delivered and less toxicity has been reported. Furthermore, during the accumulation phase there is a more rapid accretion of nuclide, when the antibody is already in place, which could contribute to an increased initial dose rate. Furthermore, the low molecular weight of the nuclide-conjugate in the final step, makes a very rapid excretion possible, and typically more than 70% may appear within some hours in the urine. Despite several phase I trials, a few phase II trials have been performed with dosimetric evaluation. A ^{90}Y-DOTA-biotin-conjugate, linked to the antibody NR-LU-10 IgG-streptavidin, focusing on advanced colorectal cancer, was found to deliver 5 and 29 Gy in only 2 patients out of 25, and no significant responses were observed [116, 117]. Paganelli et al. however were able to demonstrate 25% clinical response in glioblastoma or astrocytoma patients given two injections with the "three-step" pretargeting procedure, using biotinylated antibodies against tenascin, followed by ^{90}Y-DOTA-biotin [57].

Conclusions

The history of radioimmunotherapy, in a 50 years perspective, contains more than just findings of suitable target antigens and the generation of initially monoclonal and later recombinant, tailored antibodies. While treatment of non-Hodgkin's lymphomas has evolved from an appealing concept to an established treatment modality, the treatment of solid tumours has not yet really outgrown the preclinical stage. Most of the patients with solid tumours, irrespective of tumour type or localization, still present progressive disease during treatment, but occasionally partial responses or stable disease can appear, which is promising.

An obvious trend, typically observed for CEA, being the most used target antigen for radioimmunotherapy of solid tumours so far, is the switch from intact murine or chimeric/humanized antibodies to multivalent/bispecific antibodies, which can be engineered to contain multivalent binding sites for the target, but also specific binding sites for the nuclides. These different approaches to tailor multivalent antibodies with specific binding sites for both targets and nuclides seem to increase. The antibodies and different types of clearing molecules have also gained wider interest. They can be combined in "two-step" or "three step" pretargeting trials, which can improve tumour to non-tumour ratios rapidly. These approaches also gain wider acceptance.

The rapidly expanding scenario of different cell deaths (chapter 12) offers new putative ways to gain synergistic effects, which not yet have been fully explored or employed. Not only necrosis or apoptosis are involved, but also mitotic catastrophes, autophagy and senescence induction are in operation. Combinations with chemotherapy or even external beam radiation have in preclinical settings been favourable, but remains to be more explored in the clinic.

Locoregional therapy and pretargeting "multi-step" procedures today offers the best potential, and bring some optimism for future targeting inventions. Also the use of antiidiotypic antibodies or other clearing devices or techniques still need further exploration. The selection of patients may also affect the outcome of treatment. Minimal disease or locoregional therapy offers the best clinical settings for positive results, since much lower objective response rates usually are seen with bulky disease, with too low accretion of nuclide to exert tumouricidal effects.

Some of the limits in gaining wider acceptance clinically might also partially be related to the necessity of a multidisciplinary approach. A number of disciplines, including immunology, radiochemistry, radiation medicine, medical oncology and nuclear medicine have to collaborate in order to control the chain of judgements necessary for each patient. All these requirements may not always be available or easy to accomplish. This is a management paradigm shift, which usually would take some time. Maybe the time now has come when clinical radioimmunotherapy is added to standard regimens and could position this treatment modality for the future.

Acknowledgements Financial support from the Swedish Cancer Society, the County of Västerbotten and the Medical Faculty at Umeå University is acknowledged.

References

1. Goldenberg DM: Targeted therapy of cancer with radiolabeled antibodies. J Nucl Med 2002; 43:693–713.
2. Boswell CA, Brechbiel MW: Development of radioimmunotherapeutic and diagnostic antibodies: An inside-out view. Nucl Med Biol 2007; 34:757–778.
3. Goldenberg DM, Sharkey RM: Advances in cancer therapy with radiolabeled monoclonal antibodies. Q J Nucl Med Mol Imaging 2006; 50:248–264.

4. Imam SK: Status of radioimmunotherapy in the new millennium. Cancer Biother Radiopharm 2001; 16:237–256.
5. Oriuchi N, Higuchi T, Hanaoka H, Iida Y, Endo K: Current status of cancer therapy with radiolabeled monoclonal antibody. Ann Nucl Med 2005; 19:355–365.
6. Goldenberg DM: The role of radiolabeled antibodies in the treatment of non-hodgkin's lymphoma: The coming of age of radioimmunotherapy. Crit Rev Oncol Hematol 2001; 39:195–201.
7. Silverman DH, Delpassand ES, Torabi F, Goy A, McLaughlin P, Murray JL: Radiolabeled antibody therapy in non-hodgkins lymphoma: Radiation protection, isotope comparisons and quality of life issues. Cancer Treat Rev 2004; 30:165–172.
8. Russeva MG, Adams GP: Radioimmunotherapy with engineered antibodies. Expert Opin Biol Ther 2004; 4:217–231.
9. Bethge WA, Sandmaier BM: Targeted cancer therapy and immunosuppression using radiolabeled monoclonal antibodies. Semin Oncol 2004; 31:68–82.
10. Koppe MJ, Postema EJ, Aarts F, Oyen WJ, Bleichrodt RP, Boerman OC: Antibody-guided radiation therapy of cancer. Cancer Metastasis Rev 2005; 24:539–567.
11. Vose JM: Bexxar: Novel radioimmunotherapy for the treatment of low-grade and transformed low-grade non-Hodgkin's lymphoma. Oncologist 2004; 9:160–172.
12. Gordon LI, Witzig T, Molina A, Czuczman M, Emmanouilides C, Joyce R, Vo K, Theuer C, Pohlman B, Bartlett N, Wiseman G, Darif M, White C: Yttrium 90-labeled ibritumomab tiuxetan radioimmunotherapy produces high response rates and durable remissions in patients with previously treated b-cell lymphoma. Clin Lymphoma 2004; 5:98–101.
13. Milenic DE, Brady ED, Brechbiel MW: Antibody-targeted radiation cancer therapy. Nat Rev Drug Discov 2004; 3:488–499.
14. Walsh G: Biopharmaceutical benchmarks 2006. Nat Biotechnol 2006; 24:769–776.
15. DeNardo GL, Kennel SJ, Siegel JA, Denardo SJ: Radiometals as payloads for radioimmunotherapy for lymphoma. Clin Lymphoma 2004; 5(Suppl 1):S5–S10.
16. Press OW: Radioimmunotherapy for non-Hodgkin's lymphomas: A historical perspective. Semin Oncol 2003; 30:10–21.
17. Macklis RM, Pohlman B: Radioimmunotherapy for non-Hodgkin's lymphoma: A review for radiation oncologists. Int J Radiat Oncol Biol Phys 2006; 66:833–841.
18. Linden O, Hindorf C, Cavallin-Stahl E, Wegener WA, Goldenberg DM, Horne H, Ohlsson T, Stenberg L, Strand SE, Tennvall J: Dose-fractionated radioimmunotherapy in non-hodgkin's lymphoma using dota-conjugated, 90y-radiolabeled, humanized anti-cd22 monoclonal antibody, epratuzumab. Clin Cancer Res 2005; 11:5215–5222.
19. DeNardo GL, Kukis DL, Shen S, DeNardo DA, Meares CF, DeNardo SJ: 67cu-versus 131i-labeled lym-1 antibody: Comparative pharmacokinetics and dosimetry in patients with non-Hodgkin's lymphoma. Clin Cancer Res 1999; 5:533–541.
20. Beatty JD, Williams LE, Yamauchi D, Morton BA, Hill LR, Beatty BG, Paxton RJ, Merchant B, Shively JE: Presurgical imaging with indium-labeled anti-carcinoembryonic antigen for colon cancer staging. Cancer Res 1990; 50:922s–926s.
21. Bischof-Delaloye A, Delaloye B, Buchegger F, Gilgien W, Studer A, Curchod S, Givel JC, Mosimann F, Pettavel J, Mach JP: Clinical value of immunoscintigraphy in colorectal carcinoma patients: A prospective study. J Nucl Med 1989; 30:1646–1656.
22. Blumenthal RD, Sharkey RM, Kashi R, Goldenberg DM: Comparison of therapeutic efficacy and host toxicity of two different 131i-labelled antibodies and their fragments in the gw-39 colonic cancer xenograft model. Int J Cancer 1989; 44:292–300.
23. Liersch T, Meller J, Kulle B, Behr TM, Markus P, Langer C, Ghadimi BM, Wegener WA, Kovacs J, Horak ID, Becker H, Goldenberg DM: Phase II trial of carcinoembryonic antigen radioimmunotherapy with 131i-labetuzumab after salvage resection of colorectal metastases in the liver: Five-year safety and efficacy results. J Clin Oncol 2005; 23:6763–6770.
24. Wong JY, Chu DZ, Williams LE, Yamauchi DM, Ikle DN, Kwok CS, Liu A, Wilczynski S, Colcher D, Yazaki PJ, Shively JE, Wu AM, Raubitschek AA: Pilot trial evaluating an

123i-labeled 80-kilodalton engineered anticarcinoembryonic antigen antibody fragment (ct84.66 minibody) in patients with colorectal cancer. Clin Cancer Res 2004; 10:5014–5021.
25. Wong JY, Shibata S, Williams LE, Kwok CS, Liu A, Chu DZ, Yamauchi DM, Wilczynski S, Ikle DN, Wu AM, Yazaki PJ, Shively JE, Doroshow JH, Raubitschek AA: A phase I trial of 90y-anti-carcinoembryonic antigen chimeric t84.66 radioimmunotherapy with 5-fluorouracil in patients with metastatic colorectal cancer. Clin Cancer Res 2003; 9:5842–5852.
26. Chong G, Lee FT, Hopkins W, Tebbutt N, Cebon JS, Mountain AJ, Chappell B, Papenfuss A, Schleyer P, Paul U, Murphy R, Wirth V, Smyth FE, Potasz N, Poon A, Davis ID, Saunder T, O'Keefe G J, Burgess AW, Hoffman EW, Old LJ, Scott AM: Phase I trial of 131i-hua33 in patients with advanced colorectal carcinoma. Clin Cancer Res 2005; 11:4818–4826.
27. Scott AM, Lee FT, Jones R, Hopkins W, MacGregor D, Cebon JS, Hannah A, Chong G, Paul U, Papenfuss A, Rigopoulos A, Sturrock S, Murphy R, Wirth V, Murone C, Smyth FE, Knight S, Welt S, Ritter G, Richards E, Nice EC, Burgess AW, Old LJ: A phase I trial of humanized monoclonal antibody a33 in patients with colorectal carcinoma: Biodistribution, pharmacokinetics, and quantitative tumor uptake. Clin Cancer Res 2005; 11:4810–4817.
28. Buchsbaum D, Khazaeli MB, Liu T, Bright S, Richardson K, Jones M, Meredith R: Fractionated radioimmunotherapy of human colon carcinoma xenografts with 131i-labeled monoclonal antibody cc49. Cancer Res 1995; 55:5881s–5887s.
29. Tempero M, Leichner P, Baranowska-Kortylewicz J, Harrison K, Augustine S, Schlom J, Anderson J, Wisecarver J, Colcher D: High-dose therapy with 90yttrium-labeled monoclonal antibody cc49: A phase I trial. Clin Cancer Res 2000; 6:3095–3102.
30. DeNardo SJ, Kramer EL, O'Donnell RT, Richman CM, Salako QA, Shen S, Noz M, Glenn SD, Ceriani RL, DeNardo GL: Radioimmunotherapy for breast cancer using indium-111/yttrium-90 bre-3: Results of a phase I clinical trial. J Nucl Med 1997; 38:1180–1185.
31. DeNardo SJ, Kukis DL, Miers LA, Winthrop MD, Kroger LA, Salako Q, Shen S, Lamborn KR, Gumerlock PH, Meares CF, DeNardo GL: Yttrium-90-dota-peptide-chimeric l6 radioimmunoconjugate: Efficacy and toxicity in mice bearing p53 mutant human breast cancer xenografts. J Nucl Med 1998; 39:842–849.
32. Schrier DM, Stemmer SM, Johnson T, Kasliwal R, Lear J, Matthes S, Taffs S, Dufton C, Glenn SD, Butchko G, et al.: High-dose 90y mx-diethylenetriaminepentaacetic acid (dtpa)-bre-3 and autologous hematopoietic stem cell support (ahscs) for the treatment of advanced breast cancer: A phase I trial. Cancer Res 1995; 55:5921s–5924s.
33. Behr TM, Sharkey RM, Juweid ME, Dunn RM, Vagg RC, Ying Z, Zhang CH, Swayne LC, Vardi Y, Siegel JA, Goldenberg DM: Phase I/II clinical radioimmunotherapy with an iodine-131-labeled anti-carcinoembryonic antigen murine monoclonal antibody igg. J Nucl Med 1997; 38:858–870.
34. Ebeling FG, Stieber P, Untch M, Nagel D, Konecny GE, Schmitt UM, Fateh-Moghadam A, Seidel D: Serum cea and ca 15-3 as prognostic factors in primary breast cancer. Br J Cancer 2002; 86:1217–1222.
35. Burke PA, DeNardo SJ, Miers LA, Kukis DL, DeNardo GL: Combined modality radioimmunotherapy. Promise and peril. Cancer 2002; 94:1320–1331.
36. Burke PA, DeNardo SJ, Miers LA, Lamborn KR, Matzku S, DeNardo GL: Cilengitide targeting of alpha(v)beta(3) integrin receptor synergizes with radioimmunotherapy to increase efficacy and apoptosis in breast cancer xenografts. Cancer Res 2002; 62:4263–4272.
37. DeNardo SJ, Kukis DL, Kroger LA, O'Donnell RT, Lamborn KR, Miers LA, DeNardo DG, Meares CF, DeNardo GL: Synergy of taxol and radioimmunotherapy with yttrium-90-labeled chimeric l6 antibody: Efficacy and toxicity in breast cancer xenografts. Proc Natl Acad Sci USA 1997; 94:4000–4004.
38. Bander NH: Technology insight: Monoclonal antibody imaging of prostate cancer. Nat Clin Pract Urol 2006; 3:216–225.
39. Raj GV, Partin AW, Polascik TJ: Clinical utility of indium 111-capromab pendetide immunoscintigraphy in the detection of early, recurrent prostate carcinoma after radical prostatectomy. Cancer 2002; 94:987–996.

40. Meredith RF, Bueschen AJ, Khazaeli MB, Plott WE, Grizzle WE, Wheeler RH, Schlom J, Russell CD, Liu T, LoBuglio AF: Treatment of metastatic prostate carcinoma with radiolabeled antibody cc49. J Nucl Med 1994; 35:1017–1022.
41. Vallabhajosula S, Goldsmith SJ, Kostakoglu L, Milowsky MI, Nanus DM, Bander NH: Radioimmunotherapy of prostate cancer using 90y- and 177lu-labeled j591 monoclonal antibodies: Effect of multiple treatments on myelotoxicity. Clin Cancer Res 2005; 11:7195s–7200s.
42. O'Donnell RT, DeNardo SJ, Miers LA, Lamborn KR, Kukis DL, DeNardo GL, Meyers FJ: Combined modality radioimmunotherapy for human prostate cancer xenografts with taxanes and 90yttrium-dota-peptide-chl6. Prostate 2002; 50:27–37.
43. Epenetos AA, Hird V, Lambert H, Mason P, Coulter C: Long term survival of patients with advanced ovarian cancer treated with intraperitoneal radioimmunotherapy. Int J Gynecol Cancer 2000; 10:44–46.
44. Buijs WC, Tibben JG, Boerman OC, Molthoff CF, Massuger LF, Koenders EB, Schijf CP, Siegel JA, Corstens FH: Dosimetric analysis of chimeric monoclonal antibody cmov18 igg in ovarian carcinoma patients after intraperitoneal and intravenous administration. Eur J Nucl Med 1998; 25:1552–1561.
45. Buist MR, Molthoff CF, Kenemans P, Meijer CJ: Distribution of ov-tl 3 and mov18 in normal and malignant ovarian tissue. J Clin Pathol 1995; 48:631–636.
46. Coliva A, Zacchetti A, Luison E, Tomassetti A, Bongarzone I, Seregni E, Bombardieri E, Martin F, Giussani A, Figini M, Canevari S: 90y labeling of monoclonal antibody mov18 and preclinical validation for radioimmunotherapy of human ovarian carcinomas. Cancer Immunol Immunother 2005; 54:1200–1213.
47. Nicodemus CF, Berek JS: Monoclonal antibody therapy of ovarian cancer. Expert Rev Anticancer Ther 2005; 5:87–96.
48. Breitz HB, Weiden PL, Beaumier PL, Axworthy DB, Seiler C, Su FM, Graves S, Bryan K, Reno JM: Clinical optimization of pretargeted radioimmunotherapy with antibody-streptavidin conjugate and 90y-dota-biotin. J Nucl Med 2000; 41:131–140.
49. Machac J, Krynyckyi B, Kim C: Peptide and antibody imaging in lung cancer. Semin Nucl Med 2002; 32:276–292.
50. Forero A, Meredith RF, Khazaeli MB, Shen S, Grizzle WE, Carey D, Busby E, LoBuglio AF, Robert F: Phase I study of 90y-cc49 monoclonal antibody therapy in patients with advanced non-small cell lung cancer: Effect of chelating agents and paclitaxel co-administration. Cancer Biother Radiopharm 2005; 20:467–478.
51. Arista A, Sturiale C, Riva P, Tison V, Frattarelli M, Moscatelli G, Franceschi G, Spinelli A: Intralesional administration of i-131 labelled monoclonal antibodies in the treatment of malignant gliomas. Acta Neurochir (Wien) 1995; 135:159–162.
52. Bigner DD, Brown M, Coleman RE, Friedman AH, Friedman HS, McLendon RE, Bigner SH, Zhao XG, Wikstrand CJ, Pegram CN, et al.: Phase I studies of treatment of malignant gliomas and neoplastic meningitis with 131i-radiolabeled monoclonal antibodies anti-tenascin 81c6 and anti-chondroitin proteoglycan sulfate me1-14f (ab')2–a preliminary report. J Neurooncol 1995; 24:109–122.
53. Reardon DA, Akabani G, Coleman RE, Friedman AH, Friedman HS, Herndon JE, 2nd, Cokgor I, McLendon RE, Pegram CN, Provenzale JM, Quinn JA, Rich JN, Regalado LV, Sampson JH, Shafman TD, Wikstrand CJ, Wong TZ, Zhao XG, Zalutsky MR, Bigner DD: Phase II trial of murine (131)i-labeled antitenascin monoclonal antibody 81c6 administered into surgically created resection cavities of patients with newly diagnosed malignant gliomas. J Clin Oncol 2002; 20:1389–1397.
54. Reardon DA, Akabani G, Coleman RE, Friedman AH, Friedman HS, Herndon JE, 2nd, McLendon RE, Pegram CN, Provenzale JM, Quinn JA, Rich JN, Vredenburgh JJ, Desjardins A, Gururangan S, Badruddoja M, Dowell JM, Wong TZ, Zhao XG, Zalutsky MR, Bigner DD: Salvage radioimmunotherapy with murine iodine-131-labeled antitenascin monoclonal antibody 81c6 for patients with recurrent primary and metastatic malignant brain tumors: Phase II study results. J Clin Oncol 2006; 24:115–122.

55. Quang TS, Brady LW: Radioimmunotherapy as a novel treatment regimen: 125i-labeled monoclonal antibody 425 in the treatment of high-grade brain gliomas. Int J Radiat Oncol Biol Phys 2004; 58:972–975.
56. Grana C, Chinol M, Robertson C, Mazzetta C, Bartolomei M, De Cicco C, Fiorenza M, Gatti M, Caliceti P, Paganelli G: Pretargeted adjuvant radioimmunotherapy with yttrium-90-biotin in malignant glioma patients: A pilot study. Br J Cancer 2002; 86:207–212.
57. Paganelli G, Bartolomei M, Ferrari M, Cremonesi M, Broggi G, Maira G, Sturiale C, Grana C, Prisco G, Gatti M, Caliceti P, Chinol M: Pre-targeted locoregional radioimmunotherapy with 90y-biotin in glioma patients: Phase I study and preliminary therapeutic results. Cancer Biother Radiopharm 2001; 16:227–235.
58. Rossi Norrlund R, Ullen A, Sandstrom P, Holback D, Johansson L, Stigbrand T, Hietala SO, Riklund Ahlstrom K: Dosimetry of fractionated experimental radioimmunotargeting with idiotypic and anti-idiotypic anticytokeratin antibodies. Cancer 1997; 80:2681–2688.
59. Stigbrand T, Ullen A, Sandstrom P, Mirzaie-Joniani H, Sundstrom B, Nillson B, Arlestig L, Norrlund RR, Ahlstrom KR, Hietala S: Twenty years with monoclonal antibodies: State of the art–where do we go? Acta Oncol 1996; 35:259–265.
60. Radford IR, Murphy TK, Radley JM, Ellis SL: Radiation response of mouse lymphoid and myeloid cell lines. Part II. Apoptotic death is shown by all lines examined. Int J Radiat Biol 1994; 65:217–227.
61. Abend M: Reasons to reconsider the significance of apoptosis for cancer therapy. Int J Radiat Biol 2003;79:927–941.
62. Eriksson D, Joniani HM, Sheikholvaezin A, Lofroth PO, Johansson L, Riklund Ahlstrom K, Stigbrand T: Combined low dose radio- and radioimmunotherapy of experimental hela hep 2 tumours. Eur J Nucl Med Mol Imaging 2003; 30:895–906.
63. Eriksson D, Lofroth PO, Johansson L, Riklund KA, Stigbrand T: Cell cycle disturbances and mitotic catastrophes in hela hep2 cells following 2.5 to 10Gy of ionizing radiation. Clin Cancer Res 2007; 13:5501s–5508s.
64. Koral KF, Kaminski MS, Wahl RL: Correlation of tumor radiation-absorbed dose with response is easier to find in previously untreated patients. J Nucl Med 2003; 44:1541–1543; author reply 1543.
65. Sgouros G, Squeri S, Ballangrud AM, Kolbert KS, Teitcher JB, Panageas KS, Finn RD, Divgi CR, Larson SM, Zelenetz AD: Patient-specific, 3-dimensional dosimetry in non-Hodgkin's lymphoma patients treated with 131i-anti-b1 antibody: Assessment of tumor dose-response. J Nucl Med 2003; 44:260–268.
66. Sharkey RM, Brenner A, Burton J, Hajjar G, Toder SP, Alavi A, Matthies A, Tsai DE, Schuster SJ, Stadtmauer EA, Czuczman MS, Lamonica D, Kraeber-Bodere F, Mahe B, Chatal JF, Rogatko A, Mardirrosian G, Goldenberg DM: Radioimmunotherapy of non-Hodgkin's lymphoma with 90y-dota humanized anti-cd22 igg (90y-epratuzumab): Do tumor targeting and dosimetry predict therapeutic response? J Nucl Med 2003; 44:2000–2018.
67. Witzig TE, Gordon LI, Cabanillas F, Czuczman MS, Emmanouilides C, Joyce R, Pohlman BL, Bartlett NL, Wiseman GA, Padre N, Grillo-Lopez AJ, Multani P, White CA: Randomized controlled trial of yttrium-90-labeled ibritumomab tiuxetan radioimmunotherapy versus rituximab immunotherapy for patients with relapsed or refractory low-grade, follicular, or transformed b-cell non-Hodgkin's lymphoma. J Clin Oncol 2002; 20:2453–2463.
68. Gordon LI, Molina A, Witzig T, Emmanouilides C, Raubtischek A, Darif M, Schilder RJ, Wiseman G, White CA: Durable responses after ibritumomab tiuxetan radioimmunotherapy for cd20 + b-cell lymphoma: Long-term follow-up of a phase I/II study. Blood 2004; 103:4429–4431.
69. Davis TA, Kaminski MS, Leonard JP, Hsu FJ, Wilkinson M, Zelenetz A, Wahl RL, Kroll S, Coleman M, Goris M, Levy R, Knox SJ: The radioisotope contributes significantly to the activity of radioimmunotherapy. Clin Cancer Res 2004; 10:7792–7798.
70. Mone AP, Huang P, Pelicano H, Cheney CM, Green JM, Tso JY, Johnson AJ, Jefferson S, Lin TS, Byrd JC: Hu1d10 induces apoptosis concurrent with activation of the akt survival pathway in human chronic lymphocytic leukemia cells. Blood 2004; 103:1846–1854.

71. Leonard JP, Coleman M, Ketas JC, Chadburn A, Ely S, Furman RR, Wegener WA, Hansen HJ, Ziccardi H, Eschenberg M, Gayko U, Cesano A, Goldenberg DM: Phase I/II trial of epratuzumab (humanized anti-cd22 antibody) in indolent non-Hodgkin's lymphoma. J Clin Oncol 2003; 21:3051–3059.
72. Dechant M, Bruenke J, Valerius T: Hla class II antibodies in the treatment of hematologic malignancies. Semin Oncol 2003; 30:465–475.
73. Liu C, DeNardo G, Tobin E, DeNardo S: Antilymphoma effects of anti-hla-dr and cd20 monoclonal antibodies (lym-1 and rituximab) on human lymphoma cells. Cancer Biother Radiopharm 2004; 19:545–561.
74. Kaminski MS, Tuck M, Estes J, Kolstad A, Ross CW, Zasadny K, Regan D, Kison P, Fisher S, Kroll S, Wahl RL: 131i-tositumomab therapy as initial treatment for follicular lymphoma. N Engl J Med 2005; 352:441–449.
75. Press OW, Unger JM, Braziel RM, Maloney DG, Miller TP, LeBlanc M, Gaynor ER, Rivkin SE, Fisher RI: A phase II trial of chop chemotherapy followed by tositumomab/iodine i 131 tositumomab for previously untreated follicular non-hodgkin lymphoma: Southwest oncology group protocol s9911. Blood 2003; 102:1606–1612.
76. Kaminski MS, Estes J, Zasadny KR, Francis IR, Ross CW, Tuck M, Regan D, Fisher S, Gutierrez J, Kroll S, Stagg R, Tidmarsh G, Wahl RL: Radioimmunotherapy with iodine (131)i tositumomab for relapsed or refractory b-cell non-Hodgkin lymphoma: Updated results and long-term follow-up of the University of Michigan experience. Blood 2000; 96:1259–1266.
77. Gopal AK, Gooley TA, Maloney DG, Petersdorf SH, Eary JF, Rajendran JG, Bush SA, Durack LD, Golden J, Martin PJ, Matthews DC, Appelbaum FR, Bernstein ID, Press OW: High-dose radioimmunotherapy versus conventional high-dose therapy and autologous hematopoietic stem cell transplantation for relapsed follicular non-Hodgkin lymphoma: A multivariable cohort analysis. Blood 2003; 102:2351–2357.
78. Jain RK: Physiological barriers to delivery of monoclonal antibodies and other macromolecules in tumors. Cancer Res 1990; 50:814s–819s.
79. Sheikholvaezin A, Eriksson D, Ahlstrom KR, Johansson L, Stigbrand T: Tumor radioimmunolocalization in nude mice by mono- and divalent- single-chain fv antiplacental alkaline phosphatase antibodies. Cancer Biother Radiopharm 2007; 22:64–72.
80. Sheikholvaezin A, Eriksson D, Riklund K, Stigbrand T: Construction and purification of a covalently linked divalent tandem single-chain fv antibody against placental alkaline phosphatase. Hybridoma (Larchmt) 2006; 25:255–263.
81. Sheikholvaezin A, Sandstrom P, Eriksson D, Norgren N, Riklund K, Stigbrand T: Optimizing the generation of recombinant single-chain antibodies against placental alkaline phosphatase. Hybridoma (Larchmt) 2006; 25:181–192.
82. Rydh A, Riklund-Ahlstrom K, Widmark A, Bergh A, Johansson L, Tavelin B, Nilsson S, Stigbrand T, Damber JE, Hietala SO: Radioimmunotherapy of du-145 tumours in nude mice–a pilot study with e4, a novel monoclonal antibody against prostate cancer. Acta Oncol 1999; 38:1075–1079.
83. Rossi Norrlund R, Ullen A, Sandstrom P, Holback D, Johansson L, Stigbrand T, Hietala SO, Ahlstrom KR: Experimental radioimmunotargeting combining nonlabeled, iodine-125-labeled, and anti-idiotypic anticytokeratin monoclonal antibodies: A dosimetric evaluation. Cancer 1997; 80:2689–2698.
84. Behr TM, Sharkey RM, Juweid ME, Blumenthal RD, Dunn RM, Griffiths GL, Bair HJ, Wolf FG, Becker WS, Goldenberg DM: Reduction of the renal uptake of radiolabeled monoclonal antibody fragments by cationic amino acids and their derivatives. Cancer Res 1995; 55:3825–3834.
85. Behr TM, Sharkey RM, Sgouros G, Blumenthal RD, Dunn RM, Kolbert K, Griffiths GL, Siegel JA, Becker WS, Goldenberg DM: Overcoming the nephrotoxicity of radiometal-labeled immunoconjugates: Improved cancer therapy administered to a nude mouse model in relation to the internal radiation dosimetry. Cancer 1997; 80:2591–2610.
86. Jamar F, Barone R, Mathieu I, Walrand S, Labar D, Carlier P, de Camps J, Schran H, Chen T, Smith MC, Bouterfa H, Valkema R, Krenning EP, Kvols LK, Pauwels S: 86y-dota0)-d-phe1-tyr3-octreotide (smt487) – a phase I clinical study: Pharmacokinetics, biodistribution and renal protective effect of different regimens of amino acid co-infusion. Eur J Nucl Med Mol Imaging 2003; 30:510–518.

87. Bodei L, Cremonesi M, Zoboli S, Grana C, Bartolomei M, Rocca P, Caracciolo M, Macke HR, Chinol M, Paganelli G: Receptor-mediated radionuclide therapy with 90y-dotatoc in association with amino acid infusion: A phase I study. Eur J Nucl Med Mol Imaging 2003; 30:207–216.
88. Moll S, Nickeleit V, Mueller-Brand J, Brunner FP, Maecke HR, Mihatsch MJ: A new cause of renal thrombotic microangiopathy: Yttrium 90-dotatoc internal radiotherapy. Am J Kidney Dis 2001; 37:847–851.
89. Cybulla M, Weiner SM, Otte A: End-stage renal disease after treatment with 90y-dotatoc. Eur J Nucl Med 2001; 28:1552–1554.
90. van Eerd JE, Vegt E, Wetzels JF, Russel FG, Masereeuw R, Corstens FH, Oyen WJ, Boerman OC: Gelatin-based plasma expander effectively reduces renal uptake of 111in-octreotide in mice and rats. J Nucl Med 2006; 47:528–533.
91. Vegt E, Wetzels JF, Russel FG, Masereeuw R, Boerman OC, van Eerd JE, Corstens FH, Oyen WJ: Renal uptake of radiolabeled octreotide in human subjects is efficiently inhibited by succinylated gelatin. J Nucl Med 2006; 47:432–436.
92. Jaggi JS, Seshan SV, McDevitt MR, Sgouros G, Hyjek E, Scheinberg DA: Mitigation of radiation nephropathy after internal alpha-particle irradiation of kidneys. Int J Radiat Oncol Biol Phys 2006; 64:1503–1512.
93. Barone R, Borson-Chazot F, Valkema R, Walrand S, Chauvin F, Gogou L, Kvols LK, Krenning EP, Jamar F, Pauwels S: Patient-specific dosimetry in predicting renal toxicity with (90)y-dotatoc: Relevance of kidney volume and dose rate in finding a dose-effect relationship. J Nucl Med 2005; 46 Suppl 1:99S–106S.
94. Nilsson R, Lindgren L, Lilliehorn P: Extracorporeal immunoadsorption therapy on rats. In vivo depletion of specific antibodies. Clin Exp Immunol 1990; 82:440–444.
95. Martensson L, Nilsson R, Ohlsson T, Sjogren HO, Strand SE, Tennvall J: Reduced myelotoxicity with sustained tumor concentration of radioimmunoconjugates in rats after extracorporeal depletion. J Nucl Med 2007; 48:269–276.
96. Martensson L, Nilsson R, Sjogren HO, Strand SE, Tennvall J: A nonsurgical technique for blood access in extracorporeal affinity adsorption of antibodies in rats. Artif Organs 2007; 31:312–316.
97. Johansson A, Sandstrom P, Ullen A, Behravan G, Erlandsson A, Levi M, Sundstrom B, Stigbrand T: Epitope specificity of the monoclonal anticytokeratin antibody ts1. Cancer Res 1999; 59:48–51.
98. Stigbrand T, Andres C, Bellanger L, Bishr Omary M, Bodenmuller H, Bonfrer H, Brundell J, Einarsson R, Erlandsson A, Johansson A, Leca JF, Levi M, Meier T, Nap M, Nustad K, Seguin P, Sjodin A, Sundstrom B, van Dalen A, Wiebelhaus E, Wiklund B, Arlestig L, Hilgers J: Epitope specificity of 30 monoclonal antibodies against cytokeratin antigens: The isobm td5-1 workshop. Tumour Biol 1998; 19:132–152.
99. Ullen A, Ahlstrom KR, Heitala S, Nilsson B, Arlestig L, Stigbrand T: Secondary antibodies as tools to improve tumor to non tumor ratio at radioimmunolocalisation and radioimmunotherapy. Acta Oncol 1996; 35:281–285.
100. Ullen A, Nilsson B, Ahlstrom KR, Makiya R, Stigbrand T: In vivo and in vitro interactions between idiotypic and antiidiotypic monoclonal antibodies against placental alkaline phosphatase. J Immunol Methods 1995; 183:155–165.
101. Ullen A, Riklund Ahlstrom K, Makiya R, Stigbrand T: Syngeneic anti-idiotypic antibodies eliminate excess radiolabeled idiotypes at experimental radioimmunolocalization. Cell Biophys 1995; 27:31–45.
102. Ullen A, Sandstrom P, Ahlstrom KR, Sundstrom B, Nilsson B, Arlestig L, Stigbrand T: Use of anticytokeratin monoclonal anti-idiotypic antibodies to improve tumor:Nontumor ratio in experimental radioimmunolocalization. Cancer Res 1995; 55:5868s–5873s.
103. Erlandsson A, Holm P, Ullen A, Stigbrand T, Sundstrom BE: Studies of the interactions between the anticytokeratin 8 monoclonal antibody ts1, its antigen and its anti-idiotypic antibody alphats1. J Mol Recognit 2003; 16:157–163.
104. Erlandsson A, Eriksson D, Johansson L, Riklund K, Stigbrand T, Sundstrom BE: In vivo clearing of idiotypic antibodies with antiidiotypic antibodies and their derivatives. Mol Immunol 2006; 43:599–606.

105. Johansson A, Erlandsson A, Eriksson D, Ullen A, Holm P, Sundstrom BE, Roux KH, Stigbrand T: Idiotypic-anti-idiotypic complexes and their in vivo metabolism. Cancer 2002; 94:1306–1313.
106. Goldenberg DM, Sharkey RM, Paganelli G, Barbet J, Chatal JF: Antibody pretargeting advances cancer radioimmunodetection and radioimmunotherapy. J Clin Oncol 2006; 24:823–834.
107. Boerman OC, van Schaijk FG, Oyen WJ, Corstens FH: Pretargeted radioimmunotherapy of cancer: Progress step by step. J Nucl Med 2003; 44:400–411.
108. Hnatowich DJ, Virzi F, Rusckowski M: Investigations of avidin and biotin for imaging applications. J Nucl Med 1987; 28:1294–1302.
109. Axworthy DB, Reno JM, Hylarides MD, Mallett RW, Theodore LJ, Gustavson LM, Su F, Hobson LJ, Beaumier PL, Fritzberg AR: Cure of human carcinoma xenografts by a single dose of pretargeted yttrium-90 with negligible toxicity. Proc Natl Acad Sci USA 2000; 97:1802–1807.
110. Zhang M, Zhang Z, Garmestani K, Schultz J, Axworthy DB, Goldman CK, Brechbiel MW, Carrasquillo JA, Waldmann TA: Pretarget radiotherapy with an anti-cd25 antibody-streptavidin fusion protein was effective in therapy of leukemia/lymphoma xenografts. Proc Natl Acad Sci USA 2003; 100:1891–1895.
111. Sato N, Hassan R, Axworthy DB, Wong KJ, Yu S, Theodore LJ, Lin Y, Park L, Brechbiel MW, Pastan I, Paik CH, Carrasquillo JA: Pretargeted radioimmunotherapy of mesothelin-expressing cancer using a tetravalent single-chain fv-streptavidin fusion protein. J Nucl Med 2005; 46:1201–1209.
112. Cheung NK, Modak S, Lin Y, Guo H, Zanzonico P, Chung J, Zuo Y, Sanderson J, Wilbert S, Theodore LJ, Axworthy DB, Larson SM: Single-chain fv-streptavidin substantially improved therapeutic index in multistep targeting directed at disialoganglioside gd2. J Nucl Med 2004; 45:867–877.
113. Forero-Torres A, Shen S, Breitz H, Sims RB, Axworthy DB, Khazaeli MB, Chen KH, Percent I, Besh S, LoBuglio AF, Meredith RF: Pretargeted radioimmunotherapy (rit) with a novel anti-tag-72 fusion protein. Cancer Biother Radiopharm 2005; 20:379–390.
114. Buchsbaum DJ, Khazaeli MB, Axworthy DB, Schultz J, Chaudhuri TR, Zinn KR, Carpenter M, LoBuglio AF: Intraperitoneal pretarget radioimmunotherapy with cc49 fusion protein. Clin Cancer Res 2005; 11:8180–8185.
115. Paganelli G, Magnani P, Zito F, Villa E, Sudati F, Lopalco L, Rossetti C, Malcovati M, Chiolerio F, Seccamani E, et al.: Three-step monoclonal antibody tumor targeting in carcinoembryonic antigen-positive patients. Cancer Res 1991; 51:5960–5966.
116. Knox SJ, Goris ML, Tempero M, Weiden PL, Gentner L, Breitz H, Adams GP, Axworthy D, Gaffigan S, Bryan K, Fisher DR, Colcher D, Horak ID, Weiner LM: Phase II trial of yttrium-90-dota-biotin pretargeted by nr-lu-10 antibody/streptavidin in patients with metastatic colon cancer. Clin Cancer Res 2000; 6:406–414.
117. Breitz HB, Fisher DR, Goris ML, Knox S, Ratliff B, Murtha AD, Weiden PL: Radiation absorbed dose estimation for 90y-dota-biotin with pretargeted nr-lu-10/streptavidin. Cancer Biother Radiopharm 1999; 14:381–395.

Chapter 5
Antibody Fragments Produced by Recombinant and Proteolytic Methods

Gregory P. Adams

Summary While monoclonal antibodies provide the means to specifically target radioisotopes to tumors, the initial clinical radioimmunotherapy trials were largely unsuccessful. In the past decade, the field of molecular biology has matured to the point where we can re-engineer antibodies to overcome the limitations that were likely responsible for the early failures of radioimmunotherapy. In this chapter the wide variety of engineered and proteolytically produced antibody fragments are described along with their potential benefits for radioimmunotherapy.

Introduction

Koehler and Milstein's seminal development of hybridoma technology in the 1970s enabled the production of defined, clonal populations of antibodies (monoclonal antibodies or MAbs) [1]. This ushered in an era where products of the immune system could be exploited for a more focused delivery of cytotoxic agents, such as radioisotopes, to sites of tumor. While radioimmunotherapy (RAIT) with intact MAbs clearly is associated with effective treatment of diffuse or liquid malignancies, these successes have not extended to solid tumors. This is likely due to the prolonged retention in circulation and slow tumor penetration of intact antibodies. These properties arise from the natural role of antibodies – to protect the body from infections. As such, evolutionary pressures have resulted in the inclusion of sequences that are targeted by a range of Fc receptors on circulating immune effector cells, to direct these cells to foreign targets and on other tissues, such as the endothelium, to maintain constant levels of antibodies in the circulation. It should therefore come as no surprise that modifications of these antibodies will be necessary if they are to be used to target cytotoxic payloads to tumor without leading to undue normal tissue toxicity.

Department of Medical Oncology, Fox Chase Cancer Center, 333 Cottman Ave, Philadelphia, PA 19111, USA

T. Stigbrand et al. (eds.) *Targeted Radionuclide Tumor Therapy*,

Antibody Engineering

The prolonged retention of radiolabeled MAbs in circulation is a major concern as the delivery of doses sufficient to mediate an anti-tumor effect to the tumor can expose sensitive normal tissues, such as the bone marrow, to lethal levels of radiation. Additionally, tumor cells are relatively inaccessible to antibodies due to increased interstitial pressure in the tumor microenvironment resulting from a lack of draining lymphatics. Small, novel antibody-based molecules that are rapidly cleared from the circulation and do not interact with Fc receptors can be employed to address these issues (Table 5.1).

Reducing the size of antibody molecules to less than about (65 kDa) makes them susceptible to first pass renal elimination via the glomerulus, a three-layer filtration membrane (filtration barrier) in the kidneys [2]. In contrast, larger molecules with molecular weights of about 70 kDa or greater can not pass through the filtration barrier and remain in circulation. In order to identify an optimal antibody-based structure for RAIT, it is necessary to consider both the location of the target and the decay properties of the therapeutic nuclide that will be coupled to the antibody. A critical question is whether rapid elimination through the kidneys is desired or if prolonged circulation of the immunoconjugate is necessary for optimal therapeutic efficacy. Additionally, the conformation and electrical charge of an antibody fragment can impact on its glomerular permeability. Ellipsoid molecules filter more readily than round molecules and negatively charged molecules can be repulsed by the filtration barrier which also has a net negative charge [2].

For the purpose of simplicity, we have divided antibodies into two broad classes, intact antibodies and antibody fragments. The first class contains murine MAbs, chimeric MAbs that contain both murine and human domains, humanized MAbs that were converted through antibody engineering techniques into intact human immunoglobulins, and "natural" human MAbs produced from human hybridomas or from transgenic mice, which have human immunoglobulin genes in place of the mouse genes. In general, these molecules were developed to avoid the induction of

Table 5.1 Biological properties of antibody-based molecules

Antibody-based molecule	Size (kDa)	Valence	T 1/2 alpha	T 1/2 beta (h)	Reference
scFv	28	1	2.4–12 min	1.5–3.9	[44–46]
$scFv_2$	56	2	13 min	2.4	[47]
bs-scFv	56	2	–	–	[48]
Diabody	55	2	40 min	6.4	[15]
Flex minibody	80	2	35.2 min	5.3	[23]
LD minibody	80	2	72.6 min	4.8	[23]
$[sc(Fv)_2]_2$	120	4	2.1 h	–	[49]
$F(ab')_2$	100	2	0.4 h	6–12	[50]
Domain-deleted MAb: delta C_H2	130	2	1.7 h	7.8	[51]
IgG	150	2	0.7–2.6 h	50–113	[50]

human anti-mouse antibody, HAMA, responses in patients. This class of molecules is addressed at length in chapter 4 in this volume.

The second class contains classic antibody fragments that are produced by enzymatic cleavage and bioengineered antibody-based structures that are not found in nature. These molecules can be created by deleting domains (to change the size or the propensity to interact with receptors), altering structure, combining antigen-binding arms with different antigen specificities, or modifying charge to alter the in vivo distribution or clearance rate. While the intact antibodies in the first class have been effective in the RAIT of diffuse malignancies, their slow elimination and poor tumor penetration have spurred the development of the second class of molecules.

The basic structure of an intact IgG molecule and selected promising derivatives are presented in Fig. 5.1. All antibody-based engineered fragments contain a series of highly variable loops known as complementarity determining regions (CDRs). These contain the residues that form the contact with the target antigen and therefore define the antibody's specificity. Intact IgG molecules contain two antigen-binding domains, one on the end of each Fab (fragment antigen-binding) "arm". Each Fab "arm" has six CDRs, three on the variable light (V_L) chain and three on the variable heavy (V_H) chain.

Enzymatically produced antibody fragments (e.g., Fab, Fab' and F[ab']$_2$ molecules) maintain the function and orientation of the CDRs that were dictated by the

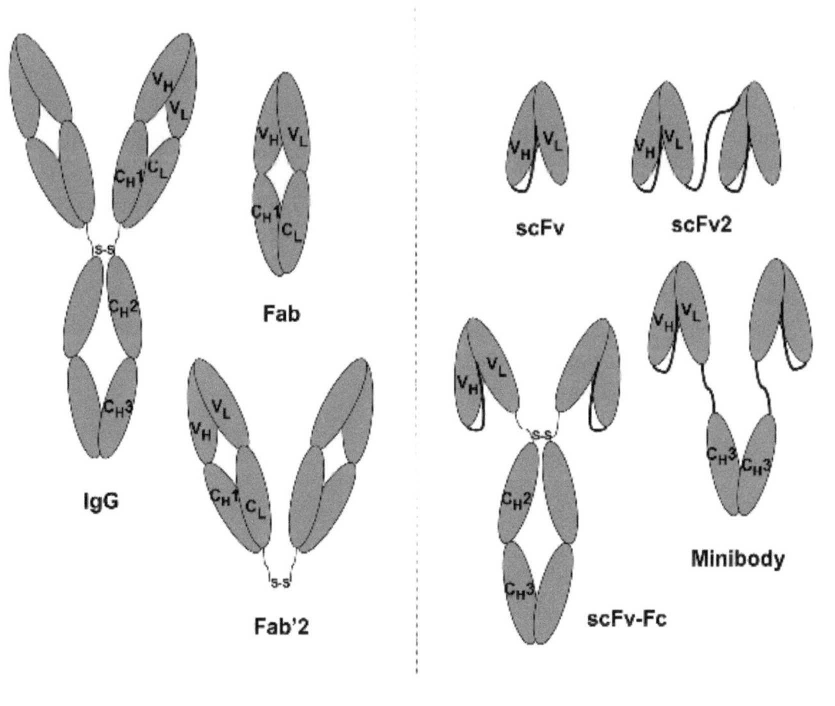

Fig. 5.1 Schematic diagram of the structures of antibody-based molecules. Engineered molecules are on the right side of the line

parent IgG molecule. In contrast, engineered fragments can suffer from a loss of affinity (antigen binding strength) or specificity if the orientation of the CDRs is changed. While there are six CDRs, most interactions with antigen actively involve only a few of them and the CDR3 of the light or heavy chain is typically considered to play the most dominant role. The remainder of the V_H and V_L regions exhibits greater sequence conservation and are known as the framework regions. The primary function of the framework regions is to support the CDR loops and to maintain the antibody structure. Modifications to the amino acid sequence can also effect affinity and specificity of the molecule and many affinity maturation techniques are based upon rational or random amino acid substitutions in the CDRs or the underlying framework regions [3, 4].

The heavy and light chains of an intact IgG molecule also contain constant, or highly conserved, regions. The light chain has only one constant region (C_L), while the heavy chain has three constant regions: C_H1, C_H2 and C_H3. The constant regions closest to the variable (C_H1 and C_L) maintain the orientation of the V_H and V_L domains and facilitate antibody/antigen interactions. The variable domains and the first constant domains of the light and heavy chains form the Fab region. In an IgG molecule C_H1 is connected to the Fc (fragment crystallisable, composed of the C_H2 and C_H3 regions) domain via a proline rich "hinge" region.

The hinge provides conformational flexibility for the two Fab domains, allowing the Ab to bind bivalently to cell surface antigens (each Fab arm is capable of binding to one target epitope of an antigen). The hinge region also allows independent mobility of the Fc region allowing the engagement of effector ligands, such as C1 component of complement or membrane bound Fc receptors. While engagement of effector mechanisms is not typically considered to play a major response in the therapeutic efficacy of RAIT, the Fc domain plays a critical role in the trafficking and the half-life of the IgG molecule.

When IgGs bind to FcRn (salvage receptor), they are protected (or salvaged) from lysosomal degradation, which is the major mechanism behind the regulation of serum IgG levels (reviewed in [5]). The FcRn-IgG interaction has been shown to take place at a highly conserved portion of the C_H2-C_H3 domain interface (reviewed in [5]). By reengineering this sequence on IgG, the affinity for FcRn can be altered, allowing one to tailor the serum half-life and transport of an antibody to be compatible with a variety of therapeutic radioisotopes.

Structures

In the section below we will briefly review the types of engineered antibody-based fragments in order of increasing size that are available for use as RAIT agents. Intact native, chimeric and humanized MAbs are reviewed in chapter 4 in this book.

Single-chain Fv. The basic building block of most engineered antibody fragments that are useful for RAIT is the single-chain Fv molecule (scFv). This 26–28 kDa binding protein is produced from the variable light and heavy chains of an antibody molecule, joined together by a peptide linker. Typically a 15 amino acid hydrophilic sequence is used [6], but the linker length can range from 10–25 amino acid residues depending on the desired flexibility. scFv molecules can be produced from genes isolated from hybridomas [7, 8], or can be selected (isolated) from a combinatorial scFv phage display library [9]. While single domain antibody fragments that consist of a single variable light or variable heavy domain have been successfully produced [10], these are considered to be too small for RAIT applications.

The scFv often can possesses the full binding affinity and specificity of each of its intact parent antibody's Fab arms. However, the utility of scFv molecules in RAIT and other applications, where avidity is important, is often limited by the short association between these monovalent molecules and their target antigens. While they are seldom used directly as vehicles for RAIT, scFv molecules are the most commonly used building blocks in the construction of a number of novel antibody-based molecules with therapeutic potential. These structures include dimers $(scFv)_2$, diabodies, bispecific (bs)-scFv, minibodies, tetramers and scFv-Fc fusion proteins (Fig. 5.1) that have higher molecular weight and increased functional affinity (avidity).

scFv$_2$. Dimeric versions of scFv molecules (e.g., scFv2) can be created using disulfide linkages by producing an scFv with a carboxy-terminal cysteine residue [11], or by engineering a single-gene construct encoding two scFv connected by a peptide spacer [12]. With two tandem scFv molecules, these dimers achieve greater binding avidity (increased functional affinity) and somewhat reduced rates of systemic elimination. Together, this often results in enhanced tumor retention, with similar or better in vivo tumor-targeting specificity than was achieved with the parent scFv molecule.

bsAb. Bispecific antibodies (bsAbs) are most commonly created from scFv molecules (bs-scFv) or Fab' fragments. bs-scFv are similar to the $scFv_2$ described above except that each scFv arm is specific for a different target. In RAIT applications, these molecules can be employed to increase tumor specificity by co-targeting two different tumor-associated antigens [13] or to serve in pretargeted radioimmunotherapy (PRIT) by targeting the tumor with one "arm" and a conjugated radioisotope with the other "arm" [14].

In the former application, the incorporation of two antigen binding domains (e.g., Fabs or scFvs), each with a low affinity for a tumor associated antigen, can result in a higher avidity interaction with tumor cell that expresses both antigens and lower affinity (monovalent binding) to normal tissues that only express one antigen. This could provide increased selectivity in tumor targeting, thereby reducing normal tissue toxicity resulting from RAIT applications.

In the latter application, a bispecific scFv (or Fab) with a high affinity arm that is specific for a tumor antigen is administered and allowed to localize in the tumor (pretarget). After allowing the unbound antibody to clear from the circulation, a conjugate of the therapeutic nuclide and the target ligand of the bsAb's second "arm" is administered and retention of this agent primarily occurs in tissues where the bsAb has previously localized.

Diabody. The diabody is a dimeric scFv that has been associated with promising preclinical RAIT studies. Diabodies are stable non-covalent scFv dimers produced by reducing the length of the intra-scFv peptide linkers to less than 8 amino acid residues. This prohibits the V_H and V_L domains of a single chain from associating with each other to form a functional scFv, as the V_H and V_L domains have a high affinity for each other. The most stable conformation is a non-covalent dimer in which the V_H and V_L domain from one scFv pairs with the V_H and V_L domain of a second scFv to form a functional structure with two binding pockets (Fig. 5.1) [15–17]. Diabodies have been found to be very effective as vehicles for the RAIT of human tumor xenografts growing in immunodeficient mice [18, 19]. Further reduction of the intra-scFv linker length to less than 3 amino acid residues leads to the formation of a non-covalent tripod-shaped trimer called a triabody [20–22].

Minibody. Minibodies are engineered divalent molecules that are produced through the genetic fusion of an scFv molecule and a C_H3 domain of a human IgG molecule [23]. In an intact antibody, noncovalent bonds between C_H3 domains serve to hold the two heavy chains in close proximity thereby stabilizing the structure of the antibody. The presence of the C_H3 domains in minibodies leads to the dimerization of two scFv-C_H3 fusion proteins to yield the (scFv-$C_H3)_2$ minibody structure. The lack of an intact Fc domain prevents minibodies from interacting with FcRn, thereby promoting an accelerated systemic clearance. However, based on their molecular weight alone, these molecules are large enough to exceed the renal threshold for first pass elimination yet are still small enough to exhibit better tumor penetration properties than intact MAbs [24]. They are therefore expected to be promising vehicles for RAIT.

ScFv-Fc. These molecules are very similar to the minibody discussed above, except that they incorporate an intact Fc domain instead of a single CH3 dimerization domain [25, 26]. The presence of an intact Fc domain allows scFv-Fc molecules to interact with FcRn, the Ig salvage receptor. This prolongs their residence in circulation, which facilitates effective conjugation to longer-lived RAIT nuclides. The functional Fc domain also allows scFv-Fc molecules to interact with the host immune system in eliciting antibody directed cellular cytotoxicity (ADCC), which is often believed to play a significant role in many antibody-based therapeutic regimens.

Domain-deleted MAbs. Another approach that has recently been used to produce antibody-based agents with in vivo properties that will be associated with efficacy of RAIT has been the selective deletion of unnecessary or unfavorable domains. For example, by deleting the C_H2 domain from an IgG molecule, the overall size of the molecule is diminished and the sequences on the MAb that are responsible for interaction with Fc receptors are eliminated [27]. This increases the systemic elimination rate and reduces the retention of the MAbs by immune effector cells and tissues of the reticuloendothelial system (liver and spleen). A delta C_H2 form of CC49, a humanized MAb specific for the TAG-72 pan carcinoma antigen, has been produced and has been recently been employed in a clinical trial (discussed elsewhere in this volume).

Fab fragments. Functional fragments of antibodies have been produced for many years through the use of proteolytic enzymes. Fab fragments, composed of a single binding arm of an Ig molecule are produced by digestion with papain which digests the Ig hinge region, yielding two Fab fragments and an intact Fc domain that can be removed by protein A chromatography. While Fab fragments have most commonly been produced by enzymatic digestion of IgG molecules, recombinant forms of these molecules can also be expressed in large bacteriophage libraries [28]. These molecules can be used in the construction of larger molecules, such as F(ab')$_2$ or even intact Ig molecules. Fab fragments are eliminated from the circulation very rapidly, rendering them more useful for imaging applications than for RAIT.

F(ab')$_2$ fragments. These divalent fragments are composed of two identical Fab' fragments connected by a disulfide linker. F(ab')$_2$ fragments are produced by proteolytic digestion with the enzyme pepsin. Pepsin digests the Ig molecule below the disulfide bonds that hold the heavy chains together, yielding a divalent F(ab')$_2$ fragment and numerous peptides derived from the Fc region. With a molecular weight 100 to 110kDa, F(ab')$_2$ fragments are more suitable to RAIT applications than monovalent Fab fragments. Furthermore, their divalent nature increases the avidity of their interactions with targeted cancer cells, thereby prolonging their retention in the tumor.

Isolation of Unique Antibody Clones

There are a number of methods that can be employed to isolate antibodies that specifically bind to a desired antigen. While the classic immunization strategies that have been employed for many years are still in use, they have more recently been used to generate a desired immune response in transgenic mice that are capable of producing fully-human antibodies [29]. These antibodies can then be manipulated by enzymatic or genetic means to generate the antibody-based structures described above.

In vitro selection methodologies have also been used to isolate desired antibody genes from large libraries. The most commonly used method utilizes large non-immune or immune phage display libraries that are composed of bacterophage or phagemid particles, each containing the gene encoding a unique scFv or Fab fragment and expressing that molecule on its surface as a fusion with a coat protein [30, 31]. Other methods for selection of antibody clones from combinatorial libraries include yeast display [32, 33], ribosome display [34] and E. coli display [35]. Yeast display is particularly useful for the isolation of antibody clones with altered affinity from libraries that were created by adding directed or spontaneous mutations to a clone with a desired specificity.

Functional Groups

The development of novel antibody-based structures for RAIT applications has been driven by the inherent properties of antibodies. While intact antibodies provide high-avidity binding to target cells, their large size (150kDa) impedes tumor penetration and leads to prolonged retention in blood and normal tissues. The rate of diffusion of intact IgG molecules into a solid tumor xenograft is to a large extent limited by hydrostatic pressure and the composition of the extracellular matrix and the penetration seems to be less than one mm in two days [36]. This can be a major limitation when antibodies are used to deliver nuclides as it increases the potential for damage to normal tissues.

Fusion proteins composed of biologically active agents and antibodies offer a unique method to alter the tumor penetration properties of antibodies. While a number of cytokines are capable of effecting the circulatory system, many fail to retain this ability when they are part of a functional fusion protein. For example, novel VEGF-scFv fusion protein exhibited decreased tumor targeting as compared with that observed with the parental scFv, instead of the expected increase [37]. In contrast, fusion proteins composed of antibody-based molecules and Interleukin-2 (IL-2) [38] or tumor necrosis factor alpha (TNFα) [39] have both led to significant improvements in tumor uptake.

With the IL-2 fusion proteins this effect is believed to be due in part to a vascular leak syndrome, VLS. However, as VLS, is associated with damage to vascular endothelial cells, extravasation of fluids, interstitial edema and organ failure, these effects can lead to significantly more difficulties in the clinic that are commonly associated with non-targeted toxicities stemming from RAIT. While efforts are being made to eliminate the sequences that trigger VLS, it is unclear if these modified fusion proteins will still be associated with increased tumor retention.

As noted above, antibody-based molecules with low molecular weights display the most promising tumor penetration properties and could therefore deliver therapeutic nuclides to a greater portion of the tumor than larger intact antibodies. However, engineered antibodies with molecular weights below the renal threshold for first pass elimination (approximately 65 kDa) are rapidly removed from the circulation by glomerular filtration [40]. This not only limits the therapeutic efficacy of these agents but can also result in significant renal toxicity when radiometals are employed. To address this, Tarburton et al modified the isoelectric point (pI) of antibody fragments with the intent of altering the degree of retention in the kidneys. Acetylation of Fab' fragments significantly reduced renal retention, but unfortunately also reduced their immunoreactivity by 50% [41]. With the same goal in mind, Pavlinkova et al. introduced negatively charged amino acids to the carboxy terminus of the V_H region of a scFv [42]. This resulted in the production of two scFvs with pIs of 5.8 and 5.2, both significantly lower than that of the parent scFv (pI = 8.1). Unfortunately, all three molecules exhibited the same renal retention and rates of clearance from the blood pool. The tumor uptake of all three forms of the scFv were also similar with a peak levels at 0.5 h: 5.59 percent injected dose per gram (%ID/g), 4.87%ID/g and 5.29%ID/g, for the scFvs with pIs of 5.2, 5.8 and 8.1, respectively. As charge-based repulsion was expected between the negatively charged glomerular cells and the negatively charged scFv constructs (pI 5.2 and 5.8), these results are difficult to explain. However, it is possible that charge modifications need to be considered across the whole molecule rather than on a specific region.

Another approach to alter the clearance properties of an engineered antibody fragment was attempted by Dennis et al. In this study, the authors attempted to promote prolonged retention in the circulation of a normally rapidly cleared Fab fragment by engineering in a sequence that would promote interactions with serum albumin [43]. They identified a series of peptides with the core sequence DICLPRWGCLW that specifically binds with a high affinity to serum albumin from multiple species. The addition of peptides based upon this sequence to Fab fragments mediated a 26-fold enhancement in the serum half-life in mice, exceeding the half-life of $F(ab')_2$ fragments that have molecular weights greater than the renal threshold for first pass elimination. It is hoped that small fragments with this sequence will exhibit prolonged serum retention while maintaining the ability to readily penetrate into solid tumors.

Conclusions

Genetic engineering of antibody fragments and intact antibodies has facilitated the creation of a variety of novel molecules with promising properties for RAIT. As we are now capable of varying the size, affinity and valence of such molecules, it is now possible to improve the pharmacokinetic and tumor targeting properties that will best pair with a selected nuclide and therapeutic indication.

References

1. Kohler, G. and Milstein, C. Continuous cultures of fused cells secreting antibody of predefined specificity. Nature, 256: 495–497, 1975.
2. Holechek, M. J. Glomerular filtration: an overview. Nephrol Nurs J, 30: 285–290; quiz 291–282, 2003.
3. Schier, R., Bye, J., Apell, G., McCall, A., Adams, G. P., Malmqvist, M., Weiner, L. M., and Marks, J. D. Isolation of high-affinity monomeric human anti-c-erbB-2 single chain Fv using affinity-driven selection. J Mol Biol, 255: 28–43, 1996.
4. Schier, R., McCall, A., Adams, G. P., Marshall, K. W., Merritt, H., Yim, M., Crawford, R. S., Weiner, L. M., Marks, C., and Marks, J. D. Isolation of picomolar affinity anti-c-erbB-2 single-chain Fv by molecular evolution of the complementarity determining regions in the center of the antibody binding site. J Mol Biol, 263: 551–567, 1996.
5. Ghetie, V. and Ward, E. S. Multiple roles for the major histocompatibility complex class I-related receptor FcRn. Annu Rev Immunol, 18: 739–766, 2000.
6. Kortt, A. A., Lah, M., Oddie, G. W., Gruen, C. L., Burns, J. E., Pearce, L. A., Atwell, J. L., McCoy, A. J., Howlett, G. J., Metzger, D. W., Webster, R. G., and Hudson, P. J. Single-chain Fv fragments of anti-neuraminidase antibody NC10 containing five- and ten-residue linkers form dimers and with zero-residue linker a trimer. Protein Eng, 10: 423–433, 1997.
7. Bird, R. E., Hardman, K. D., Jacobson, J. W., Johnson, S., Kaufman, B. M., Lee, S. M., Lee, T., Pope, S. H., Riordan, G. S., and Whitlow, M. Single-chain antigen-binding proteins. Science, 242: 423–426, 1988.

8. Huston, J. S., Levinson, D., Mudgett-Hunter, M., Tai, M. S., Novotny, J., Margolies, M. N., Ridge, R. J., Bruccoleri, R. E., Haber, E., Crea, R., et al. Protein engineering of antibody binding sites: recovery of specific activity in an anti-digoxin single-chain Fv analogue produced in Escherichia coli. Proc Natl Acad Sci USA, 85: 5879–5883, 1988.
9. Marks, J. D., Hoogenboom, H. R., Bonnert, T. P., McCafferty, J., Griffiths, A. D., and Winter, G. By-passing immunization. Human antibodies from V-gene libraries displayed on phage. J Mol Biol, 222: 581–597, 1991.
10. Ward, E. S., Gussow, D., Griffiths, A. D., Jones, P. T., and Winter, G. Binding activities of a repertoire of single immunoglobulin variable domains secreted from Escherichia coli. Nature, 341: 544–546, 1989.
11. Adams, G. P., McCartney, J. E., Tai, M. S., Oppermann, H., Huston, J. S., Stafford, W. F., 3rd, Bookman, M. A., Fand, I., Houston, L. L., and Weiner, L. M. Highly specific in vivo tumor targeting by monovalent and divalent forms of 741F8 anti-c-erbB-2 single-chain Fv. Cancer Res, 53: 4026–4034, 1993.
12. Beresford, G. W., Pavlinkova, G., Booth, B. J., Batra, S. K., and Colcher, D. Binding characteristics and tumor targeting of a covalently linked divalent CC49 single-chain antibody. Int J Cancer, 81: 911–917, 1999.
13. Robinson, M. K., Hodge, K., Sundberg, A. L., Russeva, M., Horak, E., Shaller, C., von Mehren, M., Simmons, H. H., Marks, J. D., and Adams, G. P. Targeting ErbB2 and ErbB3 with a bispecific-single chain Fv enhances targeting selectivity and induces a therapeutic effect in vitro. Br J Cancer Unpublished data, 2008.
14. Goldenberg, D. M., Chatal, J. F., Barbet, J., Boerman, O., and Sharkey, R. M. Cancer imaging and therapy with bispecific antibody pretargeting. Update Cancer Ther, 2: 19–31, 2007.
15. Adams, G. P., Schier, R., McCall, A. M., Crawford, R. S., Wolf, E. J., Weiner, L. M., and Marks, J. D. Prolonged in vivo tumour retention of a human diabody targeting the extracellular domain of human HER2/neu. Br J Cancer, 77: 1405–1412, 1998.
16. Holliger, P., Prospero, T., and Winter, G. 'Diabodies': small bivalent and bispecific antibody fragments. Proc Natl Acad Sci, 90: 6444–6448, 1993.
17. Yazaki, P. J., Wu, A. M., Tsai, S. W., Williams, L. E., Ikler, D. N., Wong, J. Y., Shively, J. E., and Raubitschek, A. A. Tumor targeting of radiometal labeled anti-CEA recombinant T84.66 diabody and t84.66 minibody: comparison to radioiodinated fragments. Bioconjug Chem, 12: 220–228, 2001.
18. Adams, G. P., Shaller, C. C., Dadachova, E., Simmons, H. H., Horak, E. M., Tesfaye, A., Klein-Szanto, A. J., Marks, J. D., Brechbiel, M. W., and Weiner, L. M. A single treatment of yttrium-90-labeled CHX-A"-C6.5 diabody inhibits the growth of established human tumor xenografts in immunodeficient mice. Cancer Res, 64: 6200–6206, 2004.
19. Robinson, M. K., Shaller, C., Garmestani, K., Plascjak, P. S., Hodge, K. M., Yuan, Q. A., Marks, J. D., Waldmann, T. A., Brechbiel, M. W., and Adams, G. P. Effective treatment of established human breast tumor xenografts in immunodeficient mice with a single dose of the alpha-emitting radioisotope astatine-211 conjugated to anti-HER2/neu diabodies. Clin Cancer Res, 14: 875–882, 2008.
20. Lawrence, L. J., Kortt, A. A., Iliades, P., Tulloch, P. A., and Hudson, P. J. Orientation of antigen binding sites in dimeric and trimeric single chain Fv antibody fragments. FEBS Lett, 425: 479–484, 1998.
21. Le Gall, F., Kipriyanov, S. M., Moldenhauer, G., and Little, M. Di-, tri- and tetrameric single chain Fv antibody fragments against human CD19: effect of valency on cell binding. FEBS Lett, 453: 164–168, 1999.
22. Pei, X. Y., Holliger, P., Murzin, A. G., and Williams, R. L. The 2.0-A resolution crystal structure of a trimeric antibody fragment with noncognate VH-VL domain pairs shows a rearrangement of VH CDR3. Proc Natl Acad Sci USA, 94: 9637–9642, 1997.
23. Hu, S., Shively, L., Raubitschek, A., Sherman, M., Williams, L. E., Wong, J. Y., Shively, J. E., and Wu, A. M. Minibody: A novel engineered anti-carcinoembryonic antigen antibody fragment (single-chain Fv-CH3) which exhibits rapid, high-level targeting of xenografts. Cancer Res, 56: 3055–3061, 1996.

24. Wu, A. M. and Yazaki, P. J. Designer genes: recombinant antibody fragments for biological imaging. Q J Nucl Med, 44: 268–283, 2000.
25. Kenanova, V., Olafsen, T., Williams, L. E., Ruel, N. H., Longmate, J., Yazaki, P. J., Shively, J. E., Colcher, D., Raubitschek, A. A., and Wu, A. M. Radioiodinated versus radiometal-labeled anti-carcinoembryonic antigen single-chain Fv-Fc antibody fragments: optimal pharmacokinetics for therapy. Cancer Res, 67: 718–726, 2007.
26. Powers, D. B., Amersdorfer, P., Poul, M., Nielsen, U. B., Shalaby, M. R., Adams, G. P., Weiner, L. M., and Marks, J. D. Expression of single-chain Fv-Fc fusions in Pichia pastoris. J Immunol Methods, 251: 123–135, 2001.
27. Mueller, B. M., Reisfeld, R. A., and Gillies, S. D. Serum half-life and tumor localization of a chimeric antibody deleted of the CH2 domain and directed against the disialoganglioside GD2. Proc Natl Acad Sci USA, 87: 5702–5705, 1990.
28. Lu, D., Shen, J., Vil, M. D., Zhang, H., Jimenez, X., Bohlen, P., Witte, L., and Zhu, Z. Tailoring in vitro selection for a picomolar-affinity human antibody directed against VEGF receptor 2 for enhanced neutralizing activity. J Biol Chem, 2003.
29. Green, L. L. Antibody engineering via genetic engineering of the mouse: XenoMouse strains are a vehicle for the facile generation of therapeutic human monoclonal antibodies. J Immunol Methods, 231: 11–23, 1999.
30. Clackson, T., Hoogenboom, H. R., Griffiths, A. D., and Winter, G. Making antibody fragments using phage display libraries. Nature, 352: 624–628, 1991.
31. Winter, G., Griffiths, A. D., Hawkins, R. E., and Hoogenboom, H. R. Making antibodies by phage display technology. Annu Rev Immunol, 12: 433–455, 1994.
32. Feldhaus, M. J. and Siegel, R. W. Yeast display of antibody fragments: a discovery and characterization platform. J Immunol Methods, 290: 69–80, 2004.
33. Swers, J. S., Kellogg, B. A., and Wittrup, K. D. Shuffled antibody libraries created by in vivo homologous recombination and yeast surface display. Nucleic Acids Res, 32: e36, 2004.
34. Hanes, J. and Pluckthun, A. In vitro selection and evolution of functional proteins by using ribosome display. Proc Natl Acad Sci USA, 94: 4937–4942, 1997.
35. Harvey, B. R., Georgiou, G., Hayhurst, A., Jeong, K. J., Iverson, B. L., and Rogers, G. K. Anchored periplasmic expression, a versatile technology for the isolation of high-affinity antibodies from Escherichia coli-expressed libraries. Proc Natl Acad Sci USA, 101: 9193–9198, 2004.
36. Davies Cde, L., Berk, D. A., Pluen, A., and Jain, R. K. Comparison of IgG diffusion and extracellular matrix composition in rhabdomyosarcomas grown in mice versus in vitro as spheroids reveals the role of host stromal cells. Br J Cancer, 86: 1639–1644, 2002.
37. Halin, C., Niesner, U., Villani, M. E., Zardi, L., and Neri, D. Tumor-targeting properties of antibody-vascular endothelial growth factor fusion proteins. Int J Cancer, 102: 109–116, 2002.
38. Carnemolla, B., Borsi, L., Balza, E., Castellani, P., Meazza, R., Berndt, A., Ferrini, S., Kosmehl, H., Neri, D., and Zardi, L. Enhancement of the antitumor properties of interleukin-2 by its targeted delivery to the tumor blood vessel extracellular matrix. Blood, 99: 1659–1665, 2002.
39. Halin, C., Gafner, V., Villani, M. E., Borsi, L., Berndt, A., Kosmehl, H., Zardi, L., and Neri, D. Synergistic therapeutic effects of a tumor targeting antibody fragment, fused to interleukin 12 and to tumor necrosis factor alpha. Cancer Res, 63: 3202–3210, 2003.
40. Wochner, R. D., Strober, W., and Waldmann, T. A. The role of the kidney in the catabolism of Bence Jones proteins and immunoglobulin fragments. J Exp Med, 126: 207–221, 1967.
41. Tarburton, J. P., Halpern, S. E., Hagan, P. L., Sudora, E., Chen, A., Fridman, D. M., and Pfaff, A. E. Effect of acetylation on monoclonal antibody ZCE-025 Fab': distribution in normal and tumor-bearing mice. J Biol Response Mod, 9: 221–230, 1990.
42. Pavlinkova, G., Beresford, G., Booth, B. J., Batra, S. K., and Colcher, D. Charge-modified single chain antibody constructs of monoclonal antibody CC49: generation, characterization, pharmacokinetics, and biodistribution analysis. Nucl Med Biol, 26: 27–34, 1999.
43. Dennis, M. S., Zhang, M., Meng, Y. G., Kadkhodayan, M., Kirchhofer, D., Combs, D., and Damico, L. A. Albumin binding as a general strategy for improving the pharmacokinetics of proteins. J Biol Chem, 277: 35035–35043, 2002.

44. Huston, J. S., George, A. J., Adams, G. P., Stafford, W. F., Jamar, F., Tai, M. S., McCartney, J. E., Oppermann, H., Heelan, B. T., Peters, A. M., Houston, L. L., Bookman, M. A., Wolf, E. J., and Weiner, L. M. Single-chain Fv radioimmunotargeting. Q J Nucl Med, 40: 320–333, 1996.
45. Kang, N., Hamilton, S., Odili, J., Wilson, G., and Kupsch, J. In vivo targeting of malignant melanoma by 125Iodine- and 99mTechnetium-labeled single-chain Fv fragments against high molecular weight melanoma-associated antigen. Clin Cancer Res, 6: 4921–4931, 2000.
46. Fang, J., Jin, H. B., and Song, J. D. Construction, expression and tumor targeting of a single-chain Fv against human colorectal carcinoma. World J Gastroenterol, 9: 726–730, 2003.
47. Weiner, L. M., Houston, L. L., Houston, J. C., McCartney, J. E., Tai, M. S., Apell, G., Stafford, W. F., Bookman, M. A., Gallo, J., and Adams, G. P. Improving the tumor-selectve delivery of single-chain Fv molecules. Tumor Targeting: 51–60, 1995.
48. Adams, G. P., Tai, M. S., McCartney, J. E., Marks, J. D., Stafford, W. F., 3rd, Houston, L. L., Huston, J. S., and Weiner, L. M. Avidity-mediated enhancement of in vivo tumor targeting by single-chain Fv dimers. Clin Cancer Res, 12: 1599–1605, 2006.
49. Goel, A., Colcher, D., Baranowska-Kortylewicz, J., Augustine, S., Booth, B. J., Pavlinkova, G., and Batra, S. K. Genetically engineered tetravalent single-chain Fv of the pancarcinoma monoclonal antibody CC49: improved biodistribution and potential for therapeutic application. Cancer Res, 60: 6964–6971, 2000.
50. Milenic, D. E., Yokota, T., Filpula, D. R., Finkelman, M. A., Dodd, S. W., Wood, J. F., Whitlow, M., Snoy, P., and Schlom, J. Construction, binding properties, metabolism, and tumor targeting of a single-chain Fv derived from the pancarcinoma monoclonal antibody CC49. Cancer Res, 51: 6363–6371, 1991.
51. Slavin-Chiorini, D. C., Horan Hand, P. H., Kashmiri, S. V., Calvo, B., Zaremba, S., and Schlom, J. Biologic properties of a CH2 domain-deleted recombinant immunoglobulin. Int J Cancer, 53: 97–103, 1993.

Chapter 6
Novel Alternative Scaffolds and Their Potential Use for Tumor Targeted Radionuclide Therapy

Fredrik Y. Frejd[1,2]

Summary The class of macromolecules referred to as "Alternative Scaffolds" is reviewed in this chapter. A general introduction to alternative scaffolds is presented, and groups of alternative scaffolds are described according to structural folds. The properties of these biomolecules as molecular recognition tools are presented, scaffolds of special interest for targeted radionuclide therapy are highlighted and tumor targeting data is discussed.

Introduction

In the aftermath of sequencing the human genome, our society is beginning to harvest the fruits of the many genomic and proteomic efforts undertaken the last decades. Our increasing knowledge in the rich interplay between gene-expression and protein abundance in malignant cells has deepened our understanding of the complexity of cancer. Introduction of new medical disciplines like molecular and medical imaging, targeted therapy and personalized medicine has evolved from this. In this context, specific imaging of protein structures in the body, e.g. receptors overexpressed on cancer cells, provides an instrumental opportunity to tap some of the information available about the disease process in a single patient. The information can also be used for monitoring patient response to targeted therapy.

Traditional cytotoxic cancer therapies often cause significant toxicity also to normal cells, and this may hamper the treatment efficacy as it limits the total therapeutic dose that can be administered. Other options like surgery and external beam radiation may be efficient when treating localized and accessible tumors, but do not suffice for disseminated disease. However, by targeting a cell-killing agent like a radionuclide to tumor associated structures, using a molecular recognition vehicle

[1]Unit of Biomedical Radiation Sciences, Department of Oncology, Radiology and Clinical Immunology, Rudbeck Laboratory, Uppsala University, SE-751 85, Uppsala, Sweden

[2]Affibody AB, Voltavägen 13, Box 20137, SE-161 02 Bromma, Sweden

T. Stigbrand et al. (eds.) *Targeted Radionuclide Tumor Therapy*,

as carrier, it is possible to combine the therapeutic efficacy of radiation with the opportunity of systemic treatment, as the targeting would increase the concentration of the cytotoxic agent in the tumors while reducing its levels in normal tissues. Clinically, there is a growing appreciation of the potential of targeted imaging and therapy using different vehicles, but the tools of today are not always optimal. There is a need to increase the traditional molecular toolbox with new suitable carriers. Such new carriers should be able to specifically recognize malignant lesions and to deliver diagnostic or therapeutic payloads even to very small metastases. The various kinds of radioactive nuclides that can be utilized are described in depth later in this book (chapter 7). This chapter will focus on new molecular carriers that can serve as affinity recognition tools in targeted radionuclide tumor therapy with special focus on a class denoted "alternative scaffolds", i.e. molecular recognition tools that are based on an underlying robust scaffold with desirable properties, but which are not antibodies or fragments thereof.

Background

Criterias for Molecular Recognition Tools

When using affinity structures for targeted delivery of radionuclides, it is important to find a molecule with a 3D-shape that will fit specifically onto a patch on the target antigen, for example an oncogene product. The targeting structure should display comparatively high binding strength (affinity) in order to recognize structures less abundant *in vivo*. It should not bind to any other protein except the intended target protein in order to be able to specifically localize to the relevant pathologic structure and avoid normal tissue [1, 2]. The structure should not be too immunogenic, as this could limit repeated administrations, even if one should keep in mind that the protein doses used for targeted radionuclide therapy generally are very low and that the number of administrations are low compared to chronic treatment. Furthermore the structure should be heat stable, resist various harsh chemical environments as such conditions often are required for labeling procedures

In addition, for ***medical imaging*** applications, the affinity structure should quickly find its target in the patient whereas unbound molecules should be rapidly excreted, thus facilitating high contrast tumor imaging and reducing the time between injection and examination. This is typically a feature of comparatively small molecules [3–5].

In contrast, for ***targeted therapeutic*** applications, the total dose to the tumor should be high compared to normal tissues, and this may require longer circulations times to allow the vehicle to find the tumor. Longer circulation times may also reduce the total need of administered radioactivity. Too long circulation time however causes radiation exposure of normal organs and tissues, especially bone marrow. Thus, for targeted radiotherapy, the possibility to tailor the plasma half life is of importance [6].

Antibodies

Antibodies are commonly used tools for molecular recognition of different targets. More than 23 monoclonal antibodies have been approved by the FDA and many more are in clinical development. A vast number of antibodies are used in basic research and for *in vitro* diagnostic applications. Furthermore, a large number of antibodies are in clinical and pre-clinical testing for targeting various nuclides to tumors, including two approved by the FDA for treatment of non-Hodgkin's lymphoma: Tositumomab (Bexxar) and Ibritumomab tiuxetan (Zevalin) [7]. See also chapter 4.

A key step to reach this success level was the development of the hybridoma monoclonal technology by Kohler and Milstein [8]. The first antibodies, of murine origin, evoke an immune response in the patients, limiting their potential. Later however, techniques for humanization of murine parental antibodies, or isolation of human monoclonal antibodies from mice transgenic for the human IgGs, presented a solution to the immunogenicity problem. A large number of such antibodies are now in clinical trials for various indications. In general however, full size antibodies may not be the best molecules for *in vivo* delivery of radionuclides to tumors. The clinical use of antibodies for molecular imaging and radioimmunotherapy is still limited by intrinsic properties like insufficient tumor penetration, inadequate therapeutic doses delivered to tumors, transport to, or targeting of, normal organs, and occurrence of unwanted side-effects e.g. interaction via the Fc-receptor or induction of receptor signaling due to the bivalent nature of a native antibody.

Antibodies display very long circulation half-lives in plasma (typically days to weeks) with slow blood compartment clearance, which obscures the contrast for imaging and induces negative side-effects. Interestingly, the two antibodies approved for radioimmunotherapy by the FDA are both of murine origin, and are comparatively rapidly cleared from blood, thereby reducing bone marrow toxicity.

Fragments of Antibodies

By use of recombinant and proteolytic methods, antibodies can be reshaped, maintaining the molecular recognition function within a smaller size (reviewed in [9]). A range of different antibody fragment formats are now in use (see chapter 5), and many of the intrinsic drawbacks of full size monoclonal antibodies may be avoided. Small engineered fragments like scFv's (size 27 kDa) or their dimers (diabodies, size 54 kDa) are rapidly cleared via the kidneys and seem suitable for imaging applications [10, 11], whereas larger fragments like minibodies or small immunoproteins (size ca 80 kDa) have intermediate clearance rates, reach higher tumor uptakes, and are thus better suited therapeutically [12, 13]. In addition, by including the neonatal Fc receptor (FcRn) binding site in the minibodies, and by introducing mutants of this binding site with different affinities for the receptor, modulation of the clearance rate of such antibody fragments is possible [14]. This makes this class of molecules very attractive for therapeutic applications and warrants further investigations.

The basic properties of the antibody structure are however retained, and even the smallest fragment, the scFv, contains two polypeptide chains, linked via a peptide linker, and two disulphide bridges. The yield of such constructs, when produced in E. coli is not very high and the problem of chemical modifications (labeling) to homogeneity still exists, i.e. it is difficult to perform site specific modifications using maleimide chemistry due to the intrinsic disulphide bond. The stability is comparatively poor, which may make certain labeling procedures difficult. In addition, considering that tissue penetration, tumor targeting and body clearance will increase with decreasing size, it would be attractive to consider even smaller recognition structures for tumor targeting. Recently, a new class of antibody derivatives consisting of only the Fv portion and only half the size (11–15 kDa) of the scFv's has been described. As these do not any longer retain the antigen binding capacity of a traditional monoclonal antibody, and since they share a lot of the characteristics of alternative scaffold proteins, they are described later in this chapter.

Peptides

Another approach has been to use linear or cyclic peptides. As described in chapter 7, regulatory peptide receptors are often overexpressed in certain human cancers and radiolabeled derivatives of their natural ligands can be used for tumor targeting. The most advanced peptide targeting system is based on somatostatin analogues [15], with the ligand Octreoscan® approved for diagnosis of neuroendocrine tumors, and many other somatostatin derivatives have been tested, including some for peptide receptor radiation therapy (PRRT) in humans [16]. Peptides have many advantages as they can be synthesized chemically, allowing well controlled site-specific incorporation of chelating groups, and they have very small size, allowing rapid kinetics and very good tissue penetration. In addition, they can generally withstand harsh chemical conditions during labeling and are comparatively easy to manufacture under GMP-conditions. A drawback with peptide derivatives of natural ligands is that they are limited to cases where a natural ligand exists. There are for example many structures that are good tumor targets but not receptors, for which there are no ligands, e.g. adhesion molecules like EpCAM and CEA, or extracellular matrix proteins like the extra domain B of fibronectin (ED-B) or domain C of tenascin. Other important targets are receptors with no known ligands, for example the human epidermal growth factor receptor 2 (HER2). While peptides thus seem to be very promising, a clear need to find new peptides that can bind to different kinds of protein targets exist.

In spite of substantial efforts, there are not many examples of new high affinity, monomeric peptide ligands that have been selected to bind interesting tumor targets and the binding efficacy and specificity of such novel peptides is seldom comparable to larger affinity proteins, like antibodies and their fragments. In most cases, the peptides that have been isolated often bind proteins containing a receptor cleft or a groove into which they can fit, and it seems more problematic to find peptides binding to globular proteins without such features. To improve the binding affinity, multimerisation strategies are often employed, which makes the molecules larger and more complex. In addition, peptides may need modifications to remain stable in plasma, and due to their small size, different labeling methods may have a substantial impact on the *in vivo* distribution and clearance of the peptide.

One attempt to combine the advantages of antibody recognition and the favorable kinetics of peptides, is to apply different pretargeting strategies. Pretargeting of e.g. bispecific antibodies followed by administration of radiolabeled small peptides have presented high tumor signal intensity, improved tumor-to-blood (T/B) ratio, and contrast [17]. However, since pretargeting is a multistep process, the practical clinical use may be hampered by the prolonged treatment regimes required before injection of the radiolabeled second step reagent.

Introduction to Alternative Scaffolds

Taking established classes of affinity ligands together it can be concluded that antibodies, antibody fragments and peptides indeed constitute useful radiopharmaceutical reagents. There are a number of such molecules tested and even approved in the clinic and there are new candidates in the drug development pipeline. However, these are not always optimal for all applications and they display limitations in radionuclide based applications. These affinity ligands, especially antibodies, have been used for some time for other purposes than radioimmunotargeting. Since external beam radiation clearly has demonstrated the benefits of using radiation as cancer treatment, it is striking that there are still comparatively few clinical examples of targeted radioimmunotherapy.

The remaining part of this chapter is dedicated to investigate alternative scaffolds as an alternative class of binding structures that may complement the established classes of binding molecules as tumor targeting agents for radionuclide based diagnosis and therapy.

During the last decade, this new class of recognition units has boomed, and from engineering point of view the many different alternatives have been subjected to a number of reviews [18–23], see also Table 6.1. Usually, alternative scaffolds are much smaller than antibodies but larger than peptides, with potential properties to display high affinity binding suitable for radionuclide targeting. It is however an extremely diverse class of binding molecules with only one common denominator: they are all discovered and engineered as binding tools based on molecular scaffolds with advantageous biochemical, biophysical, biological and commercial properties.

The goal of strategies using affinity structures for targeting is to identify a molecule with a 3D-shape that will fit onto a patch on the target antigen, for example an

Table 6.1 Selected examples of protein scaffolds with potential for tumor targeting

Scaffold	Acronym	Randomization size	Example of target proteins	Tumor targeting data	Company reference
Human Fv fragments	Domain antibody dAb	Different loops 12–15 kDa	TNF-alpha, albumin, CD40L	No	GSK/Domantis [36]
Camel Fv fragments	Nanobody cAb	Different loops ca 15 kDa	CEA, TNF-alpha, albumin	Yes	Ablynx [35]
^{10}Fn3 Fibronectin	Adnectin	Different loops, 21/94 aa	VEGFR, TNF-alpha, integrin	No	Adnexus [43]
CTLA-4	Evibody	6–9/136 aa	Integrin	No	Evogenix [46]
Apolipoprotein D	Anticalin	Four loops 24/178 aa	CTLA-4 VEGF	No	Pieris Proteolab [108]
T-cell receptor	mTCR	Different loops /250 aa	Peptide/MHC complexes	No	Medigene/Avidex [47]
Protein A domain	Affibody molecule	13/58 aa	HER2, EGFR, CD33, TNF-alpha, albumin	Yes	Affibody [57]
Ankyrin repeats	DARPin	7–21 for 1–3 repeats/100–166 (size is 67 + n·33)	HER2, AcrB, caspase-2	Yes	Molecular partners [68]
Ldl receptor domain A	Avimer	Up to 28/40 aa per domain, normally two to three domains (80–120 aa)	Il-6, cMet, CD28	No	Avidia [66]
Min-23	Microbody/Knottin	10/23 aa	Mabs, HIV-1 Nef, AMA-1	No	[77]
Fyn Src homology domain 3	Fynomer	12/63 aa	Extra domain B of fibronectin, albumin	Yes	Covagen [89]

oncogene product, specific for or upregulated in the tumor. Alternative scaffolds generally consist of a selected protein structure/scaffold with suitable basic properties onto which topographic variation has been built in. It is very important that the protein structure is stable enough to tolerate introduction of a vast array of specific solvent exposed amino acid positions, subjected to recombinant engineering methods. Small size is often desired, in part to facilitate production but also to increase the engineering freedom of making multimeric constructs, bispecific constructs or tailoring plasma half life by *increasing* the apparent size. Often claimed to combine the advantages of antibodies and peptides, the list of desirable basic properties can be made very long, but the most frequently mentioned properties are:

- Cheap production at high yields, preferably in *Escherichia coli*
- Highly soluble protein
- No or few intrinsic disulphide bonds, facilitating site directed chemical modification by introduction of a single cystein and maintaining stability in reducing environment.
- Low or no immunogenicity, allowing repeated administration
- Small size
- Genetic manipulation of fusion constructs possible if bispecificity or bivalency or additional effector functions would be desirable
- Favorable IP-situation which is mandatory for the technology if translated into the clinic and to patients as a marketed product

Some different basic protein structure variations that have been used to create alternative scaffolds will be described (see Fig. 6.1).

Regardless of which class of molecules to use, a molecule with a certain set of binding characteristics has to be found. Strategies need to be designed on how to find suitable binders. Using various molecular methods, a vast repertoire – a library – of individual molecules is created with each member slightly different from the other [24].

A protein library, per definition, contains up to billions of molecules consisting of the underlying constant scaffold and randomized variable regions that differ from each other. Typically, the library is mixed with an immobilized antigen in a selection process, schematically depicted in Fig. 6.2. By washing away unbound affinity molecules, only the ones with binding properties remain on the immobilized antigen and can be collected. If a very specific binding is desired, and there may be similar variants of the target, it is possible to add a subtraction step in the selection procedure, removing the molecules binding both to the unwanted target and the desired one. Following target encounter, washing and collecting, it is a challenge to characterize the isolated molecules. The trick is to couple the information of how they are built to each of the library members when creating the library. This is made by physically linking the 3D-structure, the phenotype, with the information of the design, the genotype, to each of the library members before the selections. To date, the strategy has been to link the gene encoding the molecule to the expressed affinity protein.

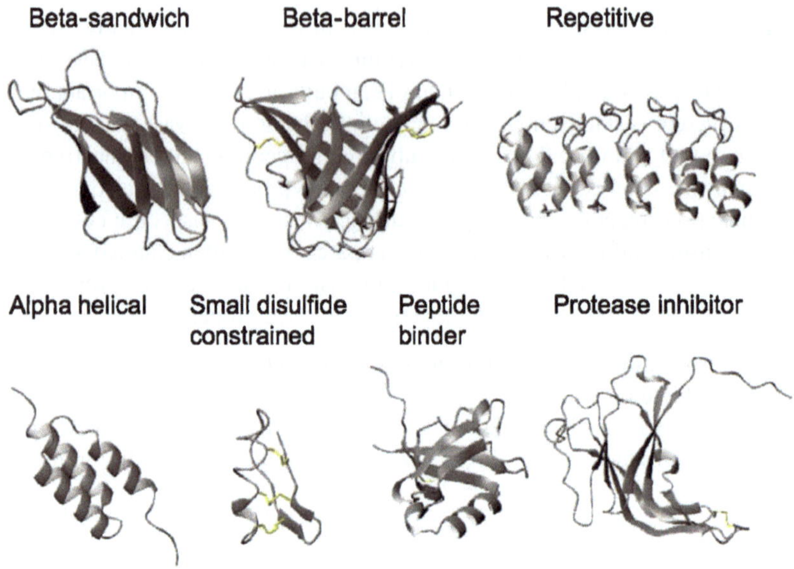

Fig. 6.1 Examples of different protein structures used as scaffolds. Typical representatives of each group are depicted. Beta-sandwich (fibronectin); beta-barrel (lipocalin); three-helix bundle (affibody molecule); repetitive proteins (ankyrin repeat protein); peptide binders (PDZ domain); protease inhibitors (ecotin); and disulfide-bonded scaffolds (scorpion toxin) (The figure was adapted with modification from [20]. With permission from Elsevier)

There are a number of strategies to link genotype and phenotype for selections. The standard has been a method called phage display, in which the gene of the scaffold protein is integrated in the phage genome in such a way that the corresponding gene product, the scaffold protein library member, appears fused to a surface coat protein on the bacterial virus (phage) [25]. While phage display is still very much in use, a number of other approaches are applied today, such as ribosome display (reviewed in [26]), yeast display [27] bacterial display [28, 29], various oil emulsions for compartmentalization [30], microbead selections [31] and many more (reviewed in [24]).

Basic Types of Scaffolds

It is possible to classify alternative scaffold proteins by many different properties like size, method of production, species of origin (there are scaffolds from species like llama, shark, man, camel, butterfly and bacteria), protein fold/structure or biological function. I have chosen to classify according to structure, because the underlying protein fold, the "scaffold" structure, may transfer biological properties also

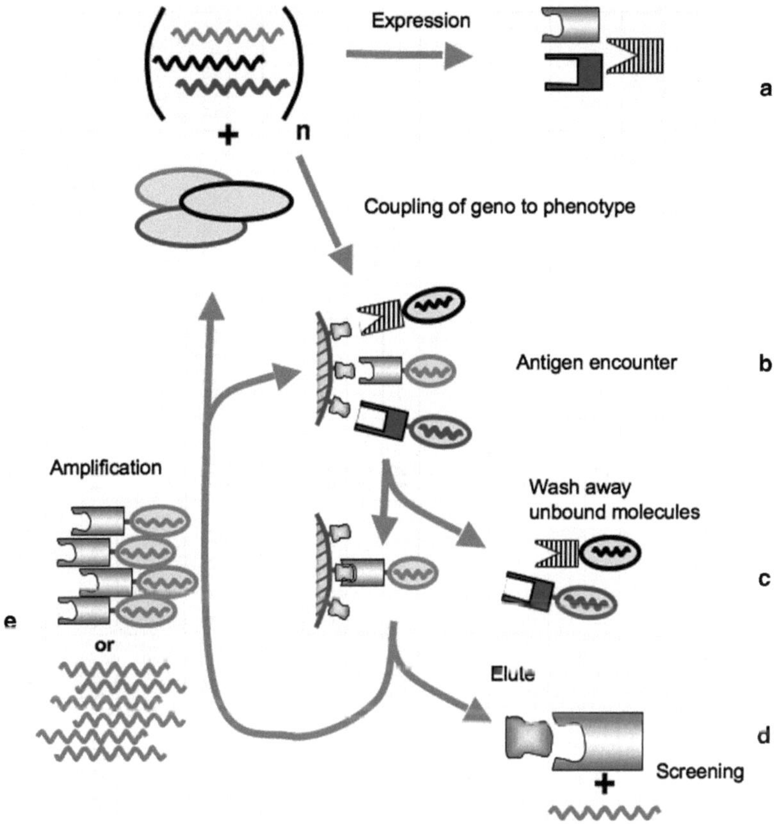

Fig. 6.2 Schematic drawing of a typical selection scheme. (**A**) Library diversity is created from synthetic genes or shuffling procedures. The size typically ranges from 10^8 to 10^{15} members. Each gene can be expressed as a specific protein. Next, the genes of the library are attached into/onto a molecular carrier, host particle, which can be fused or coupled to the gene product after translation of the gene to a protein. As a result, each host particle displays (expresses) a unique binding protein on its surface. (**B**) The library encounters an immobilized antigen. (**C**) Only the particles that display a binding protein can recognize the antigen with sufficient affinity at the conditions at which the selection takes place and remain in place, while the other molecules are washed away. (**D**) The molecules that bind are eluted, the gene is recovered and translated to protein and subjected to screening procedures. (**E**) Binders with desirable properties can be enriched by repeating the selection process after amplifying the eluted binders or genes

to the derived new binders. Focus has been on scaffolds for which *in vivo* data are available, especially if there is tumor targeting data, examples which are summarized in Table 6.2.

Alternative scaffold proteins may be divided into structures with beta-sandwich/barrel fold with randomized loops, often structural antibody mimetics or even antibody-derived, or into non-antibody like scaffolds. The non-antibody like scaffolds are very diverse, but can be subgrouped into alpha helical proteins, repetitive protein

Table 6.2 Selected scaffolds for which tumor targeting data are available. A reference means that the activity has occurred (e.g. imaging) – marks no reported activity. As many scaffolds have been tested at different time intervals, time and data are shown separately for each study in the table

Scaffold	Specificity	Size (kDa)	Affinity (K_D)	Biodistribution mice/nuclide	Biodistribution Hours post inj. T/B ratio			Biodistribution Hours p.i. Tumor uptake %ID/g			Imaging/ nuclide	Radio-immuno-therapy/ nuclide
Nanobody monomer	Lysozyme[a]	15	2 nM	Cortez-Retamozo et al. 2002 ^{125}I [39]	**2 h**	**8 h**		**2 h**	**8 h**		–	–
					3.7	15.1		2.7	0.4			
Nanobody monomer	Lysozyme[a]	15	65 nM	Cortez-Retamozo et al. 2002 ^{125}I [39]	3.2	10.4		2.7	0.3		–	–
Nanobody dimer	Lysozyme[a]	33	11 nM	Cortez-Retamozo et al. 2002 ^{125}I [39]	2.6	8.6		2.2	0.3		–	–
Nanobody	EGFR	15	5 nM (IC_{50})	Huang et al. 2008 ^{99m}Tc [40]	**3 h**			**3 h**			Huang et al. 2008 ^{99m}Tc [40]	
					7.4[b]			5.2				
Nanobody-beta-lactamase fusion	CEA	54	0.34 nM	Cortez-Retamozo et al. 2004 ^{125}I [38]	**6 h**	**24 h**	**48 h**	**6 h**	**24 h**	**48 h**	–	–
					2[d]	10[d]	10[d]	2.8[d]	1.0[d]	1.0[d]		
Affibody dimer-ABD fused molecule	HER2	17 kDa, with albumin ca 82 kDa	n.d.	Tolmachev et al. 2007 ^{177}Lu [6]	**24 h**	**48 h**	**72 h**	**24 h**	**48 h**	**72 h**	Tolmachev et al. 2007 ^{177}Lu [6]	Tolmachev et al. 2007 ^{177}Lu [6]
					2.0	4.7	6	19	26	21		
Affibody molecule	HER2	7	22 pM	Orlova et al. 2006 ^{125}I [58]	**1 h**	**4 h**	**24 h**	**1 h**	**4 h**	**24 h**	Orlova et al. 2006 ^{125}I [58]	–
					2	38	103	8.2	9.5	4.1		
Affibody molecule	HER2	7	22 pM	Tolmachev et al. 2006 ^{111}In [60]	**1 h**	**4 h**	**24 h**	**1 h**	**4 h**	**24 h**	Tolmachev et al. 2006 ^{111}In [60]	
					5.7	100	215	12	12	8.6		

Synthetic Affibody Molecule	HER2	7	200 pM	Engfeldt et al. 2007 [61, 62] ^{99m}Tc	**2 h**	**4 h**	**6 h**	**2 h**	**4 h**	**6 h**	Engfeldt et al. 2007a, b ^{99m}Tc [61, 62]	–
					12.5	23.8	39.3	7	7	7		
Synthetic Affibody molecule	HER2	7	65 pM	Orlova et al. 2007 ^{111}In [63]	**1 h**	**4 h**	**24 h**	**1 h**	**4 h**	**24 h**	*Clinical*: Feldwish et al. 2007 ^{111}In, ^{68}Ga [64]	
					8	12	47	23	13	15		
Affibody molecule	EGFR	7	25 nM	Nordberg et al. 2006 ^{125}I [109]	**4 h**	**8 h**		**4 h**	**8 h**		Nordberg et al. 2006 ^{125}I [109]	–
					9.1	–		3.8	2.0			
Affibody molecule	EGFR	7	5 nM	Friedman et al. 2008 ^{111}In [110]	**4 h**	**24 h**		**4 h**	**24 h**			
					5.5[d]							
DARPin[c]	HER2	10	90 pM	Stumpp 2006 ^{99m}Tc [73]	**1 h**	**4 h**	**24 h**	**1 h**	**4 h**	**24 h**	Stumpp 2006 ^{99m}Tc [73]	–
					~8[d]	~22[d]	–	8.5[d]	11[d]	8[d]		
Fynomer monomer	ED-B	8	85 nM	Grabulovski et al. 2007 ^{125}I [89]	**4 h**		**24 h**	**4 h**	**24 h**		–	–
					1.1		5.8	5.6	0.7			
Fynomer dimer	ED-B	15	4.5 nM apparent	Grabulovski et al. 2007 ^{125}I [89]	1.0		8.7	3.4	2.6		–	–

[a]The tumour cell line was transfected with and expressed lysozyme.
[b]Tumor to Background ratio.
[c]The DARPin data are so far only presented at conferences.
[d]Numerical values are estimated from graphs.

structures, small disulphide-constrained scaffolds, and others, with specialized functions like protease inhibition, peptide binding or exerting their function as enzymes useful for signaling upon binding. Finally, there are binding molecules addressing the same problems as alternative scaffolds, but not included in the group because they are not being based on an underlying stable scaffold structure. One exception is aptamers, that will be included in this chapter as there are some pre-clinical reports on imaging using these molecules.

Antibody Derivatives

Antibody fragments that resemble alternative scaffold proteins and alternative scaffold proteins that are mimicking antibody fragments do exist. In an attempt to profit from the advantageous properties of antibodies, but trying to reduce size and enhance engineering possibilities further, researchers have taken advantage of the modular construction of the recognition units of antibodies and isolated specifically one of the two molecular recognition units making up the binding pocket of an antibody. This occurs naturally in certain species e.g. camelids [32] and sharks [33, 34], in which both normal antibodies and antibodies with only the heavy variable chain is present, the smallest antigen recognizing unit being called a V_{HH} fragment. This was pioneered for camel antibodies but some other species were identified to express natural single domain antibodies as well and also these have been exploited to create repertoires of protein binders. Most advanced is the technology based on camel antibodies originally discovered by professor Hamers and co-workers [32]. There are several examples of the use of camel antibodies including imaging of inflammation and blocking of TNF-alpha effects in transgenic mice [35], a phase I trial for acute thrombosis (www.ablynx.com) and tumor targeting applications, see below.

Another approach was initiated by researchers at MRC, Cambridge, where they developed the use of fragments of normal human single chain Fv-fragments, separating the heavy and light chains and screening for fragments that were soluble, stable and bound to the desired antigen [36]. Solubility and stability issues were thought to hamper the development of such human ligands, but the researchers at the company Domantis (now GSK) have proven that these domain antibodies can act as TNF-alpha blockers. These binders should also be able to target tumors *in vivo* but no published data are presently available.

Camel V_{HH} domains: Nanobodies. Camels synthesize naturally occurring heavy-chain antibodies devoid of light chain and the CH1 domain. This observation enabled the generation of functional single-domain antibody fragments binding to a variety of antigens. By simply immunizing e.g. llamas or dromedars and either conventionally screen hybridomas or collect their antibody gene repertoire, and subject the repertoire to phage display and panning procedures, high affinity, stable monomeric 15 kDa size binders have been isolated to several antigens (for review see [37]).

Fusion constructs have been made with an anti-CEA VHH-domain and the enzyme beta-lactamase for targeted enzyme prodrug therapy with cures of established xenografts [38] and targeting of radionuclides to tumors have been reported. In a first tumor targeting study, the impact of affinity and valency was investigated in an artificial tumor model overexpressing the enzyme lysozyme [39]. Two different radioiodinated camel antibody fragments (cAb) of monomeric K_D of 2 or 65 nM, and a dimeric version (33 kDa) of the 65 nM variant were tested both in mice bearing subcutaneous tumors, as well as a pulmonary metastases model.

There were small differences between the low affinity monomeric or dimeric variants in uptake of radioactivity in the solid tumors at 2 h (2.69 versus 2.15%ID/g respectively), but the tumor to blood contrast (T/B), was higher for the monomeric construct (tumor to blood ratio of 3.22 as compared to 2.64 for the dimer), suggesting that small size is of advantage for high contrast imaging. Interestingly, the high affinity variant had an almost identical tumor uptake as the low affinity one (2.65% ID/g), but better T/B ratio (3.70). Eight hours following injection, the tumor uptake and T/B contrast was highest for the high affinity monomer (0.41%ID/g and T/B 15.05) whereas the low affinity monomer and dimer had almost identical tumor uptake (0.30 and 0.29%ID/g respectively), though the blood contrast remained better for the monomeric construct. At all time points, the kidney values were much higher than the tumor values, as could be expected from small, kidney cleared proteins.

In a later prodrug therapy publication, CEA-expressing LS174T xenografts were targeted in a biodistribution study using a radioiodinated (125-I) CEA-specific cAb fused to the enzyme beta-lactamase [38]. The in vivo distribution was assessed at 6, 24 and 48 h, with the highest tumor uptake at 6 h with approx. 2.8%ID/g in the tumor and 1.4%ID/g in blood. The tumor and blood levels remained stable at approx. 1%ID/g and ca 0.12%ID/g respectively throughout the study. Interestingly, and in contrast to previous investigations, the tumor uptake was at all time points higher than in the kidney, with tumor to kidney ratio at 48 h of 2.7:1, probably reflecting the larger size of the fusion protein. This indicates a modulation in both the kinetics and the distribution profile. The radioactivity in the kidneys did not correlate with any catalytic activity, suggesting that the protein was degraded in the kidneys.

Recently, imaging using an EGFR-specific, ^{99m}Tc-labeled Nanobody has been presented [40]. Three hours following injection in normal mice, there is a substantial uptake in liver (19.6%ID/g), as can be expected due to the high EGFR-expression in this organ. Kidney uptake was also high as expected for small proteins, 139.5–143%ID/g. Imaging quantification demonstrated uptake in A431 tumors at 3 h p.i. with 5.2%ID/cm^3 in tumors compared to liver and kidney values of 15.6 and 53.6%ID/g respectively. Gamma camera images could clearly visualize the xenografts, along with kidney and liver.

Antibody Mimetics: The Beta Sandwich/Barrel Fold

A number of protein folds resemble the structure of antibody Fv fragments with stabilizing beta-sandwich sheets in which the molecular recognition is localized to randomized loops. As is the case with Fv-fragments, many do also contain a stabilizing disulphide bond, more or less restricting these molecules to applications in which antibodies are used, but with a much better intellectual property-situation.

Examples of such scaffolds include tendamistat [41], fibronectin [42–45], cytotoxic T-lymphocyte-associated antigen 4 (CTLA-4) [46], T-cell receptors [47] and neocarzinostatin [48]. Fibronectin for example has an antibody-like structure and even display complementarity determining region (CDR)-like loops. As one of the few if not the only scaffold in this class, fibronectin is free of a stabilizing cystein, permitting modifications for site specific labeling.

Interestingly however, researchers have recently reported the introduction of a cystein also into the fibronectin scaffold to improve stability [49]. This demonstrates one of the limitations with antibody mimetics if it is desirable to obtain fully disulphide-free molecules. Furthermore, it suggests the need of other types of scaffolds to avoid cysteins. Nevertheless, they are good scaffolds and hold promise for *in vivo* applications. The similarity to antibodies may be an advantage for the translation of products into the clinic if they can be shown to maintain similar *in vivo* properties as antibodies.

One of the most advanced alternative scaffold products in this class is based on the 10th fibronectin type III domain and binds with high affinity and specificity to VEGFR2. It is currently in phase I clinical trials in patients with solid tumors or non-Hodgkin's lymphoma (former Adnexus, now part of Bristol-Myers Squibb). These so called Adnectins have been reported against other targets including TNF-alpha and the scaffold should be suited for tumor targeting applications. So far however, no quantitative tumor targeting data are available for the fibronectin fold, nor for the other folds within this class.

A special form of scaffold using beta-strands for stabilization is the beta-barrel type scaffold. The best example probably is the lipocalin-family, comprised by members that form conical beta-barrel proteins with a ligand-binding pocket surrounded by four loops [50]. The four loops can be randomized in analogy with the loops of antibody CDRs and may allow isolation of lipocalin members specific not only for the natural type of antigen, small molecules, but also for larger proteins. The company Pieris AG is developing lipocalin family members denoted anticalins [51]. Preclinical testing of anticalin binding digoxin, blocking VEGF and CTLA-4 action is ongoing, demonstrating capability of binding protein targets [52]. The anticalins however contain a number of disulphides and are not much smaller than antibody fragments, which may limit their use for targeted radionuclide therapy of tumors.

Alpha Helical Proteins

Although proteins built by helix bundles belong to a very abundant protein class of motifs, the number of alternative scaffolds based on alpha-coil structure is minute compared to the numerous examples for beta-sheet frameworks. The most advanced class of alternative scaffolds used for radionuclide tumor targeting however is a three helix protein belonging to a group, Affibody molecules, described below. Other members of this group include proteins like the *E. Coli* colichin E7 immunity protein (ImmE7) [53], or the immunity protein 9 (Im9) [54], or Cytochrome b562, in which the two loops connecting the alpha-helical framework were randomized, but no *in vivo* data have yet been reported for these proteins.

Protein A derivatives: Affibody molecules. Affibody molecules are derived from the B-domain in the Ig binding region of staphylococcal protein A [55]. Libraries of this cysteine-free, three-helix bundle, 58 amino acid residues domain were generated by combinatorial randomization of the 13 amino acid positions in helices 1 and 2, which make up the Fc-binding surface of the domain Z, thereby destroying the Fc interaction [56]. Affibody molecules that selectively bind to a range of different proteins, including insulin, fibrinogen, transferrin, tumor necrosis factor-alpha, IL-8, gp120, CD28, human serum albumin, IgA, IgE, IgM, HER2 and epidermal growth factor receptor [EGFR] have been identified (for review, see [57]). As for other scaffold proteins, the affinity of the primary constructs can be improved by affinity maturation, if the initial affinity is not sufficient. Affibody molecules were obtained with very high binding strength (K_D 22 pM) to the breast cancer antigen HER2 [58]. Given the small size of the Affibody molecules, 6 kDa, they should be good candidates for *in vivo* applications [59].

To evaluate the usefulness of this class of molecules for tumor imaging, a number of biodistribution and gamma camera studies have been performed using a high affinity, iodine labeled Affibody molecule, $Z_{HER2:342}$ (see Fig. 6.3). The tumor uptake of 9.5% injected dose per gram (ID/g) and tumor to blood ratio of 38 at 4 h following injection (post injection, p.i.) indicated that the performance was comparable or better than the best antibody fragments specific for HER2 [58]. High contrast gamma camera images were obtained 6 h p.i. Biodistribution studies using Indium-111 labeled $Z_{HER2:342}$, chelated by benzyl-DTPA resulted in a tumor uptake of 12%ID/g 4 h after administration and an impressive tumor to blood ratio of approximately 100 at this time point [60]. The molecules were labeled with Technetium-99 m, with tumor to blood ratio of 12, 24 and 40 after 2, 4 and 6 h respectively [61, 62].

After these initial investigations, the Affibody molecule $Z_{HER2:342}$ was produced in vitro by peptide synthesis, generating a fully synthetic molecule with a specifically attached DTPA-chelate site for incorporation of the diagnostic radiometal Indium-111. The molecule was carefully tested in animal studies, with high contrast imaging of small xenografted tumors in mice as early as 1 h p.i. in combination with a very high tumor uptake of the radionuclide (23%ID/g) at that time point and still 15%ID/g in the tumor after 24 h [63]. This molecule is now being developed by the company Affibody AB and is in clinical testing for women with metastasized breast cancer. Early results reveal that high contrast imaging of patient tumor metastases expressing the HER2 antigen is possible within a few hours after injection of the agent, and that both SPECT (using Indium-111) and PET (using Gallium-68) is possible [64].

To explore options for targeted radionuclide therapy using the HER2-specific Affibody molecule, a dimer of $Z_{HER2:342}$ was fused to a Albumin Binding Domain

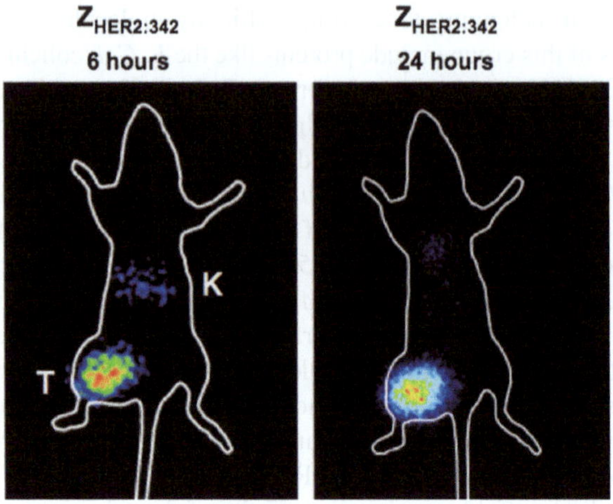

Fig. 6.3 Affibody-mediated tumor imaging of xenografted mice after injection of the Iodine-125 labeled $Z_{HER2:342}$ Affibody molecule. Pictures were taken 6 or 24 h after injection. Only kidneys, K, and the tumor, T, are detectable. The intensity of color corresponds to nuclide accumulation, blue is low and yellow represents high accumulation. The tumor uptake of $Z_{HER2:342}$ was stable up to at least 24 h p.i. (Figure adapted from [58])

(ADB) [65] to increase its apparent size by binding to the 67 kDa serum albumin protein, which is present in plasma at high concentrations and with long residence time in the circulation. The kidney uptake was decreased 25 times and the tumor dose increased three to five fold, making targeted radionuclide therapy using the beta-emitter Lutetium-177 (^{177}Lu) as cytotoxic molecule possible. Treatment of HER2-expressing SKOV-3 micro-xenografts with ^{177}Lu labeled ABD-fused $Z_{HER2:342}$-dimer completely prevented formation of tumors, while tumors were established in control animals treated with PBS (median tumor free-survival of 43 days) or a non-targeting, ^{177}Lu labeled, ABD-fused Z_{abeta} Affibody molecule carrying the same amount of radioactivity (median tumor free-survival of 43 days) and having the same plasma kinetic profile [6]. This is the first example of radionuclide therapy using an alternative scaffold protein, and of using non-covalent association to albumin as a modulator of the plasma kinetics in a radiotherapeutic setting.

Repetitive Protein Scaffolds

One way to increase binding strength of molecules is simply to enlarge the binding surface by combining two or more domains in the same molecule, with the aim to create avidity (simultaneous binding and as a consequence a larger binding interaction) or at least increase the functional concentration of binding molecules (without enlargement of the binding interaction). Native antibodies for example, combine two identical binding sites in each antibody to create a strong avid binding. In fact, it is quite common in nature to increase binding strength by positioning antigen binding repetitive small structural domains consecutively.

An example of engineering increased binding was demonstrated by Silverman, Stemmer and colleagues, taking a cystein rich protein module derived from human A-domains as the basic structure [66]. A-domains occur as strings of multiple domains in several cell surface receptors and have been shown to bind a range of different proteins in their natural context. They are very small, 4 kDa, and typically very robust as they contain three disulphide bonds in each subunit, even if the many cysteins may create problems during E. Coli expression and purification or when site specific labeling is desired. Even though as many as 28 of totally 40 amino acid residues can be randomized, the affinity of the monomers seems to be low. Instead, the increased binding surface was engineered into the finally created molecule by adding one or more domains to the initially weakly binding subunit in a stepwise manner, assuring that each additional binder would find a new, adjacent epitope to the earlier ones, generating a large molecular recognition surface.

In this way, dimers and trimers with picomolar binding strength to proteins such as Il-6, cMet, CD28, CD40L and BAFF were obtained. The constructs have been denoted "avimers". Especially a trimeric avimer binding Il-6, with a blocking IC50 value of 0.8 pM, is interesting as this molecule have proven *in vivo* efficacy in mice. This molecule is now in an Amgen sponsored phase I clinical trial as AMG220 (www.amgen.com), with the aim to treat Crohn's disease. As molecules of this class can be very small (4–8–12 kDa), it would be interesting to investigate a tumor specific avimer for tumor targeting.

Repeat Proteins

Another way to enlarge the binding surface is to exploit natures approach to combine repetitive small structural recognition units, each binding adjacent to its neighbor, to form a single binding epitope in a single fold, like repeat proteins do. Repeat proteins comprise consecutive copies of small structural units of ca 20–40 amino acid residues each, stacked together to form a binding domain. Among examples in nature of such proteins are Ankyrin repeats, Armadillo repeats, leucine rich repeats and tetratricopeptide repeat proteins [67]. Recently, ankyrin repeats have been subjected to protein engineering to form Designed Ankyrin-Repeat Proteins (DARPins).

Ankyrin repeats: DARPins. Designed ankyrin-repeat protein libraries were designed from a consensus-designed 33 amino acid residue ankyrin repeat (AR) module (reviewed in [68]). Randomizing seven amino acids per such repeat, and normally using approximately two to three basic repeats per domain, plus a N- and C-capping repeat to shield the hydrophobic core of the protein, AR protein libraries have been used for the generation of a number of binding molecules [69]. Nanomolar to picomolar affinity binder have been isolated against proteins such as maltose binding protein (MBP), the eukaryotic kinases JNK2 and p38, caspase-2

[70], the citrate symporter CitS of Klebsiella pneumoniae, the multidrug exporter AcrB [71] and recently a 90 pM affinity HER2 binder [72]. The basic unit is only 33 amino acids, but as there is a need of two capping domains, the smallest functional size of the protein is thus approx. 100 amino acids, and more common with two to three repetitive units, 133–166 amino acid residues or 10–20 kDa. This is still quite small and it would be interesting to investigate this scaffold for tumor targeting applications, for example using the HER2-binder, as HER2 targeting data for other scaffold proteins are available.

Some initial tests have been done, the DARPin binder has been shown to bind immunohistochemically, and biodistribution studies using the technetium-99 m labeled DARPin G3 indicated tumor targeting [73]. One hour following administration, the concentration of radioactivity in the tumor was approx. 8%ID/g and increased to approx. 11%ID/g 4 h later and decreased to 8%ID/g after 24 h. Blood level at 1 h was approx. 1%ID/g which rapidly decreased, reflecting the rapid half life of the G3 DARPin (alpha 2.6 min and beta 1.6 h). Four hours following administration, gamma camera images were obtained clearly presenting subcutaneous HER2 expressing SKOV-3 xenografts. This scaffold thus seems to be useful for *in vivo* tumor targeting and imaging applications and warrants further investigations in this field.

Small Cystein-Constrained Scaffolds

Even if a scaffold without cysteins is desirable, it can be difficult to obtain very small scaffolds, stable enough to allow for the necessary modifications. On the other hand, with two or three cystein bonds, a very small 4 kDa size scaffold of 40 amino acids, like the human A-domains, can accept randomization of 28 residues, with only 12 residues to maintain the structure [66]. Because rapid kinetics, good tissue penetration and highly stable proteins are important factors in targeted radionuclide therapy of tumors, this class of alternative scaffolds, often referred to as miniproteins, is interesting as it may provide the smallest possible binders having a very stable protein structure.

For example, serine proteinase inhibitors from the squash family, with only about 30 amino acids and three disulfide bridges, are among the smallest rigid structures available [74]. Their specific arrangement with three disulfide bridges is present in many proteins with no apparent evolutionary relationship, called knottins from their knot-like cysteine structure, including protease inhibitors, toxins from plants and animals, hormone-like peptides, or insect antimicrobials [75]. One engineered example is the trypsin inhibitor EETI-II, in which six residues in the first loop were randomized and the library screened using ribosome display [76]. A minimal 23-residue peptide library (Min-23) containing only two disulfide bonds was designed from EETI-II [77] by insertion of 10 random amino acids into the second alpha-turn of Min-23. Binders to various mAbs, AMA-1, Tom70 and HIV-1 Nef were isolated, with one Min-23 protein binding in the low nanomolar range.

Another engineering example from the Knottin group is the cellulose binding domain (CBD) derived from the cellobiohydrolase Cel7A from Trichoderma reesei as starting scaffold [78]. A combinatorial library was constructed by randomization of 11 positions located at the domain surface and distributed over three separate beta-sheets of the domain which should allow binding also to flat protein surfaces [79]. Low affinity binders for the target, the enzyme porcine alpha-amylase (PPA) were isolated and two CBD variants could block the enzyme activity. There are further examples of small, disulphide-stabilized binding miniproteins including scorpion charybdotoxin derivatives specific for HIV gp120 [80] and scylla- and alpha-conotoxin [20] but so far, use for tumor targeting has not been reported.

Other Scaffold Structures

It is possible to generate alternative scaffolds of a range of different proteins, many more than can be classified into the groups described above. Below are some further examples of alternative scaffolds that have been described in the literature.

Kunitz type protease inhibitors. Protease inhibitors are important in many pharmacologically relevant processes e.g. blood clotting and were therefore among the first scaffolds to be chosen for molecular engineering. Kunitz domain inhibitors constitute a group of small irregular serine protease inhibitors with few secondary structures, but with three disulfide bonds stabilizing the molecule, allowing for large loops to be randomized when making libraries. Examples of such scaffolds include Alzheimer's amyloid beta-protein precursor inhibitor (APPI) [81] or human pancreatic secretory trypsin inhibitor (PSTI) [82]. The human lipoprotein associated coagulation inhibitor (LACI), has been used to develop a drug candidate, inhibiting plasma kallikrein, DX-88 [83], currently in Phase III clinical trials for treatment of hereditary angioedema (HAE) (www.dyax.com June 2007).

Large scaffolds or enzymes presenting constrained peptides. Another approach has been to take a rather large protein as carrier molecule, and graft peptides known to bind to certain targets in order to improve half-life in plasma, gain stability of a targeting peptide, maintain enzyme reporter function, or other desired properties. One example is the 80 kDa human serum transferrin, which provides one or two loop domains onto which interesting peptides can be grafted. The company Biorexis (now part of Pfizer) has developed a GLP-1 receptor agonist by fusing the GLP-1 peptide to transferrin with the aim to treat diabetes. The approach is interesting also for tumor targeting as there is clinical evidence of the favorable properties of transferrin conjugated with chemotherapy, when the natural receptor was used as target for the treatment of malignant gliomas. Another example is the TEM-1 beta-lactamase, in which variants with new binding specificities to monoclonal antibodies, streptavidin or ferritin were isolated after two loops around its active site [84]. After maturation, affinities of K_D in the low nanomolar region could be obtained, sufficient for tumor targeting.

Peptide binding scaffolds. One group of proteins display properties that they bind peptides in their functional context. Since it is usually quite difficult to isolate binders to peptides with molecules other than antibodies or their fragments, the SH3, SH2 and PDZ domains are interesting. SH2 domains have been used to identify binders for phosphorylated proteins [85] and SH3 domains to bind to proline-rich peptides [86, 87]. PDZ domains preferably bind to the C-terminal end of target proteins and are believed to link these target proteins into functional signaling networks. Artificial PDZ domains were selected via a mutagenesis screen *in vivo* to recognize a different C-terminal peptide and they were shown to bind their target in different subcellular compartments [88]. It is however important to remember that alternative scaffold proteins are synthetic and not always restricted to bind to similar targets as they originally did in their natural context. One striking example is the recent engineering of a Fyn SH3 domain.

SH3 Fyn domains: Fynomers. Src homology 3 domains are approx. 60-residue recognition protein modules, present in larger proteins generally involved in the regulation of dynamic processes occurring at the plasma membrane. The protein modules can be isolated and the SH3 domains of Hck and Abl have been used to generate novel binding proteins. So far however, SH3 derived proteins have been used only for generation of binders against known SH3 ligands. The 63 residue SH3 domain of the Fyn tyrosine kinase is composed of two antiparallel beta-sheets and contains two flexible loops (the RT- and n-src-loop), which interact with other proteins. Grabulovski and coworkers recently engineered a human Fyn SH3 library randomizing these two loops [89], and isolated a binder to the extra domain B (ED-B) of fibronectin, a marker of angiogenesis [90]. As angiogenesis is an important component of aggressive tumor growth, ED-B can serve as a tumor target. An ED-B specific binder D3, denoted Fynomer, was isolated with a monomeric binding strength of K_D 85 nM, and a dimer version of that protein had an apparent binding strength of 4.5 nM. *In vitro* specificity was shown in Biacore and on cryosections of F9 teratocarcinoma tumors, in which the D3 molecule stained neovascular structures.

Biodistribution experiments were performed using radioiodinated proteins in subcutaneous xenografts of the F9 teratocarcinoma in mice. Monomers and dimers were compared at 4 and 24 h, both accumulated in the tumors while radioiodinated wild type Fyn SH3 domains did not accumulate in the tumor. At 4 h, the D3 monomer had a higher tumor uptake than the dimer, with 5.6%ID/g compared to 3.44%ID/g for the dimer. Tumor to blood ratios at that time point was however ca 1 for both constructs, indicating also higher blood levels for the monomer. Kidney uptake was just above the tumor uptake with ca 6.7%ID/g for both constructs. At 24 h, the tumor uptake was much higher for the dimer (2.62%ID/g) than for the monomer (0.69%ID/g), with tumor to blood ratios of 8.7 for the dimer and 5.8 for the monomer. This would enable imaging,, even though 24 h is a too long time to be appreciated in the clinic. Recently, a fynomer binding to mouse serum albumin was reported [91], and could obviously be used to modulate the kinetic profile of tumor targeting fynomers, if they would be fused to it.

Non-scaffold Structural Molecules: Aptamers

Aptamers [92], and peptide aptamers [93] are examples of small structures (8–12 kDa) that address many of the problems that the alternative scaffold proteins do, but which are not derived from a predefined scaffold with favorable properties. They are short DNA or RNA oligonucleotides or peptides that assume a specific and stable three-dimensional shape *in vivo*, thereby providing specific tight binding to protein targets. In the selection process, the oligonucleotide or peptide chain will spontaneously adopt secondary structures that aid the display of recognition epitopes that interact with the target protein.

There are very advanced DNA aptamers, for example Pegatinib which is already approved in the clinic for use in AMD [94], AS1411 which is a human nucleolin-binding aptamer in phase I clinical trials for treating patients with solid tumors [95], preclinical efficacy data on PDFG-R blocker [96] and aptamers binding tumor associated antigens like alpha v beta 3, MUC1, PSMA, Tenascin C, HER3 and other antigens [97].

Aptamers may have certain advantages over proteins, they are fully synthetic, allowing site specific modifications, and furthermore highly negatively charged which seems to correspond to reduced liver and low or no kidney uptake. They have also been reported to lack immunogenicity [97]. Unmodified aptamers are rapidly degraded in blood due to nuclease activity and they need secondary modifications to overcome this problem. Initial experiments to investigate the usefulness of aptamers for *in vivo* imaging of inflammation have been reported [98] as have experiments studying oligonucleotide biodistribution properties [99, 100].

An aptamer specific for the tumor associated extracellular matrix protein Tenascin-C (Tn-C) was selected: TTA1 [101]. Tumor targeting with the 99m-Technetium labeled anti-Tenascin C aptamer and a control aptamer was performed in xenografted mice [102]. Blood clearance was extremely rapid, dropping from 50 to 18%ID/g in the initial 2 min and to 0.1%ID/g at 60 min. The tumor uptake maximized after 10 min p.i. with 5.9%ID/g compared to the non-specific aptamer with 3.9%ID/g uptake. TTA1 was retained on the tumor with 2.7%ID/g after 1 h, when tumor to blood ratio was 24 and after 3 h, the tumor to blood ratio of TTA1 surpassed 50. Kidney values decreased rapidly, reflecting renal clearance but not uptake, but also the intestines presented high levels, indicating hepatobiliar excretion as well. *In vivo* imaging was possible after 3 h, with prominent intestinal signals, but also clearly visible tumor. In images taken at 18 h, radioactivity had almost entirely cleared the body, and the tumor was the brightest structure visualized.

Discussion

Alternative scaffold proteins represent a rapidly growing class of binding molecules with different and advantageous properties. Over the last decade, such molecules have been developed for a wide range of biotechnological and biopharmaceutical applications, with use in affinity chromatography columns or employed as capturing molecules on protein chips to efficient blockers of TNF-alpha mediated inflammatory responses or blood clotting mechanisms *in vivo*. The purpose of this chapter on alternative scaffolds for targeted radionuclide diagnosis and therapy of tumors is not to list every existing scaffold and its putative applications, but rather to give an overview on validated alternative scaffolds with a focus on scaffolds that may be of special interest for tumor targeting.

Interestingly, even if there are more than 30 different alternative scaffolds described [20], only a few are substantiated by *in vivo* data and even fewer by tumor targeting data. This may mirror properties and quality of the scaffolds, but also that this molecular class is still quite young with a lot of initial findings not yet translated into *in vivo* applications. In addition, targeted radionuclide diagnosis and therapy diagnosis are quite specialized activities and to enter this field people skilled in radiochemistry and applications of in animal experimental models are required. Many initial academic findings may stay on an *in vitro* biotechnological proof-of concept level because the people developing the technology for new scaffolds may not always be the same as those who will do the animal studies and push a drug candidate into the clinic. In fact, many of the more advanced alternative scaffold molecules now act as a technological base in companies focused on translating the technological findings into preclinical data and clinical products.

Among novel scaffold proteins that have been tested for radionuclide targeting of tumors, the Affibody technology is the most advanced, with preclinical biodistribution data in xenografted mice, high contrast gamma- and PET-camera imaging of grafted tumors and efficacious radionuclide based therapy experiments in xenografted animal models. In addition, several breast cancer patients have been injected with a HER2-specific, fully synthetic Affibody molecule and had their HER2-expressing metastases visualized using Indium-111 and gamma camera or Gallium-68 and PET. Other interesting scaffolds are camel V_{HH}-antibody fragments (cAb) and designed ankyrin repeats (DARPins) which both provided good tumor targeting data with a quality which should be sufficient for future *in vivo* diagnostic imaging.

One of the latest alternative scaffolds developed, the SH3 domains of the Fyn protein, or the so called ED-B specific Fynomer, was developed and directly tested for tumor targeting purposes. In contrast, many other scaffold proteins were developed for non-tumor targeting indications like inflammatory diseases, blood clotting, angiogenesis blocking, rheumatoid arthritis. Even though the data of the Fynomer may need to be improved somewhat before this targeting agent can be developed for imaging purposes, it hopefully reflects a trend towards the development of more tumor targeting agents.

When developing agents for targeting of radionuclides to tumors for cancer diagnostics and therapy, a dilemma today is that the easy task is to develop a diagnostic targeting ligand, but it can be very difficult to sell as a product, as the clinical need is less well defined or not yet developed. Furthermore, to develop a radiotherapeutic agent not taken up by any normal tissues, with display of a perfect kinetic profile and which is compatible with a therapeutic radionuclide, is a difficult task from an engineering perspective. The concept of molecular imaging is attractive, but as long as there are few therapeutic treatment decisions influenced by molecular information on receptor expression, there will be a limited clinical demand for such products and therefore few new molecular tools for the development of such novel treatments.

Which other alternative scaffolds would be optimal for tumor targeting? Given that the four examples above are all derived from different binding classes, this is difficult to predict. Very small scaffolds with long protruding loops e.g. protease inhibitors like the Kunitz domains may face similar difficulties as constrained peptides and may thus be limited to a few special antigens. For molecular imaging, small size is the key and the very small cystein-knot constrained scaffolds may be ideal. So far however, there are not very many examples of such scaffolds with high affinity binding to globular proteins. The camel V_{HH}-antibody fragments performed well, and it may therefore be fair to expect also other antibody-like beta-sandwich proteins as for example Adnectins to function as carrier proteins for tumor targeting. Larger proteins, onto which peptide loops have been grafted, may not have the fast kinetics necessary for imaging, but may be acceptable for therapy.

Alternative scaffolds are generally small, which is of advantage for molecular imaging, but may be questionable for therapy. Clearance may be too quick to allow for sufficient tumor accumulation of the radionuclide, unless very high doses are administered.

There may also be unwanted accumulation of small radiolabeled molecules in the kidneys. Different avenues to modify and prolong the biological plasma half life have been investigated. Pegylation is a well validated method with several approved pegylated products on the market [103, 104]. Pegylation is however not unproblematic and requires costly process optimization to meet regulatory standards.

Many biotech companies developing alternative scaffolds have therefore investigated alternative approaches, like scaffold association to abundant plasma proteins. By hitchhiking with a protein like the abundant long lived serum albumin, the plasma half life of the targeting molecule may be altered dramatically. Especially reversible non-covalent association by use of albumin binding proteins, fused with the targeting agent into one single molecule, omits difficult albumin conjugating procedures or cumbersome recombinant expression of large albumin-alternative scaffold fusion proteins. In addition, by modulating the affinity to albumin, the albumin association and thus the half-life of the molecule may be tailored [105].

A small albumin-binding peptide was fused to a HER2-specific Fab-fragment rendering the antibody fragment full size antibody properties in terms of total tumor uptake, but provided more rapid clearance and therefore better contrast for gamma camera imaging [106]. Many biotech companies are indeed developing albumin binders using their own scaffold proteins [91]. The most advanced example for radionuclide targeting is modulation of the kinetic profile using the 5 kDa albumin binding domain of streptococcal protein G described already in 1991 [107]. It was recently used to optimize the kinetics of a HER2-specific Affibody molecule in a curative preclinical targeted radionuclide therapy study using Lutetium-177 [6].

For antibodies, there is only one class of scaffold, the Ig-fold, and the size may vary. In contrast to antibodies, alternative scaffolds do not constitute a homogenous group with similar and predictable properties. A challenge in the development of novel tumor targeting alternative scaffold-binders is that this class of proteins is very young and very diverse and it is today difficult to predict if there is a special type of alternative scaffold that is better suited for targeting applications than another. Therefore, alternative scaffold molecules deserve an open mind for further investigations and development in the clinic.

References

1. Behr TM, Gotthardt M, Barth A, Behe M (2001) Imaging tumors with peptide-based radioligands. Q J Nucl Med 45:189–200
2. Britz-Cunningham SH, Adelstein SJ (2003) Molecular targeting with radionuclides: state of the science. J Nucl Med 44:1945–61
3. Russeva MG, Adams GP (2004) Radioimmunotherapy with engineered antibodies Expert Opin Biol Ther 4:217–31
4. Batra SK, Jain M, Wittel UA (2002) Pharmacokinetics and biodistribution of genetically engineered antibodies. Curr Opin Biotechnol 13:603–8. Review
5. Heppeler A, Froidevaux S, Eberle AN, Maecke HR (2000) Receptor targeting for tumour localisation and therapy with radiopeptides. Curr Med Chem 7:971–94
6. Tolmachev V, Orlova A, Pehrson R, et al. (2007) Radionuclide therapy of HER2-positive microxenografts using a 177Lu-labeled HER2-specific Affibody molecule. Cancer Res 67:2773–82
7. Milenic DE, Brady ED, Brechbiel MW (2004) Antibody-targeted radiation cancer therapy. Nat Rev Drug Discov 6:488–99. Review
8. Kohler G, Milstein C (1975) Continuous cultures of fused cells secreting antibody of predefined specificity. Nature 256:495–7
9. Holliger P, Hudson PJ (2005) Engineered antibody fragments and the rise of single domains. Nat Biotechnol 9:1126–36. Review
10. Robinson MK, Doss M, Shaller C (2005) Quantitative immuno-positron emission tomography imaging of HER2-positive tumor xenografts with an iodine-124 labeled anti-HER2 diabody. Cancer Res 65:1471–8
11. Adams GP, Tai MS, McCartney JE (2006) Avidity-mediated enhancement of in vivo tumor targeting by single-chain Fv dimers. Clin Cancer Res 12:1599–605
12. Olafsen, T et al. (2004) Characterization of engineered anti-p185HER-2 (scFv-CH3)2 antibody fragments (minibodies) for tumor targeting. Protein Eng Des Sel 17:315–23
13. Tijink BM, Neri D, Leemans CR, et al. (2006) Radioimmunotherapy of head and neck cancer xenografts using 131I-labeled antibody L19-SIP for selective targeting of tumor vasculature. J Nucl Med 47:1127–35
14. Olafsen T, Kenanova VE, Wu AM (2006) Tunable pharmacokinetics: modifying the in vivo half-life of antibodies by directed mutagenesis of the Fc fragment. Nat Protoc 1:2048–60
15. De Jong M, Valkema R, Jamar F (2002) Somatostatin receptor-targeted radionuclide therapy of tumors: preclinical and clinical findings. Semin Nucl Med Apr; 32(2):133–40. Review
16. Reubi JC, Mäcke HR, Krenning EP (2005) Candidates for peptide receptor radiotherapy today and in the future. J Nucl Med 46 (Suppl 1):67S–75S. Review
17. Sharkey RM, Cardillo TM, Rossi EA, et al. (2005) Signal amplification in molecular imaging by pretargeting a multivalent, bispecific antibody. Nat Med 11:1250–5

18. Hey T, Fiedler E, Rudolph R, Fiedler M (2005) Artificial, non-antibody binding proteins for pharmaceutical and industrial applications. Trends Biotechnol 23:514–22
19. Hosse RJ, Rothe A, Power BE (2006) A new generation of protein display scaffolds for molecular recognition. Protein Sci 15:14–27. Review
20. Binz HK, Amstutz P, Pluckthun A (2005) Engineering novel binding proteins from nonimmunoglobulin domains. Nat Biotechnol 23:1257–68. Review
21. Binz HK, Pluckthun A (2005) Engineered proteins as specific binding reagents. Curr Opin Biotechnol 16:459–69. Review
22. Nygren PA, Skerra A (2004) Binding proteins from alternative scaffolds. J Immunol Methods 290:3–28. Review
23. Nygren PA, Uhlen M (1997) Scaffolds for engineering novel binding sites in proteins. Curr Opin Struct Biol7:463–9. Review
24. Hoogenboom HR (2005) Selecting and screening recombinant antibody libraries. Nat Biotechnol 23:1105–16. Review
25. Hoogenboom HR (2002) Overview of antibody phage-display technology and its applications. Methods Mol Biol 178:1–37. Review
26. Lipovsek D, Plückthun A (2004) In-vitro protein evolution by ribosome display and mRNA display. J Immunol Methods 290:51–67
27. Boder ET, Wittrup KD (1997) Yeast surface display for screening combinatorial polypeptide libraries. Nat Biotechnol 15:553–7
28. Samuelson P, Gunneriusson E, Nygren PA, Stahl S (2002) Display of proteins on bacteria. J Biotechnol 96(2):129–54. Review
29. Chen G, Hayhurst A, Thomas JG (2001) Isolation of high-affinity ligand-binding proteins by periplasmic expression with cytometric screening (PECS). Nat Biotechnol 19:537–42
30. Bertschinger J, Neri D (2004) Covalent DNA display as a novel tool for directed evolution of proteins in vitro. Protein Eng Des Sel 17:699–707
31. Sepp A, Tawfik DS, Griffiths AD (2002) Microbead display by in vitro compartmentalisation: selection for binding using flow cytometry FEBS Lett 532:455–8
32. Hamers-Casterman C, Atarhouch T, Muyldermans S (1993) Naturally occurring antibodies devoid of light chains. Nature 363:446–8
33. Greenberg AS, Avila D, Hughes M et al. (1995) A new antigen receptor gene family that undergoes rearrangement and extensive somatic diversification in sharks. Nature 374(6518):168–73
34. Nuttall SD, Krishnan UV, Hattarki M, De Gori R, Irving RA, Hudson PJ (2001) Isolation of the new antigen receptor from wobbegong sharks, and use as a scaffold for the display of protein loop libraries. Mol Immunol 38:313–26
35. Coppieters K, Dreier T, Silence K, et al. (2006) Formatted anti-tumor necrosis factor alpha VHH proteins derived from camelids show superior potency and targeting to inflamed joints in a murine model of collagen-induced arthritis. Arthritis Rheum 54:1856–66
36. Holt LJ, Herring C, Jespers LS, et al. (2003) Domain antibodies: proteins for therapy. Trends Biotechnol 11:484–90. Review
37. Revets H, De Baetselier P, Muyldermans S (2005) Nanobodies as novel agents for cancer therapy. Expert Opin Biol Ther 5:111–24. Review
38. Cortez-Retamozo V, Backmann N, Senter PD, et al. (2004) Efficient cancer therapy with a nanobody-based conjugate. Cancer Res 64:2853–7
39. Cortez-Retamozo V, Lauwereys M, Hassanzadeh Gh G, et al. (2002) Efficient tumor targeting by single-domain antibody fragments of camels. Int J Cancer 98:456–62
40. Huang L, Gainkam LO, Caveliers V, et al. (2008) SPECT imaging with (99 m)Tc-labeled EGFR-specific nanobody for in vivo monitoring of EGFR expression. Mol Imaging Biol Feb 23; 1:31–41
41. Li R, Hoess RH, Bennett JS, DeGrado WF (2003) Use of phage display to probe the evolution of binding specificity and affinity in integrins. Protein Eng 16:65–72
42. Xu L, Aha P, Gu K (2002) Directed evolution of high-affinity antibody mimics using mRNA display. Chem Biol 9:933–42

43. Parker MH, Chen Y, Danehy F (2005) Antibody mimics based on human fibronectin type three domain engineered for thermostability and high-affinity binding to vascular endothelial growth factor receptor two. Protein Eng Des Sel 18:435–44
44. Koide A, Koide S (2007) Monobodies: antibody mimics based on the scaffold of the fibronectin type III domain. Methods Mol Biol 352:95–109
45. Karatan E, Merguerian M, Han Z, et al. (2004) Molecular recognition properties of FN3 monobodies that bind the Src SH3 domain. Chem Biol June; 11:835–44
46. Hufton SE, van Neer N, van den Beuken T (2000) Development and application of cytotoxic T lymphocyte-associated antigen 4 as a protein scaffold for the generation of novel binding ligands. FEBS Lett 475:225–31
47. Li Y, Moysey R, Molloy PE (2005) Directed evolution of human T-cell receptors with picomolar affinities by phage display. Nat Biotechnol 23:349–54
48. Heyd B, Pecorari F, Collinet B (2003) In vitro evolution of the binding specificity of neocarzinostatin, an enediyne-binding chromoprotein. Biochemistry 42:5674–83
49. Lipovsek D, Lippow SM, Hackel BJ (2007) Evolution of an interloop disulfide bond in high-affinity antibody mimics based on fibronectin type III domain and selected by yeast surface display: molecular convergence with single-domain camelid and shark antibodies. J Mol Biol 368:1024–41
50. Beste G, Schmidt FS, Stibora T, Skerra A (1999) Small antibody-like proteins with prescribed ligand specificities derived from the lipocalin fold. Proc Natl Acad Sci USA 96:1898–903
51. Schlehuber S, Skerra A (2005a) Anticalins as an alternative to antibody technology. Expert Opin Biol Ther 5:1453–62. Review
52. Schlehuber S, Skerra A (2005b) Lipocalins in drug discovery: from natural ligand-binding proteins to "anticalins". Drug Discov Today 10:23–33. Review
53. Juraja SM, Mulhern TD, Hudson PJ, et al. (2006) Engineering of the Escherichia coli Im7 immunity protein as a loop display scaffold. Protein Eng Des Sel 19:231–44.
54. Bernath K, Magdassi S, Tawfik DS (2005) Directed evolution of protein inhibitors of DNA-nucleases by in vitro compartmentalization (IVC) and nano-droplet delivery. J Mol Biol 345:1015–26
55. Nilsson B, Moks T, Jansson B, et al. (1987) A synthetic IgG-binding domain based on staphylococcal protein A. Protein Eng 1(2):107–13
56. Nord K, Gunneriusson E, Ringdahl J (1997) Binding proteins selected from combinatorial libraries of an alpha-helical bacterial receptor domain. Nat Biotechnol 15:772–7
57. Nilsson FY, Tolmachev V (2007) Affibody molecules: new protein domains for molecular imaging and targeted tumor therapy. Curr Opin Drug Discov Devel 10:167–75. Review
58. Orlova A, Magnusson M, Eriksson TL, et al. (2006) Tumor imaging using a picomolar affinity HER2 binding affibody molecule. Cancer Res 66:4339–48
59. Tolmachev V, Orlova A, Nilsson FY, et al. (2007) Affibody molecules: potential for in vivo imaging of molecular targets for cancer therapy. Expert Opin Biol Ther 7:555–68
60. Tolmachev V, Nilsson FY, Widstrom C, et al. (2006) 111In-benzyl-DTPA-ZHER2:342, an affibody-based conjugate for in vivo imaging of HER2 expression in malignant tumors. J Nucl Med May; 47(5):846–53
61. Engfeldt T, Tran T, Orlova A, et al. (2007a) (99 m)Tc-chelator engineering to improve tumour targeting properties of a HER2-specific Affibody molecule. Eur J Nucl Med Mol Imaging 34:1843–53
62. Engfeldt T, Orlova A, Tran T, et al. (2007b) Imaging of HER2-expressing tumours using a synthetic Affibody molecule containing the (99 m)Tc-chelating mercaptoacetyl-glycyl-glycyl-glycyl (MAG3) sequence. Eur J Nucl Med Mol Imaging 34:722–33
63. Orlova A, Tolmachev V, Pehrson R, et al. (2007) Synthetic affibody molecules: a novel class of affinity ligands for molecular imaging of HER2-expressing malignant tumors. Cancer Res 67:2178–86
64. Feldwisch J, Orlova A, Tolmachev V, Baum RP (2006) Clinical and pre-clinical application of HER2-specific Affibody molecules for diagnosis of recurrent HER2 positive breast cancer by SPECT or PET/CT. Mol Imaging 5(ID045):215

65. Makrides SC, Nygren PA, Andrews B, et al. (1996) Extended in vivo half-life of human soluble complement receptor type 1 fused to a serum albumin-binding receptor. J Pharmacol Exp Ther 277:534–42
66. Silverman J, Liu Q, Bakker A (2005) Multivalent avimer proteins evolved by exon shuffling of a family of human receptor domains. Nat Biotechnol 23(12):1556–61
67. Forrer P, Stumpp MT, Binz HK, Pluckthun A (2003) A novel strategy to design binding molecules harnessing the modular nature of repeat proteins. FEBS Lett 539:2–6
68. Stumpp MT, Amstutz P (2007) DARPins: a true alternative to antibodies. Curr Opin Drug Discov Devel 10:153–9. Review
69. Binz HK, Amstutz P, Kohl A, et al. (2004) High-affinity binders selected from designed ankyrin repeat protein libraries. Nat Biotechnol 22:575–82
70. Schweizer A, Roschitzki-Voser H, Amstutz P, et al. (2007) Inhibition of caspase-2 by a designed ankyrin repeat protein: specificity, structure, and inhibition mechanism. Structure 15:625–36
71. Sennhauser G, Amstutz P, Briand C, et al. (2006) Drug export pathway of multidrug exporter AcrB revealed by DARPin inhibitors. PLoS Biol 5:106–13
72. Zahnd C, Wyler E, Schwenk JM (2007) A designed ankyrin repeat protein evolved to picomolar affinity to her2. J Mol Biol 369:1015–28
73. Stumpp, MT (2006) Oral presentation at IBC's 2nd Annual International conference on Protein Engineering, December 12–14
74. Otlewski J, Krowarsch D (1996) Squash inhibitor family of serine proteinases. Acta Biochim Pol 43:431–44
75. Gelly JC, Gracy J, Kaas Q, et al. (2004) The KNOTTIN website and database: a new information system dedicated to the knottin scaffold. Nucleic Acids Res 32:D156–9
76. Baggio R, Burgstaller P, Hale SP, et al. (2002) Identification of epitope-like consensus motifs using mRNA display. J Mol Recognit 15(3):126–34
77. Souriau C, Chiche L, Irving R, Hudson P (2005) New binding specificities derived from Min-23, a small cystine-stabilized peptidic scaffold. Biochemistry 44:7143–55
78. Smith GP, Patel SU, Windass JD (1998) Small binding proteins selected from a combinatorial repertoire of knottins displayed on phage. J Mol Biol Mar 27; 277(2):317–32
79. Lehtiö J, Teeri TT, Nygren PA (2000) Alpha-amylase inhibitors selected from a combinatorial library of a cellulose binding domain scaffold. Proteins 41:316–22.
80. Li C, Dowd CS, Zhang W, Chaiken IM (2001) Phage randomization in a charybdotoxin scaffold leads to CD4-mimetic recognition motifs that bind HIV-1 envelope through non-aromatic sequences. J Pept Res 57:507–18.
81. Dennis MS, Lazarus RA (1994) Kunitz domain inhibitors of tissue factor-factor VIIa. I. Potent inhibitors selected from libraries by phage display. J Biol Chem 269:22129–36
82. Rottgen P, Collins J (1995) A human pancreatic secretory trypsin inhibitor presenting a hypervariable highly constrained epitope via monovalent phagemid display. Gene 164:243–50
83. Williams A, Baird LG (2003) DX-88 and HAE: a developmental perspective. Transfus Apher Sci 29:255–8
84. Legendre D, Vucic B, Hougardy V, et al. (2002) TEM-1 beta-lactamase as a scaffold for protein recognition and assay. Protein Sci 11:1506–18
85. Malabarba MG, Milia E, Faretta M (2001) A repertoire library that allows the selection of synthetic SH2s with altered binding specificities. Oncogene 20(37):5186–94
86. Panni S, Dente L, Cesareni G (2002) In vitro evolution of recognition specificity mediated by SH3 domains reveals target recognition rules. J Biol Chem 277:21666–74
87. Hiipakka M, Saksela K (2007) Versatile retargeting of SH3 domain binding by modification of non-conserved loop residues. FEBS Lett 581:1735–41
88. Schneider S, Buchert M, Georgiev O, et al. (1999) Mutagenesis and selection of PDZ domains that bind new protein targets. Nat Biotechnol 17:170–5
89. Grabulovski D, Kaspar M, Neri D (2007) A novel, non-immunogenic Fyn SH3-derived binding protein with tumor vascular targeting properties. J Biol Chem 282:3196–204

90. Castellani P, Viale G, Dorcaratto A, et al. (1994) The fibronectin isoform containing the ED-B oncofetal domain: a marker of angiogenesis. Int J Cancer 59:612–8
91. Bertschinger J, Grabulovski D, Neri D (2007) Selection of single domain binding proteins by covalent DNA display. Protein Eng Des Sel 20:57–68
92. Brody EN, Gold L (2000) Aptamers as therapeutic and diagnostic agents. Rev Mol Biotechnol 74:5–13. Review
93. Hoppe-Seyler F, Crnkovic-Mertens I, Tomai E, Butz K (2004) Peptide aptamers: specific inhibitors of protein function. Curr Mol Med 4:529–38. Review
94. Ng EW, Shima DT, Calias P, et al. (2006) Pegaptanib, a targeted anti-VEGF aptamer for ocular vascular disease. Nat Rev Drug Discov 5:123–32. Review
95. Ireson CR, Kelland LR (2006) Discovery and development of anticancer aptamers. Mol Cancer Ther 5:2957–62. Review
96. Pietras K, Rubin K, Sjöblom T (2002) Inhibition of PDGF receptor signaling in tumor stroma enhances antitumor effect of chemotherapy. Cancer Res 62:5476–84
97. Pestourie C, Tavitian B, Duconge F (2005) Aptamers against extracellular targets for in vivo applications. Biochimie 87:921–30. Review
98. Charlton J, Sennello J, Smith (1997) In vivo imaging of inflammation using an aptamer inhibitor of human neutrophil elastase D. Chem Biol 4:809–16
99. Zhang YM, Liu N, Zhu ZH, Rusckowski M, Hnatowich DJ (2000) Influence of different chelators (HYNIC, MAG3 and DTPA) on tumor cell accumulation and mouse biodistribution of technetium-99 m labeled to antisense DNA. Eur J Nucl Med 27:1700–7
100. Tavitian B, Terrazzino S, Kuhnast B, et al. (1998) In vivo imaging of oligonucleotides with positron emission tomography. Nat Med 4:467–71
101. Hicke BJ, Marion C, Chang YF, et al. (2001) Tenascin-C aptamers are generated using tumor cells and purified protein. J Biol Chem 276:48644–54
102. Hicke BJ, Stephens AW, Gould T (2006) Tumor targeting by an aptamer. J Nucl Med 47:668–78
103. Matthews SJ, McCoy C (2004) Peginterferon alfa-2a: a review of approved and investigational uses. Clin Ther 26:991–1025. Review
104. Veronese FM, Pasut G (2005) PEGylation, successful approach to drug delivery. Drug Discov Today 10:1451–8. Review
105. Nguyen A, Reyes AE 2nd, Zhang M (2006) The pharmacokinetics of an albumin-binding Fab (AB.Fab) can be modulated as a function of affinity for albumin. Protein Eng Des Sel 19:291–7
106. Dennis MS, Jin H, Dugger D, et al. (2007) Imaging tumors with an albumin-binding Fab, a novel tumor-targeting agent. Cancer Res 67:254–61
107. Nygren PA, Uhlén M, Flodby P, et al. (1991) In vivo stabilization of a human recombinant CD4 derivative by fusion to a serum-albumin-binding receptor. Vaccines 91:363–8
108. Vogt M, Skerra A (2004) Construction of an artificial receptor protein ("anticalin") based on the human apolipoprotein D. Chembiochem Feb 6; 5(2):191–9.
109. Nordberg E, Friedman M, Nilsson F, et al. (2006) Biological characterization in vitro and in vivo of a new EGFR binding Affibody molecule. Eur J Nucl Med Mol Imaging 33 (Suppl 14):S284.
110. Friedman M, Orlova A, Johansson E, et al. (2008) Directed evolution to low nanomolar affinity of a tumor-targeting epidermal growth factor receptor-binding affibody molecule. J Mol Biol Mar 7; 376:1388–402

Chapter 7
Peptides for Radionuclide Therapy

Marion de Jong, Suzanne M. Verwijnen, Monique de Visser, Dik J. Kwekkeboom, Roelf Valkema, and Eric P. Krenning

Summary Somatostatin receptor-targeting peptides are widely being used for imaging and therapy of neuroendocrine tumors. Peptide receptor radionuclide therapy (PRRT) with e.g. ^{177}Lu labeled somatostatin analogues in neuroendocrine tumor patients has resulted in symptomatic improvement, prolonged survival and enhanced quality of life. Yet, much profit can be gained from improving the receptor-targeting strategies available and developing new strategies, e.g. targeting other tumor-specific receptors, such as gastrin-releasing peptide (GRP) receptors and gastrin/cholecystokinin (CCK) receptors, and combining PRRT with other treatment strategies like chemotherapy or co-treatment with radiosensitizers.

This chapter presents an overview of several options to optimize receptor-targeted imaging and also radionuclide therapy. It outlines the efforts currently underway to develop optimized radiopharmaceuticals, increase the target density and combine treatment strategies.

Introduction

Peptide receptor radionuclide therapy (PRRT) with radiolabelled peptide analogues is a relatively new and promising treatment modality for patients with inoperable or metastasised tumours. The presentation below is partly overlapping the section on "Somatostatin Receptor Therapy" in chapter 20 (Clincal Radionuclide Therapy).

The discovery that certain tumor types overexpress receptors for peptide hormones dates back to the mid-1980s. For evaluation of tumor receptor expression, radiolabeled peptide analogues such as somatostatin, bombesin, neurotensin and gastrin analogues, have been introduced. The most commonly used receptor-targeting agents are a variety of analogues of somatostatin. Treatment with unlabeled somatostatin analogues including octreotide and lanreotide can reduce hormonal overproduction in neuroendocrine tumors and results in symptomatic

Department of Nuclear Medicine, Erasmus MC, Rotterdam, The Netherlands

T. Stigbrand et al. (eds.) *Targeted Radionuclide Tumor Therapy*,

relief in most patients with metastatic disease. However, tumor size reduction with somatostatin analogue treatment is seldom achieved.

Radiolabeled receptor-binding peptides are powerful tools for both imaging and therapy of tumors expressing receptors specifically binding these peptides. Such radiolabelled peptide analogues therefore serve as "thera-nostics", as they can be applied for imaging as well as for therapy, dependent on the radionuclide being attached to the peptide moiety. Especially analogues of somatostatin appeared suitable for receptor-targeted localization, staging and treatment of somatostatin receptor (sst)-expressing neuroendocrine tumors [1]. Structures of somatostatin analogues currently used for PRRT are shown in Fig. 7.1.

Radionuclide Therapy Using Somatostatin Analogues, Current Status

The somatostatin receptor family consists of five receptor subtypes: sst_1-sst_5. The majority of neuroendocrine tumors features a strong over-expression of sst, mainly subtype 2 (sst_2). The introduction of radiolabeled somatostatin analogues started with the development of the sst-targeting somatostatin analogue [^{111}In-DTPA^0]octreotide (Octreoscan®). This analogue is being used to visualize sst-receptor positive tumours and their metastases [2, 3]. After the successful studies to visualise somatostatin receptor positive tumours, a logical next step was taken in trying to use radiolabelled somatostatin analogues as a treatment in these patients.

The therapeutic efficacy of [^{111}In-DTPA^0]octreotide was found promising, although no effects were found in patients with larger tumours and advanced disease [4]. Five out of 26 patients had a decrease in tumour size of in between 25%

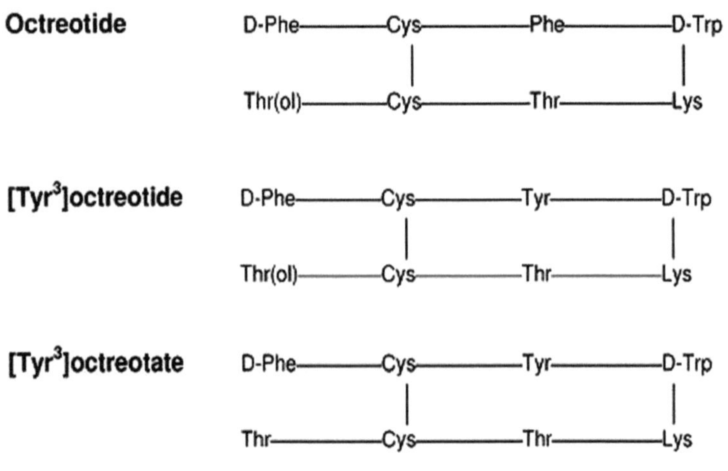

Fig. 7.1 Structures of some somatostatin analogues being used for peptide receptor radionuclide therapy (PRRT)

and 50% (minor response, MR), as measured on CT scans. They were treated with high activities of [^{111}In-DTPA^{0}]octreotide and received a total cumulative activity of at least 550 mCi (20 GBq). None, however, had partial remission (PR). Many patients were in poor clinical condition and many had progressive disease at baseline. The most common long-term side effects in both series were due to bone marrow toxicity. Serious side effects consisted of leukaemia and myelodysplastic syndrome (MDS) in three patients: they had been treated with total cumulative activities of >2.7 Ci (100 GBq) and bone marrow radiation doses were estimated to be more than 3 Gy. One of these patients had also been treated with chemotherapy previously, which may have contributed to or caused this complication. It was not surprising that CT-assessed tumour regression was observed only in rare cases: ^{111}In-coupled peptides are not ideal for PRRT because of the small particle range of Auger-electrons and therefore shorter tissue penetration compared to beta-particle emitters.

The modified somatostatin analogue [DOTA^{0},Tyr^{3}]octreotide was used in the next generation of somatostatin receptor targeted radionuclide therapy. This analogue has a higher affinity for somatostatin receptor subtype-2, and has 1,4,7,10-tetraazacyclododecane-$^{N',N'',N''',N''''}$-tetraacetic acid (DOTA) instead of DTPA as chelator. This allows a more stable binding of the intended beta-emitting radionuclide ^{90}Y. Several phase-1 and phase-2 peptide-receptor radionuclide therapy (PRRT) trials were performed using [^{90}Y-DOTA^{0}-Tyr^{3}]octreotide (^{90}Y-DOTATOC; OctreoTher®) [5–9]. Objective responses in most of the studies with [^{90}Y-DOTA^{0},Tyr^{3}]octreotide in patients with GEP tumours ranged from 9–33% [10]. These results were better than those obtained with [^{111}In-DTPA^{0}]octreotide, despite differences in the [^{90}Y-DOTA^{0},Tyr^{3}]octreotide protocols applied. Different phase-1 and phase-2 studies were performed in Switzerland in patients with neuroendocrine GEP tumours. A dose escalating scheme of up to a cumulative activity of 160 mCi (6 GBq)/m^{2} divided over four cycles was used in initial studies with amino acid infusion as renal protection in half of the patients. Four of 29 patients developed renal insufficiency. These four patients had not received renal protection. The overall response rate was 24% in patients with GEP tumours who were either treated with up to 200 mCi (7.4 GBq)/m^{2} in four cycles [8]. Dosimetric and dose-finding studies with [^{90}Y-DOTA^{0},Tyr^{3}]octreotide with and without the administration of renal protecting agents were performed in Milan, Italy [9]. They observed no major acute reactions when administering doses up to 150 mCi (5.6 GBq) per cycle. In 43% of patients injected with 140 mCi (5.2 GBq), reversible grade 3 haematological toxicity was found and this was then defined as the maximum tolerated dose per cycle. Acute or delayed kidney failure did not develop in any of the patients, although follow-up was short. This included 30 patients in the first phase of the study who received three cycles of up to 2.59 GBq per cycle without renal protection. The same group later reported the results of a phase-1 study in 40 patients with somatostatin receptor positive tumours, including 21 with GEP tumours. The treatment consisted of two treatment cycles with cumulative total activities ranging from 160 to 300 mCi (5.9–11.1 GBq). Six of 21 (29%) patients had tumour regression and median duration of the response was 9 months [9].

[^{90}Y-DOTA^0,Tyr^3]octreotide was also given as part of a multi-centre phase-1 study [6]. Sixty patients received escalating activities up to 400 mCi (14.8 GBq)/m^2 in four cycles or up to 250 mCi (9.3 GBq)/m^2 single dose, without reaching the maximum tolerated single dose. For renal protection, amino acids were administered concomitantly with [^{90}Y-DOTA^0,Tyr^3]octreotide. The cumulative radiation dose to kidneys was limited to 27 Gy based on positron emission tomography data using [^{86}Y-DOTA^0,Tyr^3]octreotide, also under concomitant amino acid infusion. In three patients dose-limiting toxicity was observed: one transient hepatic toxicity, one thrombocytopenia grade 4 ($<25^*10^9$/l), and one MDS. Fifty-eight patients had carcinoids or other GEP tumours. Seven patients had MR (12%) and five had PR (9%). Disease was stable in 29 patients (50%) and progressive in 14 (24%). Outcome could not be determined in three patients. In the subgroup of 41 patients with at least stable disease (SD) as treatment outcome, median time to progression was 29.3 months. Median overall survival since the start of therapy was 36.7 months, considering all patients.

In the same group of patients and thus using the same treatment protocol, long-term follow-up of kidney function was performed. As there is physiological renal retention of radiolabelled somatostatin analogues, the renal radiation dose is a limiting factor in the amount of radioactivity that can be safely administered. Valkema et al. [11] reported a median annual decline in creatinine clearance of 7.3% in patients treated with [^{90}Y-DOTA^0,Tyr^3]octreotide. The following factors probably contribute to the rate of this decline: cumulative renal radiation dose, renal radiation dose per cycle, age, hypertension and diabetes. In 2 of 28 patients radiation nephropathy was histologically confirmed.

[^{177}Lu-DOTA^0,Tyr^3]octreotate was the next somatostatin analogue for PRRT and is being used in our medical center since the year 2000. [DOTA^0,Tyr^3]octreotate differs from [DOTA^0,Tyr^3]octreotide in that the C-terminal threoninol of the octapeptide has been replaced with threonine. Compared with [DOTA^0,Tyr^3]octreotide, it shows considerable improvement in binding to sst$_2$-positive tissues *in vitro* and *in vivo* [12, 13]. Compared to [^{111}In-DTPA^0]octreotide and [^{177}Lu-DOTA^0,Tyr^3]octreotide, [^{177}Lu-DOTA^0,Tyr^3]octreotate represents an important improvement because of the higher absorbed radiation doses that can be achieved to most tumours with about equal radiation doses to dose-limiting organs [14, 15]. ^{90}Y and ^{177}Lu-labeled peptides have greater therapeutic potential compared to ^{111}In-labeled peptides, for their emitted β-particle range exceeds the cell diameter, enabling irradiation of neighboring tumour cells, which is favorable in case of heterogeneous receptor expression. ^{177}Lu, as compared to ^{90}Y, has a lower tissue penetration range which is favorable for treatment of small tumours, whereas ^{90}Y might be more effective in tumours with a larger diameter [16, 17]. In contrast to ^{90}Y, ^{177}Lu also emits low energy γ-rays which directly allows imaging and dosimetry following [^{177}Lu-DOTA^0,Tyr^3]octreotate therapy (see also Fig. 7.2). Treatment with [^{177}Lu-DOTA^0,Tyr^3]octreotate in patients with GEP tumours resulted in complete or partial remission in 28% of patients [18]. Median time to progression was more than 36 months in patients who had either stable disease or tumour regression after treatment. In addition, patients treated with [^{177}Lu-DOTA^0,Tyr^3]octreotate indicated a significant improvement of their quality of life [19].

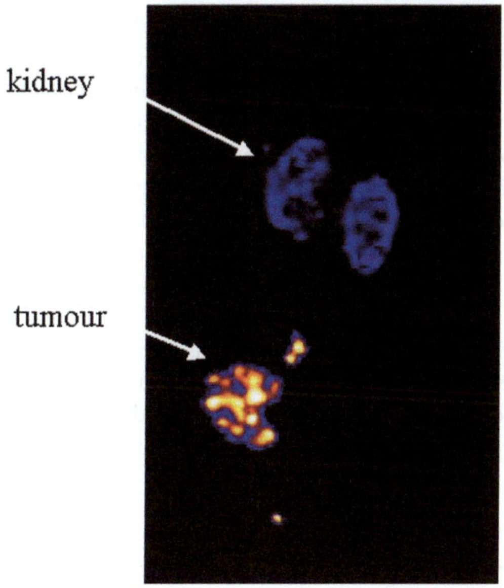

Fig. 7.2 SPECT scan (NanoSPECT, Bioscan) of a rat bearing a CA20948 tumour (expressing sst_2) showing uptake of [^{177}Lu-DOTA^0, Tyr^3]octreotate in tumour and kidneys. Scan was taken at 4 h p.i. of a therapeutic dose of [^{177}Lu-DOTA^0, Tyr^3]octreotate

In summary, PRRT with radiolabeled somatostatin analogues is a promising treatment option for patients with inoperable or metastasized neuroendocrine tumours. Tumour regression can be obtained with [^{90}Y-DOTA^0,Tyr^3]octreotide and [^{177}Lu-DOTA^0,Tyr^3]octreotate and survival improvement has been described for [^{90}Y-DOTA^0,Tyr^3]octreotide [6]. Additionally, symptomatic improvement may occur with the various ^{111}In, ^{90}Y, and ^{177}Lu-labeled somatostatin analogues being used. The side-effects of PRRT are few and mostly mild, certainly when using kidney protective agents. If more widespread use of PRRT is possible, such therapy might become the therapy of first choice in patients with metastasized or inoperable GEP tumours.

Developments

New Peptide Analogues

The native structure of peptides makes them sensitive to peptidases. They are rapidly broken down in blood and other tissues, restricting their potential use as radiopharmaceuticals. Metabolically stable analogues are therefore preferable for clinical application. Strategies to stabilize peptides include the introduction of non-biodegradable peptide bonds, stabilized amino acid derivatives replacing the natural amino acids, and cyclization.

High *in vivo* stability is advantageous but not sufficient for good target-to-non target ratios. One important factor isalso long retention time of nuclide at the tumour site and rapid clearance of nuclide from non-target tissues and blood. Internalisation of the radiolabeled peptides may lead to longer residence time of nuclide [20]. Peptide agonists often undergo receptor-mediated endocytosis enabling internalisation of the radionuclide into the tumour, whereas antagonists do most often not internalize [21]. Major research into design peptide based radiopharmaceuticals has focused on receptor-agonists. Recently, antagonistic analogues of somatostatin and bombesin were shown most suitable for receptor targeting as well [22, 23].

Subtle changes in peptide structures as described above, can have dramatic effects on the receptor-binding capacity and biodistribution of the compound. Attempts to improve the stability of the radiolabeled peptide can at the same time be fatal for its targeting abilities, e.g. due to loss of receptor-binding affinity.

SST Receptor-Targeting Peptides for Imaging and Therapy

^{99m}Tc-labeled somatostatin analogues like hydrazinonicotinamide (Hynic)-derivatised ^{99m}Tc-[Hynic-Tyr^3]octreotide, ^{99m}Tc-[Hynic-Tyr^3]octreotate [24–28], and tetraamine-functionalized derivative ^{99m}Tc-[N_4^0,Tyr^3]octreotate (Demotate 1) [29–31] can be regarded as promising new radiopharmaceuticals for sst scintigraphy. Both Hynic- and N_4-derivatized analogues were capable of detecting sst-expressing lesions in patients. Stable labeling of these analogues with the therapeutic radionuclide ^{188}Re will enable radionuclide therapy.

Compared to single-photon emission computed tomography (SPECT) imaging, clinical positron emission tomography (PET) imaging provides higher spatial resolution and the possibility to more accurately quantitate tumour and normal organ uptake. For PET imaging, peptides can be labeled with positron emitting radionuclides such as ^{68}Ga, ^{18}F, ^{64}Cu, ^{86}Y, ^{89}Zr, and ^{124}I. In contrast to other PET radionuclides, that require a cyclotron for production, ^{68}Ga can be produced in-house using a ^{68}Ge/^{68}Ga generator [32]. Antunes et al. [33] demonstrated that $^{67/68}$Ga-DOTA-octapeptides show distinctly better preclinical, pharmacological performances than the ^{111}In-labelled peptides in corresponding animal models. In addition, PET imaging using ^{68}Ga-[DOTA^0-Tyr^3]octreotide has been shown to have favorable detection characteristics [34, 35].

The radiolabeled analogues of octreotide and octreotate, including the analogues described above, have high binding-affinity for sst_2 [12], the most frequently expressed receptor subtype in neuroendocrine. tumours.In some cancers, however, sst_2 is absent or expressed only in low density whereas other subtype receptors are present [36, 37]. The heterogeneous and concomitant sst receptor subtype expression strongly pleads for tracers, or combinations of tracers, that can target more than one sst receptor *in vivo*. Ginj et al. evaluated 24 DOTA-somatostatin analogues, all based on the octreotide using a systematic modification at amino acid position 3 [38]. Two analogues, namely [DOTA^0-Nal^3]octreotide and [DOTA^0-BzThi^3]octreotide presented high binding affinity for sst_2, sst_3 and sst_5. ^{68}Ga-labeled [DOTA^0-Nal^3]octreotide has been shown to be a good tracer for primary diagnostic and follow-up studies in patients suspected from or with proven sst receptor-expressing tumours [39, 40]. Wehrmann et al. [41] found [^{177}Lu-DOTA^0-Nal^3]octreotide having a significantly higher uptake in whole-body and normal tissue as compared to ^{177}Lu-[DOTA^0-Tyr^3]octreotate, leading to a significantly higher whole-body dose. Renal and spleen uptake and radiation doses were not significantly higher. The uptake in tumor lesions and the mean absorbed tumor dose were higher for ^{177}Lu-[DOTA^0-Tyr^3]octreotate. They conclude that the high interpatient variability of their results makes an individual patient dosimetry obligatory.

As mentioned above, peptide agonists internalize into the cell after receptor-binding, which is thought to be essential for good retention of radionuclides in target cells. IGinj et al., however, recently reported promising and interesting results in a preclinical study comparing the targeting characteristics of sst_2 or sst_3 selective agonists versus antagonists [22]. They found that these labelled sst_2 and sst_3 antagonists, even though they did not internalize, presented higher accumulation in tumour cells compared to agonists, whereas the receptor affinity of agonists and antagonists was in the same range. In addition, accumulation in non-tumour tissues, except for that in the kidneys, was less for the antagonists than for agonists up to 24 hours after injection. These results suggest that antagonists may be better candidates to target tumours than agonists. The authors attribute the superior antagonist accumulation to binding to a larger variety of receptor configurations. Recently, the observation that antagonists may be preferable for receptor targeting to agonists has been translated to bombesin receptor antagonists [23]. The use of such potent radiolabeled antagonists for *in vivo* tumour targeting may considerably improve the sensitivity of future tumour imaging and PRRT efficacy.

GRP Receptor-Targeting Peptides

Overexpression of GRP receptors has been demonstrated in a large number of human tumours, including prostate and breast tumours [42], which are among the major causes of cancer death world wide [43]. Bombesin (BN) is a 14 amino acid peptide with high affinity for the GRP receptor and radiolabeled analogues of BN might therefore be useful for GRP receptor-targeted tumour imaging and therapy.

The first attempts to develop a radiolabeled BN analogue for diagnostic SPECT imaging were aimed at radioiodinated peptides. The iodine labeled compounds were found to be very unstable and iodine was rapidly cleared from the tumour cells [44]. Now, more than 10 years later several ^{111}In and ^{99m}Tc labeled BN analogues have been developed with favorable *in vivo* characteristics for SPECT imaging of GRP receptor-expressing tumours [45–50].

^{99m}Tc-labeled bombesin analogues have a tendency to accumulate in the liver and intestines as a result of their high lipophilicity. This high unspecific accumulation of nuclides interferes with detection of GRP receptor-positive lesions in the abdominal area. Much effort has been put into reducing the lipophilicity of the ^{99m}Tc-labeled BN analogues. Ferro-Flores et al. conjugated the bifunctional chelator HYNIC and the co-ligand EDDA (ethylenediamine-*N,N*-diacetic acid) to bombesin for the preparation of ^{99m}Tc-EDDA/HYNIC-[Lys^3]-BN. This conjugation of HYNIC resulted in less lipophilic properties of the peptide and consequently lower hepatobiliary and predominantly renal excretion [51]. Furthermore, Garcia Garayoa et al. recently showed that the introduction of a hydrophilic spacer between the peptide sequence and the ^{99m}Tc-binding complex can reduce the high lipophilicity, and improve tumour-to-non tumour ratios [52].

Next to tumour diagnosis, staging, and localization, ^{111}In-labeled peptide analogues are often used as surrogates to determine the biodistribution and dosimetry of therapeutic radiopharmaceuticals labeled with radiometals like ^{90}Y. DTPA and DOTA are being used as chelating systems coupled to the BN analogues for this purpose [53]. ^{111}In-DTPA-BN analogues, e.g. [^{111}In-DTPA-Pro^1,Tyr^4]BN [21, 50] have been reported to have good receptor-targeted tumour uptake and rapid clearance from non target tissues and blood via the kidneys and the urinary tract. Substitution of the DTPA chelator system in the [DTPA-Pro^1,Tyr^4]BN analogue by DOTA was previously found to have favorable effects on the receptor-binding characteristics of this radioligand [50]. We recently synthesized a new DTPA-coupled BN analogue, [^{111}In-DTPA-ACMpip^5,Tha^6,βAla^{11},Tha^{13},Nle^{14}]BN(5-14) (Cmp 3), with a marginally increased stability in human serum compared to that of [^{111}In-DTPA-Pro^1,Tyr^4]BN, but with a significantly higher GRP receptor-mediated tumour uptake *in vivo* in animal studies [54]. As ^{111}In-Cmp 3 seems promising for SPECT imaging of GRP receptor-expressing tumours, replacing the DTPA chelator by a DOTA would enable therapeutic use of the compound, and diagnostic PET imaging.

Most of the recent studies on newly developed BN peptide analogues focus on the DOTA-chelating system for its multipurpose utilization options: SPECT, PET, and PRRT [20, 55–61]. For example, DOTA-PESIN (DOTA-PEG$_4$-BN(7-14)) was demonstrated to be a very promising new compound. Although it has only a moderate affinity for the GRP receptor, it presented good *in vivo* tumour uptake in animal studies [55]. Clearance of the compound proceeded via the kidneys and the urinary tract with fast washout from GRP receptor-negative tissues but rather high accumulation in the kidneys. The high kidney retention could not be reduced by co-injection of lysine.

Another very promising DOTA-BN analogue is ^{177}Lu-AMBA [61]. This compound consists of DOTA attached to the BN(7-14) sequence by a short linker. ^{177}Lu-AMBA, like DOTA-PESIN, showed in animals high GRP receptor-mediated tumour uptake with good tumour retention, and favorable tumour-to-background ratios. *In vivo* tumour treatment with ^{177}Lu-AMBA resulted in a significantly prolonged survival of tumour-bearing mice, and decreased tumour growth rate over that of controls. Like DOTA-PESIN, ^{177}Lu-AMBA is excreted via the kidneys, and the relatively high kidney retention cannot be reduced by co-injection of lysine, which is probably due to the lack of lysine residues in these peptide sequences.

However, the accumulation of radioactivity in the kidneys is still 50% lower for the DTPA- and DOTA-derivatized BN analogues compared to that of somatostatin analogues.

PRRT using the BN analogues described above may be promising. Clinical scintigraphy with ^{99m}Tc- and ^{68}Ga-labeled BN analogues could clearly delineate tumour lesions, involved lymph nodes, and metastases [47, 62, 63]. However, also comparatively high uptake in non-targeted, GRP receptor-positive tissues such as pancreas and intestines was found, which is unfavorable for PRRT. In a pre-clinical study using ^{111}In-Cmp 3 we found that increasing amounts of injected peptide mass in tumour-bearing rats decreased uptake in receptor-positive normal tissues more than that in the tumour. Also pre-injection of excess unlabeled peptide before administration of radiolabeled compound was shown to be profitable for tumour uptake compared to that in receptor-expressing normal tissues [64]. These effects were also found with ^{177}Lu-AMBA in tumour bearing mice [61]. Thus, injection of higher peptide mass and/or pre-injection of excess BN may increase tumour-to-non tumour ratios.

Taking into account the biologic activity of BN agonists in patients and the much quicker pancreatic wash-out of radiolabelled antagonist than that of agonist [23], the use of GRP receptor antagonists for pre-injection and for radionuclide therapy might be highly preferable.

Radiolabeled BN analogues are of particular interest for PRRT of advanced prostate cancer patients who do not respond to hormone therapy. So far, the best treatment strategies available for this group of patients are only marginally effective [65, 66]. However, in a study evaluating GRP receptor-expression in human prostate cancer xenograft models representing the different stages of prostate tumour development, including the shift from androgen-dependent towards androgen-independent tumour growth, we found high GRP receptor density only in androgen–dependent prostate cancer xenografts. These results suggest high GRP receptor expression in the early, androgen-dependent, stages of prostate tumour development and not in later stages. In addition, simulation of androgen ablation treatment in the animal model (i.e. castration) strongly reduced GRP receptor-expression in androgen-dependent tumours, suggesting that GRP receptor expression in human prostate cancer is androgen-regulated [67]. Studies evaluating GRP receptor-expression on clinical prostate cancer tissue samples are underway to determine whether these results are clinically relevant.

The application of BN peptides in cancer patients is still in its infancy [47, 62, 63]. However, recent developments in the synthesis of new promising BN analogues are encouraging for further utilization in clinical studies.

NT Receptor-Targeting Peptides

Neuroendocrine pancreatic tumours can be successfully localized and treated using radiolabeled somatostatin analogues. Exocrine pancreatic cancer, however, does not express a sufficient level of somatostatin receptors for scintigraphic imaging of these tumours. Reubi et al. reported that 75% of ductal pancreatic carcinomas overexpressed neurotensin (NT) receptors, whereas normal pancreatic tissue, pancreatitis and endocrine pancreatic tumours were NT receptor-negative [68]. Neurotensin is a 13-amino acid peptide expressed both in the central nervous system and in peripheral tissues, mainly the gastrointestinal tract [69, 70]. The instability of native neurotensin prompted several groups [71–76] to synthesize neurotensin analogues less susceptible to degradation, while maintaining the binding affinity to the NT receptors. Pre-clinical studies using ^{111}In-labeled DTPA (MP2530) and DOTA (MP2656) linked NT analogues demonstrated that subtle changes by introducing non-natural amino acids on specific positions can be made in the C-terminal part of the peptide, the crucial part for binding and biological activity, without markedly affecting the binding properties [77]. These NT analogues displayed good receptor-mediated uptake in NT receptor–expressing HT29 xenografts and were thus promising tools for imaging of exocrine pancreatic tumours. PRRT using these analogues might however be hampered by the comparatively high kidney retention of the ^{111}In-NT analogues. Recently, Maes et al. [73] reported a triply-stabilized ^{99m}Tc-labeled NT (NT-XIX) analogue with a high tumour uptake and a reduced kidney uptake which led to a superior tumour-to-kidney ratio compared to the ^{111}In-labeled analogues. Also ^{99m}Tc-Demotensin 4, a doubly-stabilized NT analogue reported by Nock et al. [72], showed a favorable tumour-to-kidney ratio in the same animal model. Still, the tumour-to-intestine and tumour-to-liver ratios were considerably higher for the ^{111}In-labeled analogues, which is favorable for visualisation of the pancreatic tumours in patients [78].

Only one clinical evaluation study using a radiolabeled NT analogue has been reported [79]. This study included four exocrine pancreatic cancer patients, who were injected with the NT analogue: ^{99m}Tc-NT-XI. Scintigraphic imaging showed moderate tumour uptake in one patient whereas the other three patients showed no tumour uptake. Two out of these three patients were found to have a NT receptor-negative tumour.

CCK$_2$ Receptor-Targeting Peptides

Unlike other neuroendocrine tumours, somatostatin receptor expression is rather low in medullary thyroid cancer (MTC) and is completely absent in clinically aggressive forms of the disease [80, 81]. The presence of cholecystokinin-2 (CCK$_2$) receptors was shown in more than 90% of MTCs, and in a high percentage of small cell lung cancers, stromal ovarian cancers, astrocytomas and several other tumour types [82]. On the basis of these findings, Behr et al. [83] evaluated the suitability of radioiodinated gastrin, a specific high affinity ligand for the CCK$_2$ receptor, for targeting CCK$_2$ receptor expressing tumours *in vivo*. Their data suggested that gastrin analogues may represent a useful new class of receptor-binding peptides for diagnosis and therapy of a variety of tumour types, including MTC. Reubi et al.

[84] developed DTPA-conjugated CCK_2 receptor binding CCK analogues, evaluated their receptor-binding characteristics and obtained initial preclinical biodistribution data in non tumour-bearing rats. For the DOTA counterpart of the most promising analogue [^{111}In-DOTA^0]CCK_8, a high CCK_2 receptor affinity was found. The latter analogue could visualize CCK_2 receptor-expressing tumours *in vivo* in rats [85], and also in patients with advanced metastatic MTC, [^{111}In-DTPA^0]CCK_8 was able to visualize the tumour lesions [86]. Recently, Mather et al. [87] evaluated 34 ^{111}In-labelled compounds based on the C-terminal sequences of CCK-8 or minigastrin. Minigastrin analogs containing a pentaglutamate sequence showed the highest tumor uptake but very high renal retention. CCK analogs showed the lowest tumor and renal uptake. Interestingly, insertion of histidine residues in the sequence reduced kidney uptake by a factor of almost twofold. In AR42J tumor-bearing mice, the peptide with the sequence DOTA-HHEAYGWMDF-NH2 showed the highest tumor-to-kidney ratio of all peptides studied, making this peptide a worthwhile candidate for clinical studies.

A clinical study in MTC patients showed that most of the tumour sites could be visualized with ^{111}In-DTPA-minigastrin [83, 88]. Nock et al. synthesized ^{99m}Tc-labeled N_4-derivatized analogues of minigastrin [89]. Preclinical evaluation studies resulted in the selection of [N_4^{0-1},Gly^0,(D)Glu^1]minigastrin (Demogastrin 2) as the most promising CCK_2-targeting analogue for tumour imaging. Recent clinical studies by Gotthardt et al. [90, 91] in patients with metastatic/recurrent MTC compared the results of CCK_2 (gastrin) receptor scintigraphy (GRS), using [^{111}In-(D)Glu^1]minigastrin, with somatostatin receptor scintigraphy (SRS), CT and ^{18}F-FDG PET. They found that GRS had a higher tumour detection rate than SRS and ^{18}F-FDG PET. GRS in combination with CT was most effective in the detection of metastatic MTC. Furthermore, GRS in patients bearing neuroendocrine tumours other than MTC detected additional tumour sites that were missed in SRS in 20% of patients. The authors conclude that GRS may become the scintigraphic imaging modality of choice in MTC patients. In conclusion, preclinical and clinical studies have shown the suitability of radiolabeled CCK and gastrin analogues for scintigraphy of CCK_2 receptor expressing tumours such as MTC. PRRT using these radioligands is still preliminary, but its future is promising.

GLP-1 Receptor-Targeting Peptides

A new promising candidate for *in vivo* tumour targeting is glucagon-like peptide 1 (GLP-1) receptor, a member of the glucagon receptor family [92]. The GLP-1 receptor was recently shown to be highly overexpressed in human endocrine tumours, in particular insulinomas, gastrinomas [93], and pheochromocytomas [94].

Similar to other naturally occurring receptor-binding ligands, native GLP-1 receptor agonists are rapidly degraded in the blood [95, 96]. Therefore, Gotthardt et al. evaluated the more stable GLP-1 selective analogue exendin, which was shown to have potential for scintigraphic imaging of GLP-1 receptor-expressing tumours [97]. Recently, the exendin analogue has been further optimized, which has led to two new, ^{111}In-DTPA-conjugated, Exendin-4 analogues: ^{111}In-DTPA-Lys^{40}-exendin-4 [98] and [Lys^{40}(Ahx-DTPA-^{111}In)NH_2]exendin-4 [99]. Both analogues showed encouraging preclinical characteristics with high GLP-1 receptor-mediated uptake in target tissues and good target-to-background ratios *in vivo* in animal models. In addition, Wicky et al. showed that [Lys^{40}(Ahx-DTPA-^{111}In)NH_2]exendin-4 efficiently repressed insulinoma growth in mice [100]. Kidney toxicity was found to be the limiting factor in this treatment strategy.

No clinical study using GLP-1 receptor-targeting analogues has been reported so far. For therapeutic purposes, high kidney retention of the exendin-4 analogues could be problematic. Nevertheless, when this high accumulation in the kidneys can be overcome, high GLP-1 receptor-expression on tumours like insulinomas, in combination with the favorable *in vivo* characteristics of the recent exendin-4 analogues, gives GLP-1 receptor-targeted PRRT serious potential.

$\alpha_v\beta_3$ *Integrin-Targeting Peptides*

Cell matrix interactions are of fundamental importance for tumour invasion and formation of metastases as well as tumour-induced angiogenesis.

The $\alpha_v\beta_3$ integrin is a transmembrane protein which is preferentially expressed on proliferating endothelial cells [101], whereas it is absent on quiescent endothelial cells. For growth beyond the size of 1–2 mm in diameter, tumours require the formation of new blood vessels. The $\alpha_v\beta_3$ receptors are overexpressed on these newly formed blood vessels of actively growing tumours, and are therefore potential targets for receptor-mediated tumour imaging and therapy and for planning and monitoring of $\alpha_v\beta_3$ targeting treatment strategies.

It was found that the essential amino acid sequence for the binding of extracellular matrix proteins to $\alpha_v\beta_3$ receptors is arginine-glycine-aspartic acid (RGD) [102]. Several studies have been devoted to developing optimized $\alpha_v\beta_3$ targeting compounds. In summary, it was found that cyclic analogues of RGD containing five amino acids (RGD sequence + hydrophobic amino acid in position 4 + one additional amino acid in position 5) have the highest $\alpha_v\beta_3$ binding affinities [103, 104]. Radiolabeled analogues containing the five amino acid cyclic RGD sequence have been synthesized and evaluated for their $\alpha_v\beta_3$ targeting characteristics. Among them are DTPA and DOTA conjugated analogues radiolabelled with ^{111}In, ^{90}Y, ^{177}Lu, ^{68}Ga and ^{64}Cu, enabling SPECT and PET imaging and PRRT [105, 106]. Also ^{18}F-labeled cyclic RGD analogues for PET imaging have been characterized [106–108]. In patients, Beer et al. showed that PET imaging using the RGD analogue, ^{18}F-galacto-RGD, can effectively indicate the level of $\alpha_v\beta_3$ expression in man [109–111].

Dijkgraaf et al. [112] developed multivalent RGD peptides in an attempt to increase receptor-binding affinity. They synthesized and compared the *in vitro* and *in vivo* $\alpha_v\beta_3$ targeting characteristics of DOTA-linked monomeric, dimeric, and tetrameric RGD peptides radiolabeled with ^{111}In. They found enhanced receptor affinity *in vitro* and better tumour uptake *in vivo* for the tetrameric compound compared to its monomeric and dimeric analogues. Alternatively, they synthesized multimeric RGD peptides as dendrimers: macromolecules consisting of multiple perfectly branched monomers. Consistent with their previous results, the tetrameric RGD dendrimer showed enhanced affinity and significantly higher tumour uptake compared to its monomeric and dimeric analogues [113]. The authors ascribe the improved targeting characteristics of the multimer to the enhanced local concentration of RGD units in the vicinity of the receptor (statistical rebinding) and not to binding of the compound to multiple $\alpha_v\beta_3$ receptors. Unfortunately, the kidney retention of the mulitimeric peptides was also increased resulting in unfavorable tumour-to-kidney ratios. Introduction of a linker between the peptide moiety and the DOTA chelator, in an attempt to improve the target-to-background ratios of the peptide, led to a marginal enhancement of the tumour-to-kidney ratio only [114]. In a study evaluating the targeting potential of a cyclic RGD analogue in an intraperitoneally (i.p.) growing tumour model, Dijkgraaf et al. found that i.p. *vs* i.v injection of the radiolabeled RGD peptide resulted in markedly higher tumour uptake after i.p. administration, whereas uptake in the other organs like kidneys were unaffected by the route of administration. PRRT experiments in this model indicated that i.p. growing tumours can be inhibited significantly by i.p. injection of a therapeutic dose of ^{177}Lu-labeled RGD analogue [115].

Multimeric RGD peptides are promising tools for *in vivo* imaging of tumour angiogenesis in cancer patients. $\alpha_v\beta_3$ targeted PRRT with these compounds might particularly be used for i.p. growing tumours. Currently, ^{18}F-galacto-RGD is the only $\alpha_v\beta_3$-targeting peptide shown effective for tumour imaging in patients [111].

Receptor Density on Target Cells

By increasing the receptor density on tumour cells in patients to be treated with radiolabeled peptides, and thereby increasing radioactivity uptake in the tumour, the therapeutic window can be enlarged.

Up-Regulation

During the last three decades several reports have been published concerning hormones and growth factors inducing increased expression of receptors on tumour cells [116–124].

Up-regulation of peptide receptors on tumour cells following irradiation was first reported by Béhé et al. [125, 126], who reported that a total dose of 4 to 16 Gy of external beam irradiation led to up-regulation of both sst_2 and gastrin receptors on AR42J cells, *in vitro* as well as *in vivo*, in a time dependent way. This phenomenon was also investigated *in vitro* in NCI-H69 small cell lung cancer cells [127]. These cells were irradiated with a total dose of 4 Gy and the subsequent internalisation of [^{177}Lu-DTPA^0,Tyr^3]octreotate was 1.5–3 times increased compared to that in control cells.

Not only the use of external beam radiation, but also low therapeutic doses of radiolabeled peptides were found to induce sst_2 up-regulation. This was shown in two studies using CA20948 rat pancreatic tumour-bearing rats [128, 129]. These rats were treated with a comparatively low, non-curative dose of either [^{111}In-DTPA^0]octreotide [128] or [^{177}Lu-DOTA^0,Tyr^3]octreotate [129], and sst_2 receptor expression in different phases of the tumour response was determined versus base-line (control). Both studies revealed an increased sst_2 density on tumours re-growing after initial therapy-induced regression compared to control: treatment with [^{111}In-DTPA^0]octreotide resulted in a twofold increase, while [^{177}Lu-DOTA^0,Tyr^3]octreotate treatment presented a more pronounced effect (two- to five-fold increase). This radiation induced up-regulation of receptor expression might be important for improving the response rate in clinical PRRT. The clinical value, however, has to be determined.

Gene Therapy

In general, gene transfer methods can be applied to induce expression of a desired gene in a cell. This concept has been used for treatment of malignant diseases [130]. By using a vector, either viral or non-viral, a peptide receptor-encoding gene (or several genes) can be transferred into a tumour cell with the aim to enhance the uptake of radiolabeled peptide analogues. Gene therapy approaches in combination with PRRT might have some advantages: first, transduction of receptors is locally achieved (only in the tumour) and thereby a higher tumour-to-background ratio will be achieved. Second, constitutive receptor expression in the tumour is not required, therefore also receptor-negative tumours could theoretically be treated. And third, the therapeutic effect might be enormously increased by performing a dual gene transfer, meaning that another gene, for example a "suicide" gene, is co-transferred with the receptor gene into the tumour cell and can be simultaneously or subsequently used for treatment. On the other hand, patients with metastatic disease will be difficult to treat with gene therapy, since this requires systemic administration of gene therapy vectors, with all related risks. Therefore, mostly patients with circumscribed tumour lesions would probably benefit from gene therapy strategies, which is the case in glioblastoma and ovarian cancer patients.

Several groups have explored the possibility to increase sst expression on tumours using gene transfer modalities followed by non-invasive imaging of receptor expression or PRRT *in vitro* and *in vivo*. One of the first studies using the adenoviral vector AdCMVhSSTr2, encoding the human sst_2, was performed in intraperitoneally growing SKOV3.ip1 human ovarian cancer tumour and s.c. A-427 human non-small cell lung cancer tumour [131]. Biodistribution and gamma camera imaging showed higher uptake of various radiolabeled sst analogues in infected tumours, than in control tumours.

Zinn and Hemminki introduced the concept of dual gene transfer using a replication-incompetent adenoviral vector encoding sst_2 and a so-called "suicide gene": the herpes simplex virus type 1 thymidine kinase (HSV1-tk) [132, 133]. This gene encodes the thymidine kinase (tk) enzyme, that unlike mammalian tk, preferentially phosphorylates acycloguanosines, such as acyclovir (ACV) and ganciclovir (GCV), into monophosphate compounds. Cellular enzymes convert these monophosphates into di- and triphosphates, which are then trapped inside the cell. Zinn and co-workers showed that expression of both sst_2 and HSV1-tk following AdTKSSTR infection could be measured with ^{99m}Tc-P2045 and radioiodinated FIAU, respectively, in mice bearing an A-427 tumour [134]. In addition, it was found that sst_2 imaging *in vivo* following viral infection was more favorable than tk imaging, due to the excellent binding affinity of the sst_2 tracer [134]. These results indicate that sst_2 imaging is preferred over tk imaging, because analogues of sst_2 have high affinity and specificity for their receptor and show rapid internalisation. Prerequisite of the use of sst_2 imaging is that expression of this receptor in the surrounding tissue is low.

Using an AdTKSSTR vector, our group showed a non-homogeneous uptake of specific sst_2 and HSV1-tk tracers in U87MG human glioma-bearing nude mice intra-tumourally infected with Ad5.tk.sst_2 [135]. We used small animal SPECT/CT imaging plus *ex vivo* autoradiography and found a non-homogeneous radioactivity distribution in the viral infected tumours, probably visualizing the needle tracts of the viral injection procedure. Herewith a major hurdle of gene therapy was visualized: poor viral spread is not favorable for the therapeutic outcome.

Rogers and co-workers transfected A-427 tumours *in vivo* with adenovirus expressing sst_2, AdSSTr2. They performed therapy studies in animals, receiving AdSSTr2 infection and 400–500 μCi [^{90}Y]SMT-487 [136]. Animals that received viral infection plus radiolabeled peptide treatment showed a significantly reduced tumour quadrupling time compared to control animals, receiving no treatment or PRRT alone. In a later study by this group, sst_2 expression was effectively visualized with microPET imaging using a novel PET-tracer: ^{94m}Tc-Demotate 1 [137].

The use of molecular imaging in gene therapy experiments offers the opportunity to provide information about, for example, the location of vector delivery and the extent and magnitude of gene transfer and gene expression. Integrating imaging techniques such as SPECT and PET into these gene therapy protocols will make it possible to determine optimal treatment time points following vector administration. Furthermore, imaging might help to obtain optimized treatment protocols for gene therapy modalities.

Combination Treatment

Chemotherapeutics and Radiosensitizers

Recently, investigations have been started to combine PRRT with either chemotherapy or other radiosensitizing agents to increase therapeutic effects in patients with neuroendocrine tumours. Gotthardt et al. performed mono- and combination treatment in nude mice bearing AR42J tumours [138]. They examined [^{177}Lu-DOTA^0,Tyr^3]octreotide (^{177}Lu-DOTATOC) either alone or in combination with doxorubicin (DX) or cisplatinum (CS) during a 4-week period. They found that the combination of ^{177}Lu-DOTATOC plus DX was 14% and that of ^{177}Lu-DOTATOC plus CS was 23% more effective than ^{177}Lu-DOTATOC treatment alone, making the combination "PRRT plus chemotherapy" an effective approach to increase therapeutic efficacy in sst expressing tumours.

In patients, the radiosensitizing agent 5-fluorouracil (5-FU) was investigated in combination with high dose ^{111}In-labeled octreotide [139]. In 21 patients with neuroendocrine tumours, the efficacy and toxicity of this combination treatment was evaluated. The authors found that the combination of high dose [^{111}In-DTPA^0]octreotide and 5-FU was safe and symptomatic response rates were at least comparable to those reported for [^{111}In-DTPA^0]octreotide treatment alone. Stable disease or improvements in hormonal and functional scan abnormalities in patients with previous progression were achieved with the combination treatment. Our group recently started a pilot trial using the oral pro-drug of 5-FU, capecitabine, in combination with [^{177}Lu-DOTA^0,Tyr^3]octreotate in patients with GEP tumours to investigate the feasibility of combination treatment in these patients.

Johnson et al. recently investigated combination treatment of radiolabeled BN analogues with chemotherapy in a pre-clinical setting [59]. They examined the chemotherapeutic agents docetaxel (DC) and estramustine (EMP) in combination with ^{177}Lu labeled DOTA-8-AOC-BBN(7-14)NH_2 (^{177}Lu-BBN) in a PC-3 flank xenograft model. These chemotherapeutics were chosen since they are currently evaluated in clinical trials for the treatment of androgen independent prostate cancer. They work synergistically as microtubule inhibitors and offer an increased cytotoxic effect; they also exhibit radiosensitization properties. The results showed that mice treated with ^{177}Lu-BBN combined with either DC alone or DC + EMP showed a statistically significant longer survival, 107 and 109 days respectively, than the control animals (50 days). Furthermore, combination therapy demonstrated a significant survival advantage compared to the ^{177}Lu-BBN therapy alone. Blood was analyzed during the experiment until 2 weeks after the final therapy administration and no differences in blood cell counts were found.

Unfortunately, kidney damage was not evaluated in these studies. It is of interest to investigate the effect of chemotherapeutics combined with PRRT on radiation uptake in the kidneys and on the long term renal damage. Wild et al. reported therapy studies investigating the combination of the GLP-receptor binding analogue [^{111}In-DTPA^0]Exendin-4 and the angiogenesis inhibitor PTK in Rip1Tag2 mice. They found that combination therapy resulted in a significantly lower median tumour volume compared to monotherapy. In addition, this study did not reveal renal toxicity in the group that was treated with the combination [140].

An issue that also needs to be addressed is the effect chemotherapeutic agents might have on receptor expression on the tumour. Fueger and co-workers examined the possible influence of cytotoxic or cytostatic agents on binding characteristics of an sst ligand *in vitro* [141] and they found a reduced expression of high-affinity DOTA-lanreotide binding sites in response to the incubation with gemcitabine, camptotecin, mitomycin C and doxorubicin. In the case of gemcitabine, sst was again over-expressed after a 4-day recovery period, indicating that the down-regulation of receptor expression can be reversed. However, *in vivo* studies need to be performed to investigate the effect of chemotherapeutic agents on receptor expression, especially when combination treatment is given.

Combinations of Different Radionuclides

In pre-clinical studies, we found that the anti-tumour effect of radiolabeled sst analogues is dependent on tumour size [142, 143]. In a study comparing two radionuclides coupled to sst analogues, we demonstrated that [^{177}Lu-DOTA^{0}-Tyr^{3}]octreotate has a very good tumour cure rate in small tumours of approximately 0.5 cm^2, while larger tumours of about 7–9 cm^2 were better treated with [^{90}Y-DOTA-Tyr^{3}]octreotide [17]. These results agreed with the mathematical model proposed by O'Donoghue et al. [16]. For different radionuclide energies, the model predicts the chance of curation for different tumour diameters: according to this model, radionuclides with lower energies (e.g. ^{177}Lu) are optimal for small tumours and radionuclides with higher energies (e.g. ^{90}Y) are optimal for larger tumours. This indicates that PRRT in patients with sst_2-positive tumours of different sizes might have better potential with a combination of radionuclides with higher and lower energy β-particles. However, the feasibility of this combination treatment should be further evaluated in patients, preferably in a randomized clinical trial.

Hybrid Molecules: Apoptosis-Inducing Peptides

The receptor-targeted delivery of cytotoxic agents was first proposed to reduce toxicity of chemotherapeutic drugs in patients [144]. In order to achieve this, chemotherapeutic agents were linked to peptide analogues, resulting in the internalisation of the complete molecule into the tumour cell. It is conceivable that these hybrid peptides can be used to improve PRRT, for example in tumours with a low receptor expression or in non-responding receptor-expressing tumour types [145]. Hofland et al. and Nagy et al. have described the development and anti-tumour action of different cytotoxic sst analogues [145, 146]. Recently, new publications showed that the targeted cytotoxic analogue AN-238, a conjugate based on the sst analogue RC-121 coupled to a derivative of doxorubicin, could offer a more effective therapy than RC-121 treatment alone in mice bearing human melanoma tumours [147] or endometrial tumours [148]. In addition, the combination of targeted cytotoxic conjugates of luteinizing hormone-releasing hormone (LHRH) (AN-207), somatostatin (AN-238) and BN (AN-215) were tested in mice bearing ovarian tumours [149]. Results showed that AN-238 and AN-215 significantly inhibited tumour growth, the combination being equally effective. The authors concluded that combination treatment is feasible and effective with low toxicity risk [149]. Other studies showed that mice bearing human glioblastomas, U118MG and U87MG, could also be effectively treated with these agents. Both AN-215 and AN-238 could strongly reduce tumour growth in glioblastoma-bearing mice [150–152]. These studies show that a wide variety of receptor-expressing tumours can be treated with receptor-targeted chemotherapeutic agents, although tumour cure was not yet achieved in these animal studies. It would be of great interest to investigate the effects on tumour growth when these agents are radiolabeled with therapeutic radionuclides or combined with PRRT strategies. Meanwhile, clinical trials using these (unlabeled) targeted chemotherapeutic agents are ongoing [145, 148].

Other examples of hybrid peptides are camptothecin conjugated analogues of sst [153, 154] or BN [155, 156]. Several *in vitro* studies have shown increased efficacy of treatment with camptothecin-sst and camptothecin-BN conjugates compared to camptothecin alone [153–156]. This concept was further investigated in mice bearing NCI-H1299 human non-small cell lung tumours, which were treated with the camptothecin-BN conjugate and a camptothecin-BN analogue that does not specifically bind the receptor. Tumour growth was significantly reduced after incubation with the camptothecin-BN conjugate, demonstrating the importance of receptor-specific binding and internalisation of the conjugate to the tumour cell for therapeutic purposes [155].

Recently, we investigated the hybrid peptide [RGD-DTPA^0]octreotate radiolabeled with ^{111}In [146, 157–159]. Arg-Gly-Asp (RGD) binds the integrin receptor $\alpha_v\beta_3$ and is known as an apoptosis-inducing agent by direct activation of caspase 3 [160]. We found that [RGD-^{111}In-DTPA^0]octreotate predominantly internalizes via the sst$_2$, probably due to the higher affinity of octreotate for the sst$_2$ than that of RGD for the $\alpha_v\beta_3$ [157]. Furthermore, when [RGD-^{111}In-DTPA^0]octreotate was compared with either [^{111}In-DTPA^0]RGD or [^{111}In-DTPA^0]octreotate in a clonogenic survival assay using sst$_2$/$\alpha_v\beta_3$ expressing tumour cells [RGD-^{111}In-DTPA^0]octreotate showed the highest tumouricidal effects [158]. Caspase 3 activity assays confirmed that [RGD-^{111}In-DTPA^0]octreotate had the most pronounced activation of this executioner protease in the apoptosis pathway. Unfortunately, *in vivo* studies showed that renal uptake of [RGD-^{111}In-DTPA^0]octreotate was high, a disadvantage for PRRT [159]. However, caspase-3 activity after incubation with the unlabeled hybrid peptide was found to be higher than after RGD or DTPA-octreotide alone, making unlabeled [RGD-DTPA^0]octreotate during or after PRRT interesting as well [159].

Combinations of Different Peptides: Multi-Receptor Targeting

Many cancer types simultaneous overexpress several peptide receptors [93]. There are a number of possible advantages in utilizing multiple radiolabeled ligands for therapeutic application of neuroendocrine tumours: (1) *in vivo* application of multi-receptor targeting agents selectively increases the nuclide accumulation in tumours, (2) some of the receptors are not homogeneously expressed, and by multi-receptor targeting it is possible to achieve a higher tumouricidal effect, (3) there is a reduced risk of loss of some peptide receptors during therapy, due to tumour dedifferentiation and the subsequent loss of some peptide receptors [17].

Reubi et al. performed *in vitro* autoradiography on neuroendocrine tumours including ileal carcinoids, bronchial carcinoids, insulinomas, gastrinomas, glucagonomas and vipomas [93]. They found that all neuroendocrine tumours examined expressed two or more receptors and several combinations of peptides are of interest for optimal targeting of neuroendocrine tumours *in vivo*: (1) a combination of radiolabeled ligands for the glucagon-like peptide-1 (GLP-1) and CCK_2 receptors for insulinomas, (2) a mixture of sst_2, GLP-1 and GRP radiolabeled ligands for gastrinomas.

Radiation Protection in Normal Organs

Increasing the therapeutic window can also be achieved by reducing radiation toxicity to normal organs. In peptide(sst)-based therapy, the kidney is one of the dose-limiting organs and some clinical studies showed renal toxicity following PRRT [11, 161, 162]. It is therefore favorable to reduce the renal radiation dose, making it feasible to increase the total amount of injected radioactivity.

It has been found that radiolabeled somatostatin analogues were filtered and re-absorbed in the proximal tubules of rat kidneys [163]. Also, in the human kidney radioactivity was mostly concentrated in the cortex and the megalin/cubulin system was found to play an essential role in the re-absorption of octreotide [164, 165]. In addition, it was shown that 18% of the renal uptake of sst_2 targeting peptides can be dedicated to sst-mediated uptake [166].

Standard procedure to reduce renal uptake during PRRT using somatostatin analogues in our institution is a 4-hour infusion of a mixture of the positively charged amino acids lysine (25 g/l) and arginine (25 g/l) [18, 167]. We investigated whether oral administration of lysine could also reduce the renal uptake. In rats, we showed that oral administration of lysine reduced the radioactivity in the kidneys by 40%, which is comparable to the reduction found with intravenous administration of lysine [168].

Moreover, other agents, such as gelofusine [169, 170], colchicine [171] and the radioprotective drug amifostine [172], might improve the kidney protection strategies currently used in the clinic.

Conclusions

Many tumours over-express one or more receptors which can be targeted using receptor-specific radiolabeled peptides. So far, sst-targeting peptides are widely used for imaging and therapy of cancer patients. PRRT with ^{177}Lu labeled somatostatin analogues has resulted in symptomatic improvement, prolonged survival and enhanced quality of life of neuroendocrine tumour patients. PRS and PRRT targeting other tumour-specific receptors, such as GRP and CCK receptors, are well on their way to clinical utilization as well.

Literature shows that it is possible to increase the receptor density on tumour cells using different methods. In PRRT treatment, this would enable the administration of higher therapeutic doses to tumours, which might lead to a higher cure rate in patients.

Targeting one or several tumour-specific receptors by combinations of therapeutic agents, as well as by reducing non-target uptake of radioactivity, will enlarge the therapeutic window of PRRT. Clinical studies will provide more insight in the effects of combination treatment strategies in cancer patients.

References

1. Krenning, E. P., Teunissen, J. J., Valkema, R., et al.: Molecular radiotherapy with somatostatin analogs for (neuro-)endocrine tumors. J Endocrinol Invest 28, 146–150 (2005)
2. Krenning, E. P., Kwekkeboom, D. J., Bakker, W. H., et al.: Somatostatin receptor scintigraphy with [111In-DTPA-D-Phe1]- and [123I-Tyr3]-octreotide: the Rotterdam experience with more than 1000 patients. Eur J Nucl Med 20, 716–731 (1993)
3. Kwekkeboom, D., Krenning, E. P. and de Jong, M.: Peptide receptor imaging and therapy. J Nucl Med 41, 1704–1713 (2000)
4. Valkema, R., De Jong, M., Bakker, W. H., et al.: Phase I study of peptide receptor radionuclide therapy with [In-DTPA]octreotide: the Rotterdam experience. Semin Nucl Med 32, 110–122 (2002)
5. Bodei, L., Cremonesi, M., Zoboli, S., et al.: Receptor-mediated radionuclide therapy with 90Y-DOTATOC in association with amino acid infusion: a phase I study. Eur J Nucl Med Mol Imaging 30, 207–216 (2003)
6. Valkema, R., Pauwels, S., Kvols, L. K., et al.: Survival and response after peptide receptor radionuclide therapy with [90Y-DOTA0,Tyr3]octreotide in patients with advanced gastroenteropancreatic neuroendocrine tumors. Semin Nucl Med 36, 147–156 (2006)
7. Otte, A., Herrmann, R., Heppeler, A., et al.: Yttrium-90 DOTATOC: first clinical results. Eur J Nucl Med 26, 1439–1447 (1999)
8. Waldherr, C., Pless, M., Maecke, H. R., et al.: Tumor response and clinical benefit in neuroendocrine tumors after 7.4 GBq (90)Y-DOTATOC. J Nucl Med 43, 610–616 (2002)
9. Chinol, M., Bodei, L., Cremonesi, M., et al.: Receptor-mediated radiotherapy with Y-DOTA-DPhe-Tyr-octreotide: the experience of the European Institute of Oncology Group. Semin Nucl Med 32, 141–147 (2002)
10. van Essen, M., krenning, E. P., de Jong, M., et al.: Peptide receptor radionuclide therapy with radiolabelled somatostatin analogues in patients with somatostatin receptor positive tumours Acta Oncology, 46(6):723–34 (2007)
11. Valkema, R., Pauwels, S. A., Kvols, L. K., et al.: Long-term follow-up of renal function after peptide receptor radiation therapy with (90)Y-DOTA(0),Tyr(3)-octreotide and (177)Lu-DOTA(0), Tyr(3)-octreotate. J Nucl Med 46 (Suppl 1), 83S–91S (2005)
12. Reubi, J. C., Schar, J. C., Waser, B., et al.: Affinity profiles for human somatostatin receptor subtypes SST1-SST5 of somatostatin radiotracers selected for scintigraphic and radiotherapeutic use. Eur J Nucl Med 27, 273–282 (2000)
13. de Jong, M., Breeman, W. A., Bakker, W. H., et al.: Comparison of (111)In-labeled somatostatin analogues for tumor scintigraphy and radionuclide therapy. Cancer Res 58, 437–441 (1998)

14. Esser, J. P., Krenning, E. P., Teunissen, J. J., et al.: Comparison of [(177)Lu-DOTA(0),Tyr(3)] octreotate and [(177)Lu-DOTA(0),Tyr(3)]octreotide: which peptide is preferable for PRRT? Eur J Nucl Med Mol Imaging 33, 1346–1351 (2006)
15. Kwekkeboom, D. J., Bakker, W. H., Kooij, P. P., et al.: [177Lu-DOTAOTyr3]octreotate: comparison with [111In-DTPAo]octreotide in patients. Eur J Nucl Med 28, 1319–1325 (2001)
16. O'Donoghue, J. A., Bardies, M. and Wheldon, T. E.: Relationships between tumor size and curability for uniformly targeted therapy with beta-emitting radionuclides. J Nucl Med 36, 1902–1909 (1995)
17. de Jong, M., Breeman, W. A., Valkema, R., et al.: Combination radionuclide therapy using 177Lu- and 90Y-labeled somatostatin analogs. J Nucl Med 46 (Suppl 1), 13S–17S (2005)
18. Kwekkeboom, D. J., Teunissen, J. J., Bakker, W. H., et al.: Radiolabeled somatostatin analog [177Lu-DOTA0,Tyr3]octreotate in patients with endocrine gastroenteropancreatic tumors. J Clin Oncol 23, 2754–2762 (2005)
19. Teunissen, J. J., Kwekkeboom, D. J. and Krenning, E. P.: Quality of life in patients with gastroenteropancreatic tumors treated with [177Lu-DOTA0,Tyr3]octreotate. J Clin Oncol 22, 2724–2729 (2004)
20. Zhang, H., Chen, J., Waldherr, C., et al.: Synthesis and evaluation of bombesin derivatives on the basis of pan-bombesin peptides labeled with indium-111, lutetium-177, and yttrium-90 for targeting bombesin receptor-expressing tumors. Cancer Res 64, 6707–6715 (2004)
21. Breeman, W. A., Hofland, L. J., de Jong, M., et al.: Evaluation of radiolabelled bombesin analogues for receptor-targeted scintigraphy and radiotherapy. Int J Cancer 81, 658–665 (1999)
22. Ginj, M., Zhang, H., Waser, B., et al.: Radiolabeled somatostatin receptor antagonists are preferable to agonists for in vivo peptide receptor targeting of tumors. Proc Natl Acad Sci USA 103, 16136–16441 (2006)
23. Cescato, R., Maina, T., Nock, B., et al.: Bombesin receptor antagonists may be preferable to agonists for tumor targeting. J Nucl Med 49, 318–326 (2008)
24. Gabriel, M., Decristoforo, C., Donnemiller, E., et al.: An intrapatient comparison of 99 mTc-EDDA/HYNIC-TOC with 111In-DTPA-octreotide for diagnosis of somatostatin receptor-expressing tumors. J Nucl Med 44, 708–716 (2003)
25. Bangard, M., Behe, M., Guhlke, S., et al.: Detection of somatostatin receptor-positive tumours using the new 99 mTc-tricine HYNIC-D-Phe1-Tyr3-octreotide: first results in patients and comparison with 111In-DTPA-D-Phe1-octreotide. Eur J Nucl Med 27, 628–637 (2000)
26. Hubalewska-Dydejczyk, A., Fross-Baron, K., Golkowski, F., et al.: 99 mTc-EDDA/HYNIC-octreotate in detection of atypical bronchial carcinoid. Exp Clin Endocrinol Diabetes 115, 47–49 (2007)
27. Hubalewska-Dydejczyk, A., Fross-Baron, K., Mikolajczak, R., et al.: 99 mTc-EDDA/HYNIC-octreotate scintigraphy, an efficient method for the detection and staging of carcinoid tumours: results of 3 years' experience. Eur J Nucl Med Mol Imaging 33, 1123–1133 (2006)
28. Hubalewska-Dydejczyk, A., Szybinski, P., Fross-Baron, K., et al.: (99 m)Tc-EDDA/HYNIC-octreotate - a new radiotracer for detection and staging of NET: a case of metastatic duodenal carcinoid. Nucl Med Rev Cent East Eur 8, 155–156 (2005)
29. Gabriel, M., Decristoforo, C., Maina, T., et al.: 99 mTc-N4-[Tyr3]Octreotate versus 99 mTc-EDDA/HYNIC-[Tyr3]Octreotide: an intrapatient comparison of two novel Technetium-99 m labeled tracers for somatostatin receptor scintigraphy. Cancer Biother Radiopharm 19, 73–79 (2004)
30. Nikolopoulou, A., Maina, T., Sotiriou, P., et al.: Tetraamine-modified octreotide and octreotate: labeling with 99 mTc and preclinical comparison in AR4-2J cells and AR4-2J tumor-bearing mice. J Pept Sci 12, 124–131 (2006)
31. Decristoforo, C., Maina, T., Nock, B., et al.: 99 mTc-Demotate 1: first data in tumour patients-results of a pilot/phase I study. Eur J Nucl Med Mol Imaging 30, 1211–1219 (2003)
32. Breeman, W. A., de Jong, M., de Blois, E., et al.: Radiolabelling DOTA-peptides with 68 Ga. Eur J Nucl Med Mol Imaging 32, 478–485 (2005)

33. Antunes, P., Ginj, M., Zhang, H., et al.: Are radiogallium-labelled DOTA-conjugated somatostatin analogues superior to those labelled with other radiometals? Eur J Nucl Med Mol Imaging 34, 982–993 (2007)
34. Kowalski, J., Henze, M., Schuhmacher, J., et al.: Evaluation of positron emission tomography imaging using [68 Ga]-DOTA-D Phe(1)-Tyr(3)-Octreotide in comparison to [111In]-DTPAOC SPECT. First results in patients with neuroendocrine tumors. Mol Imaging Biol 5, 42–48 (2003)
35. Gabriel, M., Decristoforo, C., Kendler, D., et al.: 68 Ga-DOTA-Tyr3-octreotide PET in neuroendocrine tumors: comparison with somatostatin receptor scintigraphy and CT. J Nucl Med 48, 508–518 (2007)
36. Kulaksiz, H., Eissele, R., Rossler, D., et al.: Identification of somatostatin receptor subtypes 1, 2A, 3, and 5 in neuroendocrine tumours with subtype specific antibodies. Gut 50, 52–60 (2002)
37. Reubi, J. C., Waser, B., Schaer, J. C., et al.: Somatostatin receptor sst1-sst5 expression in normal and neoplastic human tissues using receptor autoradiography with subtype-selective ligands. Eur J Nucl Med 28, 836–846 (2001)
38. Ginj, M., Schmitt, J. S., Chen, J., et al.: Design, synthesis, and biological evaluation of somatostatin-based radiopeptides. Chem Biol 13, 1081–1090 (2006)
39. Wild, D., Macke, H. R., Waser, B., et al.: 68 Ga-DOTANOC: a first compound for PET imaging with high affinity for somatostatin receptor subtypes 2 and 5. Eur J Nucl Med Mol Imaging 32, 724 (2005)
40. Pettinato, C., Sarnelli, A., Di Donna, M., et al.: (68)Ga-DOTANOC: biodistribution and dosimetry in patients affected by neuroendocrine tumors. Eur J Nucl Med Mol Imaging 35, 72–79 (2008)
41. Wehrmann, C., Senftleben, S., Zachert, C., et al.: Results of individual patient dosimetry in peptide receptor radionuclide therapy with 177Lu DOTA-TATE and 177Lu DOTA-NOC. Cancer Biother Radiopharm 22, 406–416 (2007)
42. Reubi, J. C., Wenger, S., Schmuckli-Maurer, J., et al.: Bombesin receptor subtypes in human cancers: detection with the universal radioligand (125)I-[D-TYR(6), beta-ALA(11), PHE(13), NLE(14)] bombesin(6-14). Clin Cancer Res 8, 1139–1146 (2002)
43. Jemal, A., Siegel, R., Ward, E., et al.: Cancer statistics, 2007. CA Cancer J Clin 57, 43–66 (2007)
44. Breeman, W. A., de Jong, M., Bernard, B., et al.: Tissue distribution and metabolism of radioiodinated DTPA0, D-Tyr1 and Tyr3 derivatives of octreotide in rats. Anticancer Res 18, 83–89 (1998)
45. Nock, B., Nikolopoulou, A., Chiotellis, E., et al.: [(99 m)Tc]Demobesin 1, a novel potent bombesin analogue for GRP receptor-targeted tumour imaging. Eur J Nucl Med Mol Imaging 30, 247–258 (2003)
46. Nock, B. A., Nikolopoulou, A., Galanis, A., et al.: Potent bombesin-like peptides for GRP-receptor targeting of tumors with 99 mTc: a preclinical study. J Med Chem 48, 100–110 (2005)
47. Van de Wiele, C., Dumont, F., Vanden Broecke, R., et al.: Technetium-99 m RP527, a GRP analogue for visualisation of GRP receptor- expressing malignancies: a feasibility study. Eur J Nucl Med 27, 1694–1699 (2000)
48. van Bokhoven, A., Varella-Garcia, M., Korch, C., et al.: Molecular characterization of human prostate carcinoma cell lines. Prostate 57, 205–225 (2003)
49. Hoffman, T. J., Gali, H., Smith, C. J., et al.: Novel series of 111In-labeled bombesin analogs as potential radiopharmaceuticals for specific targeting of gastrin-releasing peptide receptors expressed on human prostate cancer cells. J Nucl Med 44, 823–831. (2003)
50. Breeman, W. A., de Jong, M., Erion, J. L., et al.: Preclinical comparison of (111)In-labeled DTPA- or DOTA-bombesin analogs for receptor-targeted scintigraphy and radionuclide therapy. J Nucl Med 43, 1650–1656 (2002)
51. Ferro-Flores, G., Arteaga de Murphy, C., Rodriguez-Cortes, J., et al.: Preparation and evaluation of 99 mTc-EDDA/HYNIC-[Lys 3]-bombesin for imaging gastrin-releasing peptide receptor-positive tumours. Nucl Med Commun 27, 371–376 (2006)

52. Garcia Garayoa, E., Ruegg, D., Blauenstein, P., et al.: Chemical and biological characterization of new Re(CO)(3)/[(99m)Tc](CO)(3) bombesin analogues. Nucl Med Biol 34, 17–28 (2007)
53. Reubi, J. C., Macke, H. R. and Krenning, E. P.: Candidates for peptide receptor radiotherapy today and in the future. J Nucl Med 46 (Suppl 1), 67S–75S (2005)
54. de Visser, M., Bernard, H. F., Erion, J. L., et al.: Novel (111)In-labelled bombesin analogues for molecular imaging of prostate tumours. Eur J Nucl Med Mol Imaging (2007)
55. Zhang, H., Schuhmacher, J., Waser, B., et al.: DOTA-PESIN, a DOTA-conjugated bombesin derivative designed for the imaging and targeted radionuclide treatment of bombesin receptor-positive tumours. Eur J Nucl Med 34, 1198–1208 (2007)
56. Yang, Y. S., Zhang, X., Xiong, Z., et al.: Comparative in vitro and in vivo evaluation of two 64Cu-labeled bombesin analogs in a mouse model of human prostate adenocarcinoma. Nucl Med Biol 33, 371–380 (2006)
57. Smith, C. J., Gali, H., Sieckman, G. L., et al.: Radiochemical investigations of (177)Lu-DOTA-8-Aoc-BBN[7-14]NH(2): an in vitro/in vivo assessment of the targeting ability of this new radiopharmaceutical for PC-3 human prostate cancer cells. Nucl Med Biol 30, 101–109 (2003)
58. Rogers, B. E., Bigott, H. M., McCarthy, D. W., et al.: MicroPET imaging of a gastrin-releasing peptide receptor-positive tumor in a mouse model of human prostate cancer using a 64Cu-labeled bombesin analogue. Bioconjug Chem 14, 756–763 (2003)
59. Johnson, C. V., Shelton, T., Smith, C. J., et al.: Evaluation of combined (177)Lu-DOTA-8-AOC-BBN (7-14)NH(2) GRP receptor-targeted radiotherapy and chemotherapy in PC-3 human prostate tumor cell xenografted SCID mice. Cancer Biother Radiopharm 21, 155–166 (2006)
60. Biddlecombe, G. B., Rogers, B. E., Visser, M. D., et al.: Molecular imaging of gastrin-releasing peptide receptor-positive tumors in mice using (64)Cu- and (86)Y-DOTA-(Pro(1),Tyr(4))-Bombesin(1-14). Bioconjug Chem 18, 724–730 (2007)
61. Lantry, L. E., Cappelletti, E., Maddalena, M. E., et al.: 177Lu-AMBA: Synthesis and characterization of a selective 177Lu-labeled GRP-R agonist for systemic radiotherapy of prostate cancer. J Nucl Med 47, 1144–1152 (2006)
62. Van de Wiele, C., Dumont, F., van Belle, S., et al.: Is there a role for agonist gastrin-releasing peptide receptor radioligands in tumour imaging? Nucl Med Commun 22, 5–15 (2001)
63. Baum, R., Prasad, V., Mutloka, N., et al.: Molecular imaging of bombesin receptors in various tumors by Ga-68 AMBA PET/CT: first results. J Nucl Med 48, 79P (2007)
64. de Visser, M., van Weerden, W. M., Melis, M., et al.: Radiolabeled bombesin analogs in preclinical studies. J Nucl Med 48 (Suppl 2), 24P (2007)
65. Mancuso, A., Oudard, S. and Sternberg, C. N.: Effective chemotherapy for hormone-refractory prostate cancer (HRPC): present status and perspectives with taxane-based treatments. Crit Rev Oncol Hematol 61, 176–185 (2007)
66. Oudard, S., Banu, E., Beuzeboc, P., et al.: Multicenter randomized phase II study of two schedules of docetaxel, estramustine, and prednisone versus mitoxantrone plus prednisone in patients with metastatic hormone-refractory prostate cancer. J Clin Oncol 23, 3343–3351 (2005)
67. de Visser, M., van Weerden, W. M., de Ridder, C. M., et al.: Androgen-dependent expression of the gastrin-releasing peptide receptor in human prostate tumor xenografts. J Nucl Med 48, 88–93 (2007)
68. Reubi, J. C., Waser, B., Friess, H., et al.: Neurotensin receptors: a new marker for human ductal pancreatic adenocarcinoma. Gut 42, 546–550 (1998)
69. Kuhar, M. J.: Imaging receptors for drugs in neural tissue. Neuropharmacology 26, 911–916 (1987)
70. Ehlers, R. A., Kim, S., Zhang, Y., et al.: Gut peptide receptor expression in human pancreatic cancers. Ann Surg 231, 838–848 (2000)
71. Zhang, K., An, R., Gao, Z., et al.: Radionuclide imaging of small-cell lung cancer (SCLC) using 99mTc-labeled neurotensin peptide 8-13. Nucl Med Biol 33, 505–512 (2006)

72. Nock, B. A., Nikolopoulou, A., Reubi, J. C., et al.: Toward stable N4-modified neurotensins for NTS1-receptor-targeted tumor imaging with 99mTc. J Med Chem 49, 4767–4776 (2006)
73. Maes, V., Garcia-Garayoa, E., Blauenstein, P., et al.: Novel 99mTc-labeled neurotensin analogues with optimized biodistribution properties. J Med Chem 49, 1833–1836 (2006)
74. Garcia-Garayoa, E., Maes, V., Blauenstein, P., et al.: Double-stabilized neurotensin analogues as potential radiopharmaceuticals for NTR-positive tumors. Nucl Med Biol 33, 495–503 (2006)
75. Garcia-Garayoa, E., Allemann-Tannahill, L., Blauenstein, P., et al.: In vitro and in vivo evaluation of new radiolabeled neurotensin(8-13) analogues with high affinity for NT1 receptors. Nucl Med Biol 28, 75–84 (2001)
76. Lugrin, D., Vecchini, F., Doulut, S., et al.: Reduced peptide bond pseudopeptide analogues of neurotensin: binding and biological activities, and in vitro metabolic stability. Eur J Pharmacol 205, 191–198 (1991)
77. de Visser, M., Janssen, P. J., Srinivasan, A., et al.: Stabilised 111In-labelled DTPA- and DOTA-conjugated neurotensin analogues for imaging and therapy of exocrine pancreatic cancer. Eur J Nucl Med Mol Imaging 30, 1134–1139 (2003)
78. Emami, B., Lyman, J., Brown, A., et al.: Tolerance of normal tissue to therapeutic irradiation. Int J Radiat Oncol Biol Phys 21, 109–122 (1991)
79. Buchegger, F., Bonvin, F., Kosinski, M., et al.: Radiolabeled neurotensin analog, 99mTc-NT-XI, evaluated in ductal pancreatic adenocarcinoma patients. J Nucl Med 44, 1649–1654 (2003)
80. Reubi, J. C., Chayvialle, J. A., Franc, B., et al.: Somatostatin receptors and somatostatin content in medullary thyroid carcinomas. Lab Invest 64, 567–573 (1991)
81. Kwekkeboom, D. J., Reubi, J. C., Lamberts, S. W., et al.: In vivo somatostatin receptor imaging in medullary thyroid carcinoma. J Clin Endocrinol Metab 76, 1413–1417 (1993)
82. Reubi, J. C., Schaer, J. C. and Waser, B.: Cholecystokinin(CCK)-A and CCK-B/gastrin receptors in human tumors. Cancer Res 57, 1377–1386 (1997)
83. Behr, T. M., Jenner, N., Radetzky, S., et al.: Targeting of cholecystokinin-B/gastrin receptors in vivo: preclinical and initial clinical evaluation of the diagnostic and therapeutic potential of radiolabelled gastrin. Eur J Nucl Med 25, 424–430 (1998)
84. Reubi, J. C., Waser, B., Schaer, J. C., et al.: Unsulfated DTPA- and DOTA-CCK analogs as specific high-affinity ligands for CCK-B receptor-expressing human and rat tissues in vitro and in vivo. Eur J Nucl Med 25, 481–490 (1998)
85. de Jong, M., Bakker, W. H., Bernard, B. F., et al.: Preclinical and initial clinical evaluation of 111In-labeled nonsulfated CCK8 analog: a peptide for CCK-B receptor-targeted scintigraphy and radionuclide therapy. J Nucl Med 40, 2081–2087 (1999)
86. Kwekkeboom, D. J., Bakker, W. H., Kooij, P. P., et al.: Cholecystokinin receptor imaging using an octapeptide DTPA-CCK analogue in patients with medullary thyroid carcinoma. Eur J Nucl Med 27, 1312–1317 (2000)
87. Mather, S. J., McKenzie, A. J., Sosabowski, J. K., et al.: Selection of radiolabeled gastrin analogs for peptide receptor-targeted radionuclide therapy. J Nucl Med 48, 615–622 (2007)
88. Behr, T. M., Jenner, N., Behe, M., et al.: Radiolabeled peptides for targeting cholecystokinin-B/gastrin receptor-expressing tumors. J Nucl Med 40, 1029–1044 (1999)
89. Nock, B. A., Maina, T., Behe, M., et al.: CCK-2/gastrin receptor-targeted tumor imaging with (99m)Tc-labeled minigastrin analogs. J Nucl Med 46, 1727–1736 (2005)
90. Gotthardt, M., Behe, M. P., Beuter, D., et al.: Improved tumour detection by gastrin receptor scintigraphy in patients with metastasised medullary thyroid carcinoma. Eur J Nucl Med Mol Imaging 33, 1273–1279 (2006)
91. Gotthardt, M., Behe, M. P., Grass, J., et al.: Added value of gastrin receptor scintigraphy in comparison to somatostatin receptor scintigraphy in patients with carcinoids and other neuroendocrine tumours. Endocr Relat Cancer 13, 1203–1211 (2006)
92. Mayo, K. E., Miller, L. J., Bataille, D., et al.: International Union of Pharmacology. XXXV. The glucagon receptor family. Pharmacol Rev 55, 167–194 (2003)

93. Reubi, J. C. and Waser, B.: Concomitant expression of several peptide receptors in neuroendocrine tumours: molecular basis for in vivo multireceptor tumour targeting. Eur J Nucl Med Mol Imaging 30, 781–793 (2003)
94. Korner, M., Stockli, M., Waser, B., et al.: GLP-1 Receptor Expression in Human Tumors and Human Normal Tissues: Potential for In Vivo Targeting. J Nucl Med 48, 736–743 (2007)
95. Meier, J. J. and Nauck, M. A.: Glucagon-like peptide 1(GLP-1) in biology and pathology. Diabetes Metab Res Rev 21, 91–117 (2005)
96. Hassan, M., Eskilsson, A., Nilsson, C., et al.: In vivo dynamic distribution of 131I-glucagon-like peptide-1 (7-36) amide in the rat studied by gamma camera. Nucl Med Biol 26, 413–420 (1999)
97. Gotthardt, M., Fischer, M., Naeher, I., et al.: Use of the incretin hormone glucagon-like peptide-1 (GLP-1) for the detection of insulinomas: initial experimental results. Eur J Nucl Med Mol Imaging 29, 597–606 (2002)
98. Gotthardt, M., Lalyko, G., van Eerd-Vismale, J., et al.: A new technique for in vivo imaging of specific GLP-1 binding sites: First results in small rodents. Regul Pept 137, 162–167 (2006)
99. Wild, D., Behe, M., Wicki, A., et al.: [Lys40(Ahx-DTPA-111In)NH2]exendin-4, a very promising ligand for glucagon-like peptide-1 (GLP-1) receptor targeting. J Nucl Med 47, 2025–2033 (2006)
100. Wicki, A., Wild, D., Storch, D., et al.: [Lys40(Ahx-DTPA-111In)NH2]-Exendin-4 is a highly efficient radiotherapeutic for glucagon-like peptide-1 receptor-targeted therapy for insulinoma. Clin Cancer Res 13, 3696–3705 (2007)
101. Brooks, P. C.: Role of integrins in angiogenesis. Eur J Cancer 32A, 2423–2429 (1996)
102. Plow, E. F., Haas, T. A., Zhang, L., et al.: Ligand binding to integrins. J Biol Chem 275, 21785–21788 (2000)
103. Gurrath, M., Muller, G., Kessler, H., et al.: Conformation/activity studies of rationally designed potent anti-adhesive RGD peptides. Eur J Biochem 210, 911–921 (1992)
104. Aumailley, M., Gurrath, M., Muller, G., et al.: Arg-Gly-Asp constrained within cyclic pentapeptides. Strong and selective inhibitors of cell adhesion to vitronectin and laminin fragment P1. FEBS Lett 291, 50–54 (1991)
105. van Hagen, P. M., Breeman, W. A., Bernard, H. F., et al.: Evaluation of a radiolabelled cyclic DTPA-RGD analogue for tumour imaging and radionuclide therapy. Int J Cancer 90, 186–198 (2000)
106. Chen, X., Park, R., Tohme, M., et al.: MicroPET and autoradiographic imaging of breast cancer alpha v-integrin expression using 18F- and 64Cu-labeled RGD peptide. Bioconjug Chem 15, 41–49 (2004)
107. Cai, W., Zhang, X., Wu, Y., et al.: A thiol-reactive 18F-labeling agent, N-[2-(4-18F-fluorobe nzamido)ethyl]maleimide, and synthesis of RGD peptide-based tracer for PET imaging of alpha v beta 3 integrin expression. J Nucl Med 47, 1172–1180 (2006)
108. Haubner, R., Kuhnast, B., Mang, C., et al.: [18F]Galacto-RGD: synthesis, radiolabeling, metabolic stability, and radiation dose estimates. Bioconjug Chem 15, 61–69 (2004)
109. Beer, A. J., Haubner, R., Sarbia, M., et al.: Positron emission tomography using [18F]Galacto-RGD identifies the level of integrin alpha(v)beta3 expression in man. Clin Cancer Res 12, 3942–3949 (2006)
110. Beer, A. J., Haubner, R., Wolf, I., et al.: PET-based human dosimetry of 18F-galacto-RGD, a new radiotracer for imaging alpha v beta3 expression. J Nucl Med 47, 763–769 (2006)
111. Beer, A. J., Haubner, R., Goebel, M., et al.: Biodistribution and pharmacokinetics of the alphavbeta3-selective tracer 18F-galacto-RGD in cancer patients. J Nucl Med 46, 1333–1341 (2005)
112. Dijkgraaf, I., Kruijtzer, J. A., Liu, S., et al.: Improved targeting of the alpha(v)beta (3) integrin by multimerisation of RGD peptides. Eur J Nucl Med Mol Imaging 34, 267–273 (2007)
113. Dijkgraaf, I., Rijnders, A. Y., Soede, A., et al.: Synthesis of DOTA-conjugated multivalent cyclic-RGD peptide dendrimers via 1,3-dipolar cycloaddition and their biological evaluation:

implications for tumor targeting and tumor imaging purposes. Org Biomol Chem 5, 935–944 (2007)
114. Dijkgraaf, I., Liu, S., Kruijtzer, J. A., et al.: Effects of linker variation on the in vitro and in vivo characteristics of an 111In-labeled RGD peptide. Nucl Med Biol 34, 29–35 (2007)
115. Dijkgraaf, I., Kruijtzer, J. A., Frielink, C., et al.: Alpha v beta 3 integrin-targeting of intraperitoneally growing tumors with a radiolabeled RGD peptide. Int J Cancer 120, 605–610 (2007)
116. Kimura, N., Hayafuji, C., Konagaya, H., et al.: 17 beta-estradiol induces somatostatin (SRIF) inhibition of prolactin release and regulates SRIF receptors in rat anterior pituitary cells. Endocrinology 119, 1028–1036 (1986)
117. Presky, D. H. and Schonbrunn, A.: Somatostatin pretreatment increases the number of somatostatin receptors in GH4C1 pituitary cells and does not reduce cellular responsiveness to somatostatin. J Biol Chem 263, 714–721 (1988)
118. Kimura, N., Hayafuji, C. and Kimura, N.: Characterization of 17-beta-estradiol-dependent and -independent somatostatin receptor subtypes in rat anterior pituitary. J Biol Chem 264, 7033–7040 (1989)
119. Slama, A., Videau, C., Kordon, C., et al.: Estradiol regulation of somatostatin receptors in the arcuate nucleus of the female rat. Neuroendocrinology 56, 240–245 (1992)
120. Vidal, C., Rauly, I., Zeggari, M., et al.: Up-regulation of somatostatin receptors by epidermal growth factor and gastrin in pancreatic cancer cells. Mol Pharmacol 46, 97–104 (1994)
121. Visser-Wisselaar, H. A., Van Uffelen, C. J., Van Koetsveld, P. M., et al.: 17-beta-estradiol-dependent regulation of somatostatin receptor subtype expression in the 7315b prolactin secreting rat pituitary tumor in vitro and in vivo. Endocrinology 138, 1180–1189 (1997)
122. Froidevaux, S., Hintermann, E., Torok, M., et al.: Differential regulation of somatostatin receptor type 2 (sst 2) expression in AR4-2J tumor cells implanted into mice during octreotide treatment. Cancer Res 59, 3652–3657 (1999)
123. Viguerie, N., Esteve, J. P., Susini, C., et al.: Dexamethasone effects on somatostatin receptors in pancreatic acinar AR4-2J cells. Biochem Biophys Res Commun 147, 942–948 (1987)
124. Gunn, S. H., Schwimer, J. E., Cox, M., et al.: In vitro modeling of the clinical interactions between octreotide and 111In-pentetreotide: is there evidence of somatostatin receptor downregulation? J Nucl Med 47, 354–359 (2006)
125. Behe, M., Püsken, M., Henzel, M., et al.: Upregulation of gastrin and somatostatin receptor after irradiation. Eur J Nucl Med Mol Imaging 30, S218 (2003)
126. Behe, M., Koller, S., Püsken, M., et al.: Irradiation-induced upregulation of somatostatin and gastrin receptors in vitro and in vivo. Eur J Nucl Med Mol Imaging 31, S237–S238 (2004)
127. Oddstig, J., Bernhardt, P., Nilsson, O., et al.: Radiation-induced up-regulation of somatostatin receptor expression in small cell lung cancer in vitro. Nucl Med Biol 33, 841–846 (2006)
128. Capello, A., Krenning, E., Bernard, B., et al.: 111In-labelled somatostatin analogues in a rat tumour model: somatostatin receptor status and effects of peptide receptor radionuclide therapy. Eur J Nucl Med Mol Imaging 32, 1288–1295 (2005)
129. Melis, M., Forrer, F., Capello, A., et al.: Up-regulation of somatostatin receptor density on rat CA20948 tumours escaped from low dose [177Lu-DOTA0,Tyr3]octreotate therapy. Q J Nucl Med Mol Imaging 51, 324–33 (2007)
130. Seth, P.: Vector-mediated cancer gene therapy: an overview. Cancer Biol Ther 4, 512–517 (2005)
131. Buchsbaum, D. J., Zinn, K. R. and Rogers, B. E.: Gene expression imaging with 111In- and 99mTc-labeled peptides of somatostatin receptors upregulated by adenovirus infection. Society of Nuclear Medicine, 47th Annual meeting, 246–251 (2000)
132. Zinn, K. R., Chaudhuri, T. R., Buchsbaum, D. J., et al.: Simultaneous evaluation of dual gene transfer to adherent cells by gamma-ray imaging. Nucl Med Biol 28, 135–144 (2001)
133. Hemminki, A., Belousova, N., Zinn, K. R., et al.: An adenovirus with enhanced infectivity mediates molecular chemotherapy of ovarian cancer cells and allows imaging of gene expression. Mol Ther 4, 223–231 (2001)

134. Zinn, K. R., Chaudhuri, T. R., Krasnykh, V. N., et al.: Gamma camera dual imaging with a somatostatin receptor and thymidine kinase after gene transfer with a bicistronic adenovirus in mice. Radiology 223, 417–425 (2002)
135. Verwijnen, S. M., ter Horst, M., Sillevis Smith, P. A. E., et al.: Molecular imaging following adenoviral gene transfer visualizes sst_2 and HSV1-tk expression (submitted) (2007)
136. Rogers, B. E., Zinn, K. R., Lin, C. Y., et al.: Targeted radiotherapy with [(90)Y]-SMT 487 in mice bearing human nonsmall cell lung tumor xenografts induced to express human somatostatin receptor subtype 2 with an adenoviral vector. Cancer 94, 1298–1305 (2002)
137. Rogers, B. E., Parry, J. J., Andrews, R., et al.: MicroPET imaging of gene transfer with a somatostatin receptor-based reporter gene and (94m)Tc-Demotate 1. J Nucl Med 46, 1889–1897 (2005)
138. Gotthardt, M., Librizzi, D., Wolf, D., et al.: Increased therapeutic efficacy through combination of Lu-177-DOTATOC and chemotheray in neuroendocrine tumours in vivo. Eur J Nucl Med Mol Imaging 33, S115 (2006)
139. Kong, G., Lau, E., Ramdave, S., et al.: High-dose In-111 octreotide therapy in combination with radiosensitizing 5-FU chemotherapy for treatment of SSR-expressing neuroendocrine tumors. J Nucl Med 46, 151P–152P (2005)
140. Wild, D., Wicki, A. and Christofori, G.: Combination therapy with [(lys40(Ahx-[111In-DTPA])]-Exendin-4 and VEGF-receptor tyrosine kinase inhibitor PTK in a glucagon-like-peptide-1 receptor-positive transgenic mouse tumor model. J Nucl Med 48 (Suppl 2), 83P (2007)
141. Fueger, B. J., Hamilton, G., Raderer, M., et al.: Effects of chemotherapeutic agents on expression of somatostatin receptors in pancreatic tumor cells. J Nucl Med 42, 1856–1862 (2001)
142. de Jong, M., Breeman, W. A., Bernard, B. F., et al.: [177Lu-DOTA(0),Tyr3] octreotate for somatostatin receptor-targeted radionuclide therapy. Int J Cancer 92, 628–633 (2001)
143. de Jong, M., Breeman, W. A., Bernard, B. F., et al.: Tumor response after [(90)Y-DOTA(0),Tyr(3)]octreotide radionuclide therapy in a transplantable rat tumor model is dependent on tumor size. J Nucl Med 42, 1841–1846 (2001)
144. Schally, A. V. and Nagy, A.: Cancer chemotherapy based on targeting of cytotoxic peptide conjugates to their receptors on tumors. Eur J Endocrinol 141, 1–14 (1999)
145. Nagy, A. and Schally, A. V.: Targeting cytotoxic conjugates of somatostatin, luteinizing hormone-releasing hormone and bombesin to cancers expressing their receptors: a "smarter" chemotherapy. Curr Pharm Des 11, 1167–1180 (2005)
146. Hofland, L. J., Capello, A., Krenning, E. P., et al.: Induction of apoptosis with hybrids of Arg-Gly-Asp molecules and peptides and antimitotic effects of hybrids of cytostatic drugs and peptides. J Nucl Med 46 (Suppl 1), 191S–198S (2005)
147. Keller, G., Schally, A. V., Nagy, A., et al.: Effective therapy of experimental human malignant melanomas with a targeted cytotoxic somatostatin analogue without induction of multidrug resistance proteins. Int J Oncol 28, 1507–1513 (2006)
148. Engel, J. B., Schally, A. V., Halmos, G., et al.: Targeted therapy with a cytotoxic somatostatin analog, AN-238, inhibits growth of human experimental endometrial carcinomas expressing multidrug resistance protein MDR-1. Cancer 104, 1312–1321 (2005)
149. Buchholz, S., Keller, G., Schally, A. V., et al.: Therapy of ovarian cancers with targeted cytotoxic analogs of bombesin, somatostatin, and luteinizing hormone-releasing hormone and their combinations. Proc Natl Acad Sci USA 103, 10403–10407 (2006)
150. Kanashiro, C. A., Schally, A. V., Nagy, A., et al.: Inhibition of experimental U-118MG glioblastoma by targeted cytotoxic analogs of bombesin and somatostatin is associated with a suppression of angiogenic and antiapoptotic mechanisms. Int J Oncol 27, 169–174 (2005)
151. Kiaris, H., Schally, A. V., Nagy, A., et al.: Regression of U-87 MG human glioblastomas in nude mice after treatment with a cytotoxic somatostatin analog AN-238. Clin Cancer Res 6, 709–717 (2000)
152. Szereday, Z., Schally, A. V., Nagy, A., et al.: Effective treatment of experimental U-87MG human glioblastoma in nude mice with a targeted cytotoxic bombesin analogue, AN-215. Br J Cancer 86, 1322–1327 (2002)

153. Moody, T. W., Fuselier, J., Coy, D. H., et al.: Camptothecin-somatostatin conjugates inhibit the growth of small cell lung cancer cells. Peptides 26, 1560–1566 (2005)
154. Sun, L. C., Luo, J., Mackey, L. V., et al.: A conjugate of camptothecin and a somatostatin analog against prostate cancer cell invasion via a possible signaling pathway involving PI3K/Akt, alphaVbeta3/alphaVbeta5 and MMP-2/-9. Cancer Lett 246, 157–166 (2007)
155. Moody, T. W., Sun, L. C., Mantey, S. A., et al.: In vitro and in vivo antitumor effects of cytotoxic camptothecin-bombesin conjugates are mediated by specific interaction with cellular bombesin receptors. J Pharmacol Exp Ther 318, 1265–1272 (2006)
156. Sun, L. C., Luo, J., Mackey, V. L., et al.: Effects of camptothecin on tumor cell proliferation and angiogenesis when coupled to a bombesin analog used as a targeted delivery vector. Anticancer Drugs 18, 341–348 (2007)
157. Bernard, B., Capello, A., van Hagen, M., et al.: Radiolabeled RGD-DTPA-Tyr3-octreotate for receptor-targeted radionuclide therapy. Cancer Biother Radiopharm 19, 173–180 (2004)
158. Capello, A., Krenning, E. P., Bernard, B. F., et al.: Increased cell death after therapy with an Arg-Gly-Asp-linked somatostatin analog. J Nucl Med 45, 1716–1720 (2004)
159. Capello, A., Krenning, E. P., Bernard, B. F., et al.: Anticancer activity of targeted proapoptotic peptides. J Nucl Med 47, 122–129 (2006)
160. Buckley, C. D., Pilling, D., Henriquez, N. V., et al.: RGD peptides induce apoptosis by direct caspase-3 activation. Nature 397, 534–539 (1999)
161. Lambert, B., Cybulla, M., Weiner, S. M., et al.: Renal toxicity after radionuclide therapy. Radiat Res 161, 607–611 (2004)
162. Kwekkeboom, D. J., Mueller-Brand, J., Paganelli, G., et al.: Overview of results of peptide receptor radionuclide therapy with 3 radiolabeled somatostatin analogs. J Nucl Med 46 (Suppl 1), 62S–66S (2005)
163. Melis, M., Krenning, E. P., Bernard, B. F., et al.: Localisation and mechanism of renal retention of radiolabelled somatostatin analogues. Eur J Nucl Med Mol Imaging 32, 1136–1143 (2005)
164. De Jong, M., Valkema, R., Van Gameren, A., et al.: Inhomogeneous Localization of Radioactivity in the Human Kidney After Injection of [(111)In-DTPA]Octreotide. J Nucl Med 45, 1168–1171 (2004)
165. de Jong, M., Barone, R., Krenning, E., et al.: Megalin is essential for renal proximal tubule reabsorption of (111)In-DTPA-octreotide. J Nucl Med 46, 1696–1700 (2005)
166. Rolleman, E. J., Kooij, P. P., de Herder, W. W., et al.: Somatostatin receptor subtype 2-mediated uptake of radiolabelled somatostatin analogues in the human kidney. Eur J Nucl Med 34, 1854–1860 (2007)
167. Rolleman, E. J., Valkema, R., de Jong, M., et al.: Safe and effective inhibition of renal uptake of radiolabelled octreotide by a combination of lysine and arginine. Eur J Nucl Med Mol Imaging 30, 9–15 (2003)
168. Verwijnen, S. M., Krenning, E. P., Valkema, R., et al.: Oral versus intravenous administration of lysine: equal effectiveness in reduction of renal uptake of [111In-DTPA]octreotide. J Nucl Med 46, 2057–2060 (2005)
169. van Eerd, J. E., Vegt, E., Wetzels, J. F., et al.: Gelatin-based plasma expander effectively reduces renal uptake of 111In-octreotide in mice and rats. J Nucl Med 47, 528–533 (2006)
170. Vegt, E., Wetzels, J. F., Russel, F. G., et al.: Renal uptake of radiolabeled octreotide in human subjects is efficiently inhibited by succinylated gelatin. J Nucl Med 47, 432–436 (2006)
171. Rolleman, E. J., Krenning, E. P., Van Gameren, A., et al.: Uptake of [111In-DTPA0]octreotide in the rat kidney is inhibited by colchicine and not by fructose. J Nucl Med 45, 709–713 (2004)
172. Rolleman, E. J., Forrer, F., Bernard, B., et al.: Amifostine protects rat kidneys during peptide receptor radionuclide therapy with [(177)Lu-DOTA (0),Tyr (3)]octreotate. Eur J Nucl Med Mol Imaging 34, 763–771 (2007)

Chapter 8
Choice of Radionuclides and Radiolabelling Techniques

Vladimir Tolmachev

Summary Considerations on the choice of type of radionuclide suitable for tumour therapy are given. The physical properties of the radionuclides in relation to the therapy conditions are discussed as well as production and availability. Labelling methods are described in terms of direct versus indirect methods and also in terms of radioactive halogens versus radioactive metals. The influence of labelling method on the binding affinity and cellular processing of the targeting agent is discussed. Emphasis is also given to the influence of the labelling method on cellular radionuclide retention and biodistribution.

Introduction

Success in the multidisciplinary area of radionuclide therapy is dependent on good collaboration between scientists specialized in different fields such as radiochemistry, biochemistry, biotechnology, immunology, oncology, pathology, haematology, radiation physics (e.g. dosimetry) and nuclear medicine. Radiochemistry is of crucial importance since the choice of radionuclide and labelling method is as important as the choice of the targeting protein or peptide. This imposes high requirements on the radiochemists, prompting these persons not only to select the best methods for stable attachment of a given nuclide to a given protein or peptide, but also to take into account a variety of biological and pharmacological factors. These factors determine selection of the most suitable radionuclide for the considered application, and the selection of the labelling method, which provide delivery of a high radiation dose to the malignant cells while sparing healthy organs and tissues.

Department of Biomedical Radiation Sciences, Department of Oncology, Radiology and Clinical Immunology, Rudbeck Laboratory, Uppsala University, SE-751 85 Uppsala, Sweden

T. Stigbrand et al. (eds.) *Targeted Radionuclide Tumor Therapy*,

Choice of Radionuclides for Therapy

General Considerations

The main precondition for a successful radionuclide therapy is delivery of a high local radiation dose to the tumour cells and a low dose to healthy tissues. This defines the main requirement to a radionuclide: the energy emitted during its decay should be mainly deposited locally, while whole body irradiation must be as small as possible. To meet these requirements, the general demands for the physical properties of radionuclides should be (modified from [1]):

- The radionuclide should emit particulate radiation: alpha- or beta-particles, Auger and/or conversion electrons in sufficient abundance to exert cytotoxic action.
- High abundance of high-energy gamma components is undesirable since it gives whole-body irradiation, however, low abundance photons (100–200 keV) might be of advantage for imaging (e.g. dosimetry) and therapy monitoring.
- A physical half-life of 1 to 14 days, depending on in vivo pharmacokinetics of the targeting agent, seems to be optimal.
- Possibility to produce the radionuclide with a high enough amount of radioactivity with a suitable specific radioactivity.
- Possibility to produce the radionuclide in a cost-efficient way.
- The chemical properties of the radionuclide should enable high-yield labelling of proteins and peptides during relatively mild conditions and provide a conjugate, which is stable in the blood circulation.
- The radiocatabolites should be quickly excreted from the body, without too much accumulation in normal organs or tissues.

Physical Properties

The physical half-life of the radionuclide should match the biological half-life of the targeting protein. One cannot expect an efficient therapy effect on a solid tumour, if a full-length antibody, which has slow tumour penetration and long residence time in the circulation, is labelled with a nuclide with a too short half life. The main part of the radionuclides would then decay when the targeting conjugate is still outside the tumour, and possibly contribute to irradiation of healthy tissues, e.g. bone marrow. Moreover, theoretical calculations suggest that long half-life of the radionuclide is more favourable for radionuclide therapy [2], since for a given anti-tumour effect long-lived nuclides are more lenient to bone marrow. Still, considerations of logistics, costs and availability might suggest the use of rather short-lived therapeutic radionuclides for small proteins and peptides with a rapid blood clearance. Such decision should include careful dosimetric evaluations.

It has been indicated that each radionuclide can be used in an optimal way only for tumours of a certain size [3–6]. Radionuclides, which emit high-energy beta particles, are useful for treatment of bulky tumours and in this case, long range can compensate poor penetration of the targeting molecule into a tumour mass and overcome a possible heterogeneity of target expression. On the other hand, high energy beta particles are inefficient for destroying single cancer cells or small micrometastases, because most of the energy associated with the radioactive decay is deposited outside the malignant cell. Taking into account that the minimal residual disease is considered as a most suitable target for radionuclide therapy [7], there is a growing interest to nuclides, which emit beta-particles with low energy, e.g. ^{177}Lu, ^{161}Tb, ^{67}Cu [1, 8]. Nuclear properties of some beta-emitting nuclides of therapy interest are listed in Table 8.1.

Low-energy Auger electrons, which are emitted during electron capture or isomeric transition decay, are also considered as suitable particles for inactivation of single spread malignant cells. These particles, due to their high yield per decay, are extremely radiotoxic if their tracks hit DNA. Then, there is very high probability to

Table 8.1 Nuclear properties of some beta-emitting radionuclides, considered for radionuclide therapy (Data compilation from [1, 8], and Table of Radioactive Isotopes on-line (http://nucleardata.nuclear.lu.se/nucleardata/toi/nucSearch.asp)). Photons with abundance of more than 5% are presented

Nuclide	Half-life (days)	Average β energy (MeV)	Average range (mm)	Photon radiation (keV)
High-energy beta-emitters				
^{188}Re	0.71	0.764	3.5	155 (15%)
^{166}Ho	1.1	0.666	3.2	80.5 (6.7%)
^{90}Y	2.7	0.935	3.9	–
^{76}As	1.1	1.0	5.0	559 (45%) 657 (6.2%)
Medium-energy beta-emitters				
^{77}As	1.6	0.228	1.2	–
^{153}Sm	1.9	0.229	1.2	103 (30%)
^{186}Re	3.7	0.362	1.8	137 (9.4%)
Low-energy beta-emitters				
^{67}Cu	2.6	0.141	0.71	91 (7%) 93 (16%) 185 (49%)
^{131}I	8.0	0.181	0.91	364 (82%)
^{161}Tb	6.9	0.154	0.77	75 (10%)
^{177}Lu	6.7	0.133	0.67	113 (6%) 208 (11%)

induce a severe double-strand break, and, hence, inactivate the cell [9–11]. The major challenge in the use of Auger electrons for therapy is their short range, which makes them efficient only if the radioactive decay occurs in the close proximity to DNA. For this reason, a targeting agent, labelled with an Auger emitter should be internalized into malignant cell, translocated into nucleus and, ideally, incorporated into DNA. Alpha-emitting nuclides are considered as potentially attractive for radionuclide therapy of single malignant cells, since alpha-particles deposit energy on a short distance causing dense ionisation along the tracks. The major problem is the relatively short half-life of most alpha-emitters that can be obtained at a reasonable cost, i.e. ^{211}At ($T_{1/2}$ = 7.2 h), ^{212}Bi ($T_{1/2}$ = 60.6 min) and ^{213}Bi ($T_{1/2}$ = 45.6 min). This complicates their use for labelling of full size IgG and creates problems even for the use of short peptides as targeting molecules. To overcome the problem with a short half-life, the concept of in vivo generators has been proposed. In this case, a long-lived alpha-emitter, such as e.g. ^{225}Ac ($T_{1/2}$ = 10 days) or ^{227}Th ($T_{1/2}$ = 18.7 h), decaying to a chain of short-lived alpha-emitting daughter nuclides, is tried [12].

"Radionuclide Cocktails"

It should be noted, that though micrometastases are considered as the main target for radionuclide therapy, it is very likely that, in practice, patients have tumour clusters of various sizes such as small subclinical metastases, macroscopic metastases and bulky tumours. This means that the use of a single type of radionuclide would not be efficient to eradicate all tumour cells. For this reason, the use of a "radionuclide cocktail", i.e. concurrent use of several therapeutic radionuclides has been proposed [6].

This concept was tried in preclinical studies in rats [13] bearing both large and small tumours. The study demonstrated that a combination of ^{90}Y and ^{177}Lu-labelled somatostatin analogues provides better survival than the use of a single radionuclide. This information has a direct implication for the radiochemist. If several radionuclides with different nuclear properties are necessary for a given targeting agent, than the labelling method should be universal enough to enable the use of different radionuclides.

A promising way is to use such a versatile chelator, as DOTA. This would allow labelling with e.g. both the high-energy beta emitter ^{90}Y and the low-energy beta emitter ^{177}Lu. Moreover, this chelator provides good stability with a variety of lanthanides, such as e.g. ^{166}Ho ($T_{1/2}$ = 26.8 h), ^{149}Pm ($T_{1/2}$ = 53.1 h), and ^{153}Sm ($T_{1/2}$ = 46.3 h). Taken into account, that radiolanthanides are numerous and possess a large variety of decay schemes and half-lives, the use of DOTA-derivatives would make possible, in principle, a selection of custom-made "radionuclide cocktails" for different tumour sizes.

Availability of Radionuclides

To be suitable for routine clinical use, the radionuclides should be readily available and, if possible, inexpensive. However, both the basic nuclear physics and available production techniques give certain limitations on the possibilities to produce radionuclides in an economically sound way. Generally speaking, the closer the radionuclide is to the stability line in the nuclide chart, the easier it is to produce by direct nuclear reactions.

Reactor based production. Beta-emitting nuclides are neutron-rich and are typically produced in nuclear reactors, either by neutron irradiation or by fission of nuclear fuel. An advantage of reactor irradiations is that this production route is relatively cheap, at least cheaper than the use of charged particle accelerators. However, the use of neutrons for radionuclide production has limitations. The most straightforward and high yield way for production is the reaction based on thermal neutrons, by (n, γ)-reactions. The problem is that an isotope of the same element as the target material is formed by this reaction. Since different isotopes of the same element possess the same chemical properties, they cannot be separated from each other by chemical means. This limits the specific radioactivity of the product, because it contains both a radioactive product isotope and the stable isotope of the target material. At the same time, therapy requires typically high specific radioactivity. For this reason (n, γ)-reactions can be reasonably well applied at reactors with high neutron flux and for high cross-section reactions, such as e.g. ^{176}Lu (n, γ) ^{177}Lu [14].

The nuclear reactions, where neutron capture causes expelling of charged particles, such as (n, p)- or (n, α)-reactions, a radionuclide with a different charge of the nucleus than the irradiated target material, i.e. an isotope of a different chemical element, is produced. The problem is that the cross-section (probability) of such reactions are usually lower by several orders of magnitude in comparison with cross-sections of (n, γ) reactions. Therefore (n, p)- or (n, α)-reactions are not often used in production of therapeutic radionuclides. In some cases, the use of indirect production methods can enable high specific radioactivity production of beta emitters. For example, ^{177}Lu can be produced even as a no-carrier added nuclide [15]. In this case, a neutron irradiation of ^{176}Yb causes formation of ^{177}Yb ($T_{½}$ = 1.9 h), which decays to ^{177}Lu. Since the product nuclide differs in chemical properties from the target material, an efficient separation leading to a high specific radioactivity is possible. Another example of the use of a (n, γ)-reaction for production of a no-carrier-added radionuclide is the production of the Auger emitter ^{125}I. In this case, ^{125}Xe ($T_{½}$ = 16.9 h) is formed when isotopically enriched ^{124}Xe is used as a target. Electron capture decay of ^{125}Xe, which is stored together with the irradiated target material in a cold trap, generates ^{125}I. Unfortunately, such an opportunity is unusual for nuclides of interest for radionuclide therapy.

The fission reactions of nuclear fuel can produce high yield radionuclides, which have an atomic weight approximately equal to one third or two thirds of the atomic weight of uranium. This is the reason why the radionuclide ^{131}I is so readily available and relatively cheap. Some limitation is that stable ^{127}I is also co-produced in this way, which reduces a specific radioactivity of ^{131}I.

Generator based production. An attractive way for production of no-carrier-added beta- and alpha- emitting isotopes are generators [16]. Generator systems include a relatively long-lived mother nuclide, which decays to a more short-lived daughter. Due to different chemical properties of the mother and daughter nuclides, the daughter can be separated. Radionuclide generators present relatively cheap and available equipment for supplying radionuclides for a hospital radiopharmacy. The most well known generator system is, of course, ^{99}Mo ($T_{½}$ = 65.9 h)/^{99m}Tc ($T_{½}$ = 6 h), which is the main supplier of ^{99m}Tc for single-photon imaging. However, this technology has a potential also for production of therapeutic nuclides. ^{188}Re ($T_{½}$ = 17 h) can be produced in a no-carrier added state from ^{188}W ($T_{½}$ = 69.4 days). The daughter radionuclide can be eluted with ammonium acetate daily form the mother immobilised on a alumina column. After concentration on ion-exchange cartridges, ^{188}Re can be used for radiopharmaceutical labelling [17]. Several companies produce this generator.

Fission produced ^{90}Sr ($T_{½}$ = 28.8 years) decays to the high-energy beta-emitter ^{90}Y ($T_{½}$ = 64 h), which can be separated with a high specific radioactivity. Several methods are suitable for separation of ^{90}Y in the hospital radiopharmacy. In spite of that, this nuclide is most often supplied as a ready for labelling [^{90}Y]yttrium chloride solution from a centralised dispensary.

Accelerator based production. Production of neutron-deficient nuclides, such as Auger emitters, requires the use of charged particle irradiation. The charged-particle-induced ^{209}Bi(α, 2n)^{211}At reaction is required for production of the interesting alpha-emitter, ^{211}At. An advantage of the use of charged particles is that the produced radionuclide is a different chemical element, than the target material. This creates an opportunity for efficient chemical separation and to obtain the radionuclides with high specific radioactivity. An accelerator, e.g. cyclotron, is required for such production.

In order to ensure availability of Auger-emitting radionuclides and astatine-211 for radionuclide therapy, a concept of *a*ccelerator-*b*ased *c*entre for *r*adio*n*uclide *t*herapy, ABC RNT, has been proposed [18]. The concept of such centre is similar to the concept of the PET centre (which includes cyclotron, radiochemical laboratory and PET cameras). In the case of ABC RNT, the centre should include a cyclotron capable to accelerate alpha-particles for 28–30 MeV for astatine production, a radiochemical laboratory/radiopharmacy and, isolated hospital beds for patients.

Similarly to PET centres, ABC RNT should preferably be placed in large regional hospitals. Arrangement of such a centre should solve logistical problems associated with transport of short-lived ($T_{½}$ = 7.2 h) astatine-111. Besides, such centre could produce long-lived positron emitters, such as ^{55}Co ($T_{½}$ = 17.53 h), ^{64}Cu ($T_{½}$ = 12.7 h), ^{66}Ca ($T_{½}$ = 9.49 h), ^{76}Br ($T_{½}$ = 16.2 h), ^{72}As ($T_{½}$ = 26.0 h), ^{86}Y ($T_{½}$ = 14.7 h), ^{89}Zr ($T_{½}$ = 78.4 h), ^{124}I ($T_{½}$ = 4.18 days) or radiopharmaceuticals labelled with these nuclides, for distribution to regional satellite PET-centra. The therapeutic radionuclides, which are currently commercially available, are listed in the Table 8.2.

General Requirements for Labelling

Radiochemical Requirements

There are general radiochemical requirements, which should be met, whatever labelling strategy has been selected:

Table 8.2 Commercially available radionuclides of interest for radionuclide therapy

Nuclide	Half-life	Emitted radiation	Production route/specific radioactivity
^{67}Cu	61.9 h	Low-energy beta	Accelerator produced. Limited availability. High specific radioactivity
^{90}Y	64 h	High-energy beta	Generator, based of fission –produced ^{90}Sr. High specific radioactivity
^{111}In	67.2 h	Auger and conversion electrons. Abundant gamma emission	Cyclotron produced. High specific radioactivity
^{125}I	60 days	Auger electrons	Indirect reactor production with high specific radioactivity
^{131}I	8 days	Low-energy beta. Abundant gamma emission	Fission production. Relatively high specific radioactivity
^{153}Sm	46.3 h	Medium-energy beta emitter	Direct reactor production. Moderate specific radioactivity
^{186}Re	3.7 days	Low-energy beta	Direct reactor production. Moderate specific radioactivity
^{188}Re	17 h	High-energy beta	Generator, high specific radioactivity
^{177}Lu	6.7 days	Low-energy beta	Direct reactor production. Moderate specific radioactivity

- The yield of the labelling procedure should be maximized, since the cost of radionuclides contribute significantly to the overall price of a targeting therapeutic conjugate.
- The specific radioactivity of the conjugate should meet the requirements of a given application. In the case of radionuclide therapy this would, most likely, mean that the specific radioactivity should be as high as possible.
- The labelling and purification methods should provide high radiochemical purity, typically higher than the radiochemical purity that is acceptable for conjugates for diagnostics.
- The labelling methods should provide preserved target specificity.
- The labelling method should provide adequate stability of conjugates during storage, transportation and in blood circulation.
- Taken into account high radioactivity levels, it is advisable, that labelling and purification should be performed automatically or under remote control [19, 20]. The experience, which has been obtained in preparation of PET-radiopharmaceuticals, may be very helpful.
- To facilitate introduction into clinical practice, the radionuclide should be cheap and readily available from commercial sources.

It should be noted, that these requirements, might to some degree be in conflict with each other. For example, high yield usually requests more or less prolonged reaction times, since no chemical reaction, including binding of a radionuclide to a protein, can occur instantly. At the same time, this requires high concentration of all reagents, including the radionuclide. Long incubation times with a high concentration of radionuclide increases risk of radiolysis. The risk of radiolytical damages is high for proteins, which activity is dependent on integrity of their structure, especially in the case of therapeutic nuclides, when the major part of energy associated with the radioactive decay is deposited in a small volume. For this reason, development of labelling methods for therapeutic applications require a high degree of optimization.

Distribution Strategy

Selection of labelling methods is also dependent on the distribution strategy and there might be two approaches:

- Labelling of a conjugate at a central dispensary with its subsequent distribution to hospitals (e.g. ^{131}I-tositumomab (Bexxar))
- Distribution of labelling kits to hospitals, where they will be labelled immediately before patient treatment (e.g. ^{90}Y- irbitumomab tiuxetan (Zevalin))

The last approach provides more flexibility and minimizes influence of radiolysis. At the same time, it should be taken into account that radionuclide therapy might, so far, be relatively infrequent. For this reason, a person at a hospital pharmacy would be inevitably less trained than a person of a centralized dispensary for radiolabelled conjugates. The requirement is that the labelling procedure should be robust and minimize the probability of human errors. Such robustness can be achieved by minimization of technological steps: e.g. the number of solution transfers should be minimized, heating and purification steps should should be avoided as much as possible.

Radiolysis

Radiolytic degradation must always be taken into account during development of radiolabelled conjugates for therapeutic purposes. Radiolysis requires attention also in the case of development of peptide conjugates for imaging [21]. In the case of therapy applications, when the radioactivity level in a preparation is high and the emitted energy is absorbed locally, the radiolysis may turn the conjugate more or less non-functional [22–24].

A radiochemist, when designing a radiolabelling approach, must be aware of this and design necessary tests for preserved specific binding of the conjugate, and give strategies for radiolysis prevention during labelling, storage and transportation. An excellent example of optimising labelling and purification conditions for high dose ^{131}I-labelling of monoclonal antibody has been presented by Visser and coworkers [25]. The most challenging is, of course, the radiolysis during labelling, since the radioactivity concentration is highest at this step. It has been shown that ascorbic and gentisic acids protect efficiently antibodies during labelling with radiometals, even with alpha-emitters [23, 26–28]. An advantage of ascorbic acid is that it is an approved drug and it does not interfere with metal chelation. However, it is not an option for direct radioiodination.

Generally, radiolysis protection is simpler during storage than during labelling, since high radionuclide concentration is not required. Dilution of the radiolabelled conjugate reduces radiolysis appreciably [19, 29]. Additionally, freezing seems to be an acceptable solution for storage of radiolabelled proteins [30, 31]. Adding of ascorbic acid [25, 32] and human serum albumin [25, 33, 34] is also a good way to protect radiolabelled proteins during storage.

Labelling Methods

Radioiodination

Originally, radioimmunotherapy was mainly tried using the radionuclide ^{131}I. The chemistry of radioiodination is well-studied and a number of excellent reviews are published [35, 36]. Generally, one can distinguish between direct and indirect radioiodination. In the case of direct radioiodination (see Fig. 8.1), [^{131}I]iodide is in situ oxidized generating electrophilic iodine (+1), which attacks activated aromatic residues of amino-acids of the proteins or peptides. If the labelling is performed at physisological pH, radioiodine would be attached mainly to tyrosine and, to less extent, to histidine or tryptophane. Several oxidants, such as Chloramine-T, Iodogen (1,3,4,6-tetrachloro-3,6-diphenylglycouril), or N-halosuccinimides, have been proposed for in-situ oxidation of radioiodide. Direct radioiodination is a rapid and robust method, providing high yields and high specific radioactivities. A general problem with direct radioiodination is that catabolism of proteins and peptides causes accumulation of radioactivity in thyroid and stomach. Though such accumulation is reduced by giving a patient non-radioactive iodide, such blocking

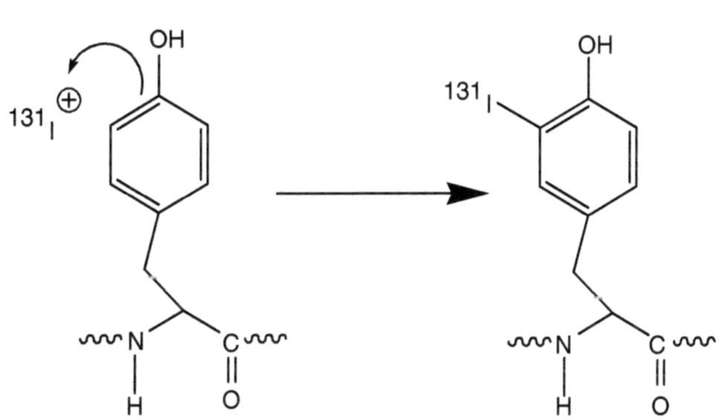

Fig. 8.1 Direct radioiodination

is never complete, which causes unnecessary irradiation of healthy tissues. Some other limitations of direct radioiodination will be discussed below. A good protocol for direct radioiodination is provided by Behr and co-workers [37].

Indirect iodination can be applied if direct labelling is not suitable because tyrosine is involved in the antigen recognition, or crucial disulphide bonds are vulnerable to red-ox condition. Direct labelling is of course also impossible in the case of molecules that does not contain tyrosine. In cases when direct labelling is not possible, intermediate linker molecules are used for labelling. Such linkers should contain two functional moieties, one provides quick and efficient radioiodination (e.g. an activated phenolic ring or an aromatic ring with a suitable leaving group), and the other enables rapid and efficient coupling to proteins, e.g. to amino groups at the N-terminus or at lysine, or to the thiol group of a cysteine. An additional advantage of indirect iodination is that the biological properties of the conjugate, e.g. intracellular retention or excretion pathway of radiocatabolites, can be manipulated by selection of an appropriate linker. Besides, accumulation of the radioactivity in thyroid and stomach is usually reduced in the case of the indirect radioiodination. The limitations of indirect radioiodination are lower yield and specific radioactivity in comparison with direct radioiodination. A detailed protocol for preparation of non-labelled linker and indirect radioiodination using N-succinimidyl 3-[*I]iodobenzoate has been provided by Vaidyanathan and Zalutsky [38]. Fig. 8.2 shows an example of indirect radioiodination.

Labelling Methods for Radioactive Metals

A majority of radionuclides have a metallic nature and metals are typically incapable to form stable covalent bonds with elements presented in proteins and peptides.

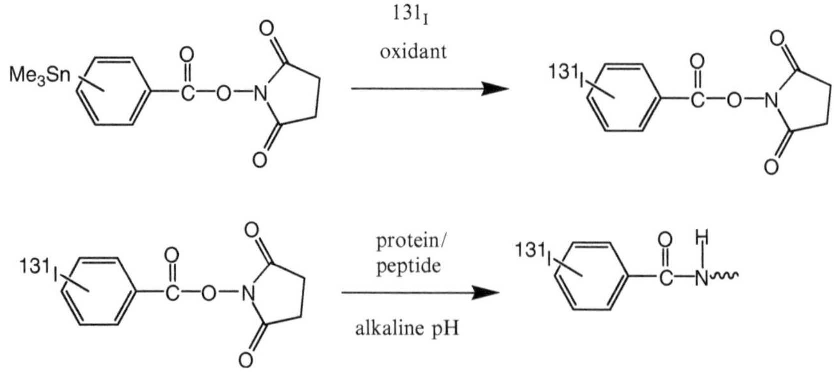

Fig. 8.2 Indirect radioiodination using N-succiniildyl trimetylstanny-benzoate. The linker molecule is radioiodinated first in acidic conditions and then coupled to free amine (N-terminal of ω-amino group of lysine) in alkaline conditions. Both meta- and para-iododerivatives of benzoate have been described in the literature

For this reason, labelling of proteins and peptides with radioactive metals is performed with the use of chelators, multydentate ligands, which form non-covalent compounds with the metal, called chelates. To be used for labelling, the chelator should be bi-functional, i.e. contain both functional moieties for chelation and for coupling to functional groups available on proteins and peptides. Most frequently, coupling to amino groups is used, although binding to thiol groups of cysteine has also been described. There might be two approaches for the use of chelators: pre-labelling and post-labelling. The post-labelling includes first a conjugation of a chelator to a peptide or protein, and then labelling with the radionuclides. In the majority of cases, a well-optimized post-labelling provides a labelling efficiency of about 100%, which excludes necessity of an additional purification. Pre-labelling is performed similarly to indirect radioiodination, i.e. the chelator is labelled with a radiometal first and then conjugated to a targeting protein. The problem with this approach is lower radionuclide yield in comparison with post-labelling. For this reason, pre-labelling is only used if the chelating conditions are so harsh (e.g. include heating, extreme pH), that they can damage the peptide or protein.

In principle, a formation of chelates is a reversible process. A measure of chelate stability is the dissociation constant, which is expressed as Kd = [M][L]/[ML], where [M],[L], and [ML] are concentrations of free metal, free chelator and metal-chelator complex, respectively, at equilibrium.

Besides thermodynamically stability, kinetic inertness versus lability plays an important role. More inert chelates possess both more slow dissociation and association rates. They are generally more stable *in vivo*, though their labelling require more harsh conditions, e.g. elevated temperature. Requirements of stability are generally high, since a number of blood plasma proteins, such as e.g. transferrin or ceruoplasmin possess also chelating properties and constantly challenge, i.e. try to "steal" the radionuclide from chelates on the therapeutic conjugates. Taken into account that the concentration of natural chelating proteins is much higher in the blood than the concentration of the labelled protein, the stability of radiometal-bifunctional chelator complex should be several orders of magnitude higher than the stability of radiometal complex with blood plasma proteins. Different groups of metals exhibit different preferences in their complex formation chemistry and require different chelators to provide the most stable labelling.

Polyaminopolycarboxylate chelators are suitable for lanthanides (such as ^{177}Lu, ^{153}Sm, or ^{166}Ho), ^{90}Y and ^{111}In [39]. One can distinguish two classes of polyamino-polycarboxylate chelators: macrocyclic and acyclic. The most commonly used macrocyclic chelators for radiolanthanides are different derivatives of DOTA (1,4,7,10-tetraazacyclododecane-1,4,7,10-tetraacetic acid), see Fig. 8.3. The high kinetical inertness, i.e. slow rate of dissociation, of DOTA favours stable attachment of the radionuclide, however, elevated temperatures are required for labelling due to slow association rate. For this reason, DOTA derivatives are widely used for labelling of short peptides, which are relatively insensitive to heating to 60–90 °C. The most commonly used acyclic polyaminopolycarboxylate chelators are different derivatives of DTPA (diethylenetriaminepentaacetic acid), Fig. 8.4. It has been found, that backbone-modified semirigid variants of DTPA provide adequate stabil-

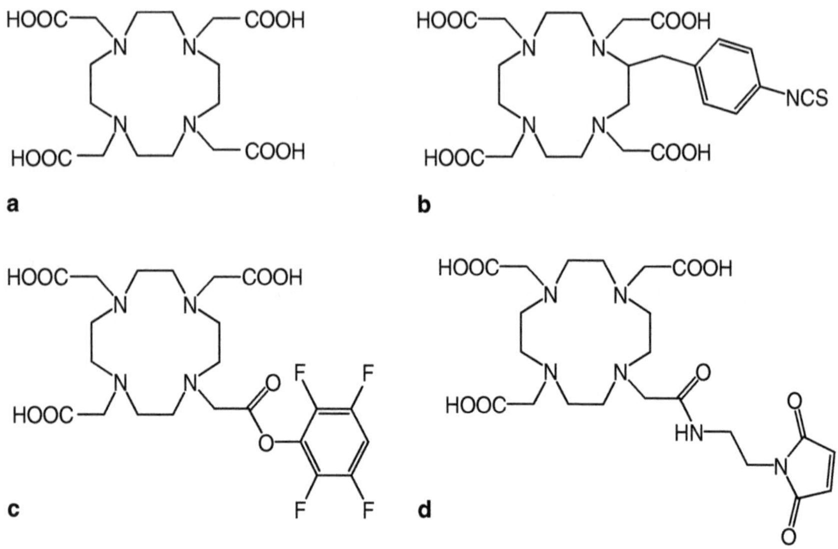

Fig. 8.3 Macrocyclic chelators for radiolanthanides, ^{90}Y and ^{111}In: DOTA (A) and its derivatives. Amino-reactive 4-Isothiocyanatobenzyl-DOTA (B) and DOTA-TFP-ester (C) and thiol-reactive maleimido-mono-amide-DOTA (D)

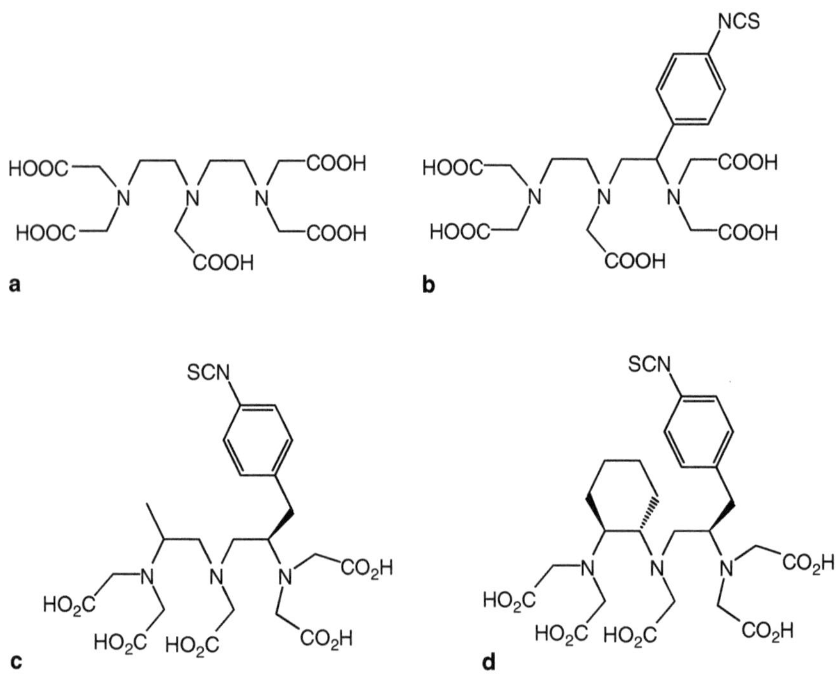

Fig. 8.4 Acyclic chelators for radiolanthanides, ^{90}Y and ^{111}In: DTPA (A) and its amino-reactive derivatives: isothiocyanatobenzyl-DTPA (B) and semirigid 2-(*para*-isothiocyanatobenzyl)-6-methyl-DTPA (lB4M) (C) CHX-A-DTPA (D)

ity for labelling with ^{90}Y of e.g. Zevalin. Though acyclic chelators are less inert, and consequently, less stable than macrocyclic ones, their labelling is rapid enough even at ambient temperature. For this reason, they might be preferred for labelling of monoclonal antibodies, which cannot tolerate heating. Detailed protocols for coupling of polyaminopolycarboxylate chelators to targeting proteins and peptides have been published [40, 41].

There are two isotopes of rhenium, which are of interest for targeted therapy, the medium-energy beta emitter ^{186}Re and the high-energy beta emitter ^{188}Re. Similarly to radioiodination, labelling with rhenium may be performed directly or indirectly [42]. For direct labelling, endogenous disulphide bonds of monoclonal antibodies are reduced, thus creating natural chelators. Though several scientific reports have been published on successful use of such an approach, this method is potentially damaging for antibodies. Besides, the labelling is site-unspecific and often unstable. For this reason, an indirect approach, which involves pre-labelling of a chelator with its subsequent coupling to an antibody, seems to be more reliable. A detailed protocol of labelling of antibodies with ^{186}Re has been published [32]. This protocol includes chelation of rhenium by mercaptoacetyltryglucine (MAG3) chelator, formation of an active ester and it's coupling to the antibody. Depending on amount of protein, the labelling yield is 40–60%.

The low-energy beta emitter copper-67 has potential as a therapeutic radionuclide [43]. Since complexes of copper with acyclic chelators are not stable enough, different macrocyclic chelators have been evaluated such as $^{64/67}Cu$-DOTA-conjugates. However, DOTA does not protect copper enough from bioreduction, and the resulting Cu(I) is not retained firmly in the chelator and is accumulated in the liver. Two other macrocyclic chelators, TETA (1,4,8,11-tetraazacyclododecane-1,4,8,11-tetraacetic acid) and CB-TE2A (4,11-bis(carboxymethyl)-1,4,8,11-tetraazabicyclo[6.6.2]hexadecane) provide better stability of the ^{67}Cu complex (Fig. 8.5). A detailed protocol for labelling with TETA- and CB-TE2A has been published [44]. Cu-CB-TE2A is more stable, but requires warming to 95 °C. For this reason, it is suitable for labelling of robust peptides that can stand high temperature. Stability of TETA-complex of Cu is lower, but the labelling is possible at ambient temperature.

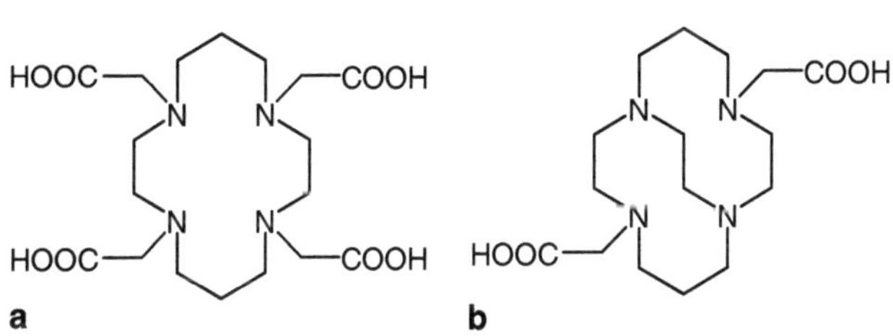

Fig. 8.5 Macrocyclic chelators for ^{64}Cu and ^{67}Cu: TETA (A) and CB-TE2A (B)

Influence of Labelling Method on Targeting Properties

Influence on Cellular Processing and Retention

Radiohalogens versus radiometals. Initial work on characterization of antibodies for radionuclide tumour targeting has been performed using iodine isotopes, predominantly ^{131}I. Introduction in the early eighties of metal chelators and indium-111 labels revealed major differences between antibodies labelled using radiohalogens versus radiometals, when comparison was performed in animal models. Typically, the tumour uptake of radionuclides was higher for indium-labelled antibodies, but uptake in normal tissues, particularly in liver, was also higher [45–51]. Besides, renal accumulation was higher in the case of indium-labelled antibody fragments [51, 52].

The same differences, e.g. higher accumulation of indium-111 in liver, and differences in radioactivity excretion (iodine via urine, indium via bile) have been observed in clinical studies [53]. It has been suggested [54] that the biodistribution of indium-111 labelled monoclonal antibodies is more similar to the biodistribution of antibodies labelled internally, by incubation of hybridoma with radioactive 75 se selenomethionine, (biosynthesis based labelling) than to the biodistribution of iodine-125 labelled antibodies. Since biosynthesis based labelling should affect the biodistribution to the least extent, the authors suggested that some features of indium-111 labelled antibodies, such as higher accumulation in tumours and liver are inherited from the natural biokinetics of immunoglobulins.

In order to explain the difference between antibodies labelled with radioiodine versus radiometals, a deiodination hypothesis was suggested [55, 56]. Since direct oxidative iodination results in attachment of iodine to tyrosine residues, and since iodotryrosine has structural similarity to thyroid hormones, it was suggested that deiodinating enzymes can remove radioiodine from immunoglobulins, thus preventing its delivery to tumours. A decrease of iodine uptake in the thyroid, when applying indirect labelling was taken as a confirmation of the concept. This was the case when monoclonal antibodies were indirectly labelled using linkers dissimilar to iodotyrosine, such as *N*-succinimidyl esters of 3-iodobenzoate [57, 58], 2,4-dimethoxy-3-iodobenzoate [59], 4- and 3-hydroxy-3-iodobenzoate [60, 61], 4-methyl-3-iodobenzoate [62].

It was found later, however, that the reduction of tumour uptake of radiohalogens in comparison with radiometals has a different explanation. It has been revealed, that most antibodies binding to the cell surface are internalized, either by clathrin-dependent endocytosis or due to the normal turnover of cell surface constituents via non-clathrin-dependent endocytosis [63, 64]. Internalisation and transfer to the lysosomal compartment are followed by proteolytic degradation of the immunoglobulins. In vitro studies have demonstrated that the fate of a radionuclide after proteolytic degradation depends on the physico-chemical properties of the obtained radiocatabolites [65–67]. Lipophilic catabolites can diffuse through phospholipide lysosomal and cellular membranes, and leak from the cells. This is the case for iodotyrosine and lysine adducts of halobenzoic acid, typical catabolites of radioiodinated antibodies.

Radiocatabolites of radiometal-labelled antibodies are bulky, hydrophilic and, often, charged compounds due to presence of metal chelates. They can not dissolve in the phospholipide membranes, and diffuse through them. Therefore, they stay trapped intracellularly. They can leave the cells by externalisation (exocytosis), which is slower than diffusion. An improved cellular retention is considered nowadays to be the main reason of better accumulation of radiometals in tumours. Examples of intracellular traffic of radionuclides are schematically shown in Fig. 8.6.

Residualizing properties. Radionuclides and non-degradeable linkers, which remain trapped intracellular, after the targeting protein is internalized and degraded, have so-called residualizing properties. Radionuclides for radionuclide therapy should possess good residualizing properties. Radionuclides such as ^{177}Lu, ^{90}Y, ^{225}Ac, ^{213}Bi, ^{213}Bi and a number of other potential therapeutic nuclides of metallic nature possess residualizing properties, at least when attached to proteins or peptides with stable chelators.

The understanding of the mechanism behind the reduced accumulation of radioiodine in tumours triggered efforts to develop residualizing principles for radiohalogens. This because ^{131}I has been considered an attractive radionuclide for therapy. The fission production in nuclear reactors makes ^{131}I cheap and readily available and rather high specific radioactivity can be obtained. In addition, a long-lived positron emitting counterpart ^{124}I ($T_{½}$ = 4.18 days) makes it possible to perform

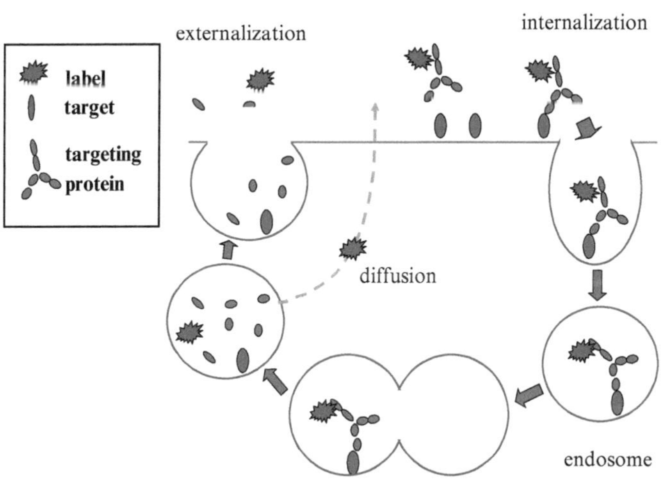

Fig. 8.6 Schematic drawing of the cellular processing of a radiolabelled conjugate after binding to a cell-surface molecular target. After binding, a conjugate-target complex is internalized and transported to lysosomes. In the lysosome, the protein is degraded by proteolytical enzymes. If the radiocatabolites are lipophilic, they can quickly diffuse through membranes and leak out from the cell. If the radiocatabolites are not soluble in phospholipids, they will be trapped inside the cell until excretion by the relatively slow externalization (exocytosis) process

patient specific dosimetry before radionuclide therapy. Moreover, due to similarities in chemistry of heavy halogens, the radioiodination methods could be relatively easy translated for the use with radioactive isotopes of bromine and astatine [35, 36]. This might further increase the flexibility in selection of radionuclides for both radionuclide therapy and non-invasive diagnostics (imaging).

Development of residualizing iodine labelling has so far included the use of bulky non-charged hydrophilic carbohydrate-based linkers, the use of positively charged linkers and the use of negatively charged linkers [68]. The carbohydrate-based linkers include a proteolytically stable carbohydrate part, typically a di-, tetra- or oligosaccharide, which is conjugated to a moiety providing substrate to electrophilic radioiodination, typically tyramine or tyrosine [69, 70].

Originally, residualizing principles have been developed for biological research, in order to identify sites of in vivo catabolism of blood plasma proteins, since the leakage of catabolites from cells was the major problem in these studies. Later, the use of residualizing radioiodinated tyramine cellobiose has been proposed for tumour targeting [71]. Biological studies demonstrated improvement of tumour targeting using antibodies labelled via tyramine cellobiose or tyramine glucose in comparison with directly radioiodinated antibodies [72]. Further studies demonstrated utility of carbohydrate-based residualizing principles for improvement of cellular retention of radioiodine [66, 73–78]. It should be noted, that the carbohydrate-based residualizing linkers are first radiolabelled and then conjugated, often with a low efficiency, which is the main disadvantage. Thus, Stein et al. [79] stated that the delivery of absorbed dose using [^{131}I]dilactitol-tyramine was limited by the low conjugation efficiency of pre-labelled linker. Low conjugation yields, 30–40%, and a possible aggregation of antibodies when using tyramine-cellobiose has been observed [73].

Positively charged linkers include basic prosthetic moieties, such as halopyridinecarboxylate or guanidinomethyl-halobenzoate. The use of these linkers demonstrated improvement of cellular retention in comparison with the use of direct radiohalogenation or non-polar neutral linkers [73–75, 80–86]. Further development of this concept included the use of proteolytically stable D-amino acid containing basic peptides, such as D-Lys-D-Arg-D-Tyr-D-Arg-D-Arg (D-KRYRR) as linker for radioiodine [87, 88]. This approach enabled to further increase charge and molecular weight of a residualizing moiety, which improved cellular retention of radioactivity both in vitro and in vivo in comparison with iodopyridinecarboxylate linkers and the direct Iodogen labelling method. Tumour uptake and retention in the case of D-KRYRR-labelling were quite comparable with retention of radiometal labelled antibodies. A disadvantage of D-KRYRR was an elevated uptake and retention of radioactivity in kidneys and liver.

The use of negatively charged linkers might solve problem of elevated kidney uptake of radioiodine. There are several approaches for creating negatively charged linkers: the use of polyhedral boron anions derivatives, such as closo-dodecaborate, closo-decaborate, and carborates [89–92], the use of phosponic acid derivatives, such as e.g. *N*-succinimidyl 3-[^{131}I]iodo-4-phosphonomethylbenzoate [93], and D-peptides with elevated negative charge due to including of glutamate [94] or coupling to DTPA [95, 96].

The residualizing properties are even more important, if the targeting agent is an agonistic, rapidly internalizing peptide. This has been shown for, e.g. radiolabelled EGF conjugates [77, 78, 97, 98], melanocyte-stimulating hormone (MSH) [99] and bombesin analogues [100]. This may be associated with a quick lysosomal degradation of short peptides. Thus, the use of a residualizing tyrosine-dextran instead of direct radioiodination increases the radiation dose to the nucleus of a cancer cell 100-fold [78]. It should be emphasized, however, that a residualizing principle increases retention of the radioactivity not only in tumours, but also in healthy tissues, if the targeting molecule is internalized.

Some Aspects of Uptake in Normal Tissues

Uptake in kidneys is often a problem for targeting peptides and smaller proteins, such as Fab-fragments, scFv fragments and their derivatives, with a molecular weight of less than 60 kDa, which can pass the glomerular membrane [101]. Even appreciably bigger $(Fab')_2$ fragments seem to be filtered to a certain degree. The use of small antibody fragments and peptide ligands is often considered as a promising alternative to monoclonal antibodies for radionuclide therapy, since a short residence time in the blood reduces haematological toxicity. A substantial part of such proteins and peptides may be reabsorbed in proximal tubule of kidneys after glomerular filtration. Recently, a role of the "scavenger" receptor megalin in such reabsorption has been elucidated [102, 103]. However, there are indications on existence of several different mechanisms, which are involved in kidney uptake of radiolabelled proteins and peptides [104]. It is likely, that renal re-absorption occurs for a given protein with approximately the same rate, independent on the labelling method, at least in the case of larger proteins.

However, the renal retention is different when applying residualizing and non-residualizing labelling methods. It has been shown that residualizing radiometals accumulate to a much higher extent in kidneys in comparison with iodine in the case of $(Fab')_2$ [52, 105], Fab [52, 105], and scFv fragments [106] and their derivatives [107, 108]. High accumulation of the residualizing radionuclides in kidneys may force to select non-residualizing principles for therapy, even if it gives low accumulation in the tumour [107]. In many cases, the renal uptake might be appreciably reduced after pre- or co-injection of basic amino acids, e.g. lysine [109–111], gelatin-based plasma expanders [112, 113], or polyglutamic acid [114]. Still, the reduction of renal retention is seldom complete, and in some cases the radioactivity concentration cannot be reduced below the concentration in the tumours.

An interesting approach to reduce radioactivity uptake in the kidneys is based on attachment of chelators and pendant groups to proteins or peptides via cleavable linkers. The idea is that the radionuclide, together with a chelator or a prosthetic group, will be cleaved off by specific brush-border enzymes in kidneys before internalisation in the proximal tubulae [115]. The use of glycyl-lysine containing linkers provided impressive reduction of renal uptake of ^{131}I- labelled [116, 117] or

^{188}Re-labelled Fabs [118]. The use of the same principle for coupling of DOTA enabled more than two times decrease of radioactivity in kidneys after injection of ^{111}In-labelled diabodies [119]. These examples illustrate how the understanding of biological mechanisms enables the radiochemist to overcome intrinsic shortcomings by clever design of a linker to the radionuclide.

Influence of Labelling Method on Binding Affinity

Besides influence on cellular processing, the labelling methods may have an appreciable influence on binding affinity of targeting agents, such as monoclonal antibodies, to their antigens. This can be caused by two factors:

- Distortion of the molecular three-dimensional structure that is optimal for binding to the target
- Chemical modification of amino-acids, which are critical for binding to the target

The affinity of binding of antibodies, their fragments and derivatives, to an antigen depends, among other on their tertiary structure. The tertiary structure depends, in turn, often on disulfide bridges. A cleavage of a crucial disulfide bridge may, in some antibodies, cause loss or significant decrease of binding capacity. There are two procedures, which are intrinsically prone to generate such defects: direct rhenium labelling and direct radioiodination.

Direct labelling with rhenium isotopes, ^{186}Re and ^{188}Re utilize the thiophilic nature of this element [120, 121]. Free thiol groups are generated in antibodies by treatment with mercaptoethanol [122, 123], stannous ion [123, 124] or ascorbic acid [125]. Direct iodination is also potentially damaging for the tumour targeting molecule. Exposure to an oxidant can convert cysteine in disulfide bonds into sulfonic derivatives, and quenching of the reaction by a reducing agent can cleave such a bond with formation of free cysteine. As a result, the structure of the antibody might be distorted and its binding properties diminished. This effect can be reduced by the use of a milder oxidizing agent, such as Iodogen [25]. It should be emphasized, that we are pointing out here only the risk of diminished antigen binding strength. It has, in fact, been demonstrated that these labelling methods can produce, after careful optimization, well working radiolabelled conjugates. However, the radiochemist should be aware about the necessity of optimization.

Another problem, crucial for the protein or peptide binding to the antigen, can be associated with modification of amino acids. Direct radioiodination at pH 7.4 causes attachment of radioiodine mainly to tyrosine residues [35] and it was demonstrated [126, 127] that tyrosine residues are over-represented in complementary determining regions (CDR) of antibodies. Iodination of such tyrosines can decrease the antigen binding capacity of Mabs or ruin it. In fact, such effect have been observed even during the use of mild Iodogen labelling, where impairment of the immunoreactive fraction with increasing specific activity was found [128]. On the other hand, lysines are presented in CDR to much lesser extent [129], and indirect radioiodination directed to amino groups of lysines provides most often better immunoreactivity of the conjugate, and thereby better tumour accumulation. Thus, the use of indirect methods enabled to keep the affinity of anti-CD44v6 antibody U36 about three-fold higher in comparison with direct radioiodination [130].

The influence of labelling methods on target-binding properties of short, 8-to-12 amino acids, peptides can be much more profound, since a prosthetic group will always be close to the binding site. The labelling can cause conformational changes, which influence appreciably the binding affinity. Such an influence might be an explanation why short peptides, which have been selected for targeting using conventional combinatorial libraries, i.e. without the use of robust scaffolds, often do not have enough affinity for radionuclide targeting purposes. Strong influence of the choice of labelling method on binding capacity and biodistribution of such kinds of potential targeting agents has been shown [131]. The most striking is, however, the finding that even different types of radionuclides coupled via the same type of chelator could affect affinity of short peptides to the target, as has been shown for somatostatin analogues [132]. In an excellent comprehensive paper, these authors have demonstrated that the gallium radionuclides provides higher affinity to somatostatin receptor type 2 than indium, yttrium and lutetium radionuclides for DOTA-derivatives. This was demonstrated for somatostatin analogues such as DOTA-octreotide, DOTA-NOC, DOTA-BOC, DOTA-NOC-ATE, DOTA-BOC-ATE, DOTA-TOC, and DOTA-TATE. This finding sends a clear signal that, for short peptides, an evaluation of several labelling methods, combined with application of several different radionuclides, is necessary to select the method providing the best affinity.

The influence of labelling methods on affinity of large peptides (5–15 kDa), is much less studied. Potential targeting peptides of this size are larger than peptide receptor ligand analogues (1–2 kDa), but smaller than scFv (25 kDa). For this reason, experience obtained for short peptides or antibody fragments, can be translated only cautiously to labelling of large peptides. The appearance of novel targeting agents, e.g. scaffold affinity proteins, such as Affibody molecules [133], necessitates such studies.

Affibody molecules are small (7 kDa) robust affinity proteins, derived from B-domain scaffold of staphylococcal protein-A. It was found that with ^{125}I using a para-iodobenzoate linker, or ^{111}In using benzyl-DTPA, had almost no influence on the affinity of the anti-HER2 Affibody molecule $Z_{HER2:342}$. Despite that both methods attach the radionuclides to lysine, and one of the lysines is present in the binding site of $Z_{HER2:342}$, the affinities remain close to the affinity of non-modified $Z_{HER2:342}$, i.e. 22 pM [134, 135]. On the other hand, modifications of the N-terminal in order to incorporate chelators for ^{99m}Tc caused significant changes in dissociation constants of this Affibody molecule [136–138].

Variable influence of labelling method on affinity was found for another intermediate size (6.5 kDa) peptide, epidermal growth factor (EGF). This natural ligand to epidermal growth factor receptor (EGFR) is considered as a possible targeting protein for radionuclide therapy of glioblastoma [139]. The use of DTPA, benzyl-DTPA or DOTA, as well as ^{111}In, ^{177}Lu or ^{68}Ga did not influence the affinity, the dissociation constant was of about 2 nM in all cases [98, 140, 141]. On the other hand, coupling of HYNIC and labelling with ^{99m}Tc, reduced the affinity to 9.3 nM, when EDDA was used as a co-ligand [142].

Influence of Labelling Method on Blood Kinetics and Excretion

Above, we described that the use of different labelling methods influence the distribution of radioactivity after injection of monoclonal antibodies. The described differences were mainly caused by differences in cellular retention and biodistribution of radiocatabolites in tumours and sites of antibody catabolism, but we did not discuss blood kinetics and biodistribution of the targeting agents. An "overmodification" of antibodies, i.e. coupling of a large number of chelators or linker moieties may, change the blood kinetics and clearance of the proteins, as demonstrated in the case of ^{186}Re-labelled antibodies [143]. In the case of a modest modification, the blood kinetics of intact antibodies is much less sensitive to what radiolabelling method that is applied and which radionuclide that is attached. This fact was the reason for development of so-called surrogate radiolabelled conjugates for patient-specific dosimetry. In this case, a radionuclide which emits radiation convenient for detection or quantification, is used for labelling of a conjugate instead of the therapeutic radionuclide. Biodistribution data for a given patient could then be used to estimate the individual radiation dose of the therapeutic conjugate to both the tumour and to normal organs. Furthermore, it can be used to judge if the given patient is eligible for radioimmunotherapy using a particular conjugate.

It has been found that when para-halobenzoate was used as a linker for attachment of ^{211}At, ^{125}I and ^{76}Br to the anti-A33 antibody, blood kinetics, as well as uptake in kidney, liver, bone and muscle was very similar for all three radioactive halogens in a rat model [144]. Higher accumulation of astatine was found in stomach, spleen and thyroid in that study, which can be explained by the differences in re-distribution of the radiocatabolites. In clinics, labelling with ^{111}In of ibritumomab tiuxetan (Zevalin) is used for prediction of the biodistribution of conjugate labelled with therapeutic ^{90}Y. Close similarity in blood kinetics was found, even when such different labels as direct $^{125/131}I$, MAG-^{186}Re, ITC-DTPA-$^{88/90}Y$ and ITC-DTPA-^{177}Lu [145], or sucDf-^{89}Zr and tiuxetan- ^{90}Y [146, 147] have been compared. These and numerous other studies show, that the major attention in the selection of labelling method for intact IgG antibodies should be paid to cellular processing and not to influence on blood kinetics.

On the opposite, overall kinetics and excretion pathways of small targeting agents, such as radiolabelled somatostatin analogues, are largely influenced by labelling methods. A nuclide, together with a pendant group or chelator, is a substantial part of the conjugate in this case, and influences its physico-chemical properties, such as overall charge and lipophilicity. A classical example is the use of DTPA for labelling of octreotide. Initial evaluation of octreotide for tumour targeting was performed with radioiodine directly labelled on Tyr^3. Coupling of DTPA and labelling with ^{111}In made a kit formulation possible, which improved availability of the tracer. Importantly, increased hydrophilicity due to coupling of DTPA switched excretion pathway from hepatobiliary to renal, which enabled to reduce interfering radioactivity in abdominal area [148, 149]. Thus, a change of labelling method opened an avenue for wide clinical application of octreotide.

Multiple other studies demonstrate that the use of more polar or charged chelators for labelling can shift an excretion pathway of short peptides from hepatobiliary to renal [150–152]. Even for much larger (7 kDa) scaffold peptides, such as Affibody molecules, increase of charge or hydrophilicity on the chelator decreases liver accumulation [153] or reduces abdominal radioactivity accumulation [137]. Besides, the use of different linkers, such as PEG, between the targeting peptide and the chelator enables to modulate an overall lipophilicity of the conjugate and manipulate the excretion pathway [154]. This opens an additional possibility to adjust biodistribution of tumour targeting peptides.

A Few Practical Considerations on the Selection of Labelling Method

The considerations listed above indicate that a radiochemist should take into account biological properties of both the target and the targeting agent during selection of the labelling method for a given application. If the target antigen internalises slowly or not at all (which might be the case, when the target is in the extracellular matrix), a non-residualizing ^{131}I labelling method might be preferable for intact IgG antibodies, since this would reduce the dose to excretory organs, such as the liver. Non-residualizing labelling methods might also be of advantage for smaller targeting agents capable to penetrate glomerular membrane, if the degree of renal reabsorption is high. In the case, when the antibody-antigen complex is rapidly internalized (which is often the case when the antigen is a receptor), the use of a residualizing radiometal will be preferable. Interestingly, it seems that the rhenium radionuclides has residualizing properties "in between" halogens and lanthanides [145], which provides certain additional possibilities for a fine tuning of the retention in the tumour and excretory organs. A good understanding of biology, associated with high knowledge of radiochemistry, will make the developmental work successful.

Acknowledgements The author acknowledges the Swedish Cancer Society for a research grant related to the content of this chapter. The author also thanks Professor Jörgen Carlsson, Professor Hans Lundqvist and Dr. Anna Orlova (Unit of Biomedical Radiation Sciences, Uppsala University) for valuable advices when concerning preparation of this chapter.

References

1. Srivastava S, Dadachova E (2001) Recent advances in radionuclide therapy. Semin Nucl Med 31:330–341
2. Howell RW, Goddu SM, Rao DV (1998) Proliferation and the advantage of longer-lived radionuclides in radioimmunotherapy. Med Phys 25:37–42
3. Howell RW, Rao DV, Sastry KS (1989) Macroscopic dosimetry for radioimmunotherapy: nonuniform activity distributions in solid tumors. Med Phys 16:66–74
4. Wheldon TE, O'Donoghue JA (1990) The radiobiology of targeted radiotherapy. Int J Radiat Biol 58:1–21
5. Wheldon TE, O'Donoghue JA, Barrett A, Michalowski AS (1991) The curability of tumours of differing size by targeted radiotherapy using ^{131}I or ^{90}Y. Radiother Oncol 21:91–99
6. O'Donoghue JA, Bardies M, Wheldon TE (1995) Relationships between tumor size and curability for uniformly targeted therapy with beta-emitting radionuclides. J Nucl Med 36:1902–1909
7. Milenic DE, Brady ED, Brechbiel MW (2004) Antibody-targeted radiation cancer therapy. Nat Rev Drug Discov 3:488–499
8. Zweit J (1996) Radionuclides and carrier molecules for therapy. Phys Med Biol 41:1905–1914
9. O'Donoghue JA, Wheldon TE (1996) Targeted radiotherapy using Auger electron emitters. Phys Med Biol 41:1973–1792
10. Adelstein SJ, Kassis AI, Bodei L, Mariani G (2003) Radiotoxicity of iodine-125 and other auger-electron-emitting radionuclides: background to therapy. Cancer Biother Radiopharm 18:301–316
11. Buchegger F, Perillo-Adamer F, Dupertuis YM, Delaloye AB (2006) Auger radiation targeted into DNA: a therapy perspective. Eur J Nucl Med Mol Imaging 33:1352–1363
12. Couturier O, Supiot S, Degraef-Mougin M, Faivre-Chauvet A, Carlier T, Chatal JF, Davodeau F, Cherel M (2005) Cancer radioimmunotherapy with alpha-emitting nuclides. Eur J Nucl Med Mol Imaging 32:601–614
13. de Jong M, Breeman WA, Valkema R, Bernard BF, Krenning EP (2005) Combination radionuclide therapy using ^{177}Lu- and ^{90}Y-labeled somatostatin analogs. J Nucl Med 46(Suppl 1):13S–17S
14. Volkert WA, Goeckeler WF, Ehrhardt GJ, Ketring AR (1991) Therapeutic radionuclides: production and decay property considerations. J Nucl Med 32:174–185
15. Lebedev NA, Novgorodov AF, Misiak R, Brockmann J, Rösch F (2000) Radiochemical separation of no-carrier-added ^{177}Lu as produced via the ^{176}Yb(n,gamma)^{177}Yb– > ^{177}Lu process. Appl Radiat Isot 53:421–425
16. Knapp FF Jr., Mirzadeh S (1994) The continuing important role of radionuclide generator systems for nuclear medicine. Eur J Nucl Med 21:1151–1165
17. Guhlke S, Beets AL, Oetjen K, Mirzadeh S, Biersack HJ, Knapp FF (2000) Simple new method for effective concentration of 188Re solutions from alumina-based ^{188}W-^{188}Re generator. J Nucl Med 41:1271–1278
18. Tolmachev V, Carlsson J, Lundqvist H (2004) A limiting factor for the progress of radionuclide-based cancer diagnostics and therapy – availability of suitable radionuclides. Acta Oncol 43:264–275
19. Weadock KS, Sharkey RM, Varga DC, Goldenberg DM (1990) Evaluation of a remote radioiodination system for radioimmunotherapy. J Nucl Med 31:508–511
20. Govindan SV, Griffiths GL, Stein R, Andrews P, Sharkey RM, Hansen HJ, Horak ID, Goldenberg DM (2005) Clinical-scale radiolabeling of a humanized anticarcinoembryonic antigen monoclonal antibody, hMN-14, with residualizing ^{131}I for use in radioimmunotherapy. J Nucl Med 46:153–159
21. Goedemans WT, de Jong MTM, Deutz E, Miller KM, Brodack J, Ensing GJ (1991) Development of an In-111 labelled somatostatin analogue: Octreoscan 111. Eur J Nucl Med 18:532

22. Bakker WH, Breeman WA, van der Pluijm ME, de Jong M, Visser TJ, Krenning EP (1996) Iodine-131 labelled octreotide: not an option for somatostatin receptor therapy. Eur J Nucl Med 23:775–781
23. Chakrabarti MC, Le N, Paik CH, De Graff WG, Carrasquillo JA (1996) Prevention of radiolysis of monoclonal antibody during labeling. J Nucl Med 37:1384–1388
24. DeNardo GL, DeNardo SJ, Wessels BW, Kukis DL, Miyao N, Yuan A (2000) ^{131}I-Lym-1 in mice implanted with human Burkitt's lymphoma (Raji) tumors: loss of tumor specificity due to radiolysis. Cancer Biother Radiopharm 15:547–560
25. Visser GW, Klok RP, Gebbinck JW, ter Linden T, van Dongen GA, Molthoff CF (2001) Optimal quality ^{131}I-monoclonal antibodies on high-dose labeling in a large reaction volume and temporarily coating the antibody with IODO-GEN. J Nucl Med 42:509–519
26. McDevitt MR, Finn RD, Ma D, Larson SM, Scheinberg DA (1999) Preparation of alpha-emitting 213Bi-labeled antibody constructs for clinical use. J Nucl Med 40:1722–1727
27. Liu S, Edwards DS (2001) Stabilization of ^{90}Y-labeled DOTA-biomolecule conjugates using gentisic acid and ascorbic acid. Bioconjug Chem 12:554–558
28. Liu S, Ellars CE, Edwards DS (2003) Ascorbic acid: useful as a buffer agent and radiolytic stabilizer for metalloradiopharmaceuticals. Bioconjug Chem 14:1052–1056
29. Eary JF, Press OW, Badger CC, Durack LD, Richter KY, Addison SJ, Krohn KA, Fisher DR, Porter BA, Williams DL, Martin PL, Appelbaum FR, Levy R, Brown SL, Miller RA, Neip WB, Bernstein ID (1990) Imaging and treatment of B-cell lymphoma. J Nucl Med 31:1257–1268
30. Wahl RL, Wissing J, del Rosario R, Zasadny KR (1990) Inhibition of autoradiolysis of radiolabeled monoclonal antibodies by cryopreservation. J Nucl Med 31:84–89
31. Huang WS, Cherng SC, Jen TK, Yu MH, Yeh MY (2000) Effects of temperature on radiochemical purity and immunoreactivity of radiolabeled monoclonal antibody 1H10. Nucl Med Technol 28:182–185
32. Visser GW, Gerretsen M, Herscheid JD, Snow GB, van Dongen G (1993) Labeling of monoclonal antibodies with rhenium-186 using the MAG3 chelate for radioimmunotherapy of cancer: a technical protocol. J Nucl Med 34:1953–1963
33. Kishore R, Eary J, Krohn KA, et al. (1986) Autoradiolysis of iodinated monocional antibody preparations. Int J Nucl Med Biol 13:457–459
34. Salako QA, O'Donnell RT, DeNardo SJ (1998) Effects of radiolysis on yttrium-90-labeled Lym-1 antibody preparations. J Nucl Med 39:667–670
35. Wilbur DS (1992) Radiohalogenation of proteins: an overview of radionuclides, labeling methods, and reagents for conjugate labeling. Bioconjug Chem 3:433–470.
36. Adam MJ, Wilbur DS (2005) Radiohalogens for imaging and therapy. Chem Soc Rev 34:153–163
37. Behr TM, Gotthardt M, Becker W, Béhé M (2002) Radioiodination of monoclonal antibodies, proteins and peptides for diagnosis and therapy. A review of standardized, reliable and safe procedures for clinical grade levels kBq to GBq in the Göttingen/Marburg experience. Nuklearmedizin 41:71–79
38. Vaidyanathan G, Zalutsky MR (2006) Preparation of N-succinimidyl 3-[*I]iodobenzoate: an agent for the indirect radioiodination of proteins. Nat Protoc 1:707–713
39. Liu S, Edwards DS (2001) Bifunctional chelators for therapeutic lanthanide radiopharmaceuticals. Bioconjug Chem 12:7–34.
40. Cooper MS, Sabbah E, Mather SJ (2006) Conjugation of chelating agents to proteins and radiolabeling with trivalent metallic isotopes. Nat Protoc 1:314–317
41. Sosabowski JK, Mather SJ (2006) Conjugation of DOTA-like chelating agents to peptides and radiolabeling with trivalent metallic isotopes. Nat Protoc 1:972–976
42. Liu G, Hnatowich DJ (2007) Labeling biomolecules with radiorhenium: a review of the bifunctional chelators. Anticancer Agents Med Chem 7:367–377
43. Novak-Hofer I, Schubiger PA (2002) Copper-67 as a therapeutic nuclide for radioimmunotherapy. Eur J Nucl Med Mol Imaging 29:821–830
44. Wadas TJ, Anderson CJ (2006) Radiolabeling of TETA- and CB-TE2A-conjugated peptides with copper-64. Nat Protoc 1:3062–3068

45. Rainsbury R, Westwood J (1982) Tumour localisation with monoclonal antibody radioactivity labelled with metal chelate rather than iodine. Lancet 2:1347–1348
46. Halpern SE, Hagan PL, Garver PR, Koziol JA, Chen AW, Frincke JM, Bartholomew RM, David GS, Adams TH (1983) Stability, characterization, and kinetics of ^{111}In-labeled monoclonal antitumor antibodies in normal animals and nude mouse-human tumor models. Cancer Res 43:5347–5255
47. Pimm MV, Perkins AC, Baldwin RW (1985) Differences in tumour and normal tissue concentrations of iodine- and indium-labelled monoclonal antibody. II. Biodistribution studies in mice with human tumour xenografts. Eur J Nucl Med 11:300–304
48. Hagan PL, Halpern SE, Chen A, Krishnan L, Frincke J, Bartholomew RM, David GS, Carlo D (1985) In vivo kinetics of radiolabeled monoclonal anti-CEA antibodies in animal models. J Nucl Med 26:1418–1423
49. Khaw BA, Cooney J, Edgington T, Strauss HW (1986) Differences in experimental tumor localization of dual-labeled monoclonal antibody. J Nucl Med 27(8):1293–1299
50. Thedrez P, Blottiere H, Chatal JF, Grzyb J, Douillard JY (1986) Comparison between ^{131}I and ^{111}In as radiolabels for monoclonal antibodies in immunoscintigraphy of tumor bearing nude mice. Tumour Biol 7:137–145
51. Sakahara H, Endo K, Nakashima T, Koizumi M, Kunimatsu M, Kawamura Y, Ohta H, Nakamura T, Tanaka H, Kotoura Y (1987) Localization of human osteogenic sarcoma xenografts in nude mice by a monoclonal antibody labeled with radioiodine and indium-111. J Nucl Med 28:342–348
52. Brown BA, Comeau RD, Jones PL, Liberatore FA, Neacy WP, Sands H, Gallagher BM (1987) Pharmacokinetics of the monoclonal antibody B72.3 and its fragments labeled with either ^{125}I or ^{111}In. Cancer Res 47:1149–1154
53. Yokoyama K, Carrasquillo JA, Chang AE, Colcher D, Roselli M, Sugarbaker P, Sindelar W, Reynolds JC, Perentesis P, Gansow OA (1989) Differences in biodistribution of indium-111-and iodine-131-labeled B72.3 monoclonal antibodies in patients with colorectal cancer. J Nucl Med 30:320–327
54. Koizumi M, Endo K, Watanabe Y, Saga T, Sakahara H, Konishi J, Yamamuro T, Toyama S (1989) Pharmacokinetics of internally labeled monoclonal antibodies as a gold standard: comparison of biodistribution of ^{75}Se-, ^{111}In-, and ^{125}I-labeled monoclonal antibodies in osteogenic sarcoma xenografts in nude mice. Cancer Res 49:1752–1757
55. Zalutsky MR, Noska MA, Colapinto EV, Garg PK, Bigner DD (1989) Enhanced tumor localization and in vivo stability of a monoclonal antibody radioiodinated using N-succinimidyl 3-(tri-n-butylstannyl)benzoate. Cancer Res 49:5543–5549
56. Zalutsky MR, Garg PK, Narula AS (1990) Labeling monoclonal antibodies with halogen nuclides. Acta Radiol 374(Suppl):141–145
57. Zalutsky MR, Narula AS (1987) A method for the radiohalogenation of proteins resulting in decreased thyroid uptake of radioiodine. Int J Rad Appl Instrum [A] 38:1051–1055
58. Zalutsky MR, Narula AS (1988) Radiohalogenation of a monoclonal antibody using an N-succinimidyl 3-(tri-n-butylstannyl)benzoate intermediate. Cancer Res 48:1446–1450
59. Vaidyanathan G, Zalutsky MR (1990) Radioiodination of antibodies via N-succinimidyl 2,4-dimethoxy-3-(trialkylstannyl)benzoates. Bioconjug Chem 1:387–393
60. Vaidyanathan G, Affleck DJ, Zalutsky MR (1993) Radioiodination of proteins using N-succinimidyl 4-hydroxy-3-iodobenzoate. Bioconjug Chem 4:78–84.
61. Vaidyanathan G, Affleck DJ, Zalutsky MR (1997) Method for radioiodination of proteins using N-succinimidyl 3-hydroxy-4-iodobenzoate. Bioconjug Chem 8:724–729
62. Garg PK, Garg S, Zalutsky MR (1993) N-succinimidyl 4-methyl-3-(tri-n-butylstannyl)benzoate: synthesis and potential utility for the radioiodination of monoclonal antibodies. Nucl Med Biol 20:379–387
63. Geissler F, Anderson SK, Venkatesan P, Press O (1992) Intracellular catabolism of radiolabeled anti-mu antibodies by malignant B-cells. Cancer Res 52:2907–2915
64. Kyriakos RJ, Shih LB, Ong GL, Patel K, Goldenberg DM, Mattes MJ (1992) The fate of antibodies bound to the surface of tumor cells in vitro. Cancer Res 52:835–842

65. Mattes MJ, Griffiths GL, Diril H, Goldenberg DM, Ong GL, Shih LB (1994) Processing of antibody-radioisotope conjugates after binding to the surface of tumor cells. Cancer 73:787–793
66. Shih LB, Thorpe SR, Griffiths GL, Diril H, Ong GL, Hansen HJ, Goldenberg DM, Mattes MJ (1994) The processing and fate of antibodies and their radiolabels bound to the surface of tumor cells in vitro: a comparison of nine radiolabels. J Nucl Med 35:899–908
67. Press OW, Shan D, Howell-Clark J, Eary J, Appelbaum FR, Matthews D, King DJ, Haines AM, Hamann P, Hinman L, Shochat D, Bernstein ID (1996) Comparative metabolism and retention of iodine-125, yttrium-90, and indium-111 radioimmunoconjugates by cancer cells. Cancer Res 56:2123–2129
68. Tolmachev V, Orlova A, Lundqvist H (2003) Approaches to improvement of cellular retention of radiohalogen labels delivered by internalizing tumor targeting proteins and peptides. Curr Med Chem 10:2447–2460
69. Strobel JL, Baynes JW, Thorpe SR (1985) ^{125}I-glycoconjugate labels for identifying sites of protein catabolism in vivo: effect of structure and chemistry of coupling to protein on label entrapment in cells after protein degradation. Arch Biochem Biophys 240:635–645
70. Pittman RC, Carew TE, Glass CK, Green SR, Taylor CA Jr., Attie AD (1983) A radioiodinated, intracellularly trapped ligand for determining the sites of plasma protein degradation in vivo. Biochem J 212:791–800
71. Ali SA, Eary JF, Warren SD, Badger CC, Krohn KA (1988) Synthesis and radioiodination of tyramine cellobiose for labeling monoclonal antibodies. Int J Rad Appl Instrum B 15:557–561
72. Ali SA, Warren SD, Richter KY, Badger CC, Eary JF, Press OW, Krohn KA, Bernstein ID, Nelp WB (1990) Improving the tumor retention of radioiodinated antibody: aryl carbohydrate adducts. Cancer Res 50(3 Suppl):783s–788s.
73. Reist CJ, Archer GE, Kurpad SN, Wikstrand CJ, Vaidyanathan G, Willingham MC, Moscatello DK, Wong AJ, Bigner DD, Zalutsky MR (1995) Tumor-specific anti-epidermal growth factor receptor variant III monoclonal antibodies: use of the tyramine-cellobiose radioiodination method enhances cellular retention and uptake in tumor xenografts. Cancer Res 55:4375–4382
74. Reist CJ, Archer GE, Wikstrand CJ, Bigner DD, Zalutsky MR (1997) Improved targeting of an anti-epidermal growth factor receptor variant III monoclonal antibody in tumor xenografts after labeling using *N*–succinimidyl 5-iodo-3-pyridinecarboxylate. Cancer Res 57:1510–1515
75. Zalutsky MR, Xu FJ, Yu Y, Foulon CF, Zhao XG, Slade SK, Affleck DJ, Bast RC Jr. (1999) Radioiodinated antibody targeting of the HER-2/neu oncoprotein: effects of labeling method on cellular processing and tissue distribution. Nucl Med Biol 26:781–790
76. Stein R, Goldenberg DM, Thorpe SR, Basu A, Mattes MJ (1995) Effects of radiolabeling monoclonal antibodies with a residualizing iodine radiolabel on the accretion of radioisotope in tumors. Cancer Res 55:3132–3239
77. Carlsson J, Blomquist E, Gedda L, Liljegren A, Malmstrom PU, Sjostrom A, Sundin A, Westlin JE, Zhao Q, Tolmachev V, Lundqvist H (1999) Conjugate chemistry and cellular processing of EGF-dextran. Acta Oncol 38:313–321
78. Sundberg AL, Blomquist E, Carlsson J, Steffen AC, Gedda L (2003) Cellular retention of radioactivity and increased radiation dose. Model experiments with EGF-dextran. Nucl Med Biol 30:303–315
79. Stein R, Goldenberg DM, Thorpe SR, Mattes M J (1997) Advantage of a residualizing iodine radiolabel for radioimmunotherapy of xenografts of human nonsmall-cell carcinoma of the lung. J Nucl Med 38:391–395
80. Garg S, Garg PK, Zalutsky MR (1991) *N*–succinimidyl 5-(trialkylstannyl)-3-pyridine-carboxylates: a new class of reagents for protein radioiodination. Bioconjug Chem 2:50–56
81. Garg S, Garg PK, Zhao XG, Friedman HS, Bigner DD, Zalutsky MR (1993) Radioiodination of a monoclonal antibody using *N*–succinimidyl 5-iodo-3-pyridinecarboxylate. Nucl Med Biol 20:835–842

82. Reist CJ, Batra SK, Pegram CN, Bigner DD, Zalutsky MR (1997) In vitro and in vivo behavior of radiolabeled chimeric anti-EGFRvIII monoclonal antibody: comparison with its murine parent. Nucl Med Biol 24:639–647
83. Kuan CT, Reist CJ, Foulon CF, Lorimer IA, Archer G, Pegram CN, Pastan I, Zalutsky MR, Bigner DD (1999) ^{125}I-labeled anti-epidermal growth factor receptor-vIII single-chain Fv exhibits specific and high-level targeting of glioma xenografts. Clin Cancer Res 5:1539–1549
84. Vaidyanathan G, Affleck DJ, Li J, Welsh P, Zalutsky MR (2001) A polar substituent-containing acylation agent for the radioiodination of internalizing monoclonal antibodies: *N*–succinimidyl 4-guanidinomethyl-3-[^{131}I]iodobenzoate ([^{131}I]SGMIB). Bioconjug Chem 12:428–438
85. Vaidyanathan G, Affleck DJ, Bigner DD, Zalutsky MR (2002) Improved xenograft targeting of tumor-specific anti-epidermal growth factor receptor variant III antibody labeled using *N*–succinimidyl 4-guanidinomethyl-3-iodobenzoate. Nucl Med Biol 29:1–11
86. Vaidyanathan G, Affleck DJ, Bigner DD, Zalutsky M (2003) *N*–succinimidyl 3-[^{211}At]astato-4-guanidinomethylbenzoate: an acylation agent for labeling internalizing antibodies with alpha-particle emitting ^{211}At. Nucl Med Biol 30:351–359
87. Foulon CF, Reist CJ, Bigner DD, Zalutsky MR (2000) Radioiodination via D-amino acid peptide enhances cellular retention and tumor xenograft targeting of an internalizing anti-epidermal growth factor receptor variant III monoclonal antibody. Cancer Res 60: 4453–4460
88. Foulon CF, Welsh PC, Bigner DD, Zalutsky MR (2001) Positively charged templates for labeling internalizing antibodies: comparison of *N*–succinimidyl 5-iodo-3-pyridinecarboxylate and the D-amino acid peptide KRYRR. Nucl Med Biol 28:769–777
89. Tolmachev V, Koziorowski J, Sivaev I, Lundqvist H, Carlsson J, Orlova A, Gedda L, Olsson P, Sjöberg S, Sundin A (1999) Closo-dodecarborate (2-) as a Linker for Iodination of Macromolecules. Aspects on Conjugation Chemistry and Biodistribution. Bioconjug Chem 10: 338–345
90. Wilbur DS, Hamlin DK, Srivastava RR, Chyan MK (2004) Synthesis, radioiodination, and biodistribution of some nido- and closo-monocarbon carborane derivatives. Nucl Med Biol 31:523–530
91. Orlova A, Bruskin A, Sivaev I, Sjöberg S, Lundqvist H, Tolmachev V (2006) Radioiodination of monoclonal antibody using isothiocyanato derivative of *closo*-dodecaborate ([^{125}I]Iodo-DABI). Anticancer Res 26:1217–1224
92. Steffen AC, Almqvist Y, Ming-Kuan Chyan, Lundqvist H, Tolmachev V, Wilbur DS, Carlsson J (2007) Biodistribution and dose calculations for ^{211}At labeled HER-2 binding affibody molecules. Oncology Rep 17:1141–1147
93. Shankar S, Vaidyanathan G, Affleck D, Welsh PC, Zalutsky MR (2003) N-succinimidyl 3-[^{131}I]iodo-4-phosphonomethylbenzoate ([^{131}I]SIPMB), a negatively charged substituent-bearing acylation agent for the radioiodination of peptides and mAbs. Bioconjug Chem 14:331–341
94. Vaidyanathan G, Alston KL, Bigner DD, Zalutsky MR (2006) Nepsilon-(3-[*I]Iodobenzoyl)-Lys5-Nalpha-maleimido-Gly1-GEEEK ([*I]IB-Mal-D-GEEEK): a radioiodinated prosthetic group containing negatively charged D-glutamates for labeling internalizing monoclonal antibodies. Bioconjug Chem 17:1085–1092
95. Govindan SV, Mattes MJ, Stein R, McBride BJ, Karacay H, Goldenberg DM, Hansen HJ, Griffiths GL (1999) Labeling of monoclonal antibodies with diethylenetriaminepentaacetic acid-appended radioiodinated peptides containing D-amino acids. Bioconjug Chem 10:231–240
96. Stein R, Govindan SV, Mattes MJ, Chen S, Reed L, Newsome G, McBride BJ, Griffiths GL, Hansen HJ, Goldenberg DM (2003) Improved iodine radiolabels for monoclonal antibody therapy. Cancer Res 63:111–118
97. Orlova A, Bruskin A, Sjostrom A, Lundqvist H, Gedda L, Tolmachev V (2000) Cellular processing of ^{125}I- and ^{111}In-labeled epidermal growth factor (EGF) bound to cultured A431 tumor cells. Nucl Med Biol 27:827–835

98. Sundberg AL, Orlova A, Bruskin A, Gedda L, Carlsson J, Blomquist E, Lundqvist H, Tolmachev V (2003) [^{111}In]Bz-DTPA-hEGF: preparation and in vitro characterization of a potential anti-glioblastoma targeting agent. Cancer Biother Radiopharm 18:643–654
99. Chen J, Cheng Z, Hoffman TJ, Jurisson SS, Quinn TP (2000) Melanoma-targeting properties of ^{99m}technetium-labeled cyclic alpha-melanocyte-stimulating hormone peptide analogues. Cancer Res 60:5649–5658
100. Lantry LE, Cappelletti E, Maddalena ME, Fox JS, Feng W, Chen J, Thomas R, Eaton SM, Bogdan NJ, Arunachalam T, Reubi JC, Raju N, Metcalfe EC, Lattuada L, Linder KE, Swenson RE, Tweedle MF, Nunn AD (2006) ^{177}Lu-AMBA: synthesis and characterization of a selective ^{177}Lu-labeled GRP-R agonist for systemic radiotherapy of prostate cancer. J Nucl Med 47:1144–1152
101. Behr TM, Goldenberg DM, Becker W (1998) Reducing the renal uptake of radiolabeled antibody fragments and peptides for diagnosis and therapy: present status, future prospects and limitations. Eur J Nucl Med 25:201–212
102. Melis M, Krenning EP, Bernard BF, Barone R, Visser TJ, de Jong M (2005) Localisation and mechanism of renal retention of radiolabelled somatostatin analogues. Eur J Nucl Med Mol Imaging 32:1136–1143
103. de Jong M, Barone R, Krenning E, Bernard B, Melis M, Visser T, Gekle M, Willnow TE, Walrand S, Jamar F, Pauwels S (2005) Megalin is essential for renal proximal tubule reabsorption of ^{111}In-DTPA-octreotide. J Nucl Med 46:1696–1700
104. Gotthardt M, van Eerd-Vismale J, Oyen WJ, de Jong M, Zhang H, Rolleman E, Maecke HR, Behe M, Boerman O (2007) Indication for different mechanisms of kidney uptake of radiolabeled peptides. J Nucl Med 48:596–601
105. Sharkey RM, Motta-Hennessy C, Pawlyk D, Siegel JA, Goldenberg DM (1990) Biodistribution and radiation dose estimates for yttrium- and iodine-labeled monoclonal antibody IgG and fragments in nude mice bearing human colonic tumor xenografts. Cancer Res 50:2330–2336
106. Schott ME, Milenic DE, Yokota T, Whitlow M, Wood JF, Fordyce WA, Cheng RC, Schlom J (1992) Differential metabolic patterns of iodinated versus radiometal chelated anticarcinoma single-chain Fv molecules. Cancer Res 52:6413–6417
107. Kenanova V, Olafsen T, Williams LE, Ruel NH, Longmate J, Yazaki PJ, Shively JE, Colcher D, Raubitschek AA, Wu AM (2007) Radioiodinated versus radiometal-labeled anti-carcino-embryonic antigen single-chain Fv-Fc antibody fragments: optimal pharmacokinetics for therapy. Cancer Res 67:718–726
108. Kobayashi H, Kao CH, Kreitman RJ, Le N, Kim MK, Brechbiel MW, Paik CH, Pastan I, Carrasquillo JA (2000) Pharmacokinetics of ^{111}In- and ^{125}I-labeled antiTac single-chain Fv recombinant immunotoxin. J Nucl Med 41:755–762
109. Behr TM, Sharkey RM, Sgouros G, Blumenthal RD, Dunn RM, Kolbert K, Griffiths GL, Siegel JA, Becker WS, Goldenberg DM (1997) Overcoming the nephrotoxicity of radiometal-labeled immunoconjugates: improved cancer therapy administered to a nude mouse model in relation to the internal radiation dosimetry. Cancer 80(12 Suppl):2591–2610
110. Bernard BF, Krenning EP, Breeman WA, Rolleman EJ, Bakker WH, Visser TJ, Macke H, de Jong M (1997) D-lysine reduction of indium-111 octreotide and yttrium-90 octreotide renal uptake. J Nucl Med 38:1929–1933
111. Rolleman EJ, Valkema R, de Jong M, Kooij PP, Krenning EP (2003) Safe and effective inhibition of renal uptake of radiolabelled octreotide by a combination of lysine and arginine. Eur J Nucl Med Mol Imaging 30:9–15
112. van Eerd JE, Vegt E, Wetzels JF, Russel FG, Masereeuw R, Corstens FH, Oyen WJ, Boerman OC (2006) Gelatin-based plasma expander effectively reduces renal uptake of ^{111}In-octreotide in mice and rats. J Nucl Med 47:528–533
113. Vegt E, Wetzels JF, Russel FG, Masereeuw R, Boerman OC, van Eerd JE, Corstens FH, Oyen WJ (2006) Renal uptake of radiolabeled octreotide in human subjects is efficiently inhibited by succinylated gelatin. J Nucl Med 47:432–436

114. Behe M, Kluge G, Becker W, Gotthardt M, Behr TM (2005) Use of polyglutamic acids to reduce uptake of radiometal-labeled minigastrin in the kidneys. J Nucl Med 46:1012–1015
115. Arano Y (1998) Strategies to reduce renal radioactivity levels of antibody fragments. Q J Nucl Med 42:262–270
116. Arano Y, Fujioka Y, Akizawa H, Ono M, Uehara T, Wakisaka K, Nakayama M, Sakahara H, Konishi J, Saji H (1999) Chemical design of radiolabeled antibody fragments for low renal radioactivity levels. Cancer Res 59:128–134
117. Fujioka Y, Arano Y, Ono M, Uehara T, Ogawa K, Namba S, Saga T, Nakamoto Y, Mukai T, Konishi J, Saji H (2001) Renal metabolism of 3 -iodohippuryl N(epsilon)-maleoyl-L-lysine (HML)-conjugated Fab fragments. Bioconjug Chem 12:178–185
118. Uehara T, Koike M, Nakata H, Hanaoka H, Iida Y, Hashimoto K, Akizawa H, Endo K, Arano Y (2007) Design, synthesis, and evaluation of [^{188}Re]organorhenium-labeled antibody fragments with renal enzyme-cleavable linkage for low renal radioactivity levels. Bioconjug Chem 18:190–198
119. Li L, Olafsen T, Anderson AL, Wu A, Raubitschek AA, Shively JE (2002) Reduction of kidney uptake in radiometal labeled peptide linkers conjugated to recombinant antibody fragments. Site-specific conjugation of DOTA-peptides to a cys-diabody. Bioconjug Chem 13:985–995
120. Griffiths GL, Goldenberg DM, Jones AL, Hansen HJ (1992) Radiolabeling of monoclonal antibodies and fragments with technetium and rhenium. Bioconjug Chem 3:91–99
121. Iznaga-Escobar N (2001) Direct radiolabeling of monoclonal antibodies with rhenium-188 for radioimmunotherapy of solid tumors–a review of radiolabeling characteristics, quality control and in vitro stability studies. Appl Radiat Isot 54:399–406
122. Griffiths GL, Goldenberg DM, Knapp FF, Callahan AP, Chang CH, Hansen HJ (1991) Direct radiolabeling of monoclonal antibodies with generator-produced rhenium-188 for radioimmunotherapy: labeling and animal biodistribution studies. Cancer Res 51:4594–4602
123. Winnard P, Virzi E, Fogarasi M, Rusckowski M, Hnatowich DJ (1996) Investigations of directly labeling antibodies with rhenium-188. Q J Nucl Med 40:151–160
124. Rhodes BA, Lambert CR, Marek MJ, Knapp FF, Harvey EB (1996) Re-188 labelled antibodies. Appl Radiat Isot 47:7–14
125. John E, Thakur ML, DeFulvio J, McDevitt MR, Damjanov I (1993) Rhenium-186-labeled monoclonal antibodies for radioimmunotherapy: preparation and evaluation. J Nucl Med 34:260–267
126. Olafsen T, Bruland OS, Zalutsky MR, Sandlie I (1996) Abundant tyrosine residues in the antigen binding site in anti-osteosarcoma monoclonal antibodies TP-1 and TP-3: Application to radiolabeling. Acta Oncol 35:297–301
127. Nikula TK, Bocchia M, Curcio MJ, Sgouros G, Ma Y, Finn RD, Scheinberg DA (1995) Impact of the high tyrosine fraction in complementarity determining regions: measured and predicted effects of radioiodination on IgG immunoreactivity. Mol Immunol 32:865–872
128. Smellie WJ, Dean CJ, Sacks NP, Zalutsky MR, Garg PK, Carnochan P, Eccles SA (1995) Radioimmunotherapy of breast cancer xenografts with monoclonal antibody ICR12 against c-erbB2 p185: comparison of iodogen and N-succinimidyl 4-methyl-3-(tri-n-butylstannyl)benzoate radioiodination methods. Cancer Res 55(23 Suppl):5842s–5846s
129. Olafsen T, Bruland OS, Zalutsky MR, Sandlie I (1995) Cloning and sequencing of V genes from anti-osteosarcoma monoclonal antibodies TP-1 and TP-3: location of lysine residues and implications for radiolabeling. Nucl Med Biol 22:765–771
130. Nestor M, Persson M, Cheng J, Tolmachev V, van Dongen G, Anniko M, Kairemo K (2003) Biodistribution of the chimeric monoclonal antibody U36 radioiodinated with a closo-dodecaborate-containing linker. Comparison with other radioiodination methods. Bioconjug Chem 14:805–810
131. Kennel SJ, Mirzadeh S, Hurst GB, Foote LJ, Lankford TK, Glowienka KA, Chappell LL, Kelso JR, Davern SM, Safavy A, Brechbiel MW (2000) Labeling and distribution of linear peptides identified using in vivo phage display selection for tumors. Nucl Med Biol 27:815–825

132. Antunes P, Ginj M, Zhang H, Waser B, Baum RP, Reubi JC, Maecke H (2007) Are radiogallium-labelled DOTA-conjugated somatostatin analogues superior to those labelled with other radiometals? Eur J Nucl Med Mol Imaging 34(7):982–993
133. Tolmachev V, Orlova A, Nilsson FY, Feldwisch J, Wennborg A; Abrahmsén L (2007) Affibody molecules: potential for *in vivo* imaging of molecular targets for cancer therapy. Expert Opin Biol Ther 7:555–568
134. Orlova A., Magnusson M, Eriksson T, Nilsson M, Larsson B, Höiden-Guthenberg I, Widström C, Carlsson J, Tolmachev V, Ståhl S, Nilsson F (2006) Tumor imaging using a picomolar affinity HER2 binding Affibody molecule. Cancer Res 66:4339–4348
135. Tolmachev V, Nilsson FY, Widström C, Andersson K, Gedda L, Wennborg A, Orlova A (2006) ^{111}In-benzyl-DTPA-$Z_{HER2:342}$, an Affibody-based conjugate for *in vivo* imaging of HER2 expression in malignant tumors. J Nucl Med 47:846–853
136. Engfeldt T, Orlova A, Tran T, Bruskin A, Widström C, Eriksson Karlström A, Tolmachev V (2007) Imaging of HER2-expressing tumours using a synthetic Affibody molecule containing the ^{99m}Tc-chelating mercaptoacetyl-glycyl-glycyl-glycyl (MAG3) sequence. Eur J Nucl Med Molec Imaging 34:722–733
137. Engfeldt T, Tran T, Orlova A, Widström C, Feldwisch J, Abrahmsen L, Wennborg A, Karlström AE, Tolmachev V (2007) ^{99m}Tc-chelator engineering to improve tumour targeting properties of a HER2-specific Affibody molecule. Eur J Nucl Med Molec Imaging 34(11):1843–1853
138. Tran T, Engfeldt T, Orlova A, Widström Ch, Bruskin A, Tolmachev V, Eriksson Karlström A (2007) Comparative in vivo evaluation of peptide-based chelators for attachment of ^{99m}Tc to HER2-targeting affibody $Z_{HER2:342}$. Biocojug Chem 18:549–558
139. Carlsson J, Ren ZP, Wester K, Sundberg ÅL, Heldin NE, Hesselager G, Persson M, Gedda L, Tolmachev V, Lundqvist H, Blomquist E, Nistér M (2006) Planning for intracavitary anti-EGFR radionuclide therapy of gliomas. Literature review and data on EGFR expression. J Neuro-Onc 77:33–45
140. Sundberg AL, Gedda L, Orlova A, Bruskin A, Blomquist E, Carlsson J, Tolmachev V (2004) [^{177}Lu]Bz-DTPA-EGF: preclinical characterization of a potential radionuclide targeting agent against glioma. Cancer Biother Radiopharm 19:195–204
141. Velikyan I, Sundberg AL, Lindhe O, Hoglund AU, Eriksson O, Werner E, Carlsson J, Bergstrom M, Langström B, Tolmachev V (2005) Preparation and evaluation of ^{68}Ga-DOTA-hEGF for visualization of EGFR expression in malignant tumors. J Nucl Med 46:1881–1888
142. Babaei MH, Almqvist Y, Orlova A, Shafii M, Kairemo K, Tolmachev V (2005) [^{99m}Tc] HYNIC-hEGF, a potential agent for imaging of EGF receptors in vivo: preparation and preclinical evaluation. Oncol Rep 13:1169–1175
143. van Gog FB, Visser GW, Stroomer JW, Roos JC, Snow GB, van Dongen GA (1997) High dose rhenium-186-labeling of monoclonal antibodies for clinical application: pitfalls and solutions. Cancer 80(12 Suppl):2360–2370
144. Orlova A, Höglund J, Lubberink M, Lebeda O, Gedda L, Lundqvist H, Tolmachev V, Sundin A (2002) Comparative biodistribution of the radiohalogenated (Br, I and At) antibody A33. Implications for in vivo dosimetry. Cancer Biother Radiopharm 17:385–396
145. Koppe MJ, Bleichrodt RP, Soede AC, Verhofstad AA, Goldenberg DM, Oyen WJ, Boerman OC (2004) Biodistribution and therapeutic efficacy of $^{125/131}$I-, ^{186}Re-, $^{88/90}$Y-, or ^{177}Lu-labeled monoclonal antibody MN-14 to carcinoembryonic antigen in mice with small peritoneal metastases of colorectal origin. J Nucl Med 45:1224–1232
146. Perk LR, Visser GW, Vosjan MJ, Stigter-van Walsum M, Tijink BM, Leemans CR, van Dongen GA (2005) ^{89}Zr as a PET surrogate radioisotope for scouting biodistribution of the therapeutic radiometals ^{90}Y and ^{177}Lu in tumor-bearing nude mice after coupling to the internalizing antibody cetuximab. J Nucl Med 46:1898–1906
147. Perk LR, Visser OJ, Stigter-van Walsum M, Vosjan MJ, Visser GW, Zijlstra JM, Huijgens PC, van Dongen GA (2006) Preparation and evaluation of ^{89}Zr-Zevalin for monitoring of ^{90}Y-Zevalin biodistribution with positron emission tomography. Eur J Nucl Med Mol Imaging 33:1337–1345

148. Bakker WH, Krenning EP, Reubi JC, Breeman WA, Setyono-Han B, de Jong M, Kooij PP, Bruns C, van Hagen PM, Marbach P (1991) In vivo application of [^{111}In-DTPA-D-Phe^{1}]-octreotide for detection of somatostatin receptor-positive tumors in rats. Life Sci 49:1593–1601
149. de Jong M, Bakker WH, Breeman WA, van der Pluijm ME, Kooij PP, Visser TJ, Docter R, Krenning EP (1993) Hepatobiliary handling of iodine-125-Tyr3-octreotide and indium-111-DTPA-D-Phe1-octreotide by isolated perfused rat liver. J Nucl Med 34:2025–2030
150. Verbeke K, Snauwaert K, Cleynhens B, Scheer W, Verbruggen A (2000) Influence of the bifuncational chelate on the biological behavior of ^{99m}Tc-labeled chemotactic peptide conjugates. Nucl Med Biol 27:769–779
151. Zhu Z, Wang Y, Zhang Y, Liu G, Liu N, Rusckowski M, Hnatowich DJ (2001) A novel and simplified route to the synthesis of N3S chelators for ^{99m}Tc labeling. Nucl Med Biol 28:703–708
152. Decristoforo C, Mather SJ (1999) Preparation, ^{99m}Tc-labeling, and in vitro characterization of HYNIC and N3S modified RC-160 and [Tyr^{3}]octreotide. Bioconjug Chem 10:431–438
153. Orlova A, Tran T, Widström Ch., Engfeldt T, Eriksson Karlström A, Tolmachev V (2007) Pre-clinical evaluation of [^{111}In]-benzyl-DOTA-Z(HER2:342), a potential agent for imaging of HER2 expression in malignant tumors. Int J Mol Med 20(3):397–404
154. Dijkgraaf I, Liu S, Kruijtzer JA, Soede AC, Oyen WJ, Liskamp RM, Corstens FH, Boerman OC (2007) Effects of linker variation on the in vitro and in vivo characteristics of an ^{111}In-labeled RGD peptide. Nucl Med Biol 34:29–35

Chapter 9
High-LET-Emitting Radionuclides for Cancer Therapy

George Sgouros

Summary During the last 15 years, alpha-particle emitting radionuclides have been investigated as a possible new class of radionuclides for targeted therapy. Alpha-particles can deposit DNA damaging energy 100 to 1,000 times greater than beta-particles. In this chapter, the background and clinical experiences of targeted alpha-particle radioimmunotherapy use are discussed.

Introduction

Linear energy transfer or LET is the average energy deposited by a particle per unit track length traversed; LET is in units of keV/μm. High LET particles are those with a LET > 10–30 keV/μm. All of the high LET emitting radionuclides used in cancer therapy emit alpha-particles. Alpha particles are charged particles made up of two protons and two neutrons (i.e., helium nuclei) whose LET ranges from 25 to 230 keV/μm, depending upon the particle energy. (High energy gives lower LET because as the particle moves faster the interaction probability is reduced and less energy is deposited per unit track length traversed.) The radiobiology of alpha particles was established in a series of articles by Barendsen and co-workers in the 1960s [1–9]. These studies first demonstrated the key features of alpha-particle irradiation. The biophysical analysis provided in the last paper of the series [10] provided theoretical support for the concept of two types of radiation induced cellular inactivation: (1) accumulation of multiple events that can be repaired at low doses (i.e., sub-lethal damage) but could saturate the cellular repair mechanisms at higher doses, yielding the characteristic linear-quadratic dose-response curve for low LET radiation and (2) lethal events for high LET radiation, yielding the log-linear cell survival curve characteristic of high LET radiation.

The Russel H. Morgan Department of Radiology and Radiological Science,
Johns Hopkins University, School of Medicine, Baltimore, Maryland, USA

T. Stigbrand et al. (eds.) *Targeted Radionuclide Tumor Therapy*,

Targeted Therapy of Cancer Using High-LET Emitters

The practical implications of the studies noted above and the distinction between alpha-particles and the more widely used beta-particle emitters for targeted radionuclide therapy is that it is possible to sterilize individual tumor cells solely from self-irradiation with alpha-particle emitters. This is, however, generally not possible with beta-particle emitters, given achievable antibody specific activity, tumor cell antigen expression levels and the need to avoid prohibitive normal organ toxicity [11]. These facts combine to provide the fundamental strength and rationale for using alpha-particle emitting radionuclides for cancer therapy. Current approaches to cancer treatment are largely inefficient once the tumor has metastasized and tumor cells are disseminated throughout the body. There is also increasing evidence that not all tumor cells are relevant targets for efficient tumor eradication and that sterilization of a putative sub-population of a small number of tumor stem cells may be critical to treatment efficacy [12]. The eradication of such disseminated tumor cells, or of a sub-population of tumor stem cells, requires a systemic targeted therapy that is minimally susceptible to chemo- or radio-resistance, that is potent enough to sterilize individual tumor cells and tumor cell clusters, even at low dose-rate, and that exhibits an acceptable toxicity profile. Alpha-particle emitting radionuclides hold the promise of addressing these critical needs.

Clinical Trials Using High-LET Emitters

The first clinical trial of an alpha-particle emitter in radiolabeled antibody therapy employed ^{213}Bi conjugated to the anti-leukemia antibody, HuM195, and was reported in 1997 [13, 14], 4 years after ^{213}Bi was first suggested for therapeutic use [15]. This was followed by a human trial of the anti-tenascin antibody, 81C6, labeled with the alpha-emitter, ^{211}At [16] in patients with recurrent malignant gliomas. In addition to these two antibody-based trials, a clinical trial of unconjugated ^{223}Ra against skeletal metastases in patients with breast and prostate cancer was recently completed [17]. More recently a patient trial of At-211 targeting ovarian carcinoma has been initiated [18]. Future trials of alpha-emitters are anticipated using antibodies against tumor neovasculature labeled with ^{211}At, ^{213}Bi or ^{225}Ac [19–22]. A conjugation methodology for ^{225}Ac was recently described [23] and a phase I trial of this radionuclide with the anti-leukemia antibody, HuM195 in leukemia patients has recently been initiated [24]. Table 9.1 summarizes clinical trials involving alpha-particle emitting radiopharmaceuticals.

Dosimetry for High LET Emitters

Absorbed dose is defined as the energy absorbed in a particular volume divided by the mass of the volume; it is the average energy density over a particular volume. The LET of alpha-particles is 100 to 1,000 times greater than the average LET of

Table 9.1 Summary of recently reported clinical trials using alpha-particle emitters

Radionuclide	Delivery vehicle	Cancer	Comments	Reference
^{211}At	Anti-tenascin IgG	Glioblastoma Multiforme (GBM)	On-going phase I using surgical cavity injection of labeled anti-tenascin IgG, median survival 60 weeks, two patients w/ recurrent GBM survived nearly 3 years	[25]
	MX35 $F(ab')_2$	Ovarian	On-going phase I using MX35 $F(ab')_2$, BM, peritoneal absorbed dose = 0.08, 8 mGy/MBq, respectively	[18]
^{213}Bi	Anti-CD33 IgG	Leukemia (AML or CML)	Phase I completed w/ no toxicity, substantial reduction in circulating and BM blasts. Phase I/II in cytoreduced patients, 4/23 very high risk patients showed lasting CRs (up to 12 months)	[13, 24]
	Anti-neurokinin receptor peptide	Glioblastoma	Two patients treated with Bi-213, one w/ oligodendroglioma treated by distillation in resection cavity alive more than 67 months	[26]
	Anti CD20 IgG (Rituximab)	Relapsed/refractory Non-Hodgkin's lymphoma (NHL)	Phase I study, nine patients treated to date	[27]
	9.2.27 IgG	Melanoma	Sixteen patients, intralesional administration led to massive tumor cell kill and resolution of lesions; significant decline in serum marker melanoma-inhibitory-activity protein (MIA) at 2 weeks post-treatment was observed	[28]
^{223}Ra	$RaCl_2$	Skeletal breast and prostate cancer metastases	On-going phase 2 randomized trial of external beam + either saline or ^{223}Ra (50 kBq/kg x 4 at 4-week intervals) injections have demonstrated a significant decrease in bone alkaline phosphatase (58% decrease vs. 47% increase with placebo; mean of 33 patients). Fifteen of 31 patients had >50% PSA reduction from baseline vs 5 of 28 in the control group	[29]
^{225}Ac	Anti-CD33 IgG	AML	Phase I trial, on-going, at first dose-level of 0.5 µCi/kg (0.01 kBq/kg), one of two patients included had elimination of peripheral blasts and a reduction in marrow blasts	[24]

beta particles. The much higher energy deposition pattern has two implications: (1) The physical quantity "mean absorbed dose" or average energy density, will not always indicate putative biological outcome in some circumstances. A microdosimetric analysis is then required to calculate a specific energy probability distribution [30]. (2) Per unit absorbed dose, the biological damage caused by alpha-particles is greater than that of beta particles or other low LET radiations [31].

In most cases a microdosimetric analysis will not be necessary for targeted therapy applications because the activity level administered and mean absorbed doses to targeted cells are beyond the classical definition of the microdosimetric realm (i.e., the stochastic deviation is expected to be substantially less than 20% of the mean). In such cases standard dosimetry methods may be applied [32, 33]. The standard approach to dosimetry calculations has been described by the Medical Internal Radionuclide Dose (MIRD) Committee [32]. In this formalism the absorbed dose to a target volume from a source region is given as the total number of disintegrations in the source region multiplied by a factor (the S value) that provides the absorbed dose to a target volume per disintegration in the source region. The sum of these products across all source regions gives the total absorbed dose to the target. MIRD cellular S values have been published for cell level dosimetry calculations for situations in which the number of disintegrations in different cellular compartments can be measured or modeled [34]. Using these S values, the absorbed dose to the nucleus may be calculated from alpha-particle emissions uniformly distributed on the cell surface, in the cytoplasm or in the nucleus. The current methodology for estimating alpha-particle absorbed dose to a particular normal organ or tumor volume is based upon the assumption that all alpha-particle disintegrations in an organ volume deposit the alpha-particle energy uniformly within the organ and that the cross-organ dose from alpha-particles and electron emissions is negligible. The dose contribution from photon emissions is calculated separately and added to the alpha-particle and electron absorbed dose. The methodology is described in detail elsewhere [33].

Conclusions

The fundamental advantage of targeted radionuclide therapy relative to external-beam radiotherapy is that the radiation dose is delivered from within to a targeted cell population that may be widely disseminated. Over the past 10 to 15 years, alpha-particle emitting radionuclides have been investigated as a possible new class of radionuclides for targeted radionuclide therapy. Aside from the ability to target cells from within, targeted delivery of alpha-emitters provides the additional fundamental advantage of a more potent, cytotoxic type of radiation. Alpha-particles are helium nuclei that deposit DNA damaging energy along their track that is 100 to 1,000 times greater than that of beta particles; the damage caused by alpha particles is predominately double-stranded DNA breaks severe enough so as to be almost completely irreparable. This means that a small number of tracks through a cell nucleus can sterilize a cell and that, because the damage is largely irreparable, alpha-particle radiation is not susceptible to resistance as seen with external radiotherapy (e.g., in hypoxic tissue). Animal and cell culture studies have demonstrated that, per unit absorbed dose, the acute biological effects of alpha-particles are three to seven times greater than the damage caused by external beam or beta-particle radiation. Clinical trials of alpha-particle emitters have demonstrated the expected hallmarks of targeted alpha-particle emitter therapy – antitumor efficacy with minimal toxicity.

References

1. Barendsen GW, Koot CJ, van Kerson GR, Bewley DK, Field SB, Parnell CJ. The effect of oxygen on the impairment of the proliferative capacity of human cells in culture by ionizing radiations of different LET. *Int J Radiat Biol.* 1966; 10:317–327.
2. Barendsen GW, Walter HMD. Effects of different ionizing radiations on human cells in tissue culture 4. Modification of radiation damage. *Radiat Res.* 1964; 21(2):314–329.
3. Barendsen GW. Modification of radiation damage by fractionation of dose anoxia + chemical protectors in relation to Let. *Ann N Y Acad Sci.* 1964; 114(A1):96–114.
4. Barendsen GW. Impairment of the proliferative capacity of human cells in culture by alpha-particles with differing linear-energy transfer. *Int J Radiat Biol Relat Stud Phys Chem Med.* 1964; 8(5):453–466.
5. Barendsen GW, Walter HMD, Bewley DK, Fowler JF. Effects of different ionizing radiations on human cells in tissue culture. 3. Experiments with cyclotron-accelerated alpha-particles and deuterons. *Radiat Res.* 1963; 18(1):106–119.
6. Barendsen GW. Dose-survival curves of human cells in tissue culture irradiated with alpha-, beta-, 20-Kv X- and 200-Kv X-radiation. *Nature.* 1962; 193(4821):1153–1155.
7. Barendsen GW, Beusker TLJ. Effects of different ionizing radiations on human cells in tissue culture. 1. Irradiation techniques and dosimetry. *Radiat Res.* 1960; 13(6):832–840.
8. Barendsen GW, Beusker TLJ, Vergroesen AJ, Budke L. Effect of different ionizing radiations on human cells in tissue culture. 2. Biological experiments. *Radiat Res.* 1960; 13(6):841–849.
9. Barendsen GW, Vergroesen AJ. Irradiation of human cells in tissue culture with alpha-rays, beta-rays and x-rays. *Int J Radiat Biol Relat Stud Phys Chem Med.* 1960; 2(4):441.
10. Goodhead DT, Munson RJ, Thacker J, Cox R. Mutation and inactivation of cultured mammalian-cells exposed to beams of accelerated heavy-ions. 4. Biophysical interpretation. *Int J Radiat Biol.* 1980; 37(2):135–167.
11. McDevitt MR, Sgouros G, Finn RD, Humm JL, Jurcic JG, Larson SM et al. Radioimmunotherapy with alpha-emitting nuclides. *Eur J Nucl Med.* 1998; 25(9):1341–1351.
12. Wicha MS. Cancer stem cells and metastasis: Lethal seeds - Commentary. *Clin Cancer Res.* 2006; 12(19):5606–5607.
13. Jurcic JG, Larson SM, Sgouros G, McDevitt MR, Finn RD, Divgi CR, et al. Targeted alpha particle immunotherapy for myeloid leukemia. *Blood.* 2002; 100(4):1233–1239.
14. Jurcic JG, McDevitt MR, Sgouros G, Ballangrud A, Finn RD, Geerlings MW, et al. Targeted alpha-particle therapy for myeloid leukemias: A phase I trial of bismuth-213-HuM195 (anti-CD33). *Blood.* 1997; 90(10):2245.
15. Geerlings MW, Kaspersen FM, Apostolidis C, van der Hout R. The feasibility of 225Ac as a source of alpha-particles in radioimmunotherapy. *Nucl Med Commun.* 1993; 14(2):121–125.
16. Zalutsky MR, Cokgor I, Akabani G, Friedman HS, Coleman RE, Friedman AH et al. Phase I trial of alpha-particle-emitting astatine-211 labeled chimeric anti-tenascin antibody in recurrent malignant glioma patients. *Proc Am Assoc Cancer Res.* 2000; 41:544.

17. Nilsson S, Larsen RH, Fossa SD, Balteskard L, Borch KW, Westlin JE, et al. First clinical experience with alpha-emitting radium-223 in the treatment of skeletal metastases. *Clin Cancer Res.* 2005; 11(12):4451–4459.
18. Hultborn R, Andersson H, Back T, Divgi C, Elgqvist J, Himmelman J, et al. Pharmacokinetics and dosimetry of (211)AT-MX35 F(AB ')(2) in therapy of ovarian cancer - Preliminary results from an ongoing phase I study. *Cancer Biother Radiopharm.* 2006; 21(4):395.
19. Kennel SJ, Mirzadeh S, Eckelman WC, Waldmann TA, Garmestani K, Yordanov AT, et al. Vascular-targeted radioimmunotherapy with the alpha-particle emitter 211At. *Radiat Res.* 2002; 157(6):633–641.
20. Kennel SJ, Mirzadeh S. Vascular targeted radioimmunotherapy with 213Bi–an alpha-particle emitter. *Nucl Med Biol.* 1998; 25(3):241–246.
21. Akabani G, McLendon RE, Bigner DD, Zalutsky MR. Vascular targeted endoradiotherapy of tumors using alpha-particle-emitting compounds: Theoretical analysis. *Int J Radiat Oncol Biol Phys.* 2002; 54(4):1259–1275.
22. Singh JJ, Henke E, Seshan SV, Kappel BJ, Chattopadhyay D, May C, et al. Selective alpha-particle mediated depletion of tumor vasculature with vascular normalization. *PLoS ONE.* 2007; 2:e267.
23. McDevitt MR, Ma D, Simon J, Frank RK, Scheinberg DA. Design and synthesis of 225Ac radioimmunopharmaceuticals. *Appl Radiat Isot.* 2002; 57(6):841–847.
24. Jurcic JG, McDevitt MR, Pandit-Taskar N, Divgi CR, Finn RD, Sgouros G, et al. Alpha-particle immunotherapy for acute myeloid leukemia (AML) with bismuth-213 and actinium-225. *Cancer Biother Radiopharm.* 2006; 21(4):396.
25. Zalutsky MR, Akabani G, Friedman HS, Cokgor I, Coleman RE, Friedman AH et al. Radioimmunotherapy of recurrent glioma patients using alpha-particle emitting astatine-211 labeled chimeric anti-tenascin monoclonal antibody. *J Nucl Med.* 2001; 42(5):121P–122P.
26. Kneifel S, Cordier D, Good S, Ionescu MCS, Ghaffari A, Hofer S, et al. Local targeting of malignant gliomas by the diffusible peptidic vector 1,4,7,10-tetraazacyclododecane-1-glutaric acid-4,7,10-triacetic acid-substance P. *Clin Cancer Res.* 2006; 12(12):3843–3850.
27. Heeger S, Moldenhauer G, Egerer G, Wesch H, Martin S, Nikula T, et al. Alpha-radioimmunotherapy of B-lineage non-Hodgkin's lymphoma using 213Bi-labelled anti-CD19-and anti-CD20-CHX-A ″-DTPA conjugates. *Abstr Pap Am Chem Soc.* 2003; 225:U261.
28. Allen BJ, Raja C, Rizvi S, Li Y, Tsui W, Graham P, et al. Intralesional targeted alpha therapy for metastatic melanoma. *Cancer Biol Ther.* 2005; 4(12):1318–1324.
29. Bruland OS, Nilsson S, Fisher DR, Larsen RH. High-linear energy transfer irradiation targeted to skeletal metastases by the alpha-emitter Ra-223: Adjuvant or alternative to conventional modalities? *Clin Cancer Res.* 2006; 12(20):6250S–6257S.
30. Humm JL, Roeske JC, Fisher DR, Chen GTY. Microdosimetric concepts in radioimmunotherapy. *Med Phys.* 1993; 20(2):535–541.
31. Feinendegen LE, McClure JJ. Meeting report, Alpha-emitters for medical therapy, Workshop of the United States Department of Energy, Denver, Colorado, May 30–31, 1996. *Radiat Res.* 1997; 148(2):195–201.
32. Loevinger R, Budinger TF, Watson EE. *MIRD Primer for Absorbed Dose Calculations, Revised Edition.* New York: Society of Nuclear Medicine,1991.
33. Sgouros G, Ballangrud AM, Jurcic JG, McDevitt MR, Humm JL, Erdi YE, et al. Pharmacokinetics and dosimetry of an alpha-particle emitter labeled antibody: 213Bi-HuM195 (anti-CD33) in patients with leukemia. *J Nucl Med.* 1999; 40(11):1935–1946.
34. Goddu SM, Howell RL, Bouchet LG, Bolch WE, Rao DV. *MIRD Cellular S Values.* Reston, VA: Society of Nuclear Medicine, 1997.

Chapter 10
Targeted High-LET Therapy of Bone Metastases

Øyvind S. Bruland[1], Dahle Jostein[2], Dag Rune Olsen[2], and Roy H. Larsen[2]

Summary Bone metastases cause pain, and may result pathological fractures, spinal cord compression and bone marrow insufficiency. External beam radiation relieves pain, but this treatment modality is limited by lack of tumor cell selectivity. Short track length bone-seeking radioisotopes associated high Linear Energy Transfer offer an attractive alternative for the treatment of bone metastases. The advantages of this approach over external beam radiation are presented and recent preclinical and clinical experience are discussed in this chapter.

Introduction

The clinical implications of skeletal metastases such as pain, pathological fractures, nerve entrapment/spinal cord compression and bone marrow insufficiency have a devastating impact on patients' quality of life [1–4]. External beam radiotherapy effectively relieves pain from localized sites of skeletal metastases [5–9], but the lack of tumor cell selectivity limits its clinical usefulness since normal cells within the target volume receive the same radiation dose as the tumor cells. Furthermore, since skeletal metastases usually are multiple and distributed throughout the axial skeleton [2–4], larger or multiple fields of irradiation are often necessary. However, external beam radiotherapy may further reduce the patient's haematopoietic capacity, already compromised due to bone marrow infiltration of metastases, and, thus, reduce the subsequent tolerance for chemotherapy.

A single fraction of external beam irradiation (8.0 Gy) should be offered to most patients when the clinical indication is pain relief [10–13]. Patients not responding, or those with new pain arising at a previously irradiated site, should be given re-treatment [6–9, 14–17]. In contrast, when the therapeutic aim is local tumor

[1]Faculty of Medicine, University of Oslo and Department of Oncology, The Norwegian Radium Hospital, Oslo, Norway [Ø.S.B.]

[2]Department of Radiation Biology, The Norwegian Radium Hospital, Oslo, Norway [J.D., DRO and R.H.L.]

T. Stigbrand et al. (eds.) *Targeted Radionuclide Tumor Therapy*,

control, such as in patients with solitary bony metastases and long life expectancy, or when medullar compression or imminent fractures are present, fractionated radiotherapy is advisable (3.0 Gy × 10 or higher) in selected cases [7, 18].

Treatment with bone-seeking radiopharmaceuticals is an intriguing alternative that will target multiple metastases simultaneously – symptomatic as well as asymptomatic foci [19]. Following i.v. injection a selective delivery of ionizing radiation to targeted areas of amplified osteoblastic activity can be obtained. The target is Ca-hydroxy-apatite in the metastasis, particularly abundant in sclerotic metastases from prostate cancer, and also present, although more heterogeneously distributed, in mixed sclerotic/osteolytic metastases from breast cancer. This is evident from a biodistribution image common to all bone-seeking radiopharmaceuticals – exemplified as "hot-spots" visualized on a routine diagnostic bone-scan (by ^{99m}Tc-MDP, a radiolabelled bisphosphonate). The clinical experiences using bone-seeking radiopharmaceuticals to relieve pain have been thoroughly reviewed [19–23]. In the commercially available formulations, the radioisotopes involved are beta-emitters: Strontium-89 dichloride (Metastron, GE Healthcare, Chalfont St. Giles, UK) and ^{153}Sm in a complex with EDTMP (Quadramet, Schering AG, Berlin, Germany, and Cytogen Co., Princeton, NJ, USA).

Published data indicate that lower dosages aimed for pain palliation result in relatively few complications in patients with sufficient bone marrow function. Following i.v. injection, the bone-marrow is, however, an innocent bystander and the dose-limiting organ, and the cross-irradiation of the bone marrow due to the millimeter range of the emitted electrons, represents an ever-present concern with beta-emitting bone-seekers. Furthermore, disease-associated bone marrow suppression already present in these patients may often result in delayed and unpredictable recovery. This severely limits the usefulness of beta-emitting radiopharmaceuticals, especially when dosages are increased to deliver potential antitumor radiation levels [22, 24] and/or repeated treatments are attempted. Only a few clinical studies have so far reported on the feasibility of combining bone-seeking radiopharmaceuticals and chemotherapy [25–30].

High-LET Radiopharmaceuticals

Dosimetric modeling and preclinical studies have indicated that alpha-emitting radionuclides could be a promising alternative to beta-emitters in the treatment of minimal residual disease by radioimmunotherapy, and there is an increasing interest to apply alpha emitters in cancer therapy [31–35]. The ranges of alpha-emitters are typically between 40 and 100 μm in tissue. These ranges are well matched with the size of micrometastases, indicating the potential for a more tumor selective irradiation [36].

In contrast to the beta-emitters, the alpha-particle-emitters deliver a much more energetic and localized radiation, classified as high-linear energy-transfer (LET) radiation [37]. Alpha-particles are relatively heavy, charged particles (helium nuclei with two positive charges) and produce densely ionizing tracks through tissue that induces predominantly non-reparable double DNA-strand breaks [38]. Patients with skeletal metastases often have chemoresistant disease and/or micrometastases with dormant clonogenic tumor cells residing in cell cycle growth phase G_0. High-LET irradiation from alpha-emitters will kill such cells at a lower dose/dose-rate than low-LET irradiation [37, 39].

Despite the fact that alpha-emitters are more toxic and mutagenic than beta-emitters, these adverse properties can be compensated for in targeted therapy because of the potential to irradiate much less volumes of normal cells when alpha-emitters are targeted against tumor cell clusters [40]. This feature helps treat skeletal metastases because the short alpha tracks would cause less dose delivered from the bone surfaces to the clonogenic bone marrow cells located within the center of bone marrow containing cavities [40]. Also the spatial distribution of the hydroxy-apatite target within an osteoblastic tumor would facilitate a volume distribution of the radionuclide and make it less likely that tumor cells evade the alpha-particles despite the limited track lengths [39].

The progress in the biomedical application of alpha emitters have been slowed down by the low availability of radionuclides with proper physical and chemical characteristics, supply limitations, and/or expenses for the most popular alpha-emitters, ^{211}At ($t_{½}$ = 7.2 h), ^{213}Bi ($t_{½}$ = 46 min) and ^{225}Ac ($t_{½}$ = 10 days) [35, 41]. Also, because of limited chemical yields and/or short half lives, the production of a final product in clinically useful quantities has been expensive and challenging.

Radium-223: From Bench to Bedside

Lately, a significant research activity has been conducted on alpha emitters that can be prepared in large quantities from long term operating generators [42, 43]. Examples of such alpha-emitters are ^{223}Ra ($t_{½}$ = 11.4 days), ^{224}Ra ($t_{½}$ = 3.7 days), ^{227}Th ($t_{½}$ = 18.7 days) and the alpha-emitter generator ^{212}Pb ($t_{½}$ = 10.6 h). The unavailability of suitable complexing agents for radium isotopes has prevented the exploration of ^{223}Ra in radioimmunotherapy [44], but methods have recently been developed to stably encapsulate ^{223}Ra and ^{225}Ac into liposomes [45–47].

Technology related to these radionuclides has recently led to a significant commercial development (see www.algeta.com) and mature clinical stage development of a new therapy against bone metastases based on radium-223 – Alpharadin® [48–50].

Like strontium, radium is a natural bone seeker that has previously been used for targeting non-malignant skeletal diseases, such as the use of ^{224}Ra for treating ankylosing spondylitis, characterized by elevated bone synthesis [51]. Radium-223 is, in our view, the most promising radium isotope, with favorable features for use in targeted radiotherapy. Radium-223 decays ($t_{½}$ = 11.4 days) via a chain of short-lived daughter radionuclides to stable lead, producing four alpha-particles (Table 10.1). In the decay of ^{223}Ra, about 94% of the total decay energy is released as alpha-particles. The noble gas first daughter ^{219}Rn has a $t_{1/2}$ of approximately 4 s, in contrast to the longer-lived radon-daughters from the other naturally occurring radium isotopes.

Radium-223 can be efficiently produced in large amounts from sources of the precursor ^{227}Ac ($t_{1/2}$ = 21.7 years) in a long-term operating generator [42]. Moreover, ^{223}Ra's half-life provides sufficient time for its preparation, distribution (including long distance shipment), and administration to patients. Its low gamma-irradiation is favorable from the point of view of handling, radiation protection, and treatment on an outpatient basis.

Alpha-particles from the first three nuclides in the decay chain are emitted almost instantaneously (Table 10.1). They are therefore likely to contribute to the radiation dose in the vicinity of the site of ^{223}Ra decay. Hence, ^{223}Ra has the potential to deliver a therapeutically relevant tumor dose from a relatively small amount of administered activity without causing unacceptable doses to non-target tissue.

Preclinical studies with ^{223}Ra. Animal data and dosimetric studies have indicated that bone-targeted alpha-emitters can deliver therapeutically relevant radiation doses to bone surfaces and skeletal metastases, at activity levels that are acceptable in terms of bone marrow radiation exposure [52]. In a comparative study of ^{223}Ra and the beta-emitter ^{89}Sr we found that ^{223}Ra and ^{89}Sr had similar bone uptake, and estimates of dose deposition in bone marrow demonstrated a clear advantage of alpha-particle emitters being bone marrow sparing [40].

A therapeutic study of ^{223}Ra in a nude rat skeletal metastases model showed a significant antitumor activity [32]. In this model, the tumor cells were resistant to

Table 10.1 Summary of effective energy and dose constants for ^{227}Ac and progeny

Nuclide	Effective energy[a] (MeV)	Dose constant Δ (Gy kg Bq^{-1} s^{-1})
^{227}Ac (21.77 years)	0.079	1.28×10^{-14}
^{227}Th (18.68 days)	6.07	9.73×10^{-13}
	5.86[b]	9.39×10^{-13}
^{223}Ra (11.43 days)	5.85	9.37×10^{-13}
	5.65[b]	9.05×10^{-13}
^{219}Rn (3.96 s)	6.81	1.09×10^{-12}
	6.75[b]	1.08×10^{-12}
^{215}Po (1.78 ms)	7.53	1.21×10^{-12}
	7.53[b]	1.21×10^{-12}
^{211}Pb (36.1 min)	0.512	8.20×10^{-14}
^{211}Bi (2.14 min)	6.73	1.08×10^{-12}
	6.67[b]	1.07×10^{-12}
^{207}Tl (4.77 min)	0.498	7.98×10^{-14}

Schematic summary of decay data extracted from the MIRD data base (http://www.nndc.bnl.gov/mird). Database version of July 2, 2007.

[a]Includes alpha, beta, photon, X-ray, and electron energies.

[b]Includes only alpha particle energies. Branching of less than 1% is not considered.

high doses of cisplatin, doxorubicin and an immunotoxin, as well as to both pamidronate (Aredia) and ^{131}I-labeled bisphosphonate treatment, suggesting that ^{223}Ra is therapeutically more effective and could be beneficial in the treatment-resistant skeletal metastases [33].

Clinical studies with ^{223}Ra. A clinical development program for $^{223}RaCl_2$ was initiated, based on these results and on approval obtained from the institutional review boards and regulatory authorities.

Phase 1A. In a phase 1 study of single-dosage administration of escalating amounts of ^{223}Ra (46, 93, 163, 213, or 250 kBq/kg) in 25 patients with bone metastases from breast and prostate cancer [49], dose-limiting hematological toxicity was not observed. Mild and reversible myelosuppression occurred, with only grade 1 toxicity for thrombocytes at the two highest dose levels. Quality of life was evaluated at baseline and at 1, 4, and 8 weeks after injection, and pain relief was observed for all time points in more than 50% of the patients [49]. Furthermore, a decline in total serum alkaline phosphatase greater than 50%, increasingly used as a prognostic marker in metastatic prostate cancer, was observed among patients with elevated pretreatment values. Radium-223 was rapidly cleared from the blood with only 12% of its initial value at 10 min after injection. It was further reduced to 6% at 1 h and to less than 1% at 24 h after infusion. In patients where gamma-camera scintigraphy was performed, ^{223}Ra accumulated in skeletal lesions similar to patterns observed in diagnostic bone scans with ^{99m}Tc-MDP [49], and a predominantly intestinal clearance was demonstrated.

Phase 1B. A small phase 1B feasibility study involving six patients with advanced prostate cancer was then performed [48] with the objective to evaluate the safety profile of repeated ^{223}Ra injections. Six prostate cancer patients were administered a total dosage of up to 250 kBq kg^{-1} body weight, either as a fractionated regimen of two injections of 125 kBq kg^{-1} bodyweight with a 6-week interval (three patients) or 50 kBq kg^{-1} body weight dosages given five times with a 3-week interval (three patients). The patients in the 50 kBq kg^{-1} × 5 group did not experience any additional toxic effects compared with the single-injection phase 1A study related to repeated treatment. It appeared that the hematological profiles were smoothed out because of the fractionation schedule compared with a single dosage totaling the same as the five fractions combined. Because of non-skeletal disease progression, only one of the patients in the 125 kBq kg^{-1} × 2 group actually got the second dosage. Of the two patients not given the 125 kBq kg^{-1} follow-up dosage, one died due to progression of liver metastases, and the other was deemed unfit for further treatment due to recurrence of a previous heart condition. Mild and reversible myelosuppression occurred, with nadir 2 to 3 weeks after injection and complete recovery during the follow-up period. The thrombocytes revealed only grade 1 toxicity, whereas neutropenia of maximum grade 3 occurred in one of the patients. Few other adverse events were seen [39, 48].

The main experience from this small phase 1B study was that repeated administration of ^{223}Ra was well tolerated, and that the time span between injections should be scheduled according to the dosages given; i.e. so that the blood cell count could normalize before a new injection was administrated.

Phase 2. Mature data from a phase 2 randomized trial, of external beam radiation plus either saline injections (four times with 4-week intervals) or four times repeated ^{223}Ra (50 kBq/kg given at 4-week intervals), has recently been published [50]. Adjuvant ^{223}Ra treatment resulted in a statistically significant decrease in bone alkaline phosphatase from baseline compared with placebo showing a particularly strong decrease in patients with elevated pre-treatment levels [50]. The median relative change during treatment for the external radiation plus ^{223}Ra group (33 patients) was –65.6% vs. +9.3% in the external beam radiation plus saline group (31 patients). This observation showed that the areas mostly affected by ^{223}Ra were the regions with an elevated bone metabolism [39]. In the external radiation plus ^{223}Ra group, 15 of 31 patients had a prostate-specific antigen decrease of more than 50% from baseline compared with only 5 of 28 patients in the group receiving external radiation plus saline. The median time to PSA progression was 26 weeks in the ^{223}Ra group and 8 weeks in the placebo group [50].

A favorable adverse event profile was confirmed with minimal bone marrow toxicity for patients who received ^{223}Ra [50]. The myelosuppression observed after ^{223}Ra treatment was minimal and seems different from that observed with the beta-emitting nuclides [19, 22, 50]. With ^{223}Ra, the neutrophils decreased more than thrombocytes, whereas for beta-emitters, thrombocytopenia are commonly dose limiting. It seems that with alpha-emitters, the endosteal bone surface receives high radiation doses, whereas fractions of the bone-marrow are spared.

Importantly, survival analyzes from this Phase 2 trial showed a significant overall survival benefit [50]. The hazard ratio for overall survival, adjusted for baseline covariates was 2.12 ($p = 0.020$, Cox regression). This finding suggests that ^{223}Ra, alone or in combined treatment strategies, should be further evaluated in future therapeutic studies aiming at further delaying disease progression and improving survival in patients with skeletal metastases from hormone-refractory prostate cancer.

Radioimmunotherapy

Actinium-227 has several attractive features as source material not only for ^{223}Ra but also for the alpha emitting radionuclide ^{227}Th. Actinium-227 can be produced relatively easily in large amounts by neutron irradiation of ^{226}Ra in reactors [53]. Its half life of 21.7 years is suitable for a long term operated generator.

Thorium is classified as an actinide although its chemical properties are slightly different from that of actinium. In aqueous solution Th exists as 4+ while Ac is present as 3+, suggesting some differences in the reactivity and stability with various complexing agents. Previously McDevitt et al. have found that DOTA was useful as chelator for ^{225}Ac giving conjugates with monoclonal antibodies, but they required a change in standard reaction conditions compared with e.g. ^{90}Y conjugates [54]. A two step reaction sequence including heating of the Ac-DOTA complex followed by cooling prior to antibody conjugation was required to obtain sufficient stability of the radioimmunoconjugate. A similar two-step reaction sequence would also conjugate ^{227}Th to antibodies [53].

As mentioned above, the mother nuclide for ^{223}Ra is ^{227}Th. This is also an alpha emitter with a half life of 18.7 days. Thus, relevant in vitro and in vivo properties have been demonstrated for monoclonal antibodies labeled with ^{227}Th via the chelator p-SCN-benzyl-DOTA [53, 55, 56]. Recently, novel translational studies in CD-20 expressing human xenografts indicating a therapeutic potential of ^{227}Th-Mabthera have recently been published [57].

A Pilot Experiment with ^{227}Th-Labeled Herceptin

Based on these observations, a pilot experiment was therefore conducted with Her-2 receptor positive BT-474 breast cancer cells. Tumor cells growing as monolayer in culture flasks, were trypsinized and diluted in growth medium (RPMI 1640, 10% FCS supplied with glutamine, streptomycin and penicillin) to about one million cells per milliliter Ten milliliter reaction tubes were added 0.5 ml of the cell suspension and half of the tubes were added 25 µg unlabeled Herceptin and incubated for 5 min at room temperature to block the antigens and act as nonbinding control cells. Thereafter antibody-blocked, as well as non-blocked cells were incubated with various amounts of ^{227}Th–radiolabeled Herceptin. After 1 h of incubation at 37 °C, the cell suspensions were diluted 1,000–5,000 times and plated into culture flasks supplied with growth medium. After 2–3 weeks colonies were fixed with ethanol, stained with methylene blue and counted using a magnifying glass and a phase contrast microscope. Colonies of more than 30 cells were counted.

Cell survival is presented in Fig. 10.1. Figure 10.2 demonstrates binding of ^{227}Th–Herceptin to BT-474 cells. The tracks made by single alpha-particles emitted from the cell surfaces and from ^{223}Ra and daughters in the medium are visualized by micro-autoradiography.

It is anticipated that similar results may be obtained by other monoclonal antibodies with specificity towards tumor-associated antigens (e.g. anti-PSMA against prostate cancer).

A Combined Treatment Strategy

When a symptomatic skeletal metastasis is treated by external beam radiotherapy, new painful foci most often arise after a short time, indicating the existence of microscopic metastases alongside the macroscopic lesions. Bone-marrow micrometastases are also present in patients both with seemingly localized breast cancer [58] and prostate cancer [59]. They may later develop into skeletal metastases, and even act as a nidus for the subsequent growth of visceral metastasis [60].

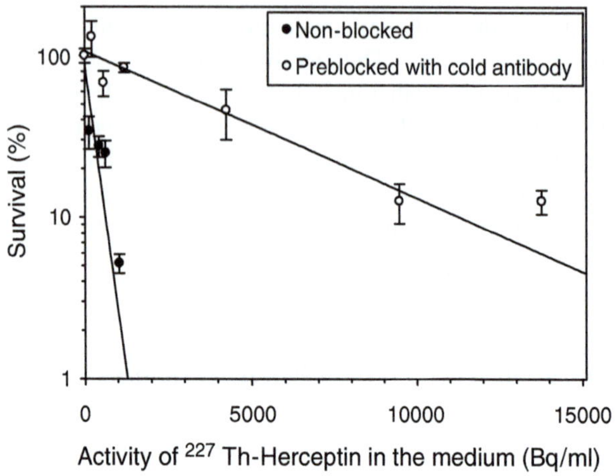

Fig. 10.1 Survival of HER-2 positive BT-474 cells treated with ^{227}Th-Herceptin (closed circles). The BT-474 cells were incubated with ^{227}Th-Herceptin for 1 h in suspension and seeded in flasks. During seeding the activity was diluted 1,000–5,000 times. The open circles represent experiments where binding of ^{227}Th-Herceptin was blocked by pre-incubation of the cells with 50 µg/ml cold Herceptin. Plating efficiency was determined using pre-blocked (open circles) or non-blocked (closed circles) cells. Treatment with 50 µg/ml cold Herceptin resulted in 76% survival. The highest concentration of Herceptin used on the cells treated with only ^{227}Th-Herceptin was 0.7 µg/ml (1,000 Bq/ml). Saturated antigen: A_{10} = 11,290 Bq/ml, A_{37} = 5,060 Bq/ml. Unsaturated antigen: A_{10} = 620 Bq/ml, A_{37} = 280 Bq/ml

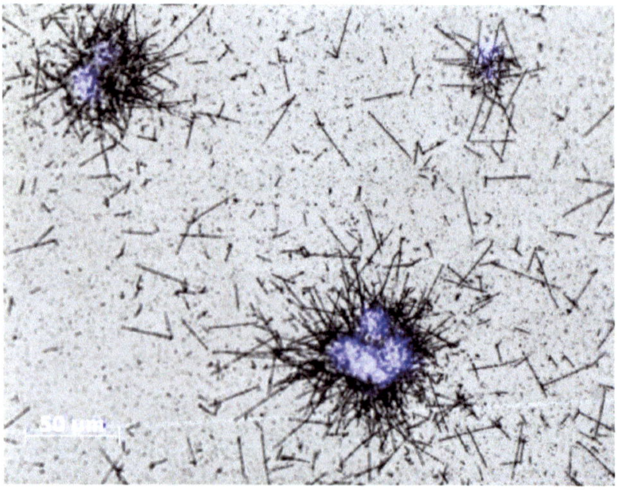

Fig. 10.2 Microautoradiograph of individual alpha tracks from ^{227}Th-Herceptin bound to BT-474 microcolonies; the lower comprising five tumor cells. The cells were seeded on slides and incubated with 10 kBq/ml ^{227}Th-Herceptin for 4 h, washed with PBS with 1% BSA and fixed in 70% ethanol before dipping in autoradiographic emulsion (Hypercoat, Amersham Biosciences, Uppsala, Sweden). After 8 days of exposure the slides were processed according to the manufacturer's instructions. Subsequently, cells were stained with Hoechst 333258, which binds to DNA, and images were acquired using brightfield settings for the alpha-tracks and UV excitation for the nuclei

Because of the dynamic nature of the developing skeletal metastases, optimal therapy should effectively deliver radiation both to multiple macroscopic foci as well as to microscopic disease, including small tumor foci and single clonogenic tumor cells.

Actinium-227 – Thorium-227 – Radium-223: A Novel Technology Platform

Solid tumor deposits have barriers to the uptake of macromolecules, such as monoclonal antibodies [61, 62], whereas radium is a small cation that easily penetrates into a sclerotic metastasis. Based on the results presented above we here propose a strategy for how this might be accomplished. Depending on the biological half life of the antibody carrier, the ^{227}Th will be an in vivo generator for the bone seeking ^{223}Ra. Thus, if conjugated to an antibody with affinity for prostate or breast cancer cells, ^{227}Th-immunoconjugates represent a dual action strategy for alpha emitter based targeted killing of bone metastases: First a cell

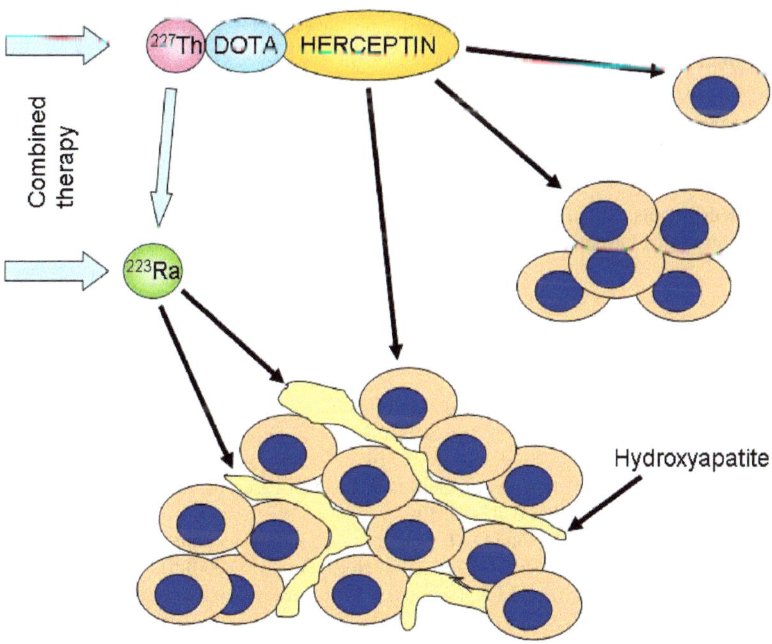

Fig. 10.3 Dual action targeted strategy: Alpharadin[R] (^{223}Ra) is a small molecule that rapidly targets hydroxyapatite in the sclerotic parts of the macroscopic skeletal metastasis. A macromolecule such as a monoclonal antibody will target single cells and may penetrate into small clusters of tumor cells – here exemplified by ^{227}Th-Herceptin that binds to the cell surface of HER2-positive breast cancer cells and microcolonies. When ^{227}Th decays, ^{223}Ra is formed and will diffuse and bind to the calcified metastasis (yellow) and the treatment continues

surface antigen targeting by ^{227}Th – then hydroxyapatite targeting by the daughter radionuclide ^{223}Ra.

Combined treatment, with dual/plural modes of action, is a firm treatment principle in cancer therapy. We here propose to utilize two alpha-emitting radiopharmaceuticals (bone-seeking radium-223 and thorium-227 conjugated to a monoclonal antibody) targeting two different targets and stages in the development cascade of skeletal metastases (Fig. 10.3):

1. Targeting of hydroxyapatite producing macroscopic metastases by radium-223 (Alpharadin^{R}).
2. Targeting of tumor single cell surface epitopes with thorium-227-labelled monoclonal antibodies which, due to their decay characteristics, will form radium-223 that is then partially trapped in the hydroxyapatite producing metastases.

Repeated dosing is the common way to use therapeutics in oncology. This is already shown to be feasible with bone-seeking radium-223 [50] and should be further exploited by two reasons. First the range of the radiation is short, and therefore repeating the treatment could improve dose homogeneity within the target. Second the bone metabolism in normal bone and calcified metastases is a dynamic process where the absorptive and resorptive zones change position over time, which would likely affect the microdistribution of the bone-seeking compound over time. Based on the low toxicity observed in Phase 1 and Phase 2 studies, the possibility seemingly exist to expand dosing further to at least six repeated monthly injections of Alpharadin.

Acknowledgements Thanks are due to the Algeta production and clinical trials teams and the clinical centers that have participated and/or are currently participating in ongoing clinical trials.

References

1. British Association of Surgical Oncology Guidelines, The management of metastatic bone disease in the United Kingdom. The Breast Specialty Group of the British Association of Surgical Oncology. Eur. J. Surg. Oncol. 25 (1999) 3–23.
2. R.E. Coleman, Clinical features of metastatic bone disease and risk of skeletal morbidity. Clin. Cancer Res. 12 (2006) 6243s–6249s.
3. W.D. Hage, A.J. Aboulafia, and D.M. Aboulafia, Incidence, location, and diagnostic evaluation of metastatic bone disease. Orthop. Clin. North Am. 31 (2000) 515–528, vii.
4. O.S. Nielsen, A.J. Munro, and I.F. Tannock, Bone metastases: pathophysiology and management policy. J. Clin. Oncol. 9 (1991) 509–524.
5. D. Hoegler, Radiotherapy for palliation of symptoms in incurable cancer. Curr. Probl. Cancer 21 (1997) 129–183.
6. S. Kaasa, E. Brenne, J.A. Lund, P. Fayers, U. Falkmer, M. Holmberg, M. Lagerlund, and O. Bruland, Prospective randomised multicenter trial on single fraction radiotherapy (8 Gy × 1) versus multiple fractions (3 Gy × 10) in the treatment of painful bone metastases. Radiother. Oncol. 79 (2006) 278–284.

7. D.E. Roos, S.L. Turner, P.C. O'Brien, J.G. Smith, N.A. Spry, B.H. Burmeister, P.J. Hoskin, and D.L. Ball, Randomized trial of 8 Gy in 1 versus 20 Gy in 5 fractions of radiotherapy for neuropathic pain due to bone metastases (Trans-Tasman Radiation Oncology Group, TROG 96.05). Radiother. Oncol. 75 (2005) 54–63.
8. E. Steenland, J.W. Leer, H. van Houwelingen, W.J. Post, W.B. van den Hout, J. Kievit, H. de Haes, H. Marijn, B. Oei, E. Vonk, E. van der Steen-Banasik, R.G. Wiggenraad, J. Hoogenhout, C. Wárlám-Rodenhuis, G. van Tienhoven, R. Wanders, J. Pomp, M. van Reijn, I. van Mierlo, and E. Rutten, The effect of a single fraction compared to multiple fractions on painful bone metastases: a global analysis of the Dutch Bone Metastasis Study. Radiother. Oncol. 52 (1999) 101–109.
9. W.B. van den Hout, Y.M. van der Linden, E. Steenland, R.G. Wiggenraad, J. Kievit, H.H. de, and J.W. Leer, Single- versus multiple-fraction radiotherapy in patients with painful bone metastases: cost-utility analysis based on a randomized trial. J. Natl. Cancer Inst. 95 (2003) 222–229.
10. E. Chow, R. Wong, G. Hruby, R. Connolly, E. Franssen, K.W. Fung, L. Andersson, T. Schueller, K. Stefaniuk, E. Szumacher, C. Hayter, J. Pope, L. Holden, A. Loblaw, J. Finkelstein, and C. Danjoux, Prospective patient-based assessment of effectiveness of palliative radiotherapy for bone metastases. Radiother. Oncol. 61 (2001) 77–82.
11. E. Chow, K. Harris, G. Fan, M. Tsao, and W.M. Sze, Palliative radiotherapy trials for bone metastases: a systematic review. J. Clin. Oncol. 25 (2007) 1423–1436.
12. W.M. Sze, M.D. Shelley, I. Held, T.J. Wilt, and M.D. Mason, Palliation of metastatic bone pain: single fraction versus multifraction radiotherapy–a systematic review of randomised trials. Clin. Oncol. (R. Coll. Radiol.) 15 (2003) 345–352.
13. J.S. Wu, R. Wong, M. Johnston, A. Bezjak, and T. Whelan, Meta-analysis of dose fractionation radiotherapy trials for the palliation of painful bone metastases. Int. J. Radiat. Oncol. Biol. Phys. 55 (2003) 594–605.
14. 8 Gy single fraction radiotherapy for the treatment of metastatic skeletal pain: randomised comparison with a multifraction schedule over 12 months of patient follow-up. Bone Pain Trial Working Party. Radiother. Oncol. 52 (1999) 111–121.
15. P.H. Blitzer, Reanalysis of the RTOG study of the palliation of symptomatic osseous metastasis. Cancer 55 (1985) 1468–1472.
16. E. Chow, J.S. Wu, P. Hoskin, L.R. Coia, S.M. Bentzen, and P.H. Blitzer, International consensus on palliative radiotherapy endpoints for future clinical trials in bone metastases. Radiother. Oncol. 64 (2002) 275–280.
17. D. Tong, L. Gillick, and F.R. Hendrickson, The palliation of symptomatic osseous metastases: final results of the Study by the Radiation Therapy Oncology Group. Cancer 50 (1982) 893–899.
18. E. Maranzano, R. Bellavita, and R. Rossi, Radiotherapy alone or surgery in spinal cord compression? The choice depends on accurate patient selection. J. Clin. Oncol. 23 (2005) 8270–8272.
19. E.B. Silberstein, Systemic radiopharmaceutical therapy of painful osteoblastic metastases. Semin. Radiat. Oncol. 10 (2000) 240–249.
20. G. Bauman, M. Charette, R. Reid, and J. Sathya, Radiopharmaceuticals for the palliation of painful bone metastasis-a systemic review. Radiother. Oncol. 75 (2005) 258–270.
21. I.G. Finlay, M.D. Mason, and M. Shelley, Radioisotopes for the palliation of metastatic bone cancer: a systematic review. Lancet Oncol. 6 (2005) 392–400.
22. V.J. Lewington, Bone-seeking radionuclides for therapy. J. Nucl. Med. 46 Suppl 1 (2005) 38S–47S.
23. G.M. Reisfield, E.B. Silberstein, and G.R. Wilson, Radiopharmaceuticals for the palliation of painful bone metastases. Am. J. Hosp. Palliat. Care 22 (2005) 41–46.
24. I. Resche, J.F. Chatal, A. Pecking, P. Ell, G. Duchesne, R. Rubens, I. Fogelman, S. Houston, A. Fauser, M. Fischer, and D. Wilkins, A dose-controlled study of 153Sm-ethylenediaminetetramethylenephosphonate (EDTMP) in the treatment of patients with painful bone metastases. Eur. J. Cancer 33 (1997) 1583–1591.

25. W. Akerley, J. Butera, T. Wehbe, R. Noto, B. Stein, H. Safran, F. Cummings, S. Sambandam, J. Maynard, R.G. Di, and L. Leone, A multiinstitutional, concurrent chemoradiation trial of strontium-89, estramustine, and vinblastine for hormone refractory prostate carcinoma involving bone. Cancer 94 (2002) 1654–1660.
26. L.C. Pagliaro, E.S. Delpassand, D. Williams, R.E. Millikan, S.M. Tu, and C.J. Logothetis, A Phase I/II study of strontium-89 combined with gemcitabine in the treatment of patients with androgen independent prostate carcinoma and bone metastases. Cancer 97 (2003) 2988–2994.
27. R. Sciuto, A. Festa, S. Rea, R. Pasqualoni, S. Bergomi, G. Petrilli, and C.L. Maini, Effects of low-dose cisplatin on 89Sr therapy for painful bone metastases from prostate cancer: a randomized clinical trial. J. Nucl. Med. 43 (2002) 79–86.
28. S.M. Tu, J. Kim, L.C. Pagliaro, F. Vakar-Lopez, F.C. Wong, S. Wen, R. General, D.A. Podoloff, S.H. Lin, and C.J. Logothetis, Therapy tolerance in selected patients with androgen-independent prostate cancer following strontium-89 combined with chemotherapy. J. Clin. Oncol. 23 (2005) 7904–7910.
29. A. Widmark, New principles in the treatment of prostate cancer–the oncologist's view. Scand. J. Urol. Nephrol. Suppl (2003) 23–27.
30. S. Nilsson, P. Strang, C. Ginman, R. Zimmermann, M. Edgren, B. Nordstrom, M. Ryberg, K.M. Kalkner, and J.E. Westlin, Palliation of bone pain in prostate cancer using chemotherapy and strontium-89. A randomized phase II study. J. Pain Symptom. Manage. 29 (2005) 352–357.
31. B.J. Allen, C. Raja, S. Rizvi, Y. Li, W. Tsui, D. Zhang, E. Song, C.F. Qu, J. Kearsley, P. Graham, and J. Thompson, Targeted alpha therapy for cancer. Phys. Med. Biol. 49 (2004) 3703–3712.
32. G. Henriksen, K. Breistol, O.S. Bruland, O. Fodstad, and R.H. Larsen, Significant antitumor effect from bone-seeking, alpha-particle-emitting (223)Ra demonstrated in an experimental skeletal metastases model. Cancer Res. 62 (2002) 3120–3125.
33. R.H. Larsen, K.M. Murud, G. Akabani, P. Hoff, O.S. Bruland, and M.R. Zalutsky, 211At- and 131I-labeled bisphosphonates with high in vivo stability and bone accumulation. J. Nucl. Med. 40 (1999) 1197–1203.
34. D.A. Mulford, D.A. Scheinberg, and J.G. Jurcic, The promise of targeted {alpha}-particle therapy. J. Nucl. Med. 46 Suppl 1 (2005) 199S–204S.
35. M.W. Brechbiel, Targeted alpha-therapy: past, present, future? Dalton Trans. (2007) 4918–4928.
36. T.E. Wheldon and J.A. O'Donoghue, The radiobiology of targeted radiotherapy. Int. J. Radiat. Biol. 58 (1990) 1–21.
37. E.J. Hall, Radiobiology for the radiologist, Lippincott, Williams & Wilkins, Philadelphia, PA (2000).
38. M.A. Ritter, J.E. Cleaver, and C.A. Tobias, High-LET radiations induce a large proportion of non-rejoining DNA breaks. Nature 266 (1977) 653–655.
39. O.S. Bruland, S. Nilsson, D.R. Fisher, and R.H. Larsen, High-linear energy transfer irradiation targeted to skeletal metastases by the alpha-emitter 223Ra: adjuvant or alternative to conventional modalities? Clin. Cancer Res. 12 (2006) 6250s–6257s.
40. G. Henriksen, D.R. Fisher, J.C. Roeske, O.S. Bruland, and R.H. Larsen, Targeting of osseous sites with alpha-emitting 223Ra: comparison with the beta-emitter 89Sr in mice. J. Nucl. Med. 44 (2003) 252–259.
41. V. Tolmachev, J. Carlsson, and H. Lundqvist, A limiting factor for the progress of radionuclide-based cancer diagnostics and therapy–availability of suitable radionuclides. Acta Oncol. 43 (2004) 264–275.
42. G. Henriksen, P. Hoff, J. Alstad, and R.H. Larsen. ^{223}Ra for endoradiotherapeutic applications prepared from an immobilized ^{227}Ac/^{227}Th source. Radiochim. Acta. 89 (2001) 661–666.

43. G. Henriksen, O.S. Bruland, and R.H. Larsen, Thorium and actinium polyphosphonate compounds as bone-seeking alpha particle-emitting agents. Anticancer Res. 24 (2004) 101–105.
44. G. Henriksen, P. Hoff, and R.H. Larsen, Evaluation of potential chelating agents for radium. Appl. Radiat. Isot. 56 (2002) 667–671.
45. T.J. Jonasdottir, D.R. Fisher, J. Borrebaek, O.S. Bruland, and R.H. Larsen, First in vivo evaluation of liposome-encapsulated 223Ra as a potential alpha-particle-emitting cancer therapeutic agent. Anticancer Res. 26 (2006) 2841–2848.
46. G. Henriksen, B.W. Schoultz, T.E. Michaelsen, O.S. Bruland, and R.H. Larsen, Sterically stabilized liposomes as a carrier for alpha-emitting radium and actinium radionuclides. Nucl. Med. Biol. 31 (2004) 441–449.
47. S. Sofou, J.L. Thomas, H.Y. Lin, M.R. McDevitt, D.A. Scheinberg, and G. Sgouros, Engineered liposomes for potential alpha-particle therapy of metastatic cancer. J. Nucl. Med. 45 (2004) 253–260.
48. S. Nilsson, L. Balteskard, S.D. Fosså, and Ø.S. Bruland. Phase I study of Alpharadin™ (^{223}Ra), and alpha-emitting bone-seeking agent in cancer patients with skeletal metastases. Eur. J. Nucl. Med. Mol. Imaging 370 Suppl (2004) 290.
49. S. Nilsson, R.H. Larsen, S.D. Fossa, L. Balteskard, K.W. Borch, J.E. Westlin, G. Salberg, and O.S. Bruland, First clinical experience with alpha-emitting radium-223 in the treatment of skeletal metastases. Clin. Cancer Res. 11 (2005) 4451–4459.
50. S. Nilsson, L. Franzen, C. Parker, C. Tyrrell, R. Blom, J. Tennvall, B. Lennernas, U. Petersson, D.C. Johannessen, M. Sokal, K. Pigott, J. Yachnin, M. Garkavij, P. Strang, J. Harmenberg, B. Bolstad, and O.S. Bruland, Bone-targeted radium-223 in symptomatic, hormone-refractory prostate cancer: a randomised, multicentre, placebo-controlled phase II study. Lancet Oncol. 8 (2007) 587–594.
51. M. Lassmann, D. Nosske, and C. Reiners, Therapy of ankylosing spondylitis with 224Ra-radium chloride: dosimetry and risk considerations. Radiat. Environ. Biophys. 41 (2002) 173–178.
52. Y. Kvinnsland, A. Skretting, and O.S. Bruland, Radionuclide therapy with bone-seeking compounds: Monte Carlo calculations of dose-volume histograms for bone marrow in trabecular bone. Phys. Med. Biol. 46 (2001) 1149–1161.
53. R.H. Larsen, J. Borrebaek, J. Dahle, K.B. Melhus, C. Krogh, M.H. Valan, and O.S. Bruland, Preparation of TH227-labeled radioimmunoconjugates, assessment of serum stability and antigen binding ability. Cancer Biother. Radiopharm. 22 (2007) 431–437.
54. M.R. McDevitt, D. Ma, J. Simon, R.K. Frank, and D.A. Scheinberg, Design and synthesis of 225Ac radioimmunopharmaceuticals. Appl. Radiat. Isot. 57 (2002) 841–847.
55. J. Dahle, J. Borrebaek, K.B. Melhus, O.S. Bruland, G. Salberg, D.R. Olsen, and R.H. Larsen, Initial evaluation of 227Th-p-benzyl-DOTA-rituximab for low-dose rate alpha-particle radioimmunotherapy. Nucl. Med. Biol. 33 (2006) 271–279.
56. K.B. Melhus, R.H. Larsen, T. Stokke, O. Kaalhus, P.K. Selbo, and J. Dahle, Evaluation of the binding of radiolabeled rituximab to CD20-positive lymphoma cells: an in vitro feasibility study concerning low-dose-rate radioimmunotherapy with the alpha-emitter ^{227}Th. Cancer Biother. Radiopharm. 22 (2007) 469–479.
57. J. Dahle, J. Borrebaek, T.J. Jonasdottir, A.K. Hjelmerud, K.B. Melhus, O.S. Bruland, O.W. Press, and R.H. Larsen, Targeted cancer therapy with a novel low-dose rate alpha-emitting radioimmunoconjugate. Blood 110 (2007) 2049–2056.
58. S. Braun, F.D. Vogl, B. Naume, W. Janni, M.P. Osborne, R.C. Coombes, G. Schlimok, I.J. Diel, B. Gerber, G. Gebauer, J.Y. Pierga, C. Marth, D. Oruzio, G. Wiedswang, E.F. Solomayer, G. Kundt, B. Strobl, T. Fehm, G.Y. Wong, J. Bliss, A. Vincent-Salomon, and K. Pantel, A pooled analysis of bone marrow micrometastasis in breast cancer. N. Engl. J. Med. 353 (2005) 793–802.
59. A. Berg, A. Berner, W. Lilleby, O.S. Bruland, S.D. Fossa, J.M. Nesland, and G. Kvalheim, Impact of disseminated tumor cells in bone marrow at diagnosis in patients with nonmetastatic prostate cancer treated by definitive radiotherapy. Int. J. Cancer 120 (2007) 1603–1609.

60. I.J. Diel, E.F. Solomayer, S.D. Costa, C. Gollan, R. Goerner, D. Wallwiener, M. Kaufmann, and G. Bastert, Reduction in new metastases in breast cancer with adjuvant clodronate treatment. N. Engl. J. Med. 339 (1998) 357–363.
61. R.K. Jain, Barriers to drug delivery in solid tumors. Sci. Am. 271 (1994) 58–65.
62. L. Eikenes, O.S. Bruland, C. Brekken, and C.L. Davies, Collagenase increases the transcapillary pressure gradient and improves the uptake and distribution of monoclonal antibodies in human osteosarcoma xenografts. Cancer Res. 64 (2004) 4768–4773.

Chapter 11
The Auger Effect in Molecular Targeting Therapy

Hans Lundqvist, Bo Stenerlöw, and Lars Gedda

Abbreviations SSB, Single-strand break (in DNA); DSB, Double-strand break (in DNA); BrdUR, Bromodeoxyuridine; IdUR, Iododeoxyuridine; RBE, Relative biological effectiveness; ER, Estrogen receptor; TFO, Triplex-forming ologonucleotides; DMSO, Dimethyl sulfoxide (radical scavenger); Mbp, Mega base pair; D_0, Cell survival parameter that describes the exponential part of a cell survival curve of type $n = n_0 * e^{-D/D_0}$; SPECT, Single photon emission computed tomography; PET, Positron emission tomography; NLS; Nuclear localizing signal

Summary Knowledge on the physical and biological aspects of Auger-electron emission is described and the major attempts to use such emitters in cancer therapy are discussed. Focus is on the need for nuclear localization of the Auger-electron emitters, i.e. preferably targeting the nuclear DNA, to have a good therapy effect. Delivery of Auger-electron emitters using nucleoside analogues, DNA-intercalators, minor groove binders, hormone receptor ligands and oligonucleotides are described as well as the need for nuclear localization signals in peptides and proteins.

Introduction

The search for the Holy Grail or the Philosophers Stone has through history been a driving force to increase our knowledge. That Isaac Newton, the father of modern science, also was an alchemist shows how the human mind is trying both rational and non-rational ways in its search for knowledge. In medicine the "magic bullet", a concept created by Paul Ehrlich in the beginning of 1900, has played this role of inspiration.

Originally, "magic bullets" were thought to be compounds that would have a specific attraction to disease-causing microorganisms. The magic bullets would seek these organisms and destroy them, avoiding other organisms and having no

Department of Oncology, Radiology and Clinical Immunology, Rudbeck Laboratory, Uppsala University, SE-751 85, Uppsala, Sweden harmful effects on the healthy tissues of the patients. In nuclear medicine the "magic bullet" concept has often been used related to the "Auger effect" caused by electrons emitted e.g. in the electron capture decay. Pierre Auger, a French physicist discovered the phenomena in 1925 [1] but not until the late 1960s the biological significance was realized. Actually, due to the small energy amount released by the Auger electrons they were usually neglected in the macroscopic dosimetry.

The pioneering work was made using ^{125}I-iododeoxyuridine (^{125}IUdR), which is incorporated into DNA as a thymidine analogue. A striking toxicity in mammalian cells was found, which could not at all be explained by the delivered absorbed dose. Furthermore, the survival curve had, similar to high LET radiation, no shoulder, which indicated that no repair was involved. This was the first experimental demonstration of what we today call the biological Auger effect, which is caused by local energy absorption of low energy electrons creating complex double-strand breaks (DSB) in the DNA.

Since then our understanding of the Auger effect and how to use it has progressed. The large improvement in DNA technology the last years has also developed new tools to analyze e.g. single and double strand breaks. Studies using simplified model systems, like synthetic DNA and plasmid DNA, have contributed with important knowledge about details in the Auger process. Still, many unresolved problems remain such as the exact delivery of the energy to the complex DNA structure in the nucleus of a living cell, how many DSBs that are created, how extended the DSBs are and to what extent non-radiation like charge contribute to the effect.

The utilization of the Auger effect in targeting radionuclide therapy is challenging. Due to the local effect within a few nanometers it is not enough to target the tumour cells but there is also a need to target the DNA in the tumour cell. In fact, to obtain the full effect, the radionuclide needs to decay within the DNA molecule either incorporated into the backbone or placed in between the strands. In this chapter we describe the current knowledge of the physical, molecular and cellular effects on Auger-electron emission and discuss briefly the major attempts to use Auger-electron emitters in cancer therapy.

Physics of the Auger Effect

The Auger effect is caused by a vacancy in the inner electron shells, preferably the K-shell, which greatly disturbs the energy stability of the atom. In the following complex process, when the energy balance is regained, a large number of low energy electrons and characteristic x-rays are emitted from the different atomic electron shells (Fig. 11.1).

The term "Auger electrons" is a conceptual name for different transitions (Auger, Coster-Kronig, and super Coster-Kronig). Generally one can say that Auger transitions takes place between the shells (L→K, M→L etc.). Since each shell with more than two electrons can be split into slightly different energy levels

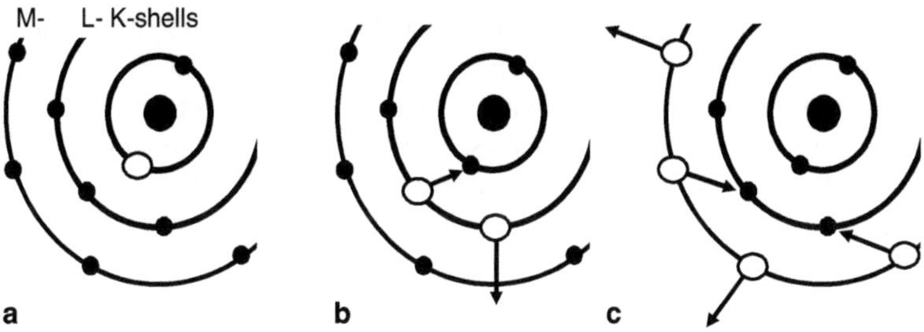

Fig. 11.1 A schematic illustration of the Auger process. (a) A hole is created in the K-shell either by electron capture decay, conversion electrons or photon irradiation. It causes energy instability in the atom and (b) one electron from the L-shell is moving inwards to an energetically more stable position. The released energy will either be emitted as characteristic X-ray or be transferred to another electron, which will be ejected from the atom (Auger electron) creating a second hole in the L-shell. (c) The holes in the L-shell will undergo the same process creating more Auger electrons and holes in the M-shell

Table 11.1 Auger electron emitting radionuclides. Only data for the Auger electrons are given. Mean energy and yields (number of electrons) are per decay. Data are mainly taken from Stepanek et al. [60,61].

Nuclide	T1/2	Mean energy (KeV)	Yield	Nuclide	T1/2	Mean energy (KeV)	Yield
^{51}Cr	27.70 d	3.97	4.68	^{114m}In	49.50 d	4.15	7.75
^{64}Cu	12.70 h	2.09	1.65	^{115m}In	4.49 h	2.85	5.04
^{67}Ga	3.26 d	7.07	7.03	^{123}I	13.20 h	7.33	12.6
^{77}Br	57.00 h	4.13	4.96	^{124}I	4.18 d	4.87	8.6
^{80m}Br	4.42 h	7.97	9.54	^{125}I	60.10 d	11.9	21.0
^{94}Tc	4.88 h	5.17	6.42	^{167}Tm	9.25 d	13.6	11.4
^{99m}Tc	6.01 h	0.96	4.67	^{193m}Pt	4.33 d	10.9	20.3
^{111}In	2.80 d	6.51	6.05	^{195m}Pt	4.02 d	21.8	31.5

(the fine structure), transitions between electrons in the same shell can also occur (the Coster-Kronig transitions). The energy of the ejected electron is equal to the energy difference between the shells that are involved. Thus, a large number of combinations will result in an Auger electron energy spectrum composed by many mono-energetic electrons of varying intensity.

Electron capture decay or internal transitions are the main sources of Auger electrons. In some radionuclides internal conversion can contribute essentially, e.g. ^{125}I (Table 11.1). Some care has to be taken when reading tables of this kind since, e.g. yields are calculated using different models that can give varying results. Still, general aspects are obvious like the increase of energy and yield with atomic number.

One radionuclide, ^{125}I, stands out from the rest due to comparatively high number of Auger electrons and since it is, as a halogen, easy to use in the labelling of bio-molecules. Most of the work related to the biological Auger effect has been performed with this single radionuclide and some more detailed understanding of how the Auger electrons are produced in this radionuclide may be of interest (Fig. 11.2).

When interpreting an experimental situation it is important to distinguish between what might be a normal increased cellular dose and the biological Auger effect. A calculated Auger electron spectrum of ^{111}In (Fig. 11.3) is given as an example. Electron energies close to the ionization potential (<30 eV) will only have a marginal effect and electrons above 5 keV with a range of about 1 µm will not contribute to the local effect. As seen in Fig. 11.3 a substantial part of the Auger electrons will have an energy of about 20 keV, which is an ideal energy to be fully deposited within the size of a mammalian cell. Thus, an unexpected high response using ^{111}In might be due to these electrons that are absorbed within the cell, but far from DNA, and they will not cause the local DNA impact that we usually associate with the biological Auger effect.

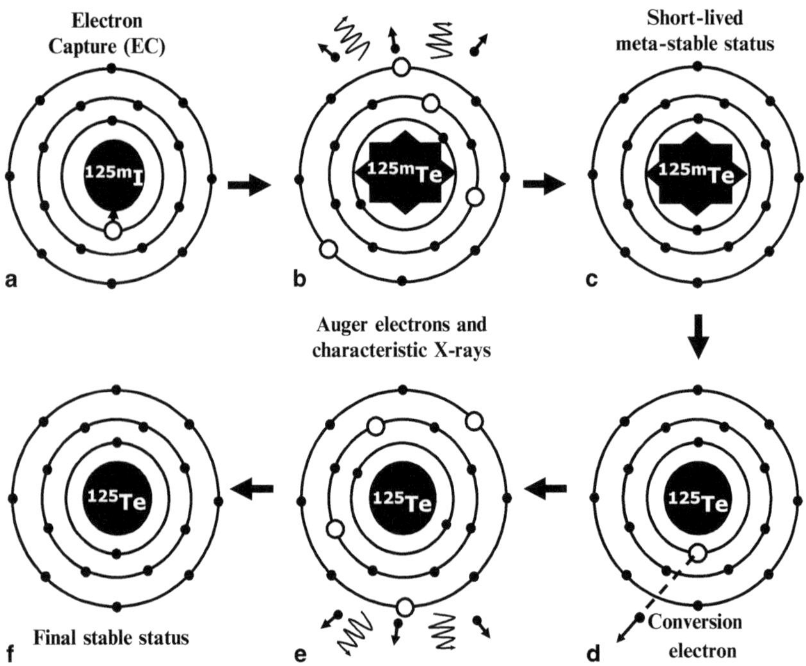

Fig. 11.2 A schematic illustration of the decay of ^{125}I. The electron capture decay (a) creates a hole and an energy imbalance in the electron shells. In the process to reach energy balance Auger electrons and characteristic X-rays are emitted (b). Following the electron capture the daughter nuclide will be left in an excited state (c). The life time of this excited state (^{125m}Te) is only a few nano-seconds but long enough to fill the electron shells. In 93% of all decays the energy in the excited state will be transferred to an orbit electron (d), which will be emitted from the atom leaving a new hole in the electron shell. A new cascade of Auger electrons and characteristic X-rays is produced (e) before finally the daughter nuclide is produced in its ground state (f)

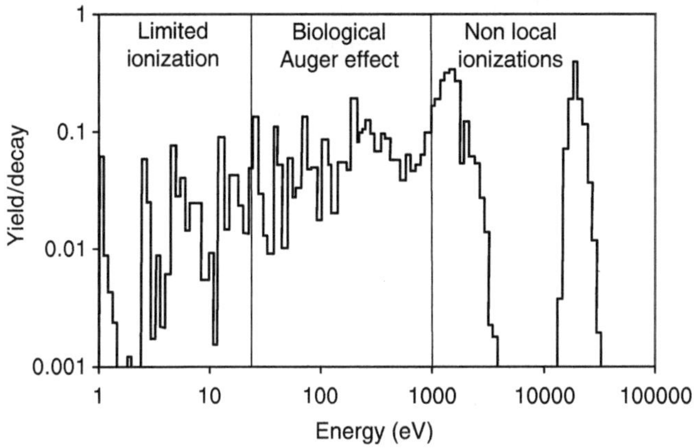

Fig. 11.3 A calculated Auger electron energy spectrum from the ^{111}In decay (Data taken from [60]). In the figure the area of electron energies that substantially contributes to the biological Auger effect is marked

Quantifying the Auger Effect

At radiation therapy we are trained to use absorbed dose (Gy) as a parameter to which we relate biological effects and therapeutic results. The use of different radiation qualities is handled with the concept of relative biological effectiveness (RBE) where the biological effect of the tested radiation is compared with that of low LET radiation. Individual electrons are mainly low-LET radiation (energy < 10 keV/μm). Only a small fraction of the Auger electrons will have LET between 10 and 30 keV/μm and a slightly increased RBE. The biological Auger effect is then explained as a collective effect of several low-LET electrons that will give a more effective production of severe double-strand breaks and hence an RBE value compared to high-LET radiation like alpha-emitters.

One problem to use absorbed dose in conjunction with the Auger effect is that we are limited to rely on calculations both of the source (yield of low energy Auger electrons) and of how the energy is absorbed since it is almost impossible to measure these parameters during physiological conditions. Most of the calculations are from free atoms i.e. without any chemical bonds or chemical and biological surrounding or in simplified systems. In the energy interval <100 eV the binding energies of the electrons will vary and so will the yields depending in which milieu the decay takes place. Furthermore, the ionization potential of the DNA molecule and the ability of the Auger electrons to create DSBs will also considerably vary depending on the chemical and physiological conditions. This means that our calculation models are still not very accurate and may give results that can differ with a factor 2 or 3.

A schematic energy distribution from the ^{125}I-decay as a function of the distance is seen in Fig. 11.4. The figure is based upon calculated energy distributions found in the literature [2]. On purpose, the y-axis is not given in an absolute energy scale since different calculation models vary with a factor of 3. However, they do reasonably well present shapes of the curves, which tells us that a central decay in DNA will give the highest absorbed dose while positioning the decay on the surface of DNA will reduce the dose with roughly a factor 2. At a distance of 3 nm the absorbed dose will be only 10% of maximum.

Beside direct ionizations and radical attacks on the DNA molecule other effects may also contribute. One such effect is referred to as the "Coulomb explosion" which was mentioned already in the early work in the 1960s. Briefly the idea is that the decay of e.g. ^{125}I releases about 20 electrons leaving a daughter nucleus that is heavily positively charged. In the neutralization processes the electrons can come from the surrounding water, but there is also a possibility that they may be recruited directly from the DNA molecule and add to the destruction of its molecular structure. In a paper by Pomplun and Sutmann in 2004 [3] it was concluded that the Coulomb explosion must be seen as a severe effect additional to and amplifying the damage induced by Auger electron radiation, at least in isolated DNA. It is obvious that more profound calculations have to be performed.

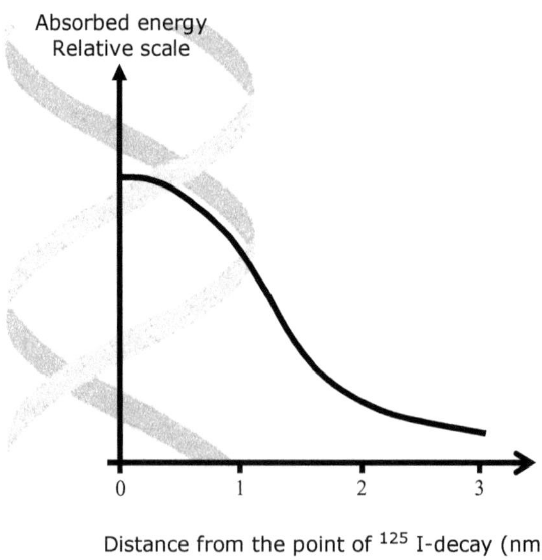

Fig. 11.4 Absorbed energy as a function of distance from the point of ^{125}I-decay. The energy distribution is related to a schematic DNA-molecule showing that the energy and hence the ability to create DSBs decreases rapidly with the distance. A central decay of ^{125}I in DNA will most likely create a large DSB caused by direct interaction of the Auger electrons. This damage is not essentially modified by radical scavengers. DNA irradiated at some distance can still develop a DSB but this damage is mainly caused by radicals and is modified by radical scavengers (Freely after [2])

The situation is somewhat more complicated than indicated in Fig. 11.4 since a decay on the surface of DNA will have a larger probability to irradiate adjacent DNA but still, measured RBE values for the ^{125}I-decay varies significantly depending on how firmly attached the radionuclide is to DNA. Thus, simulating the molecular effects of Auger decays is a challenging task, which is further complicated by the fact that measurement of DNA damage largely depends on the biological test system and assays used. Some of these aspects are discussed in the following sections.

Effects on Cells and DNA

In addition to the therapeutic potential of Auger-electron emitters, the Auger-electron emitter ^{125}I has proven to be an efficient tool in the study of radiochemical and radiobiological effects of ionizing radiation (see review by Hofer [4] and references therein). In the early days of radiobiology it became clear that DNA was the primary target for ionizing radiation and damage to DNA was closely related to cell death. In several variations on these key experiments, the cell nucleus and cytoplasm were irradiated separately. From such studies it became evident that the cellular localization of the Auger decay is critical for the cellular response: ^{125}I-decays in the cytoplasm, plasma membrane or outside the cells were relatively non-toxic, whereas decays from DNA-incorporated ^{125}I were highly efficient in cell killing [5] and showing cell survival curves similar to those obtained in high-LET experiments. This did not only prove that DNA in the cell nucleus was the primary target for radiation-induced cell death but it also demonstrated the essence of a true Auger-electron emitter – i.e. to have any significant cell killing ability it has to be located close to the DNA.

The very first results on the biological toxicity of Auger electrons were reported by Hofer and co-workers [6] followed by several other studies [7] and the first analysis of breaks on DNA was performed some years later [8, 9]. From these and later studies it is evident that Auger-electron emitters are highly efficient in inducing DSBs, although it is far from fully understood how this efficiency is influenced by cellular variations (e.g. cell cycle, localization of the decay), chemical environment (i.e. role of radical scavengers) or, sometimes, the type of radionuclide used. All these studies have contributed with important knowledge about the molecular effects of Auger-decays, but have also demonstrated that different test systems may give apparently contradictory results.

Damage to DNA

Generally, basic understanding of the biological effects of ionizing radiation is important in guiding the development of radiotherapy. For our basic understanding of the action of Auger-electron emitters on DNA and to interpret the biological consequences of Auger decays, measurements of DNA damage have been important. It was early demonstrated that ^{125}I decays in DNA induced DSBs with nearly 100% efficiency [8, 9]. This 1:1 correlation between decay and DSBs has for many years also been used to calibrate various DSB-detection assays applied on mammalian cells.

Much of our knowledge regarding DNA damage from Auger-electron emitters comes from studies using plasmid DNA or synthesized DNA. These "naked" DNA structures, lacking associated proteins or packaging, are useful tools in the molecular analysis of Auger decays at various positions in the DNA. Furthermore, in these test systems the compounds (e.g. substances labelled with Auger-electron emitters) have direct access to the DNA and the administration is independent of cellular uptake or confounding factors that might influence the delivery. Oligonucleotides are synthesized as double-stranded DNA with defined sequence and typical lengths of 20–100 bp. In their pioneer work, Martin and Haseltine [10] used such constructed DNA molecules and incorporated ^{125}I at a single known position. From these and later studies it was evident that the ^{125}I decay is highly efficient in inducing DNA strand breaks within 8–10 bases of the decay, in both the labelled and unlabelled strand, but strand breaks were detectable up to 20 bases from the ^{125}I decay.

Plasmids are double stranded and circular DNA molecules (typically 3–7 kbp long), normally present in bacteria. A single-strand break (SSB) on the supercoiled plasmid produces a relaxed DNA structure, whereas a DSB gives a linear DNA fragment and these DNA configurations can easily be separated by electrophoresis. These unique properties of plasmids have been utilized in a great number of studies on how the magnitude of DNA damage depends on the position of decay site relative to DNA [4]. In a series of experiments Kassis and Adelstein used ^{125}I-labelled substances to show that even small variations in the position of the decay site relative to DNA can have dramatic effects on the yields of SSBs and DSBs [11–13]. For example, ^{125}I-labelled substances that bind to the minor groove of DNA (e.g. Hoechst 33342) and ^{125}I that remain free in solution are equally effective in producing single-strand breaks. In contrast, the minor groove binder is five to seven times more efficient than free ^{125}I in producing DSBs. Similar types of experiments on cell killing effects of DNA-binding agents in cellular systems confirm the importance of the position of the Auger decay (see below). In summary, several SSBs are induced around the decay site but in these model systems with naked DNA there is no evidence that a single ^{125}I can induce more than one DSB.

Cellular Effects

Plasmid DNA and synthetic oligonucleotides are important tools in the investigations of basic mechanisms of radiation action on the DNA. However, DNA in a mammalian cell is bound to various associated proteins and forms a highly compact and organized structure called chromatin. This structure includes the winding of DNA around nucleosomal proteins and further compaction into a chromatin fibre that is organized into chromatin loops. This chromatin has several radio-protecting functions: besides acting as an effective radical scavenger itself, chromatin proteins also exclude water from the DNA double helix thereby reducing the radical-mediated effects from ionizing radiation. Furthermore, the compact structure may also increase the possibility that an Auger decay on one strand will damage DNA on another strand, maybe hundreds or thousands of base-pairs away (although still within a physical distance of some tens of nanometers).

The vast majority of cellular studies with Auger-electron emitters have used DNA-incorporated ^{125}I. Proliferating cells synthesize new DNA during the S-phase of the cell cycle and by adding the thymidine analogue ^{125}IdUR to the cell culture, the Auger emitting nuclide is incorporated into the DNA. In such experiments the decay-rate of the DNA-incorporated nuclide is comparatively low and cells are frozen (for days to months) to accumulate decays without the ability to repair the damage. The cells are then thawed and analysed for DNA damage or survival. Cells labelled with ^{125}IdUR for one to two cell cycles before accumulation of decays show typically high-LET dose-response where and the cell survival decreases exponentially, without shoulder, for increasing number of decays.

Indirect Radiation Action Is Important

In studies using plasmid systems the radical scavenger dimethyl sulfoxide (DMSO) is unable to protect DNA from ^{125}I decays occurring in close proximity to the DNA helix [14]. These results indicate that direct action of Auger electrons are responsible for the DNA fragmentation. In intact cells, however, the situation is more complex and factors like scavenging conditions, chromatin organization and DNA concentration may influence the action of Auger-electron emitters. Indeed, studies in mammalian (V79 hamster) cells showed a considerable effect of DMSO on both DSB yield and survival [15–17], which indicates that here the indirect action is an important contributor to the cell killing effect by Auger-electron emitters. These results could be explained by the fact that the DNA in mammalian cells, unlike naked plasmid DNA, is a highly compact and organized structure and OH-radicals from ^{125}I-decays can attack both at a local site and sites that are hundreds or thousands of base-pairs away from the decay position. Because of this, it was concluded that more than one DSB should be produced per ^{125}I-decay in the absence of scavengers. In fact, recent results show that DNA-incorporated ^{125}I can induce clusters of DSBs within 0.5 Mbp from the decay site as assessed by DNA fragmentation analysis and that this gives significantly more than one DSB per decay in an intact cell [18]. These findings support the idea that the release of >20 Auger electrons within compact and looped chromatin in intact cells may have a considerable probability of producing correlated DSBs similar to what is found after high-LET irradiation. However, since some of these DSBs, in contrary to high-LET, are affected by radical scavengers they are most likely caused by a cluster of radicals that have a longer diffusion distance than the range of the electrons creating them.

High- or Low-LET Effects

Cellular experiments using DNA-incorporated ^{125}I show typically high-LET like dose-responses. However, the so-called "pulse-chase" experiments by Hofer and co-workers [19], using short pulses of $^{125}IdUR$ to label mammalian cells clearly showed the complexity of biological responses to Auger-electron emitters. In these experiments cell synchronized in early S-phase were labelled with short pulses of $^{125}IdUR$, and were then allowed to progress in the cell cycle for different times ("chase", typically 30 min to 5 h) before cells were frozen for accumulation of decays. Remarkably, the cell killing efficiency gradually increased as the cells progressed further into the S-phase before the accumulation of ^{125}I-decays. For example, the number of decays for the same surviving fraction of cells (1/e) shifted from 135 to 42 decays/cell when the chase time was changed from about 0.5 to 5 h. The shape of the cell survival curve was also gradually shifted from a typical low-LET response to a high-LET independent of radioprotection of radical scavengers. Further, there was a corresponding shift in other cellular endpoints such as chromosomal damage assessed as micronuclei or aberrations in cells irradiated in late S-phase compared with cells irradiated in early S-phase. The interpretation of these findings was that not only the induction or repair of DNA lesions, but also radiation-induced damage to some higher-order nuclear structure(s), e.g. chromatin, nuclear matrix or the nuclear envelope, contributes to cell death, and that newly replicated DNA is not as radiosensitive to the effect of Auger electrons, as DNA allowed to associate into chromatin structures after a chase period. Recent observations partly confirm this hypothesis but link these differences to the efficiency of DNA-incorporated ^{125}I to induce DSBs: the DSB yield was four times higher in cells irradiated in late S-phase than in cells irradiated in early S-phase [20]. Thus, there is a direct link between DNA double-strand breaks and cell survival. However, the efficiency of DNA-incorporated ^{125}I-decays in inducing DSBs in mammalian cells can vary significantly depending on the chromatin structure.

Methods of Targeting Auger-Electron Emitters

Although initially not considered for therapeutic use, Auger-electron emitters are getting progressively wider recognition as radionuclides with therapy potential due to their DSB-inducing capacity in mammalian cells. The challenge is to position the nuclide as close as possible to cellular DNA and thus benefit from the biological Auger effect. Described below are some of the efforts made to target Auger-electron emitters close to DNA.

DNA Directed Agents

Nucleoside analogues. Nucleoside analogues are perhaps the most studied ligands for targeting Auger-electron emitters to DNA. The thymidine analogue 5-iodo-2′-deoxyuridine (IdUR) is the most evaluated, usually radiohalogenated with ^{125}I or ^{123}I (Fig. 11.5). The

Fig. 11.5 Molecular structures of (a) Thymidine and (b) Iodo/bromo-deoxyuridine (R=^{123}I, ^{125}I, ^{77}Br)

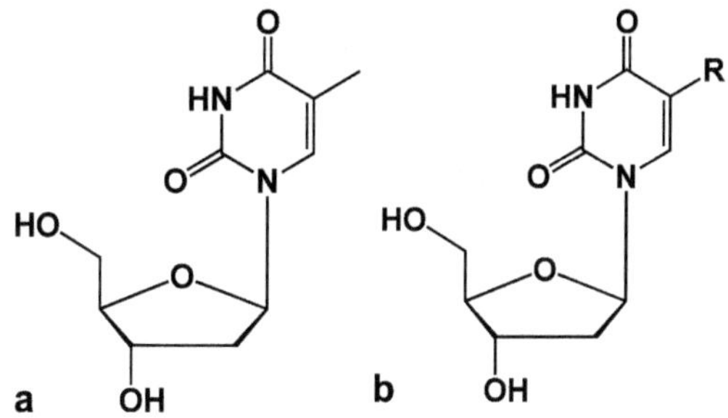

iodine atom has similar van der Waals' radius as the 5-methyl group and the compound is readily substituted for thymidine. A true advantage with this ligand is that it is directly incorporated into DNA. The analogue is built into DNA replacing thymidine during the S-phase of the cell cycle and provides a reliable and reproducible model for analyzing biological effects of Auger electrons. As described above ^{125}IdUR has commonly been used for biological studies of SSBs and DSBs of DNA demonstrating, depending on the system used, varying number of DSBs per decay.

Already in the early studies it was clear that ^{125}IdUR is highly radiotoxic to mammalian cells. Survival curves obtained from cells incorporating ^{125}IdUR were similar to those obtained using high-LET radiation, lacking the characteristic shoulder of low-LET, and indicating high RBE where less than 100 decays per cell was necessary for efficient cell killing [21]. Although the potential of ^{125}IdUR is obvious, there are problems related to its usability in a clinical situation. It is not stable *in vivo* (biological half-time <5 min), not specific to the tumour cell only, cell cycle dependent and is rapidly dehalogenated. Attempts to circumvent these problems have been suggested like locoregional distribution and inhibition of intracellular degradation of ^{125}IdUR [21–23]. This has been explored by intraperitoneal administration in mice with ovarian ascites tumours. The cell-cycle dependency was compensated by repeated i.p. injections. The tumour cell survival was reduced with up to five orders of magnitude with favourable tumour to non-tumour (T/NT) ratios [24, 25]. Similar result was also achieved with ^{123}IdUR, while ^{131}IdUR had practically no effect on tumour growth [22, 26]. The *in vivo* results also questioned the need to target every cell in a tumour to obtain a curative effect with Auger-electron emitters. Although the radiotoxic Auger effect is restricted to ^{125}IdUR pre-treated cells in a xenografted tumour there seems to be an inhibitory bystander effect on remaining surrounding non-^{125}IdUR treated tumour cells [27]. However, recently it was demonstrated that, while ^{125}IdUR had an inhibitory bystander effect, ^{123}IdUR had a stimulatory bystander effect [28] and the cause of this phenomenon is still far from understood.

As mentioned ^{123}IdUR, as well as ^{77}BrdUR, have been used to evaluate the effects of Auger-electron emitters [29, 30]. Both these compounds show exponential decrease in clonogenic survival but less steep than that of ^{125}I. The amount of decays per cell required to reach the same survival is in the order

^{77}BrdUR > ^{123}IdUR > ^{125}IdUR [22]. Although ^{77}BrdUR and ^{123}IdUR are less effective in cell inactivation per decay they could be more attractive in a clinical situation due to their shorter half-lives (57 h and 13.2 h respectively compared to 60 days for ^{125}I), which are more comparable to the tumour cell cycle times. The shorter half-lives also increases the ratio of DNA-incorporated radionuclides to those generally distributed in the body. Also, the decay-characteristics of these radionuclides make them suitable for *in vivo* imaging with SPECT.

Several clinical studies were initiated during the 1990s on the basis of the above successful *in vivo* results with ^{125}IdUR. Loco-regional administrations using ^{125}IdUR in colorectal, breast, stomach and bladder cancers have been reported presenting high T/NT ratios but rather low and heterogeneous radionuclide incorporation in the individual tumour cells [31]. Suggestions to use slow release administration of ^{125}IdUR to tumours might decrease the problem of low and heterogeneous uptake [32, 33]. However, so far no clinically successful system has been presented. Since most tumour cells need to be targeted with Auger-electron emitters, multiple injections or prolonged infusion are needed. Today the clinical interest in nucleoside analogues is low possibly due to the competition from other Auger-electron labelled targeting agents with better tumour specificity, increased tumour internalization and longer biological half-times which allow systemic bolus administration.

DNA-intercalators. Agents interacting with DNA are alternatives to molecules incorporated into the DNA. The potential use of radiolabelled aminoacridines for cancer therapy was first proposed by Martin [34]. Compounds of this type have since then been synthesized mainly to study the radiobiological properties of DNA-intercalated ^{125}I. In contrary to the nucleoside analogues that only target proliferating cells in the S-phase DNA-intercalators will target all DNA independent of the cellular status.

Acridines (e.g. aminoacridine and proflavine) are well-known DNA-intercalating agents that bind DNA by vertical interaction of the planar ring system between DNA base pairs, preferably in GC-rich regions, and have been subjects for radiohalogenation with ^{125}I. The DNA-intercalation with these ^{125}I-labelled ligands seems to be close enough to the DNA strand to generate high-LET type of damages [13, 35, 36] and the yield of DSBs per decay of an ^{125}I-acridine derivative was only about 25% less than for ^{125}IdUR [13]. However, it should be mentioned that intercalators are low molecular weight compounds and the introduction of the relatively large atom of ^{125}I can interfere with the DNA binding. Altering the position for ^{125}I-labelling in the planar ring system can be the difference between success and failure in DNA-intercalation [13].

Diamminedichlororplatinum(II) has been suggested for delivery of Auger-electron emitting platinum nuclides [37, 38]. It is based on a platinum atom surrounded by two chloride and two ammonia elements and is in its *cis*-configuration a chemotherapeutic drug that penetrates the cell membrane, docks with DNA and forms intra-strand cross-links. Several radioisotopes of platinum, ^{191}Pt, ^{193m}Pt and ^{195m}Pt, have been suggested for labelling. The large number of Auger-electrons in their decay (up to 35 electrons) will increase their probability to create DSBs in comparison with ^{125}I. Actually, cell survival studies show an RBE for ^{195m}Pt in the *trans*-configuration of 8.8, which is twice that of ^{125}I-acridine [38]. This RBE is also exceeding those of ^{125}IdUR and ^{77}BrdUR, which are 7.3 and 6.5 respectively, although they are built into DNA and should therefore be closer to the central axis of DNA [35]. Survival data also supports high-LET type of damages without any shoulder [38]. However, the production of the meta-stabile nuclides ^{193m}Pt and ^{195m}Pt is difficult and probably limits the use of them. Further, high specific radioactivity is also important to overcome the intrinsic toxicity of the platinum agent.

Two of the most used chemotherapeutic agents since the early 1970s are the anthracyclines doxorubicin and daunorubicin (Fig. 11.6a). The key mechanism of action for anthracyclines stems from their ability to intercalate with the B-form of the DNA helix through GC site-specific interactions [39]. The aglycone moiety of the anthracycline molecule intercalates with both the major (D-ring) and the minor groove (A-ring), while the aminosugar moiety is anchored within the minor groove [40]. Recently, efforts were made to iodinate daunorubicin derivatives and still preserve the DNA binding properties in order to bring ^{125}I in close contact to DNA (Fig. 11.6b). The affinity for DNA and, even more important, the ability to bind to DNA in living cells were dependent on the position of the radioactive label [41]. Modification of the aminosugar moiety was considered most appropriate and rendered approximately 0.4 DSBs per decay and might even be higher since extracted naked DNA was used (discussed earlier in this chapter). In cell cultures treated with this ^{125}I-labelled compound of high specific radioactivity vast suppression of cell growth (6 logs) was found at such low concentrations (sub-nanomolar), where neither daunorubicin, nor non-radioactive ^{127}I-derivative, had any effect. Cell killing effect could therefore be related to ^{125}I only and chemical cytotoxic effects that stem from the ability of the intercalating derivative to block DNA-, RNA-, and protein-synthesis are thus expected to be minimal for the radiolabelled compound.

Since the DNA-intercalators above have no selective binding to tumour DNA, normal tissue will also be exposed. To minimize the potential side effects and to increase the tumour specificity a delivery system is required. Suggestions have been made to use liposomal formulations for DNA-intercalator delivery [42]. In this

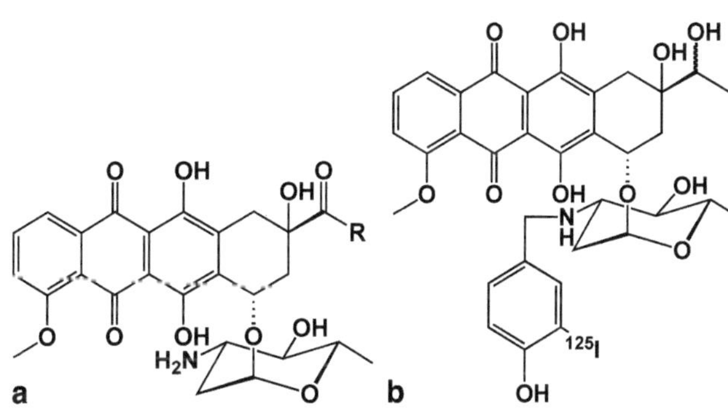

Fig. 11.6 Molecular structures of (a) Doxorubicin (R=CH_2OH), Daunorubicin (R=CH_3) and (b) ^{125}I-daunorubicin-derivative

approach, liposomes targeted against tumour cells serve as a transport vehicle to guide DNA-intercalators to their target in order to achieve tumour cell specificity.

Minor groove binding agents. Hoechst dyes are minor groove binding agents with specificity for AT-rich sequences and used for DNA quantification in living cells. They can cross the cellular membrane and are generally less toxic than the intercalators. For this reason they are considered as suitable for delivery of Auger-electron emitters to the cell nucleus. Mainly two analogues have been studied using plasmid and cellular DNA. Initially, the iodinated Hoechst compound ^{125}I-H33258 [43] (Fig. 11.7) was studied and recently it has also been labelled with ^{123}I [44]. Although ^{123}I-H33258 produces only about half the amount of DSBs per decay than ^{125}I-H33258, the shorter half-life (13.2 h vs. 60 days) is more attractive for *in vivo* use and will also provide higher specific radioactivity.

Another Hoechst dye, H33342 [45] (Fig. 11.7), which could be advantageous since it is more cell-permeable due to an additional ethyl group, has also been studied. Experimental data also support this [46]. However, the effect in terms of DSBs per decay is not expected to differ since the position of the Auger-electron emitter and the distance to the center of DNA should be similar. It was recently determined by computer-assisted molecular modelling that the distance between the central axis of double stranded DNA and the iodine atom in ^{125}I-H33342, pointing out of the groove, is 0.92 nm [47]. Estimations were made that this would give about 20% less DSBs per decay than ^{125}IdUR, where the distance is 0.57 nm. When further increasing the distance, by computational modelling of ^{125}I-H33342, to 1.09 and 1.64 nm, the DBSs per decay would decrease with about 30% and 55%, respectively [47]. This directly effect cell survival with reduced RBE and the required amount of decays per cell to reach D_0 is almost double for ^{125}I-H33342 compared to ^{125}IdUR [46]. Still the survival curve is similar to that of high-LET radiation.

So far the use of Auger-electron labelled Hoechst dyes has been focused on *in vitro* studies to understand the underlying mechanism of strand breaks in DNA. The therapeutic use in experimental systems or in man is probably limited. As for DNA-intercalators low tumour specificity can be expected and the risk for targeting any DNA-containing cell is obvious. A tumour specific delivery system is needed to avoid exposure of normal tissue.

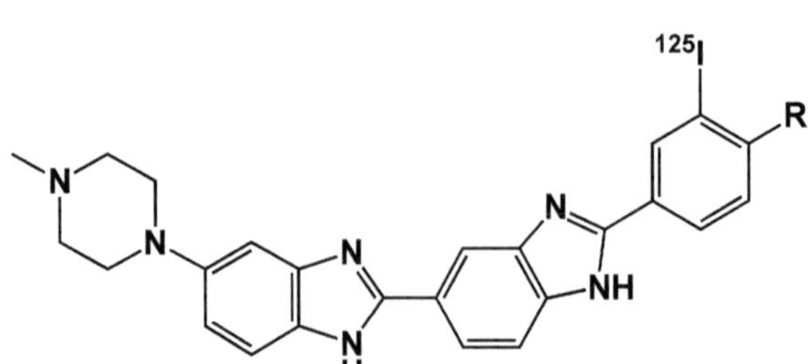

Fig. 11.7 Molecular structures of ^{125}I-H33258 (R=OH) and ^{125}I-H33342 (R=OCH_2CH_3)

Hormone Receptor Ligands

To increase tumour specificity, steroid hormones could be potential as nuclear targeting vectors for Auger-electron emitters. Over-expression of the estrogen receptor (ER) is common in breast cancer, usually referred to as "ER positive". The estrogen hormones bind to nuclear hormone receptors after passive diffusion through the phospholipids membranes of the cell. The receptor is present in the cytoplasm or the nucleus and the formed steroid-receptor complex acts as gene-specific transcription factor. This action would therefore transport Auger-electron emitters close to DNA. Early studies demonstrated that a receptor dependent exponential decrease in cell killing could be achieved with ^{125}I-estradiol [48]. It has later been suggested that the DSB yield of a ^{125}I-estradiol-derivative is almost ten times higher than for ^{125}IdUR [49]. However, the RBE for cell survival does not differ between the two ligands and it has been speculated that DSBs formed within segments of the compacted chromatin structure, like DSB cluster damages, do not necessary correlate to increased cell killing [21, 49]. This is not fully understood and future studies will hopefully clarify if the dramatic increase in DSBs by ^{125}I estradiol can be verified.

Disadvantages with estrogens are their relative short residence time in the nucleus and low receptor expression in the tumours (~10^4 ER/cell). Furthermore, ^{125}I-labelled estrogens are not considered to be efficient for tumour cell killing *in vivo* due to the long half-life of ^{125}I (60 days). Suggestions to use ^{123}I [50] and ^{80m}Br [51] have been made to increase the specific radioactivity and thereby increase the probability of tumour cell killing. The use of ^{80m}Br is limited due to short half-life (4.4 h) and hence poor availability but ^{123}I has been studied. Dose dependent reduction in survival of breast cancer cells was seen for ^{123}I-estradiol but D_0 was markedly lower than for ^{125}I-estradiol (300–600/700 vs 80 decays per cell) [50, 52].

Oligonucleotides

By using triplex-forming oligonucleotide (TFO) it is possible to target specific DNA sequences. In such an approach the target is not the total DNA but specific sequences of the genome [53]. ^{125}I-labelled TFOs targeted against the human *mdr*1, multi drug resistance gene, have been shown to generate sequence-specific DSBs that could be useful in knocking out such genes [54]. In purified genomic DNA 0.5 DSBs per decay was achieved [53]. One explanation for the lower yield compared to ^{125}IdUR could be that TFO in triple-stranded DNA is located in the major groove of the DNA duplex and thus ^{125}I is more distant from the central axis compared to incorporated ^{125}I. Moreover, in cell cultures ^{125}I-TFO generated low-LET survival curve with shoulder and the radiotoxic effect compared to ^{125}IdUR was several orders of magnitude lower [55]. Intact chromatin with nucleosomes protecting from triplex formation could be the reason for the poor outcome.

Oligonucleotides also suffer from poor *in vivo* stability as well as low tumour specificity and low rate of uptake. Not only poor cellular uptake but also limited cell nuclear uptake has been observed, controlled by yet unidentified mechanism [53]. Though, it has been demonstrated that the nuclear uptake is enhanced when adding a nuclear localizing signal (NLS) to the TFO [54].

Nuclear Localizing Signal (NLS)

Recently two research groups suggested the use of nuclear localizing signal (NLS) to transport Auger-electron emitters to the tumour cell nucleus, where different targeting agents were utilized for tumour specificity [56, 57]. The NLS of simian virus 40 (SV-40) large T antigen was used to take advantage of the nuclear pore complex that regulates the nuclear uptake of proteins with such NLS. Their innovative approaches differed and they were using a humanized antibody against CD33 in myeloid leukaemia cells [56] or synthesized somatostatin-analogues against neuro-endocrine tumour cells [57], but a clear increase in nuclear uptake of the used ^{111}In label could be seen when NLS was added. Clinical effects of the NLS approach are awaited; however, initial pre-results do not indicate a dramatic difference between treatments with and without NLS [56]. One possible drawback with NLS is that the true Auger-effect can be missed just because of the distance to DNA. The Auger-effect is active within a few cubic nanometers and without binding of the Auger-electron emitter to DNA this effect can be lost. Possibly the positive net charge of NLS could affect the association to the negatively charged DNA, but an even distribution in the nucleus is more likely. However, simply by relocating the radionuclide from the cytoplasm to the nucleus, an increase in effect should be expected, although derived from an increased macroscopic absorbed dose and not from the biological Auger effect.

Translocation of Auger-electron emitters to cell nucleus is suggested to occur for some peptides also without attachment of NLS. For both the somatostatin analogue octreotide [58] and the epidermal growth factor [59] nuclear uptake of ^{111}In is reported and was also suggested to explain an increased therapeutic effect of ^{111}In. The mechanism behind this is not fully understood but it is suggested that the epidermal growth factor receptor contains sequences similar to NLS [59].

How Magic Is the Auger Effect?

One example may demonstrate the possible benefits of Auger emitters in cancer therapy. An estimate for a patient with disseminated disease is that there is about 1 g of circulating single tumour cells or micro-metastases. Cellular studies indicate that about 60 decays of ^{125}I coupled to DNA reduce the cell survival with about 50%. If 1,000 decays can be generated in each of these cancer cells, this may create a probable cure. The total radioactivity involved corresponds to about 0.1 MBq, which when injected in the body, without attaching to cellular DNA, corresponds to about 5 mSv or approximately the yearly dose all of us get from natural sources.

The potential in the Auger-electron therapy is fascinating and a driving force to get it into the clinic. The example above emphases that Auger-electron therapy is useful in single cells and in micro-metastases mainly and might have a role in adjuvant therapy. In bulky tumours, Auger-electron therapy will not be the first choice, but may complement beta- and alpha-emitting radionuclide therapy to sterilise the tumours. However, there is a dosimetric problem, i.e. to measure the radiation dose and the biological effects of the Auger-electrons in a clinical setting. The small amount of radioactivity creating the therapeutical Auger effect will probably be drowned by the larger amount of radionuclides that will not target the tumour DNA. Macroscopic dosimetry can be used to monitor critical normal organs but will say little of the radiation effects on the targeted tumour tissue and the final judgement of the success of the therapy will have to wait for the five-year survival. Other end-points that are possible to use in the laboratory, like the number of double-strand breaks (DSB) and apoptosis, are not easily applicable in the clinics since they involve biopsies that only will give local and limited information.

The strong development of molecular imaging might in the future be of help. Now *in vivo* methods to map tumour receptor densities or other structures for targeting are developing using e.g. positron emission tomography. Such information will help in planning the Auger-electron therapy and positron-emitting markers of the therapeutic entity will at least help to understand if the first part (specific binding to tumour cells) of the targeting process is working. *In vivo* markers for apoptosis are also coming and without doubt there will be significant efforts in the future to visualize DSBs *in vivo* as well.

References

1. Auger, P. (1925) Sur les rayons b secondaires produits dans un gaz par des rayons X. In *Comptes Rendues Hebdomadaires des Seances de l'Academie des Sciences*, vol. 180, pp. 65–8.
2. Humm, J.L., Howell, R.W. and Rao, D.V. (1994) Dosimetry of Auger-electron-emitting radionuclides: report no. 3 of AAPM Nuclear Medicine Task Group No. 6. *Med Phys*, **21**, 1901–15.
3. Pomplun, E. and Sutmann, G. (2004) Is coulomb explosion a damaging mechanism for (125)IUdR? *Int J Radiat Biol*, **80**, 855–60.
4. Hofer, K.G. (2000) Biophysical aspects of Auger processes. *Acta Oncol*, **39**, 651–7.
5. Warters, R.L., Hofer, K.G., Harris, C.R. and Smith, J.M. (1978) Radionuclide toxicity in cultured mammalian cells: elucidation of the primary site of radiation damage. *Curr Top Radiat Res Q*, **12**, 389–407.
6. Hofer, K.G., Prensky, W. and Hughes, W.L. (1969) Death and metastatic distribution of tumor cells in mice monitored with 125I-iododeoxy-uridine. *J Natl Cancer Inst*, **43**, 763–73.
7. Ertl, H.H., Feinendegen, L.E. and Heiniger, H.J. (1970) Iodine-125, a tracer in cell biology: physical properties and biological aspects. *Phys Med Biol*, **15**, 447–56.

8. Krisch, R.E. and Ley, R.D. (1974) Induction of lethality and DNA breakage by the decay of iodine-125 in bacteriophage T4. *Int J Radiat Biol Relat Stud Phys Chem Med*, **25**, 21–30.
9. Painter, R.B., Young, B.R. and Burk, H.J. (1974) Non-repairable strand breaks induced by 125I incorporated into mammalian DNA. *Proc Natl Acad Sci USA*, **71**, 4836–8.
10. Martin, R.F. and Haseltine, W.A. (1981) Range of radiochemical damage to DNA with decay of iodine-125. *Science*, **213**, 896–8.
11. Adelstein, S.J. and Kassis, A.I. (1996) Strand breaks in plasmid DNA following positional changes of Auger-electron-emitting radionuclides. *Acta Oncol*, **35**, 797–801.
12. Kassis, A.I., Harapanhalli, R.S. and Adelstein, S.J. (1999) Comparison of strand breaks in plasmid DNA after positional changes of Auger electron-emitting iodine-125. *Radiat Res*, **151**, 167–76.
13. Sahu, S.K., Kortylewicz, Z.P., Baranowska-Kortylewicz, J., Taube, R.A., Adelstein, S.J. and Kassis, A.I. (1997) Strand breaks after the decay of iodine-125 in proximity to plasmid pBR322 DNA. *Radiat Res*, **147**, 401–8.
14. Kassis, A.I., Harapanhalli, R.S. and Adelstein, S.J. (1999) Strand breaks in plasmid DNA after positional changes of Auger electron-emitting iodine-125: direct compared to indirect effects. *Radiat Res*, **152**, 530–8.
15. Bishayee, A., Rao, D.V., Bouchet, L.G., Bolch, W.E. and Howell, R.W. (2000) Protection by DMSO against cell death caused by intracellularly localized iodine-125, iodine-131 and polonium-210. *Radiat Res*, **153**, 416–27.
16. Walicka, M.A., Adelstein, S.J. and Kassis, A.I. (1998) Indirect mechanisms contribute to biological effects produced by decay of DNA-incorporated iodine-125 in mammalian cells in vitro: double-strand breaks. *Radiat Res*, **149**, 134–41.
17. Walicka, M.A., Adelstein, S.J. and Kassis, A.I. (1998) Indirect mechanisms contribute to biological effects produced by decay of DNA-incorporated iodine-125 in mammalian cells in vitro: clonogenic survival. *Radiat Res*, **149**, 142–6.
18. Elmroth, K. and Stenerlow, B. (2005) DNA-incorporated 125I induces more than one double-strand break per decay in mammalian cells. *Radiat Res*, **163**, 369–73.
19. Hofer, K.G., Lin, X. and Schneiderman, M.H. (2000) Paradoxical effects of iodine-125 decays in parent and daughter DNA: a new target model for radiation damage. *Radiat Res*, **153**, 428–35.
20. Elmroth, K. and Stenerlöw, B. (2007) Influence of chromatin structure on double-strand break induction in mammalian cells irradiated with DNA-incorporated 125-I. *Radiat Res*, **168**, 312–318.
21. Kassis, A.I. (2004) The amazing world of auger electrons. *Int J Radiat Biol*, **80**, 789–803.
22. Adelstein, S.J., Kassis, A.I., Bodei, L. and Mariani, G. (2003) Radiotoxicity of iodine-125 and other auger-electron-emitting radionuclides: background to therapy. *Cancer Biother Radiopharm*, **18**, 301–16.
23. O'Donoghue, J.A. and Wheldon, T.E. (1996) Targeted radiotherapy using Auger electron emitters. *Phys Med Biol*, **41**, 1973–92.
24. Bloomer, W.D. and Adelstein, S.J. (1975) Letter: antineoplastic effect of iodine-125-labelled iododeoxyuridine. *Int J Radiat Biol Relat Stud Phys Chem Med*, **27**, 509–11.
25. Bloomer, W.D. and Adelstein, S.J. (1977) 5-125I-iododeoxyuridine as prototype for radionuclide therapy with Auger emitters. *Nature*, **265**, 620–1.
26. Baranowska-Kortylewicz, J., Makrigiorgos, G.M., Van den Abbeele, A.D., Berman, R.M., Adelstein, S.J. and Kassis, A.I. (1991) 5-[123I]iodo-2′-deoxyuridine in the radiotherapy of an early ascites tumor model. *Int J Radiat Oncol Biol Phys*, **21**, 1541–51.
27. Xue, L.Y., Butler, N.J., Makrigiorgos, G.M., Adelstein, S.J. and Kassis, A.I. (2002) Bystander effect produced by radiolabeled tumor cells in vivo. *Proc Natl Acad Sci USA*, **99**, 13765–70.
28. Kishikawa, H., Wang, K., Adelstein, S.J. and Kassis, A.I. (2006) Inhibitory and stimulatory bystander effects are differentially induced by Iodine-125 and Iodine-123. *Radiat Res*, **165**, 688–94.
29. Kassis, A.I., Adelstein, S.J., Haydock, C., Sastry, K.S., McElvany, K.D. and Welch, M.J. (1982) Lethality of Auger electrons from the decay of bromine-77 in the DNA of mammalian cells. *Radiat Res*, **90**, 362–73.

30. Makrigiorgos, G.M., Kassis, A.I., Baranowska-Kortylewicz, J., McElvany, K.D., Welch, M.J., Sastry, K.S. and Adelstein, S.J. (1989) Radiotoxicity of 5-[123I]iodo-2′-deoxyuridine in V79 cells: a comparison with 5-[125I]iodo-2′-deoxyuridine. *Radiat Res*, **118**, 532–44.
31. Bodei, L., Kassis, A.I., Adelstein, S.J. and Mariani, G. (2003) Radionuclide therapy with iodine-125 and other auger-electron-emitting radionuclides: experimental models and clinical applications. *Cancer Biother Radiopharm*, **18**, 861–77.
32. Mairs, R.J., Wideman, C.L., Angerson, W.J., Whateley, T.L., Reza, M.S., Reeves, J.R., Robertson, L.M., Neshasteh-Riz, A., Rampling, R., Owens, J., Allan, D. and Graham, D.I. (2000) Comparison of different methods of intracerebral administration of radioiododeoxyuridine for glioma therapy using a rat model. *Br J Cancer*, **82**, 74–80.
33. Reza, M.S. and Whateley, T.L. (1998) Iodo-2′-deoxyuridine (IUdR) and 125IUdR loaded biodegradable microspheres for controlled delivery to the brain. *J Microencapsul*, **15**, 789–801.
34. Martin, R.F. (1977) Induction of double-stranded breaks in DNA by binding with an 125i-labelled acridine. *Int J Radiat Biol Relat Stud Phys Chem Med*, **32**, 491–7.
35. Kassis, A.I., Fayad, F., Kinsey, B.M., Sastry, K.S. and Adelstein, S.J. (1989) Radiotoxicity of an 125I-labeled DNA intercalator in mammalian cells. *Radiat Res*, **118**, 283–94.
36. Martin, R.F., Bradley, T.R. and Hodgson, G.S. (1979) Cytotoxicity of an 125I-labeled DNA-binding compound that induces double-stranded DNA breaks. *Cancer Res*, **39**, 3244–7.
37. Areberg, J., Norrgren, K. and Mattsson, S. (1999) Absorbed doses to patients from 191Pt-, 193mPt- and 195mPt-cisplatin. *Appl Radiat Isot*, **51**, 581–6.
38. Howell, R.W., Kassis, A.I., Adelstein, S.J., Rao, D.V., Wright, H.A., Hamm, R.N., Turner, J.E. and Sastry, K.S. (1994) Radiotoxicity of platinum-195m-labeled trans platinum (II) in mammalian cells. *Radiat Res*, **140**, 55–62.
39. Chaires, J.B., Herrera, J.E. and Waring, M.J. (1990) Preferential binding of daunomycin to 5′ATCG and 5′ATGC sequences revealed by footprinting titration experiments. *Biochemistry*, **29**, 6145–53.
40. Wang, A.H., Ughetto, G., Quigley, G.J. and Rich, A. (1987) Interactions between an anthracycline antibiotic and DNA: molecular structure of daunomycin complexed to d(CpGpTpApCpG) at 1.2-A resolution. *Biochemistry*, **26**, 1152–63.
41. Ickenstein, L.M., Edwards, K., Sjoberg, S., Carlsson, J. and Gedda, L. (2006) A novel 125I-labeled daunorubicin derivative for radionuclide-based cancer therapy. *Nucl Med Biol*, **33**, 773–83.
42. Kullberg, E.B., Wei, Q., Capala, J., Giusti, V., Malmstrom, P.U. and Gedda, L. (2005) EGF-receptor targeted liposomes with boronated acridine: growth inhibition of cultured glioma cells after neutron irradiation. *Int J Radiat Biol*, **81**, 621–9.
43. Murray, V. and Martin, R.F. (1988) Sequence specificity of 125I-labelled Hoechst 33258 in intact human cells. *J Mol Biol*, **201**, 437–42.
44. Lobachevsky, P.N. and Martin, R.F. (2004) Plasmid DNA breakage by decay of DNA-associated auger emitters: experiments with 123I/125I-iodoHoechst 33258. *Int J Radiat Biol*, **80**, 915–20.
45. Harapanhalli, R.S., McLaughlin, L.W., Howell, R.W., Rao, D.V., Adelstein, S.J. and Kassis, A.I. (1996) [125I/127I]iodoHoechst 33342: synthesis, DNA binding, and biodistribution. *J Med Chem*, **39**, 4804–9.
46. Yasui, L.S., Chen, K., Wang, K., Jones, T.P., Caldwell, J., Guse, D. and Kassis, A.I. (2007) Using Hoechst 33342 to target radioactivity to the cell nucleus. *Radiat Res*, **167**, 167–75.
47. Chen, K., Adelstein, S.J. and Kassis, A.I. (2004) Molecular simulation of ligand-binding with DNA: implications for 125I-labeled pharmaceutical design. *Int J Radiat Biol*, **80**, 921–6.
48. Bronzert, D.A., Hochberg, R.B. and Lippman, M.E. (1982) Specific cytotoxicity of 16 alpha-[125I]iodoestradiol for estrogen receptor-containing breast cancer cells. *Endocrinology*, **110**, 2177–82.
49. Yasui, L., Hughes, A. and DeSombre, E. (2001) Relative biological effectiveness of accumulated 125IdU and 125I-estrogen decays in estrogen receptor-expressing MCF-7 human breast cancer cells. *Radiat Res*, **155**, 328–34.

50. DeSombre, E.R., Shafii, B., Hanson, R.N., Kuivanen, P.C. and Hughes, A. (1992) Estrogen receptor-directed radiotoxicity with Auger electrons: specificity and mean lethal dose. *Cancer Res*, **52**, 5752–8.
51. DeSombre, E.R., Harper, P.V., Hughes, A., Mease, R.C., Gatley, S.J., DeJesus, O.T. and Schwartz, J.L. (1988) Bromine-80m radiotoxicity and the potential for estrogen receptor-directed therapy with auger electrons. *Cancer Res*, **48**, 5805–9.
52. Kearney, T., Hughes, A., Hanson, R.N. and DeSombre, E.R. (1999) Radiotoxicity of Auger electron-emitting estrogens in MCF-7 spheroids: a potential treatment for estrogen receptor-positive tumors. *Radiat Res*, **151**, 570–9.
53. Panyutin, I.G. and Neumann, R.D. (2005) The potential for gene-targeted radiation therapy of cancers. *Trends Biotechnol*, **23**, 492–6.
54. Sedelnikova, O.A., Luu, A.N., Karamychev, V.N., Panyutin, I.G. and Neumann, R.D. (2001) Development of DNA-based radiopharmaceuticals carrying Auger-electron emitters for anti-gene radiotherapy. *Int J Radiat Oncol Biol Phys*, **49**, 391–6.
55. Sedelnikova, O.A., Panyutin, I.V., Neumann, R.D., Bonner, W.M. and Panyutin, I.G. (2004) Assessment of DNA damage produced by 125I-triplex-forming oligonucleotides in cells. *Int J Radiat Biol*, **80**, 927–31.
56. Chen, P., Wang, J., Hope, K., Jin, L., Dick, J., Cameron, R., Brandwein, J., Minden, M. and Reilly, R.M. (2006) Nuclear localizing sequences promote nuclear translocation and enhance the radiotoxicity of the anti-CD33 monoclonal antibody HuM195 labeled with 111In in human myeloid leukemia cells. *J Nucl Med*, **47**, 827–36.
57. Ginj, M., Hinni, K., Tschumi, S., Schulz, S. and Maecke, H.R. (2005) Trifunctional somatostatin-based derivatives designed for targeted radiotherapy using auger electron emitters. *J Nucl Med*, **46**, 2097–103.
58. Janson, E.T., Westlin, J.E., Ohrvall, U., Oberg, K. and Lukinius, A. (2000) Nuclear localization of 111In after intravenous injection of [111In-DTPA-D-Phe1]-octreotide in patients with neuroendocrine tumors. *J Nucl Med*, **41**, 1514–8.
59. Reilly, R.M., Kiarash, R., Cameron, R.G., Porlier, N., Sandhu, J., Hill, R.P., Vallis, K., Hendler, A. and Gariepy, J. (2000) 111In-labeled EGF is selectively radiotoxic to human breast cancer cells overexpressing EGFR. *J Nucl Med*, **41**, 429–38.
60. Stepanek, J., Ilvonen, S.A., Kuronen, A.A., Lampinen, J.S., Savolainen, S.E. and Valimaki, P.J. (2000) Radiation spectra of 111In, 113mIn and 114mIn. *Acta Oncol*, **39**, 667–71.
61. Stepanek, J., Larsson, B. and Weinreich, R. (1996) Auger-electron spectra of radionuclides for therapy and diagnostics. *Acta Oncol*, **35**, 863–8.

Chapter 12
Radiation Induced Cell Deaths

David Eriksson, Katrine Riklund, Lennart Johansson, and Torgny Stigbrand*

Summary The previous classification of radiation induced cell deaths into either necrosis or apoptosis is today recognized as too simplistic. New possibilities to make use of other death mechanisms, when treating malignant diseases with targeted therapy, include rapid or delayed apoptosis, mitotic catastrophes, autophagy or senescence induction. Targeted radioimmunotherapy typically delivers low doses with low dose-rate irradiation to tumors, and is able to induce this extended panorama of different death mechanisms, which will be discussed in this chapter.

Historical Aspects

The discoveries of X-rays in 1895 by Wihelm Conrad Röntgen and natural radioactivity some months later by Henry Becquerel were two important breakthroughs for new radiation based modalities to treat malignant diseases [1]. The first clinical exploration of radiation for such treatments was performed in 1896 when Emil Grubbé treated an advanced ulcerated breast cancer with X-rays [1, 2]. The field of radiation therapy began to grow in the early 1900s largely due to the pioneering work by Marie Curie, discoverer of the radioactive element radium in 1898 [1, 3]. A wide range of diseases, from cancer of the skin and breast to epilepsy and syphilis were treated [3].

This early period, which indicated that radiation could cause pronounced biological effects on cells was followed by extended investigations aiming towards better understanding of the underlying mechanisms (reviewed in [4]). The cellular radiation response, which included cell cycle effects, DNA repair and cell death induction came in focus.

Departments of Immunology, Diagnostic Radiology and Radiophysics, University of Umeå, SE-90185 Umeå, Sweden

*Address for correspondence:
Department of Immunology, Umeå University, 90185 Umeå, Sweden
E-mail: torgny.stigbrand@climi.umu.se

T. Stigbrand et al. (eds.) *Targeted Radionuclide Tumor Therapy*,

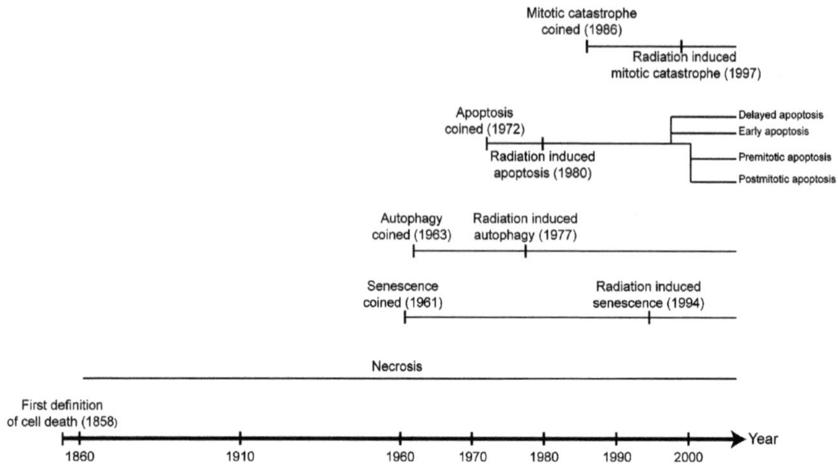

Fig. 12.1 Historical aspects of cell deaths implicated in radiation therapy

Cell death research has for long fascinated scientists and is today one of the most extensive research areas in biology (more than 123,000 publications during the last 10 years, corresponding to more than 30 publications/day) This rapid increase is driven by both the complexity and interactions between new types of deaths and the introduction of technologies making it possible in more detail to study the cellular responses to different types of cell injuries.

An overview of the historical aspects in establishing and introducing different types of cell deaths are depicted in Fig. 12.1. The early definitions of cell deaths were described by Rudolph Virchow in 1859 [5]. The first cell death to be defined was *necrosis*, a term which has been used for more than a century to describe the death of a cell or a group of cells in contact with living cells [6, 7]. Necrosis was characterized by cytoplasmic swelling, rupture of the plasma membrane and inflammatory reactions in surrounding tissues. The phenomenon of *apoptosis* was introduced 1972, when Kerr coined and characterized it as a cell death distinct from necrosis [8]. Apoptosis was established as a programmed, controlled form of cell death, whereas necrosis in contrast was considered to be an unordered accidental form of cell death. Apoptosis was morphologically defined by specific changes including reduction of cellular and nuclear volume, DNA condensation along the nucleus membrane, budding of the plasma membrane, and single cell death without inflammatory reactions.

Internucleosomal DNA fragmentation was described in irradiated lymphocytes in 1976 [9] and in 1982 the apoptotic process was used to describe radiation induced death observed in a small fraction of cells in the crypt of the small intestine [10, 11]. The increased knowledge of the complex mechanisms of different apoptotic pathways and the introduction of a cell death classified as *programmed necrosis* [12] has demonstrated that it is not as easy, as initially thought, to distinguish apoptosis and necrosis. For long time, all types of cell deaths which did not fulfil the morphological criteria of apoptosis were categorized as necrosis, which resulted in that 'necrosis' was used to refer to very different forms of cell death. Several reports also demonstrate that biochemical and morphological characteristics of both these types of cell deaths can be found in the same cell [13]. Furthermore, depending on the cell model examined and the type and intensity of the death provoking stimuli, a shift from one form of cell death to another can be observed [13]. This indicates that apoptosis and necrosis are the extremes of a continuous spectrum of cell deaths, making this area complex and challenging. Farber made the comment "There is no field of basic cell biology and cell pathology that is more confusing and more unintelligible than is the area of apoptosis versus necrosis" [14]. Radiation induced apoptosis has also been subdivided into *early apoptosis*, or *interphase apoptosis* which occurs within hours following the apoptotic stimuli, and delayed apoptosis, or *postmitotic apoptosis* which occurs days after exposure to the stimuli, during or following mitosis [15–17].

Today it is obvious that morphological features of apoptosis and necrosis are not sufficient to describe all types of cell deaths. As a consequence, the classification of cell deaths has evolved from being regarded as either apoptotic or necrotic to literally explode in new definitions describing different types of cell death, which further increases the complexity of the "cell death field" (for reviews see [18–22]). As an example *mitotic catastrophe* was introduced and originally defined to describe the cell death modality in cells prematurely forced into mitosis [23]. Today, mitotic catastrophe occupies a broader definition and includes cell deaths which appear during mitosis or as a consequence of aberrant mitoses and is close to synonymous with earlier definitions such as *mitotic death* [24, 25] and *reproductive death* [26]. In the end of 1990 mitotic catastrophe was established as an important cell death mechanism following irradiation [27, 28]. Furthermore, even though the definitions for *senescence* and *autophagy* were coined already 1961 [29] and 1963 [30] respectively and early publications implicated senescence [31, 32] and auotophagy [33, 34] as contributors of radiation induced cell death, it is only lately that they have been established as important cell death mechanisms following irradiation.

Radiation Induced Proliferative Cell Death

Ionizing irradiation at cancer therapy is being used both as external beam radiotherapy, brachytherapy, and targeted therapy with accumulating antibodies or other constructs, which deliver radionuclides to the tumor site. Ionizing irradiation deposits energy within DNA in the nucleus, producing single and double-strand breaks in DNA, which if not repaired may be lethal for the cell. Furthermore, radiation also induces damage in the cell membrane, which also may activate cell death pathways.

The characterization of death caused by radiation is a complex mission, and new death modalities continuously arise and often overlap earlier definitions. It has become apparent in the last few years that induction of apoptosis and necrosis is insufficient to alone account for the therapeutic effect of anticancer agents. Nonetheless, apparently simple questions on the very definition and classification of radiation induced cell death modalities in stereotyped patterns have not yet been solved. The Editors of Cell Death and Differentiation created in 2005 the Nomenclature Committee on Cell Death (NCCD) that was joined by a selected panel of experts [20]. The NCCD decided that the 'official' classification of cell death modalities had to rely on purely morphological criteria, owing to the absence of a clear-cut equivalence between ultrastructural alterations and biochemical cell death characteristics. We base our classification of apoptosis, necrosis, mitotic catastrophe and autophagy on the criteria that were reviewed by Galluzzi, Maiuri, Vitale, Zischka, Castedo, Zitvogel and Kroemer in [35] but also include senescence (Table 12.1).

Radiation induced cell death was early categorized into interphase death and reproductive or mitotic death based upon the time of disintegration of cells after exposure [36, 37]. Interphase death appears before entering the first mitosis after irradiation, whereas reproductive or mitotic death occurs during mitosis and one or several divisions after irradiation [37, 38]. Both interphase and reproductive death can be manifested as apoptosis and/or necrosis [39–42]. Early apoptosis is programmed, genetically controlled and rapidly induced in the interphase within single hours following irradiation, and usually occurs in cells highly sensitive to radiation, such as malignancies of hematopoietic origin [43]. Necrosis can also be executed during interphase, usually as a consequence of extensive DNA damage following high doses of irradiation.

Today it is established that the most frequent mode of cell death following irradiation is the mitotic catastrophe and together with necrosis they have traditionally been considered as passive deaths rather than controlled. However both necrosis [44] and the mitotic catastrophe [45, 46] can be genetically regulated. As pointed out by Brown and Attardi, "mitotic catastrophe is a trigger for cell death rather than a specific process by which cell death occur" [47]. Although morphologically distinct from apoptosis, the mitotic catastrophe may include activation of the apoptotic machinery [48–50]. Mitotic catastrophe is initiated during or after mitosis and is the main cell death mechanism in malignant cells of epithelial origin that often are relatively apoptosis-reluctant.

Alongside the main death mechanisms, senescence, a form of proliferative cell death can be induced following irradiation [51, 52]. Lately there is furthermore an increased interest for autophagy as a potential cell death mechanism involved in radiation induced cell death [53].

These five proliferative deaths will be described in this chapter, focusing on their relation to irradiation, their morphology and mechanisms involved in the induction and execution of cell death. Furthermore, the factors which determine these proliferative deaths induced by radiation (cell type, genotype, quality and dose of radiation) will be discussed.

Necrosis

Necrosis is generally considered to be an accidental and unregulated cell death [54] even though programmed necrosis also has been described [12].When necrosis is induced, a rapid plasma membrane permeabilization occurs, which leads to leakage

Table 12.1 Cell death pathway characteristics (Adapted from [22])

Apoptosis	Necrosis	Mitotic catastrophe	Autophagy	Senescence
Reduction of cellular and nuclear volume	Cytoplasmic swelling, swelling of cellular organelles	"Giant cell" formation	Massive vacuolization of the cytoplasm (autophagosome formation)	Flattening, increase in cell size
Blebbing, membrane integrity maintained		Mis-segregation of chromosomes during mitosis		Accumulation of heterochromatin foci
	Loss of membrane integrity			
Chromatin condensation, nuclear fragmentation, DNA laddering			Cellular content digested by lysosomal hydrolases and recycled for internal use	
				Increase in β-galactosidase activity
No immune responses	Random DNA degradation	Micronucleation, multinucleation	Granularity	
	Immune responses	Executed via delayed apoptosis or delayed necrosis		
Detection methods: Annexin staining, DNA fragmentation assays, caspase activation assays	Detection methods: Early permeability to vital dyes, electron microscopy	Detection methods: Visualization of multinucleated cells and cells with micronuclei	Detection methods: LC3 localization	Detection methods: Senescence-associated β-galactosidase activity

of cell content and induction of inflammation. Apart from that necrosis lacks specific biochemical markers and can be detected only by electron microscopy. Necrosis is usually defined in a negative fashion, as a type of cell demise that involves rupture of the plasma membrane without the hallmarks of apoptosis (pyknosis, karyorhexis, cell shrinkage and formation of apoptotic bodies) and without massive autophagic vacuolization [35]. The principal features of necrosis include a gain in cell volume (oncosis) that finally culminates in rupture of the plasma membrane, and the unorganized dismantling of swollen organelles. Radiation induced necrosis can be subdivided into early necrosis and delayed necrosis. Early necrosis is an ultra-fast cell death that is induced following particularly strong stimuli, like high doses of irradiation i.e. more than 100 Gy [39]. Delayed necrosis is a slow cell death and one of the mechanisms by which mitotic catastrophe is executed [55] (Fig. 12.3).

Apoptosis

Apoptosis is a cell death modality which is used by multicellular organisms to discard and destroy unwanted or damaged cells during very different conditions [8, 56]. Apoptosis is a regulated process, carried out in a controlled manner to ensure the safety of surrounding cells and tissues. Apoptosis involves action of proteases and nucleases, regulated with the membrane kept nearly intact [57, 58]. Apoptosis is strictly defined by morphological criteria including changes of the nucleus (chromatin condensation and margination, condensation and reduction in the size of the cell nucleus, fragmentation of the nucleus) cellular shrinkage and ruffling of the plasma membrane, called budding [54]. The DNA is furthermore fragmented in several steps to form mono- and/or oligomers of 200 base pairs [59]. Eventually the cell becomes divided in apoptotic bodies, which consist of cell organelles and/or nuclear material surrounded by an intact plasma membrane. Apoptotic bodies expose phosphatidylserine residues, that normally reside on the inner membrane leaflet, on their plasma membranes [60]. This allows for the recognition of apoptotic bodies, which are generally phagocytozed and destroyed by neighbouring cells without damage to adjacent tissue.

Apoptotic Signalling Pathways

Execution of apoptosis is closely linked to serial activation of a family of proteases called caspases [61, 62] even though caspase-independent apoptosis pathways also exist through AIF, Endonuclease G, and/or OMI/HTRA2) [63, 64]. During normal conditions these caspases exist in the cell as inactive procaspases and will be activated when the cell encounter external or internal inducers of the apoptotic machinery. Depending on the character of the initiating signal one of two major pathways involved in the activation of the caspase cascade will be triggered (reviewed in

[65]). However, irrespective of the actual route to caspase activation, both pathways will lead to the activation of the effector caspases, caspase-3, caspase-6 and caspase-7. These enzymes perform much of the proteolysis that is seen during the demolition phase of apoptosis and the targets include mediators and regulators of apoptosis, structural proteins, cellular DNA repair proteins, and cell cycle-related proteins [65].

The intrinsic pathway (Fig. 12.2), also called the mitochondrial pathway, is activated by various stress signals such as DNA damage, hypoxia, growth factor withdrawal, or transcription induction of oncogenes. Generally, irradiation induced apoptosis occurs via activation of this pathway, which involves mitochondrial outer membrane permeabilization (MOMP) that disrupts the mitochondrial function. This mitochondrial membrane permeabilization is mainly controlled and mediated by members of the Bcl-2 family. The Bcl-2 family is commonly divided into pro-apoptotic members and anti-apoptotic members. The pro-apoptotic members comprise two subfamilies, the Bax-like family (Bax, Bak, Bok) and the BH3-only proteins (Bid, Bad, Bim, Bik, Bmf, Noxa, Puma, Hrk) which both seem to be required to promote induction of apoptosis by formation of Bax-Bak pores in the

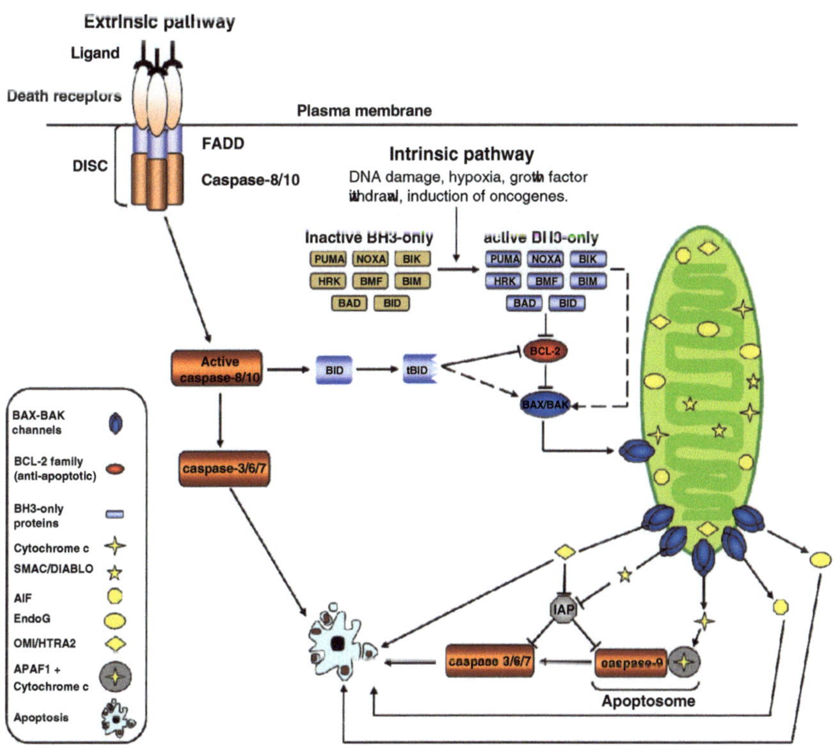

Fig. 12.2 Features of the extrinsic (death-receptor-mediated) and intrinsic (mitochondria-mediated) apoptosis signalling pathways. See text for details

mitochondrial outer membrane [65]. The anti-apoptotic members (Bcl-2, Bcl-XL, Bcl-W, Mcl1, Bcl2A1, Bcl-B) conversely block apoptosis by sequestering or neutralizing the BH3-only protein induced oligimerization of BAX and/or BAK in the outer mitochondrial membrane, which prevents pore formation and permeabilization of the outer mitochondrial membrane [66]. The ratio of anti- to pro-apoptotic members of the Bcl-2 family constitutes a rheostat that sets the threshold of susceptibility to apoptosis for the intrinsic pathway [67].

Permeabilization of the outer mitochondrial membrane releases several potentially lethal proteins from the intermembrane space into the cytoplasm [68]. Such lethal proteins include cytochrome c, SMAC/DIABLO (second mitochondria-derived activator of caspases/direct inhibitor of apoptosis (IAP)-binding protein with low pI), AIF (apoptosis inducing factor), EndoG (Endonuclease G) and OMI/HTRA2 (high temperature requirement protein A2) [61]. Cytochrome c is under many circumstances the most central of these proteins and binds and activates APAF1 and thereby changes its conformation to allow binding of ATP/dATP [69]. This formation is called the apoptosome and it will mediate the activation of caspase-9 [70, 71]. Caspase-9, as an initiator caspase, subsequently cleaves and activates effector caspases, which in turn cleave cell death substrates that collectively produce the phenotypic changes in the cell, characteristic of apoptotic cell death.

The extrinsic apoptotic pathway (Fig. 12.2), also referred to as the death receptor pathway, requires ligand dependent activation of plasma-membrane receptors from the TNF receptor superfamily (including Fas/APO-1 and Killer/DR5 also known as TRAIL). In brief, this leads to the receptor-proximal recruitment of the death inducing signalling complex (DISC). The resulting activation of caspase-8/10 cleaves and activates effector caspases (caspase-3, -6, -7), which subsequently cleave cell death substrates that collectively produce the phenotypic changes in the cell, characteristic of apoptotic cell death [66]. However, in cells where the initial level of caspase-8/10 activation is low, an amplification loop is triggered [72]. In this amplification loop, caspase-8/10 activates the pro-apoptotic Bcl-2 family member Bid, which triggers cytochrome c release from the mitochondria and subsequent activation of caspase-9 and caspase-3, strongly amplifying the initial apoptotic signal [73].

p53 and Radiation Responses

p53 is often referred to as the guardian of the genome [74–79]. P53 is a phosphoprotein known to suppress cellular transformation and tumorigenesis. The importance of p53 as a tumor suppressor is probably best emphasized by the fact that the p53 gene is mutated in more than 50% of all human cancers [80–82], which suggests that impairment of the p53 function is of advantage for tumor cells.

In normal cells the expression of p53 is low due to a short protein half-life geared by its binding to Mdm2, a ubiquitin ligase which targets p53 for proteolysis by the proteasome [83]. The default of p53 is thus "off" and p53 is only activated in response to stress or cellular damage. As an example, genotoxic stress activates

DNA damage kinases (ATM/ATR), which subsequently activates and stabilizes p53 by decreasing its degradation [84]. This elevates the concentration of p53 and enables it to exert its function. Increased levels of p53 are however not enough for induction of its transcriptional activities. The activation requires modification of p53 by phosphorylation, acetylation, glycosylation or addition of ribose modifications which changes the conformation of the protein [85].

P53 has been established as one of the most important checkpoint proteins and it plays a major role in the complex cellular responses to radiation (for reviews see [86–90]). The most important function for p53 following irradiation is as a transcription factor with transcriptional control of target genes that influence cell cycle arrest, DNA repair, apoptosis, senescence and autophagy (Fig. 12.3). However, lately evidence has emerged for transcription independent mechanisms of p53, which are important for its proapoptotic function [91]. Following irradiation, p53 will initially promote cell survival through growth arrest and DNA damage repair [88]. However, depending on cell type and the extent of damage p53 may also eliminate damaged cells by irreversible inhibition of cell growth by activation of apoptosis, autophagy and/or senescence [88]. The way p53 decides which genes to turn on or off to achieve the desirable outcome following a specific insult has been extensively studied and reviewed [92, 93]. In short, not all p53 responsive genes are equally responsive to p53 and different DNA topologies of p53 responsive elements and different binding affinities of p53 for specific p53 responsive elements contribute to diverse activation of target genes [94]. Furthermore the activation of p53 target genes is also highly predisposed by the cellular context. In cells of different origin as well as in the same cell during different conditions, the abundance of p53 partner proteins which modulate the selection of p53 targets will vary [94].

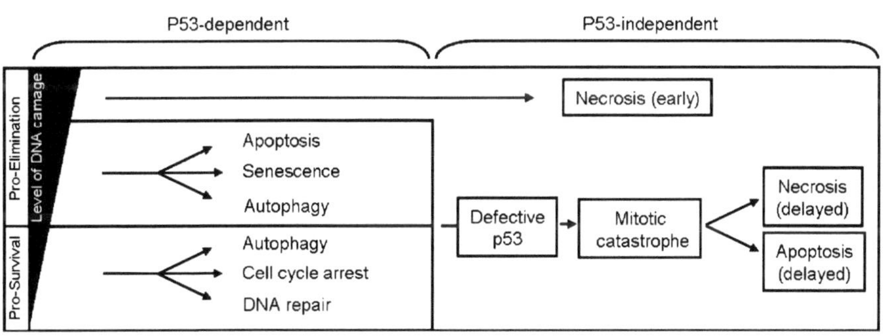

Fig. 12.3 The cell death modality induced following irradiation is dependent on the extent of DNA damage as well as p53-status of the exposed cells. Minor DNA damage induces pro-survival pathways, which include cell cycle arrest and DNA reparation. Extensive DNA damage induces pro-elimination pathways, which can be p53 dependent or p53 independent. This results in irreversible inhibition of cell proliferation by cell death (necrosis, apoptosis, mitotic catastrophe, autophagy) or senescence

p53 Dependent Apoptosis

The primary role for p53 in radiation induced apoptosis is to act as a transcriptional activator of genes encoding apoptotic effectors (Fig. 12.4). Following an apoptotic stimuli including radiation, p53 activates transcription of proapoptotic genes, the most important being members of the Bcl-2 family (Bax [95–98], PUMA [95, 99–101], Noxa [101–103]), that regulate the mitochondria dependent apoptosis. Also expression of genes encoding members of the TNF death receptor family (Fas/APO-1 [97, 104–106], Killer/DR5 [95, 107–109]) can be upregulated which subsequently activate downstream caspases both through mitochondria-dependent and

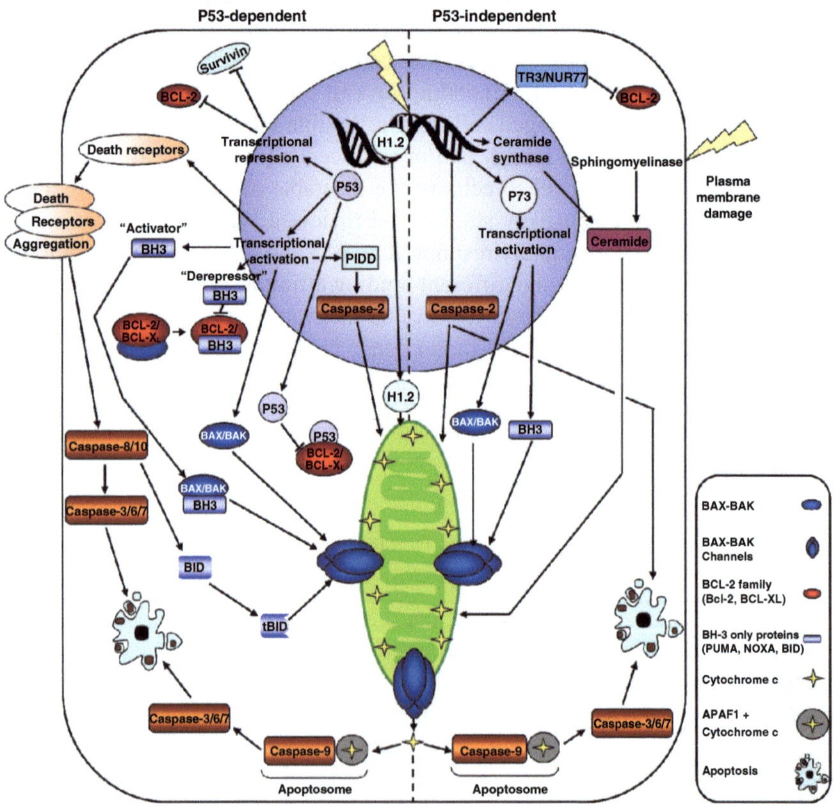

Fig. 12.4 P53 dependent and independent activation of apoptotic pathways following irradiation. P53 mediated apoptosis might be dependent on transcriptional activation of pro-apototic genes including Bcl-2 family members (Bax, PUMA, NOXA) and death receptors (Fas/APO-1, Killer/DR5). P53 can also repress transcription of the anti-apoptotic proteins Bcl-2 and survivin. P53 can translocate to the mitochondria where it neutralizes the antiapoptotic function of Bcl-2 and Bcl-X_L but promotes the pro-apoptotic function of Bax and Bak. The histone H1.2 can also be released from the nuclei, which leads to cytochrome c release. Irradiation can also activate p53-independent apoptosis pathways. These pathways might involve transduction of DNA damage or plasma membrane damage signals to the mitochondria by caspase-2, TR3/Nur77, p73 or ceramide

independent mechanisms [72, 110]. Furthermore, genes encoding proteins that localize to the cytoplasm including PIDD (p53-inducible death domain) [111] and PIGs (p53-induced genes) [112] can be transcriptionally upregulated in a p53 dependent way following an apoptotic stimuli. Finally, expression of genes that lower the apoptotic threshold to sensitize the radiosensitivity can be induced in a p53 dependent way (APAF1, caspase-6, Bid) [87]. Besides transcriptional activation of proapoptotic genes, p53 can also mediate transcriptional repression of expression of anti-apoptotic genes including the Bcl-2 gene [113, 114] and the inhibitor of apoptosis protein-family member survivin [115, 116], a down-regulation that promotes apoptosis (Fig. 12.4). Furthermore p53 itself has been reported to translocate to the mitochondria where it appears to obstruct the antiapoptotic function of Bcl-2 and Bcl-X_L directly by binding to them [117] (Fig. 12.4). P53 has also been reported to directly activate the pore-forming function of Bax [118] and Bak [119] inducing mitochondrial membrane permeabilization (MOMP) and apoptosis. Finally, the release of the nuclear histone H1.2 isoform into the cytoplasm has been shown to occur in a p53-dependent way following irradiation thereby transmitting the apoptotic signal to the mitochondria which releases cytochrome c [120]. This cytochrome c release occurred after Bak activation and was dependent on multidomain proapoptotic Bcl-2 family members [120].

p53 Independent Apoptosis

While the p53-mediated pathway for long has been established as the most important mechanism for radiation induced apoptosis [121] also p53-independent mechanisms have emerged (Fig. 12.4).

The first strategy of triggering DNA-damage induced p53-independent apoptosis involves the p53-family member p73 [122]. P53-dependent apoptosis following DNA damage has been shown to require p63 and p73 [123]. P73 conversely is proapototic following DNA damage even in the absence of p53 [122]. It is an overall assumption that p73 activates pathways following irradiation almost identical to those described for p53 [122]. P73 is able to mediate transcription of several proapoptotic members including Bax [124], PUMA [125] and NOXA [123, 126].

Lately, caspase-2 has gained increased interest as a mechanism of p53-independent apoptosis following DNA damage. Caspase-2 has been shown to be required for stress-induced apoptosis induced by several cytotoxic agents [127]. Several studies also demonstrate that caspase-2 is required, following DNA damage, before mitochondrial permeabilization and apoptosis can take place [127–130]. Furthermore a p53-independent activation of caspase-2 has also been observed by us (data not published) and others [131] during delayed apoptosis following mitotic catastrophe. However, in a recent study, DNA-damage induced apoptosis following cisplatin treatment was shown to require both functional p53 as well as caspase-2 [50].

TR3/Nur77 is an orphan steroid nuclear receptor that also has been associated with a p53-independent transduction of DNA damage signals from the nucleus to the mitochondria thereby activating an apoptotic response [113, 114, 117].

Activation via this pathway has been reported to occur when TR3/Nur77 binds and induces a Bcl-2 conformational change that results in conversion of Bcl-2 from a protector to a killer, inducing apoptosis [132].

Recent publications suggest that radiation, besides damaging nuclear DNA, can act directly on the plasma membrane of several cell types thereby activating acid sphingomyelinase, which via hydrolysis of sphingomyelin generates ceramide, a lipid second messenger acting on mitochondria to induce apoptosis [133–135]. Radiation induced DNA damage can also activate ceramide synthase, which induces de novo synthesis of ceramide and subsequent activation of apoptosis via the mitochondria [135].

Factors Influencing Induction of Early and Delayed Apoptosis

Apoptosis is considered to be one of the main cell death mechanisms following exposure to irradiation [136, 137]. There are several reports about tissues being prone to radiation induced apoptosis and about those which are not [13, 138–142]. In cells from the lymphoid and myeloid lineages, apoptosis is the main cell death mechanism induced following irradiation [143] with significantly lower levels of apoptosis induction in cells of epithelial origin. This is also observed in tumors of different histologies, where the predisposition to die by radiation induced apoptosis differs greatly [138]. In a number of tumor models, including several solid tumor types, a correlation has been established between the background level of apoptosis seen prior to irradiation and the tumor response after irradiation [138, 144]. Radiation induced early apoptosis occurs only a few hours after exposure in interphase and as a premitotic event without requirement for cell division. This mode of radiation induced apoptosis has been characterized and demonstrated to include pyknosis, cell shrinkage and internucleosomal breakage of chromatin, all of which are hallmarks of apoptotic death [16]. This apoptotic process is highly radiosensitive and most often activated in a p53-dependent way. The involvement and importance of p53 in early apoptosis was established by several studies, including those on thymocytes with either wildtype p53 or lacking functional p53 [121, 145]. In these studies, wildtype p53 thymocytes were found to be extremely radiosensitive, whereas thymocytes lacking functional p53 failed to undergo radiation induced apoptosis. The wildtype p53 genotype has been correlated to radiosensitivity [86] and cells that are made resistant to radiation induced apoptosis, either by inactivation of p53 or overexpression of Bcl-2 can demonstrate an increased clonogenic survival [121, 146, 147]. Furthermore, when the induction of radiation induced apoptosis was examined in three closely related human lymphoma cell lines (DL-40, DL-95, and DL-110) that differ in p53 status, significant differences in apoptosis induction was displayed [148].

However, the relatively low levels of radiation induced apoptosis that take place in solid tumors are generally observed much later following mitotic catastrophe. This delayed type of apoptosis has been reported to occur in association to the G2/

M arrest or as a postmitotic event [16, 28, 149, 150]. The morphology of this delayed type of radiation induced apoptosis can differ from that of classical apoptosis as it often is displayed in cells that are "giant" instead of cells with shrunken volume [48, 151]. The level of this delayed type of apoptosis can be dramatically changed by manipulation of the genes affecting apoptosis without changing the overall survival in vitro or in vivo [152]. In general, whether apoptosis matters for overall tumor response depends on how soon after treatment apoptosis occurs [153]. If it occurs early, within a few hours after treatment (tumors of lymphoid and myeloid origin), then it is more likely to be the determinant of cytotoxicity than if the apoptotic response occurs in a delayed way long after exposure (tumors of epithelial and mesenchymal origin).

Shinomiya demonstrated that in the same cell type, different doses of irradiation can induce either early or delayed apoptosis, and that the decision concerning which type of apoptosis that is induced probably reflects the magnitude of cellular damage [16, 17]. Figure 12.5 presents different fates of irradiated cells in relation to the initial damage. Following high dose irradiation and consequently extensive cellular damage to both DNA but also to proteins, enzymes and plasma membranes, early necrosis is induced within a short period of time before any apoptosis induction can occur. With lower doses the initial irradiation induced damage is reduced but still irreparable, which induces an early apoptotic cell death. In cells with impaired apoptosis induction, other cell death mechanisms like mitotic catastrophe will be induced. If the initial damage is little, pro-survival pathways will be induced, which arrest the cell cycle and promotes reparation of damaged DNA. If the reparation is successful the cell will reenter the cell cycle and continue to proliferate. However, if the reparation does not succeed, induction of mitotic catastrophe will follow, executed via delayed apoptosis or necrosis.

The reports with estimations of doses possible to deliver with targeted therapy have been comparatively few, but both fractionated administration and single bolus injection of radiolabeled antibodies have been determining the doses to up to 17 Gy [154, 155], which corresponds to levels being of significance for induction of pro-elimination pathways. By targeting antigens deposited within the tumours, accumulation peaks as late as 1 month after the initial injection with delivered doses of up to 0.44 Gy/MBq administered nuclide [156]. Fractionated approaches have been

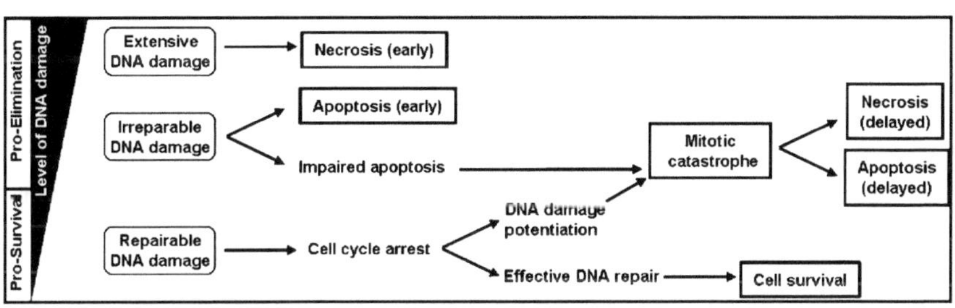

Fig. 12.5 The fate of an irradiated cell is dependent on the severity of the initial damage. See text for details (Adapted from figure by Shinomiya [16])

shown to increase delivered doses [157]. Removal of redundant labeled antibodies by use of antiidiotypic antibodies is a technique to improve tumour/non-tumour ratios [154].

Apoptotic cell death of irradiated Molt-4 cells was shifted fully to necrosis at doses higher than 100 Gy [39]. Using computerized video time-lapse microscopy (CVTL) it has also been demonstrated that following 4 Gy all ST4 cells (murine lymphoma cell line) died by early apoptosis alone (within 5–6 hours), whereas after a reduced dose of 1 Gy cells still mainly died by early apoptosis but a fraction of the cells died from apoptosis following mitosis [158]. In contrast, L5178Y-S cells (murine lymphoma cell line) and MOLT-4 cells (human lymphoid cell line) exposed to 4 Gy underwent apoptosis more slowly with only a small fraction going through apoptosis without attempting cell division. EL-4 cells have been described to display only delayed apoptosis in response to 1–40 Gy irradiation [16], which is also true for HeLa Hep2 cells exposed to different doses (0.5–15 Gy), dose-rates and types of irradiation [159, 160]. However, U937 and HL-60 cells displayed both rapid and delayed apoptosis when exposed to 1–40 Gy [16]. Following an exposure of 20 Gy, mainly rapid apoptosis was induced in these cell lines and the execution included activation of caspase-3, cleavage of PARP, 200 bp-DNA ladder formation and a reduction in the mitochondrial membrane potential which implies that the intrinsic pathway is important for this type of radiation induced apoptosis [16]. Furthermore after exposure of Molt-4 cells and M10 cells to the same dose of irradiation which caused similar clonogenic survival, apoptosis was only induced in Molt-4 cells and necrosis in M10 cells [41]. Also low dose-rate radiation has been reported to induce different amount of apoptosis depending on cell type [161]. Furthermore, an increased apoptotic response following high LET irradiation has been observed with a faster and p53-independent induction compared to low LET [162–165].

Comparison of beta- and gamma-irradiation revealed differences in the apoptosis rates at the same doses, time points and dose rates, which indicates that different types of irradiation influence the efficiency of apoptosis induction [166]. Higher apoptosis rates as well as an earlier activation of apoptosis pathways was observed following gamma-irradiation in comparison to beta-irradiation at the same dose rate [166]. Beta-irradiation and gamma-irradiation activates apoptosis pathways and caspases involving the intrinsic pathway, but also the extrinsic, death receptor pathway [166].

Although different cancer therapies kill tumour cells via apparently homogenous apoptotic pathways, they differ in their capacity to stimulate immunogenic cell death [167]. Generally apoptosis is considered to be non-immunogenic and non-inflammatory in nature. However at certain circumstances apoptosis can induce an immunogenic response [168]. Recently it was shown that exposure to irradiation induces a pre-apoptotic translocation of intracellular calreticulin to the plasma membrane surface in some but not all tumor cell lines [167]. This early calreticulin exposure allows tumor cells to be efficiently engulfed by dendritic cells and induce immunogenic cell death [167, 169].

Mitotic Catastrophe

Mitotic catastrophe was originally defined as a cell death modality in cells forced prematurely into mitosis [23]. Today, mitotic catastrophe includes cell deaths that occur during mitosis or as a result of an aberrant mitosis [35]. Abnormal mitosis may proceed through several different pathways and induces a variety of disturbances including anaphase bridging, lagging chromosomal material, and multipolar mitoses [48, 170] (Fig. 12.6). Aberrant mitosis furthermore does not produce proper chromosome segregation and cell division and leads to the formation of giant cells with aberrant nuclear morphology [48, 151, 171], multiple nuclei [48, 172] and/or several micronuclei [55], giving cells passing through a mitotic catastrophe a morphology distinct from apoptosis, necrosis and autophagy [35]. Many of these cells may divide a few times to become polyploid/aneuploid and may form abortive colonies. These cells can persist for several hours or days but eventually die either by delayed necrosis or delayed apoptosis [50, 173]. This apoptosis, however, is not always required for the lethal effects of mitotic catastrophe, since inhibition of apoptosis has demonstrated small effects on the clonogenic survival [174, 175].

Until recently, the most common mechanism to describe the way irradiation executes its lethal effect, has been by induction of apoptosis with low irradiation doses and necrosis with higher doses. This low dose induced apoptosis is mainly p53 dependent and cells with dys-functional activation of apoptosis due to p53 impairment or by other means displaying inactivated apoptotic signalling were considered resistant to irradiation. Disabling of apoptosis, which is a common feature in tumors should therefore render malignant cells less susceptible to overall radiation induced cell death, compared to normal cells and tissues. However, no such correlation could be seen in situ or in vitro [176]. Furthermore, tumors with impaired apoptotic pathways should be more resistant to DNA damage than tumors with functional apoptotic pathways. However, some reports indicate that p53 inactivation induces an enhanced sensitivity of cancer cells to DNA-damage [177–180], others have found that loss of p53 increases cellular resistance to such

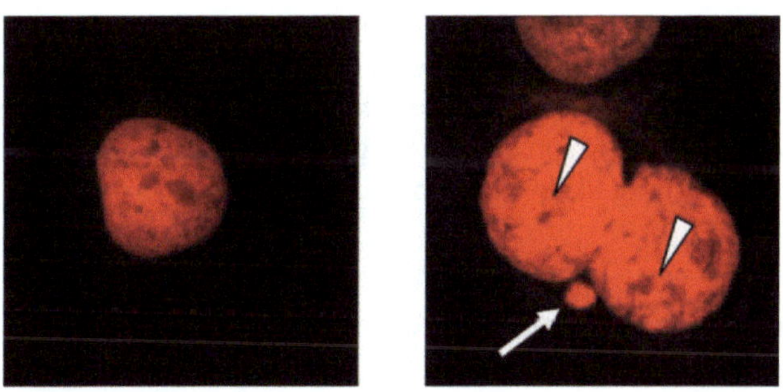

Fig. 12.6 Mitotic catastrophe following irradiation [48]. Control cells normally contain a single round nucleus (to the left). One irradiated cell with multiple nuclei (arrowheads) and micronuclei (arrow) (to the right)

agents [181, 182]. Furthermore, when Bcl-2 was overexpressed in a colon carcinoma cell line (HCT116, CDKN1A$^{-/-}$) it did not change the radiation induced therapeutic response in tumor xenografts, even though apoptosis was significantly reduced [152]. This suggests that other important cell death modalities, besides apoptosis are involved in irradiation induced cell death.

Mitosis is considered to be a critical phase in the cell cycle at which radiation induced DNA damage manifests itself and cell death has been found to occur directly as a consequence of that. This cell death modality referred to as mitotic catastrophe has been found to be the main cell death mechanism following irradiation [136] with creation of multinucleated cells, an event which is an important attribute of the mitotic catastrophe. This is frequently observed in tumors and tumor cells after irradiation [37, 48, 151, 183, 184]. The mitotic disturbances associated with mitotic catastrophe also generate cells which contain one or several micronuclei formed by nuclear membrane formation around lagging chromosomes or chromosomal material. This has also been observed in irradiated animal tumors [185]. Furthermore, an enhancement of the fraction of cells with several nuclei as well as abnormally shaped multilobulated nuclei has been observed in experimental tumors following radioimmunotherapy [151].

This mode of cell death is exhibited by most non haematopoietic cell lineages in response to ionizing radiation [31], and is considered to be the major mechanism by which the majority of solid tumors respond to clinical radiotherapy. Mitotic catastrophe is a delayed type of cell death starting days after treatment initiation, which can explain why clinical regression of solid tumors after completion of therapy is observed over many months, whereas treatment of lymphoid tumor cells, which mainly die from interphase early apoptosis may result in dramatic regression during a course of treatment [186]. This does not preclude a contribution of spontaneous and induced apoptosis in solid tumors to treatment outcome. However, there is a paucity of clinical data to indicate the true contribution of apoptosis to radiosensitivity [136]. Furthermore, several quantitative and semiquantitative studies comparing the amount of apoptosis and decrease in clonogenic survival occurring in irradiated cells indicate that in most cases, the primary mode of cell death leading to loss of reproductive integrity is associated with mitotic catastrophe, with a much smaller component being associated with apoptosis following irradiation. In almost all cases in which cell death has been studied in cells, both in culture and in vivo, apoptosis can not account for the loss of clonogenic survival that occurs after irradiation. Most of the loss of clonogenic survival (i.e. loss of reproductive integrity), occurs later after mitotic activity has resumed, and is most likely caused by mitotic catastrophe [136].

Induction of Mitotic Catastrophe

Several concepts on the induction pathways to mitotic catastrophe following irradiation has been presented. The classical explanation is that following irradiation, a premature entry into mitosis with unrepaired DNA damage induces chromosomal aberrations, which culminate in execution of the mitotic catastrophe. Several studies demonstrate that for ionizing radiation, chromosome aberrations are closely linked with cell killing [187–189]. This applies for radiations of different ionizing densities [190] and dose-rates [191]. These chromosome aberrations lead to the development of anaphase bridges and micronuclei and finally cell death. It has been demonstrated that cells containing micronuclei at the first or subsequent divisions following radiation exposure were unable to form viable colonies [192].

It has been proposed that mitotic catastrophe results from a combination of non-functional cell cycle checkpoints in combination with cellular damage [193]. Furthermore, it has been suggested that one of the cellular consequences of mutations in the tumor-suppressor gene p53 is to promote mitotic catastrophe as a mechanism for removing damaged cells following genotoxic stress [194]. P53 is important for two major DNA-damage checkpoints, especially for the one residing at the G1-S transition but also for the G2-M checkpoint by affecting the duration of arrest in G2 [89, 195]. The G2 checkpoint includes both p53-independent and p53-dependent mechanisms, with p53 playing a critical role in the maintenance of the arrest [196]. At least 50% of human tumors are p53-deficient [80–82], and some tumors also show mutations or altered expression of other components of the G2 checkpoint [55]. As a consequence tumors regularly display impaired activation of the cell cycle checkpoints after irradiation, including the G1- and G2-checkpoints [89]. Unless a damaged cell enters mitosis, such a cell cannot undergo mitotic catastrophe. This explains why abrogation of G1 and/or G2 checkpoints favours mitotic catastrophe. If cells escape G1 and G2 arrest then they will enter mitosis more rapidly, which has been shown to promote radiation induced mitotic catastrophe [55].

Mitotic catastrophe can also be a consequence of aberrant reentry into the cell cycle after prolonged G1 and G2 arrests. This form of catastrophe appears to be potentiated rather than prevented by G1 and G2 checkpoint mediators, such as p21. It remains to be determined whether tumor-specific deficiencies in mitotic checkpoints (prophase and spindle checkpoints) play a role in the susceptibility of tumor cells to delayed mitotic catastrophe.

Several groups have reported that radiation induced abnormal mitosis is associated with anomalous duplication of centrosomes [197–201]. During normal mitosis, centrosomes, the major microtubule organizing centers, exert an important function by formation of the spindle poles. The centrosomes are crucial for the number of spindle poles formed during mitosis [202, 203] and important for accurate chromosome segregation to the daughter cells. Hyperamplification of centrosomes has earlier been detected after irradiation during a prolonged G2-phase and to be dependent [204] or independent [199, 205] of a subsequent failure in cytokinesis. This centrosome hyperamplification may be a critical event contributing to the radiation induced mitotic catastrophe. We have observed hyperamplification of centrosomes in several cell lines (HeLa, HT29, Caco-2, WM-266-4) following both ^{60}Co [48] and ^{131}I-irradiation (data not published). This was followed by an increased frequency of multipolar mitotic spindles and a subsequent progression into mitotic catastrophe (Fig. 12.7).

Recently, Blagosklonny put forward an interesting theory for the induction of the mitotic catastrophe [206]. He postulates that the induction of a mitotic arrest following radiation, during which transcription is inhibited, would lead to depletion

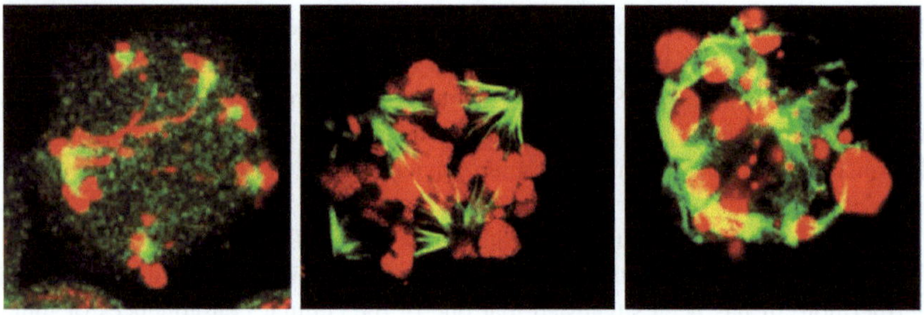

Fig. 12.7 Irradiated single cells executing a mitotic catastrophe. One irradiated cell with hyperamplified numbers of centrosomes (green colour, left), which is followed by the formation of multipolar mitotic spindles (green colour, middle). A subsequent induction of a mitotic catastrophe in a single cell with multiple micronuclei can be seen to the right (red colour)

of short-lived proteins that have short-lived RNAs. Depletion of anti-apoptotic proteins, cyclin B, and Mdm-2 can lead to delayed apoptosis, mitotic slippage and p53 stabilization respectively and can, as they discuss, explain all the complex and puzzling cell fates that are induced during a mitotic catastrophe.

Induction Pathways

Radiation induced DNA damage that occurs in cells prior to mitosis will mainly induce apoptosis in the interphase in apoptosis-prone cells. Apoptosis-prone cells would not simply have a chance to undergo mitotic catastrophe as it is a prerequisite to enter mitosis for a mitotic catastrophe to occur. Therefore, during a radiation induced mitotic catastrophe, cells most likely undergo mitotic slippage after a mitotic arrest, which is followed by an aberrant mitosis. Failure of accurate chromosome segregation and a defect cytokinesis induces formation of micronuclei and binucleated cells respectively, which is followed by non-apoptotic cell death preferentially [43], although it might include activation of the apoptotic machinery [48–50]. In other words, cells that undergo DNA-damage-induced mitotic catastrophe must be relatively apoptosis-reluctant, because otherwise DNA damage would induce apoptosis in the interphase.

The sequence of events that finally ends up in mitotic catastrophe can be schematically described as follows: After induction of a transient G2-M arrest, during which centrosome hyperamplification can occur, cells with DNA lesions enter mitosis prematurely. The mitotic checkpoint, also known as the spindle assembly checkpoint is subsequently activated and the progression through mitosis is prohibited [207]. Radiation often leads to this type of delay in mitosis [175]. This delay may be permanent and fatal. There is evidence that in some cells apoptotic pathways are activated during this arrest in mitosis, here described as delayed apoptosis type 1 (Fig. 12.8). During the mitotic catastrophe, a p53-independent death activated

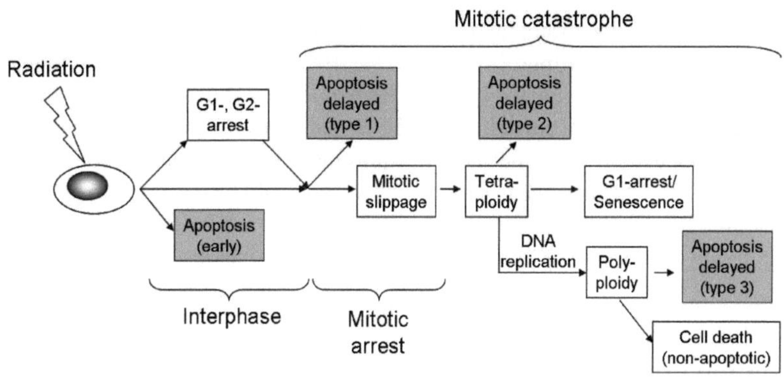

Fig. 12.8 Mitotic catastrophe is induced following irradiation in cells that are relatively reluctant to early apoptosis. Mitotic catastrophe can be executed during or after mitosis via several types of delayed apoptosis or non-apoptotic cell deaths like delayed necrosis

during metaphase results in caspase activation and subsequent mitochondrial damage [131, 171, 193]. Recently, caspase-2 has gained increased interest as an initiator caspase following DNA damage [117, 208]. Castedo et al. furthermore demonstrated that caspase-2 is important for the apoptosis-related cell death, which follows mitotic catastrophes [131]. This is in agreement with our observations of delayed apoptosis [48] and activation of caspase-2 following both ^{60}Co- and ^{131}I-irradiation (data not published). More often cells adapt to the mitotic checkpoint and exit the arrest but fail cytokinesis and enter the G1-phase with a tetraploid DNA content [209, 210]. Tumors and tumor cells are associated with weakened mitotic checkpoints and consequently have lost their ability to remain arrested in mitosis for long time [209], but if this is a prerequisite for adaptation is currently unknown. Tetraploid cells will either die in G1 via delayed apoptosis (delayed apoptosis type 2), or become reproductively dead but viable (senescent) or enter the next cell cycle [211]. Apoptosis in G1 occurs shortly after tetraploidization and unlike apoptosis in mitosis, these events are largely dependent on p53 activation of the Bax-dependent mitochondrial pathway [212]. Similarly, p53 also induces p21, which in turn induces a post-mitotic G1 arrest [213]. These multinucleated cells can survive and become senescent [55, 214, 215]. If the cells lack p53 they may proceed to another round of DNA amplification and become aneuploid/polyploid [48, 216]. These damaged cells do not necessarily die immediately, but may continue through several cycles of cell division, acquiring an increasing amount of chromosomal aberrations, finally causing cell death (delayed apoptosis type 3, delayed necrosis).

Consistent for all cell deaths that follow mitotic catastrophe is that most of these deaths occur late, 2–6 days following irradiation [175]. The mode of cell death is determined by the dose of radiation to which the cells are exposed [13]. As precisely noticed, mitotic catastrophe in apoptosis-competent cells is frequently followed by apoptosis. We have observed that a fraction of HeLa Hep2 cells exposed to different doses, dose-rates and quality of radiation die via delayed apoptosis following mitotic catastrophe [48, 151, 159, 160]. Maximal apoptosis induction was obtained between 5 and 10 Gy and at higher doses a shift towards another form of cell death modality occurred, probably in the form of delayed necrosis [159, 160]. Yet, apoptosis is not a necessary requirement for the lethal effect of mitotic catastrophe [55]. Mitotic catastrophe results in cell death by caspase-dependent and caspase-independent mechanisms. Typically, there is a mixture of apoptotic and nonapoptotic deaths during mitosis and following multinucleation.

Radiation and Senescence Induction

The concept of cellular senescence remains of significance for radiation induced mechanisms to inhibit tumor cell growth (Fig. 12.3). Senescence was initially described as a sequence of cellular metabolic changes causing irreversible growth arrest with display of characteristic phenotypic traits [29, 217]. The morphological features typical for a cell in senescence include: a flat and enlarged morphology, an increase in acidic β-galactosidase activity in the plasma membrane, chromatin condensation, changes in gene expression patterns and increased cell granularity [218, 219].

This type of growth arrest is commonly seen in normal cells and referred to as replicative senescence – with telomere size below critical range. These cells do not divide, but may remain metabolically active for longer periods (weeks and months in vitro). Various DNA stressing stimuli including irradiation may induce similar phenotypic changes, which can be analyzed and quantified in biochemical or morphological terms. One of the most used features to monitor senescence or senescence-like terminal growth arrest has been to investigate the expression of β-galactosidase.

The induction of senescense can be performed with several sorts of stress stimuli, which increase the expression or posttranscriptional activity of the tumor repressor p53 and its downstream product p16. P53 is able to activate p21 and also other members of the CIP-KIP family (cyclin-dependant kinase inhibitors) [220, 221]. Senescence can thus be induced by at least two different pathways. These cells also display significant differences in gene expression pattern, with activation of cytokine synthesis, besides factors related to the cell cycle arrest [222, 223].

Several investigations on radiation induced senescence using different tumor cell lines have been reported and doses used to reach a state with significant transformation to senescence or a senescence-like state has been reported to be in the interval 2–15 Gy. It was recently reported that glioblastoma multiforme cells, exposed to fractionated radiotherapy exposed both conventional growth arrest and senescence, but not extensive apoptosis following irradiation [224]. Similar observations have been reported for prostatic cancer cell lines, which expose significant conversion to senescence. The authors claim it to be the major mechanism to cause growth arrest, as well as a decrease in clonogenic survival for these cells [52]. Up to 90% of vascular endothelial cells expressed typical senescence markers following radiation doses of 8 Gy [225]. Also MCF-7 breast tumor cells, exposed to 10 Gy, expressed extensive induction of senescence which was related to the p53 status, but unrelated to telomer length or telomerase activity [51].

As a general conclusion from these studies it seems reasonable to accept that also transformation into senescence may be a growth retardation mechanism in operation at targeted therapy.

Radiation Induced Autophagy

The newcomer in the array of different cell deaths is autophagy. This type of cell death is characterized by an intact nucleus and an accumulation of cytoplasmatic double-membrane autophagic vacuoles called autophagosomes [226, 227]. The process is dynamic and enables delivery to the lysosomes of subcellular membranes, sequestered cytoplasm with long lived proteins and organelles, where the content is digested by lysosomal hydrolases and recycled for internal use [152].

This process could represent a survival strategy for many cells, including tumor cells, with limited supply of nutrients, but the process is also related to cell death (Fig. 12.3). It has been discussed if this mechanism is a direct death execution pathway or a defence mechanism that ultimately fails to preserve cell viability, or even a process to finally clean up cell remnants already destined for death [228]. Many of these organelles are pivotal for survival and when the degradation is too extensive, autophagic cell death may be induced. The autophagosomes may contain, besides mitochondria, polyribosomes, Golgi complex components and microtubule-associated protein light chain 3 (LC3) used as a marker for autophagy [229]. Autophagy has also been looked upon as a programmed non-apoptotic cell death [228]. Autophagy may be upregulated when apoptosis is not induced.

The signalling pathways are not completely known but may include caspase 8 and ATG7-beclin [230–232]. Also phosphatidylinositol 3-kinase (PI3K) pathways are involved [233]. Apoptosis and autophagy should not be regarded as mutually exclusive phenomena, but may represent different responses to a changing environment.

Radiation induced autophagy has been demonstrated to occur in mouse fibroblasts and several cancer cell lines (breast and lung) [234, 235]. By increasing levels of pro-autophagic proteins (beclin-1 and ATG5-ATG12 complex) an up-regulation of autophagy took place, following irradiation. Furthermore inhibition of proapoptotic proteins and induction of autophagy increased sensitivity to therapy [234]. Also malignant glioma cells, exposed to ionizing radiation are able to react on irradiation with induction of autophagy and formation of autophagosomes, but not apoptosis [236].

Conclusions

The pleomorphic cell death panorama which now is rapidly emerging and the multitude of interrelated mechanisms to induce cell death by irradiation open new avenues to more efficient gearing and tailoring of targeted therapy. The previous classification of radiation induced cell death modalities into either necrosis or apoptosis is today recognized as too simplistic.

Furthermore, the earlier consensus paradigm that "more is better" in radiotherapy when it comes to delivered doses and dose rates to tumors, both clinically and at experimental conditions, could possibly in the future be exchanged to a concept which includes benefits of continuous low-dose rate and low total doses (2–15 Gy), employing several different cell death modalities as means to improve therapy.

These requirements are possible to meet with targeted radiotherapy, which can be used to deliver different nuclides with accumulation to and long "residence time" in tumors, which may be weeks and up to months. Doses up to 15 Gy have also been possible to reach. Earlier, total delivered doses of 50–80 Gy have been desirable and considered to be optimal at external radiotherapy, when negative side effects are balanced against positive outcome of treatment. Radiosensitivity is highly dependent of mitotic frequencies, and rapidly dividing cells (as hematopoietic or intestinal cells) are very vulnerable. Slowly dividing epithelial cells and especially (cancer) stem cells display lower radiosensitivity, and may repair DNA-breaks more rapidly. This will cause accumulation of more resistant cells.

The high doses at conventional radiotherapy are usually given at high dose-rates and short time intervals. Such high doses seem to mainly cause necrosis within the tumors and also partially in surrounding tissues and to a lesser degree interphase (early) apoptosis. When doses are lowered and given during longer time intervals, as is the case with targeted therapy, other death modalities instead of necrosis take over and delayed apoptosis, mitotic catastrophe, senescence and autophagy dominate the death patterns seen. This may indicate a new discernable consensus paradigm for targeted therapy. The damage caused by these lower doses and dose-rates is less harmful with regard to side effects and does not cause immediate necrosis, but offers possibilities for the cell to repair damages, a process that however obviously is not always an easy task, and when not successful will induce the slower death modalities. The induction pattern of the interrelated pathways for the latter mechanisms is not yet fully understood, but possibilities for future elucidations of synergistic effects need to be evaluated. These latter mechanisms could furthermore be in operation simultaneously.

Targeted therapy has been most successful at treatment of haematological malignancies, when early apoptosis is induced. This has lead to the assumption that apoptosis induction should be the goal of targeted therapy. This is probably still correct for this category of malignant diseases. However, many tumors harbour a population of cells that have acquired resistance towards apoptosis and with mitotic catastrophe, autophagy and senescence as alternative cell deaths, apoptosis is no longer an obligatory and single goal. Early apoptosis is thus not the major cell death in solid tumors of epithelial and mesenchymal origin following radiation treatment. Treatment outcome of targeted therapy for solid tumors in general is poor, compared to the effects seen for radioimmunotherapy of haematological malignancies. The reason is not that apoptosis induction fails, but an overall failure to induce cell death. In this case, activation of other complementary cell death programs is beneficial and a promising therapeutic approach to complement apoptosis-based targeted therapy.

It was commonly assumed that effective radiation therapy of tumors depends on direct cytotoxic effects. Radiation induced apoptosis is generally considered to be a gentle way to dispose dying cells without activation of inflammation and such a treatment, as a consequence, has little effect on surrounding tissues. The ambition at treatment is to completely eradicate tumors and induced inflammatory reactions as well as a putatively potent immune response may be of advantage for the anti-tumor effect. Mitotic catastrophe often leads to necrosis and subsequent inflammation. Furthermore, translocation of intracellular calreticulin to the plasma membrane surface during certain types of radiation-induced apoptosis may activate an immune response against residual tumor cells indicating that also indirect effects from irradiation can be involved in the treatment response.

Even if a cell cannot undergo apoptosis, it can still die by mitotic catastrophe, autophagy and senescence. Thus, identifying the importance of different radiation induced cell deaths, their induction mechanisms and their putatively synergistic effects for the therapeutic outcome has potential and practical implications for improving targeted therapy of malignant diseases.

Acknowledgements Financial support from the Swedish Cancer Society, the County of Västerbotten and the Medical Faculty at Umeå University for research related to the content of this chapter is acknowledged.

References

1. Bernier J, Hall EJ, Giaccia A. Radiation oncology: a century of achievements. Nature Reviews 2004; 4(9):737–47.
2. Grubbé EH. Priority in the therapeutic use of X-rays. Radiology 1933; 21:156–62.
3. Cox JD. The science and art of radiation oncology after a century. International Journal of Radiation Oncology, Biology, Physics 1999; 43(1):1–2.
4. Bedford JS, Dewey WC. Radiation Research Society. 1952–2002. Historical and current highlights in radiation biology: has anything important been learned by irradiating cells? Radiation Research 2002; 158(3):251–91.
5. Virchow R. Die Cellularpathologie in ihrer Begründung auf physiologische und pathologische Gewebelehre, 2 edn. Berlin: Verlag von August Hirschwald, 1858.
6. Levin S. A toxicologic pathologist's view of apoptosis or I used to call it necrobiosis, but now I'm singing the apoptosis blues. Toxicologic Pathology 1995; 23(4):533–9
7. Levin S, Bucci TJ, Cohen SM, Fix AS, Hardisty JF, LeGrand EK, Maronpot RR, Trump BF. The nomenclature of cell death: recommendations of an ad hoc Committee of the Society of Toxicologic Pathologists. Toxicologic Pathology 1999; 27(4):484–90.
8. Kerr JF, Wyllie AH, Currie AR. Apoptosis: a basic biological phenomenon with wide-ranging implications in tissue kinetics. British Journal of Cancer 1972; 26(4):239–57.
9. Skalka M, Matyasova J, Cejkova M. Dna in chromatin of irradiated lymphoid tissues degrades in vivo into regular fragments. FEBS Letters 1976; 72(2):271–4.
10. Hendry JH, Potten CS. Intestinal cell radiosensitivity: a comparison for cell death assayed by apoptosis or by a loss of clonogenicity. International Journal of Radiation Biology and Related Studies in Physics, Chemistry, and Medicine 1982; 42(6):621–8.
11. Hendry JH, Potten CS, Chadwick C, Bianchi M. Cell death (apoptosis) in the mouse small intestine after low doses: effects of dose-rate, 14.7 MeV neutrons, and 600 MeV (maximum energy) neutrons. International Journal of Radiation Biology and Related Studies in Physics, Chemistry, and Medicine 1982; 42(6):611–20.

12. Zong WX, Thompson CB. Necrotic death as a cell fate. Genes & Development 2006; 20(1):1–15.
13. Abend M. Reasons to reconsider the significance of apoptosis for cancer therapy. International Journal of Radiation Biology 2003; 79(12):927–41.
14. Farber E. Programmed cell death: necrosis versus apoptosis. Modern Pathology 1994; 7(5):605–9.
15. Olive PL, Durand RE. Apoptosis: an indicator of radiosensitivity in vitro? International Journal of Radiation Biology 1997; 71(6):695–707.
16. Shinomiya N. New concepts in radiation-induced apoptosis: 'premitotic apoptosis' and 'postmitotic apoptosis'. Journal of Cellular and Molecular Medicine 2001; 5(3):240–53.
17. Shinomiya N, Kuno Y, Yamamoto F, Fukasawa M, Okumura A, Uefuji M, Rokutanda M. Different mechanisms between premitotic apoptosis and postmitotic apoptosis in X-irradiated U937 cells. International Journal of Radiation Oncology, Biology, Physics 2000; 47(3):767–77.
18. Broker LE, Kruyt FA, Giaccone G. Cell death independent of caspases: a review. Clinical Cancer Research 2005; 11(9):3155–62.
19. Golstein P, Kroemer G. A multiplicity of cell death pathways. Symposium on apoptotic and non-apoptotic cell death pathways. EMBO Reports 2007; 8(9):829–33.
20. Kroemer G, El-Deiry WS, Golstein P, et al. Classification of cell death: recommendations of the Nomenclature Committee on Cell Death. Cell Death and Differentiation 2005; 12(Suppl 2):1463–7.
21. Lockshin RA, Zakeri Z. Apoptosis, autophagy, and more. The International Journal of Biochemistry & Cell Biology 2004; 36(12):2405–19.
22. Ricci MS, Zong WX. Chemotherapeutic approaches for targeting cell death pathways. The Oncologist 2006; 11(4):342–57.
23. Russell P, Nurse P. cdc25 + functions as an inducer in the mitotic control of fission yeast. Cell 1986; 45(1):145–53.
24. Hopwood LE, Tolmach LJ. Deficient DNA synthesis and mitotic death in x-irradiated HeLa cells. Radiation Research 1971; 46(1):70–84.
25. Terasima T, Ohara H. Chromosome aberration and mitotic death in x-irradiated HeLa cells. Mutation Research 1968; 5(1):195–7.
26. Puck TT. Action of radiation on mammalian cells III. Relationship between reproductive death and induction of chromosome anomalies by x-irradiation of euploid human cells in vitro. Proceedings of the National Academy of Sciences of the United States of America 1958; 44(8):772–80.
27. Ianzini F, Mackey MA. Spontaneous premature chromosome condensation and mitotic catastrophe following irradiation of HeLa S3 cells. International Journal of Radiation Biology 1997; 72(4):409–21.
28. Merritt AJ, Allen TD, Potten CS, Hickman JA. Apoptosis in small intestinal epithelial from p53-null mice: evidence for a delayed, p53-independent G2/M-associated cell death after gamma-irradiation. Oncogene 1997; 14(23):2759–66.
29. Hayflick L, Moorhead PS. The serial cultivation of human diploid cell strains. Experimental Cell Research 1961; 25:585–621.
30. de Duve C. Introduced at the CIBA foundation symposium on lysosomes, 1963.
31. Chang BD, Broude EV, Dokmanovic M, et al. A senescence-like phenotype distinguishes tumor cells that undergo terminal proliferation arrest after exposure to anticancer agents. Cancer Research 1999; 59(15):3761–7.
32. Di Leonardo A, Linke SP, Clarkin K, Wahl GM. DNA damage triggers a prolonged p53-dependent G1 arrest and long-term induction of Cip1 in normal human fibroblasts. Genes & Development 1994; 8(21):2540–51.
33. Hamberg H. Cellular autophagocytosis induced by X-irradiation and vinblastine. On the origin of the segregating membranes. Acta pathologica, microbiologica, et immunologica Scandinavica 1983; 91(5):317–27.

34. Hamberg H, Brunk U, Ericsson JL, Jung B. Cytoplasmic effects of X-irradiation on cultured cells 2. Alterations in lysosomes, plasma membrane, Golgi apparatus, and related structures. Acta pathologica et microbiologica Scandinavica 1977; 85(5):625–39.
35. Galluzzi L, Maiuri MC, Vitale I, Zischka H, Castedo M, Zitvogel L, Kroemer G. Cell death modalities: classification and pathophysiological implications. Cell Death and Differentiation 2007; 14(7):1237–43.
36. Okada S. Radiation-induced cell death. In: Altman KI, Gerber GB, Okada S, eds. Radiation biochemistry, 1. New York: Academic, 1970:247–307.
37. Somosy Z. Radiation response of cell organelles. Micron 2000; 31(2):165–81.
38. Okada S. Formation of giant cells. In: Altman KI, Gerber GB, Okada S, eds. Radiation biochemistry, 1. New York: Academic, 1970:239–46.
39. Akagi Y, Ito K, Sawada S. Radiation-induced apoptosis and necrosis in Molt-4 cells: a study of dose-effect relationships and their modification. International Journal of Radiation Biology 1993; 64(1):47–56.
40. Harms-Ringdahl M, Nicotera P, Radford IR. Radiation induced apoptosis. Mutation Research 1996; 366(2):171–9.
41. Nakano H, Shinohara K. X-ray-induced cell death: apoptosis and necrosis. Radiation Research 1994; 140(1):1–9.
42. Szumiel I. Ionizing radiation-induced cell death. International Journal of Radiation Biology 1994; 66(4):329–41.
43. Jonathan EC, Bernhard EJ, McKenna WG. How does radiation kill cells? Current Opinion in Chemical biology 1999; 3(1):77–83.
44. Zong WX, Ditsworth D, Bauer DE, Wang ZQ, Thompson CB. Alkylating DNA damage stimulates a regulated form of necrotic cell death. Genes & Development 2004; 18(11):1272–82.
45. Chan TA, Hermeking H, Lengauer C, Kinzler KW, Vogelstein B. 14-3-3Sigma is required to prevent mitotic catastrophe after DNA damage. Nature 1999; 401(6753):616–20.
46. Chu K, Teele N, Dewey MW, Albright N, Dewey WC. Computerized video time lapse study of cell cycle delay and arrest, mitotic catastrophe, apoptosis and clonogenic survival in irradiated 14-3-3sigma and CDKN1A (p21) knockout cell lines. Radiation Research 2004; 162(3):270–86.
47. Brown JM, Attardi LD. The role of apoptosis in cancer development and treatment response. Nature Reviews 2005; 5(3):231–7.
48. Eriksson D, Lofroth PO, Johansson L, Riklund KA, Stigbrand T. Cell cycle disturbances and mitotic catastrophes in HeLa Hep2 cells following 2.5 to 10Gy of ionizing radiation. Clinical Cancer Research 2007; 13(18 Pt 2):5501s–8s.
49. Skwarska A, Augustin E, Konopa J. Sequential induction of mitotic catastrophe followed by apoptosis in human leukemia MOLT4 cells by imidazoacridinone C-1311. Apoptosis 2007; 12(12):2245–57.
50. Vakifahmetoglu H, Olsson M, Tamm C, Heidari N, Orrenius S, Zhivotovsky B. DNA damage induces two distinct modes of cell death in ovarian carcinomas. Cell Death and Differentiation 2008; 15(3):555–66.
51. Jones KR, Elmore LW, Jackson-Cook C, Demasters G, Povirk LF, Holt SE, Gewirtz DA. p53-Dependent accelerated senescence induced by ionizing radiation in breast tumour cells. International Journal of Radiation Biology 2005; 81(6):445–58.
52. Lehmann BD, McCubrey JA, Jefferson HS, Paine MS, Chappell WH, Terrian DM. A dominant role for p53-dependent cellular senescence in radiosensitization of human prostate cancer cells. Cell Cycle (Georgetown, TX) 2007; 6(5):595–605.
53. Moretti L, Cha YI, Niermann KJ, Lu B. Switch between apoptosis and autophagy: radiation-induced endoplasmic reticulum stress? Cell Cycle (Georgetown, TX) 2007; 6(7):793–8.
54. Kroemer G, Dallaporta B, Resche-Rigon M. The mitochondrial death/life regulator in apoptosis and necrosis. Annual Review of Physiology 1998; 60:619–42.
55. Roninson IB, Broude EV, Chang BD. If not apoptosis, then what? Treatment-induced senescence and mitotic catastrophe in tumor cells. Drug Resistance Updates 2001; 4(5):303–13.

56. Wyllie AH, Kerr JF, Currie AR. Cell death: the significance of apoptosis. International Review of Cytology 1980; 68:251–306.
57. Kroemer G, Petit P, Zamzami N, Vayssiere JL, Mignotte B. The biochemistry of programmed cell death. FASEB Journal 1995; 9(13):1277–87.
58. Thompson CB. Apoptosis in the pathogenesis and treatment of disease. Science (New York) 1995; 267(5203):1456–62.
59. Williams JR, Little JB, Shipley WU. Association of mammalian cell death with a specific endonucleolytic degradation of DNA. Nature 1974; 252(5485):754–5.
60. Savill J. Phagocyte recognition of apoptotic cells. Biochemical Society Transactions 1996; 24(4):1065–9.
61. Riedl SJ, Shi Y. Molecular mechanisms of caspase regulation during apoptosis. Nature Reviews. Molecular Cell Biology 2004; 5(11):897–907.
62. Timmer JC, Salvesen GS. Caspase substrates. Cell Death and Differentiation 2007; 14(1):66–72.
63. Chipuk JE, Green DR. Do inducers of apoptosis trigger caspase-independent cell death? Nature Reviews Molecular Cell Biology 2005; 6(3):268–75.
64. Kim R, Emi M, Tanabe K. Role of mitochondria as the gardens of cell death. Cancer Chemotherapy and Pharmacology 2006; 57(5):545–53.
65. Jin Z, El-Deiry WS. Overview of cell death signaling pathways. Cancer Biology & Therapy 2005; 4(2):139–63.
66. Taylor RC, Cullen SP, Martin SJ. Apoptosis: controlled demolition at the cellular level. Nature Reviews Molecular Cell Biology 2008; 9(3):231–41.
67. Danial NN, Korsmeyer SJ. Cell death: critical control points. Cell 2004; 116(2):205–19.
68. Wang X. The expanding role of mitochondria in apoptosis. Genes & Development 2001; 15(22):2922–33.
69. Jiang X, Wang X. Cytochrome c promotes caspase-9 activation by inducing nucleotide binding to Apaf-1. The Journal of Biological Chemistry 2000; 275(40):31199–203.
70. Li P, Nijhawan D, Budihardjo I, Srinivasula SM, Ahmad M, Alnemri ES, Wang X. Cytochrome c and dATP-dependent formation of Apaf-1/caspase-9 complex initiates an apoptotic protease cascade. Cell 1997; 91(4):479–89.
71. Rodriguez J, Lazebnik Y. Caspase-9 and APAF-1 form an active holoenzyme. Genes & Development 1999; 13(24):3179–84.
72. Scaffidi C, Fulda S, Srinivasan A, et al. Two CD95 (APO-1/Fas) signaling pathways. The EMBO Journal 1998; 17(6):1675–87.
73. Luo X, Budihardjo I, Zou H, Slaughter C, Wang X. Bid, a Bcl2 interacting protein, mediates cytochrome c release from mitochondria in response to activation of cell surface death receptors. Cell 1998; 94(4):481–90.
74. Efeyan A, Serrano M. p53: guardian of the genome and policeman of the oncogenes. Cell Cycle (Georgetown, TX) 2007; 6(9):1006–10.
75. Gottlieb TM, Oren M. p53 in growth control and neoplasia. Biochimica et biophysica acta 1996; 1287(2–3):77–102.
76. Lane DP. Cancer. p53, guardian of the genome. Nature 1992; 358(6381):15–6.
77. Marx J. Oncology. Recruiting the cell's own guardian for cancer therapy. Science (New York) 2007; 315(5816):1211–3.
78. Rodier F, Campisi J, Bhaumik D. Two faces of p53: aging and tumor suppression. Nucleic Acids Research 2007; 35:7475–84.
79. Teodoro JG, Evans SK, Green MR. Inhibition of tumor angiogenesis by p53: a new role for the guardian of the genome. Journal of Molecular Medicine (Berlin, Germany) 2007; 85(11):1175–86.
80. Hollstein M, Sidransky D, Vogelstein B, Harris CC. p53 mutations in human cancers. Science (New York) 1991; 253(5015):49–53.
81. Soussi T, Beroud C. Assessing TP53 status in human tumours to evaluate clinical outcome. Nature Reviews 2001; 1(3):233–40.

82. Soussi T, Lozano G. p53 mutation heterogeneity in cancer. Biochemical and Biophysical Research Communications 2005; 331(3):834–42.
83. Momand J, Wu HH, Dasgupta G. MDM2–master regulator of the p53 tumor suppressor protein. Gene 2000; 242(1–2):15–29.
84. Lukas J, Lukas C, Bartek J. Mammalian cell cycle checkpoints: signalling pathways and their organization in space and time. DNA Repair 2004; 3(8–9):997–1007.
85. Vogelstein B, Lane D, Levine AJ. Surfing the p53 network. Nature 2000; 408(6810): 307–10.
86. Cuddihy AR, Bristow RG. The p53 protein family and radiation sensitivity: yes or no? Cancer Metastasis Reviews 2004; 23(3–4):237–57.
87. Fei P, El-Deiry WS. P53 and radiation responses. Oncogene 2003; 22(37):5774–83.
88. Helton ES, Chen X. p53 modulation of the DNA damage response. Journal of Cellular Biochemistry 2007; 100(4):883–96.
89. Pawlik TM, Keyomarsi K. Role of cell cycle in mediating sensitivity to radiotherapy. International Journal of Radiation Oncology, Biology, Physics 2004; 59(4):928–42.
90. Vousden KH, Lu X. Live or let die: the cell's response to p53. Nature Reviews 2002; 2(8):594–604.
91. Fuster JJ, Sanz-Gonzalez SM, Moll UM, Andres V. Classic and novel roles of p53: prospects for anticancer therapy. Trends in Molecular Medicine 2007; 13(5):192–9.
92. Harris SL, Levine AJ. The p53 pathway: positive and negative feedback loops. Oncogene 2005; 24(17):2899–908.
93. Laptenko O, Prives C. Transcriptional regulation by p53: one protein, many possibilities. Cell Death and Differentiation 2006; 13(6):951–61.
94. Aylon Y, Oren M. Living with p53, dying of p53. Cell 2007; 130(4):597–600.
95. Alvarez S, Drane P, Meiller A, Bras M, Deguin-Chambon V, Bouvard V, May E. A comprehensive study of p53 transcriptional activity in thymus and spleen of gamma irradiated mouse: high sensitivity of genes involved in the two main apoptotic pathways. International Journal of Radiation Biology 2006; 82(11):761–70.
96. Findley HW, Gu L, Yeager AM, Zhou M. Expression and regulation of Bcl-2, Bcl-xl, and Bax correlate with p53 status and sensitivity to apoptosis in childhood acute lymphoblastic leukemia. Blood 1997; 89(8):2986–93.
97. Kobayashi T, Ruan S, Jabbur JR, et al. Differential p53 phosphorylation and activation of apoptosis-promoting genes Bax and Fas/APO-1 by irradiation and ara-C treatment. Cell Death and Differentiation 1998; 5(7):584–91.
98. Zhan Q, Fan S, Bae I, Guillouf C, Liebermann DA, O'Connor PM, Fornace AJ, Jr. Induction of bax by genotoxic stress in human cells correlates with normal p53 status and apoptosis. Oncogene 1994; 9(12):3743–51.
99. Erlacher M, Michalak EM, Kelly PN, et al. BH3-only proteins Puma and Bim are rate-limiting for gamma-radiation- and glucocorticoid-induced apoptosis of lymphoid cells in vivo. Blood 2005; 106(13):4131–8.
100. Jeffers JR, Parganas E, Lee Y, et al. Puma is an essential mediator of p53-dependent and -independent apoptotic pathways. Cancer Cell 2003; 4(4):321–8.
101. Villunger A, Michalak EM, Coultas L, Mullauer F, Bock G, Ausserlechner MJ, Adams JM, Strasser A. p53- and drug-induced apoptotic responses mediated by BH3-only proteins puma and noxa. Science (New York) 2003; 302(5647):1036–8.
102. Fei P, Bernhard EJ, El-Deiry WS. Tissue-specific induction of p53 targets in vivo. Cancer Research 2002; 62(24):7316–27.
103. Han J, Goldstein LA, Hou W, Rabinowich H. Functional linkage between NOXA and Bim in mitochondrial apoptotic events. The Journal of Biological Chemistry 2007; 282(22):16223–31.
104. Embree-Ku M, Venturini D, Boekelheide K. Fas is involved in the p53-dependent apoptotic response to ionizing radiation in mouse testis. Biology of reproduction 2002;66(5): 1456–61.

105. Sheard MA, Uldrijan S, Vojtesek B. Role of p53 in regulating constitutive and X-radiation-inducible CD95 expression and function in carcinoma cells. Cancer Research 2003; 63(21):7176–84.
106. Sheard MA, Vojtesek B, Janakova L, Kovarik J, Zaloudik J. Up-regulation of Fas (CD95) in human p53wild-type cancer cells treated with ionizing radiation. International Journal of Cancer 1997; 73(5):757–62.
107. Burns TF, Bernhard EJ, El-Deiry WS. Tissue specific expression of p53 target genes suggests a key role for KILLER/DR5 in p53-dependent apoptosis in vivo. Oncogene 2001; 20(34):4601–12.
108. Sheikh MS, Burns TF, Huang Y, Wu GS, Amundson S, Brooks KS, Fornace AJ, Jr., el-Deiry WS. p53-dependent and -independent regulation of the death receptor KILLER/DR5 gene expression in response to genotoxic stress and tumor necrosis factor alpha. Cancer Research 1998; 58(8):1593–8.
109. Wu GS, Burns TF, McDonald ER, 3rd, et al. KILLER/DR5 is a DNA damage-inducible p53-regulated death receptor gene. Nature Genetics 1997; 17(2):141–3.
110. Kastan M. On the TRAIL from p53 to apoptosis? Nature Genetics 1997; 17(2):130–1.
111. Lin Y, Ma W, Benchimol S. Pidd, a new death-domain-containing protein, is induced by p53 and promotes apoptosis. Nature Genetics 2000; 26(1):122–7.
112. Polyak K, Xia Y, Zweier JL, Kinzler KW, Vogelstein B. A model for p53-induced apoptosis. Nature 1997; 389(6648):300–5.
113. Haldar S, Negrini M, Monne M, Sabbioni S, Croce CM. Down-regulation of bcl-2 by p53 in breast cancer cells. Cancer Research 1994; 54(8):2095–7.
114. Miyashita T, Harigai M, Hanada M, Reed JC. Identification of a p53-dependent negative response element in the bcl-2 gene. Cancer Research 1994; 54(12):3131–5.
115. Hoffman WH, Biade S, Zilfou JT, Chen J, Murphy M. Transcriptional repression of the anti-apoptotic survivin gene by wild type p53. The Journal of Biological Chemistry 2002; 277(5):3247–57.
116. Zhou M, Gu L, Li F, Zhu Y, Woods WG, Findley HW. DNA damage induces a novel p53-survivin signaling pathway regulating cell cycle and apoptosis in acute lymphoblastic leukemia cells. The Journal of Pharmacology and Experimental Therapeutics 2002; 303(1):124–31.
117. Norbury CJ, Zhivotovsky B. DNA damage-induced apoptosis. Oncogene 2004; 23(16):2797–808.
118. Chipuk JE, Kuwana T, Bouchier-Hayes L, Droin NM, Newmeyer DD, Schuler M, Green DR. Direct activation of Bax by p53 mediates mitochondrial membrane permeabilization and apoptosis. Science (New York) 2004; 303(5660):1010–4.
119. Leu JI, Dumont P, Hafey M, Murphy ME, George DL. Mitochondrial p53 activates Bak and causes disruption of a Bak-Mcl1 complex. Nature Cell Biology 2004; 6(5):443–50.
120. Konishi A, Shimizu S, Hirota J, et al. Involvement of histone H1.2 in apoptosis induced by DNA double-strand breaks. Cell 2003; 114(6):673–88.
121. Lowe SW, Schmitt EM, Smith SW, Osborne BA, Jacks T. p53 is required for radiation-induced apoptosis in mouse thymocytes. Nature 1993; 362(6423):847–9.
122. Melino G, De Laurenzi V, Vousden KH. p73: friend or foe in tumorigenesis. Nature Reviews 2002; 2(8):605–15.
123. Flores ER, Tsai KY, Crowley D, Sengupta S, Yang A, McKeon F, Jacks T. p63 and p73 are required for p53-dependent apoptosis in response to DNA damage. Nature 2002; 416(6880):560–4.
124. Levrero M, De Laurenzi V, Costanzo A, Gong J, Wang JY, Melino G. The p53/p63/p73 family of transcription factors: overlapping and distinct functions. Journal of Cell Science 2000; 113(Pt 10):1661–70.
125. Melino G, Bernassola F, Ranalli M, et al. p73 Induces apoptosis via PUMA transactivation and Bax mitochondrial translocation. The Journal of Biological Chemistry 2004; 279(9):8076–83.

126. Flinterman M, Guelen L, Ezzati-Nik S, et al. E1A activates transcription of p73 and Noxa to induce apoptosis. The Journal of Biological Chemistry 2005; 280(7):5945–59.
127. Lassus P, Opitz-Araya X, Lazebnik Y. Requirement for caspase-2 in stress-induced apoptosis before mitochondrial permeabilization. Science (New York) 2002; 297(5585):1352–4.
128. Guo Y, Srinivasula SM, Druilhe A, Fernandes-Alnemri T, Alnemri ES. Caspase-2 induces apoptosis by releasing proapoptotic proteins from mitochondria. The Journal of Biological Chemistry 2002; 277(16):13430–7.
129. Paroni G, Henderson C, Schneider C, Brancolini C. Caspase-2 can trigger cytochrome C release and apoptosis from the nucleus. The Journal of Biological Chemistry 2002; 277(17):15147–61.
130. Robertson JD, Enoksson M, Suomela M, Zhivotovsky B, Orrenius S. Caspase-2 acts upstream of mitochondria to promote cytochrome c release during etoposide-induced apoptosis. The Journal of Biological Chemistry 2002; 277(33):29803–9.
131. Castedo M, Perfettini JL, Roumier T, et al. Mitotic catastrophe constitutes a special case of apoptosis whose suppression entails aneuploidy. Oncogene 2004; 23(25):4362–70.
132. Lin B, Kolluri SK, Lin F, et al. Conversion of Bcl-2 from protector to killer by interaction with nuclear orphan receptor Nur77/TR3. Cell 2004; 116(4):527–40.
133. Hara S, Nakashima S, Kiyono T, et al. p53-Independent ceramide formation in human glioma cells during gamma-radiation-induced apoptosis. Cell Death and Differentiation 2004; 11(8):853–61.
134. Hara S, Nakashima S, Kiyono T, Sawada M, Yoshimura S, Iwama T, Sakai N. Ceramide triggers caspase activation during gamma-radiation-induced apoptosis of human glioma cells lacking functional p53. Oncology reports 2004;12(1):119–23.
135. Kolesnick R, Fuks Z. Radiation and ceramide-induced apoptosis. Oncogene 2003; 22(37):5897–906.
136. Dewey WC, Ling CC, Meyn RE. Radiation-induced apoptosis: relevance to radiotherapy. International Journal of Radiation Oncology, Biology, Physics 1995; 33(4):781–96.
137. Verheij M, Bartelink H. Radiation-induced apoptosis. Cell and Tissue Research 2000; 301(1):133–42.
138. Meyn RE, Stephens LC, Ang KK, Hunter NR, Brock WA, Milas L, Peters LJ. Heterogeneity in the development of apoptosis in irradiated murine tumours of different histologies. International Journal of Radiation Biology 1993; 64(5):583–91
139. Rupnow BA, Knox SJ. The role of radiation-induced apoptosis as a determinant of tumor responses to radiation therapy. Apoptosis 1999; 4(2):115–43.
140. Schmitt CA, Lowe SW. Apoptosis and therapy. The Journal of Pathology 1999; 187(1):127–37.
141. Stapper NJ, Stuschke M, Sak A, Stuben G. Radiation-induced apoptosis in human sarcoma and glioma cell lines. International Journal of Cancer 1995; 62(1):58–62.
142. Steel GG. The case against apoptosis. Acta Oncologica (Stockholm, Sweden) 2001; 40(8):968–75.
143. Radford IR, Murphy TK, Radley JM, Ellis SL. Radiation response of mouse lymphoid and myeloid cell lines. Part II. Apoptotic death is shown by all lines examined. International Journal of Radiation Biology 1994; 65(2):217–27.
144. Stephens LC, Ang KK, Schultheiss TE, Milas L, Meyn RE. Apoptosis in irradiated murine tumors. Radiation Research 1991; 127(3):308–16.
145. Clarke AR, Purdie CA, Harrison DJ, Morris RG, Bird CC, Hooper ML, Wyllie AH. Thymocyte apoptosis induced by p53-dependent and independent pathways. Nature 1993; 362(6423):849–52.
146. Sentman CL, Shutter JR, Hockenbery D, Kanagawa O, Korsmeyer SJ. bcl-2 inhibits multiple forms of apoptosis but not negative selection in thymocytes. Cell 1991; 67(5):879–88.
147. Strasser A, Harris AW, Jacks T, Cory S. DNA damage can induce apoptosis in proliferating lymphoid cells via p53-independent mechanisms inhibitable by Bcl-2. Cell 1994; 79(2):329–39.

148. Ogawa Y, Nishioka A, Inomata T, *et al.* Ionizing radiation-induced apoptosis in human lymphoma cell lines differing in p53 status. International journal of molecular medicine 2000;5(2):139–43.
149. Sak A, Wurm R, Elo B, et al. Increased radiation-induced apoptosis and altered cell cycle progression of human lung cancer cell lines by antisense oligodeoxynucleotides targeting p53 and p21(WAF1/CIP1). Cancer Gene Therapy 2003; 10(12):926–34.
150. Stuschke M, Sak A, Wurm R, Sinn B, Wolf G, Stuben G, Budach V. Radiation-induced apoptosis in human non-small-cell lung cancer cell lines is secondary to cell-cycle progression beyond the G2-phase checkpoint. International Journal of Radiation Biology 2002; 78(9):807–19.
151. Eriksson D, Joniani HM, Sheikholvaezin A, Lofroth PO, Johansson L, Riklund Ahlstrom K, Stigbrand T. Combined low dose radio- and radioimmunotherapy of experimental HeLa Hep 2 tumours. European Journal of Nuclear Medicine and Molecular Imaging 2003; 30(6):895–906.
152. Wouters BG, Denko NC, Giaccia AJ, Brown JM. A p53 and apoptotic independent role for p21waf1 in tumour response to radiation therapy. Oncogene 1999; 18(47):6540–5.
153. Brown JM, Wilson G. Apoptosis genes and resistance to cancer therapy: what does the experimental and clinical data tell us? Cancer Biology & Therapy 2003; 2(5):477–90.
154. Ullen A, Sandstrom P, Ahlstrom KR, Sundstrom B, Nilsson B, Arlestig L, Stigbrand T. Use of anticytokeratin monoclonal anti-idiotypic antibodies to improve tumor:nontumor ratio in experimental radioimmunolocalization. Cancer Research 1995; 55(23 Suppl):5868s–73s.
155. Carlsson J, Eriksson V, Stenerlow B, Lundqvist H. Requirements regarding dose rate and exposure time for killing of tumour cells in beta particle radionuclide therapy. European Journal of Nuclear Medicine and Molecular Imaging 2006; 33(10):1185–95.
156. Rossi Norrlund R, Ullen A, Sandstrom P, Holback D, Johansson L, Stigbrand T, Hietala SO, Riklund Ahlstrom K. Experimental radioimmunotargeting combining nonlabeled, iodine-125-labeled, and anti-idiotypic anticytokeratin monoclonal antibodies: a dosimetric evaluation. Cancer 1997; 80(12 Suppl):2689–98.
157. Rossi Norrlund R, Ullen A, Sandstrom P, Holback D, Johansson L, Stigbrand T, Hietala SO, Riklund Ahlstrom K. Dosimetry of fractionated experimental radioimmunotargeting with idiotypic and anti-idiotypic anticytokeratin antibodies. Cancer 1997; 80(12 Suppl):2681–8.
158. Endlich B, Radford IR, Forrester HB, Dewey WC. Computerized video time-lapse microscopy studies of ionizing radiation-induced rapid-interphase and mitosis-related apoptosis in lymphoid cells. Radiation Research 2000; 153(1):36–48.
159. Mirzaie-Joniani H, Eriksson D, Johansson A, Lofroth PO, Johansson L, Ahlstrom KR, Stigbrand T. Apoptosis in HeLa Hep2 cells is induced by low-dose, low-dose-rate radiation. Radiation Research 2002; 158(5):634–40.
160. Mirzaie-Joniani H, Eriksson D, Sheikholvaezin A, Johansson A, Lofroth PO, Johansson L, Stigbrand T. Apoptosis induced by low-dose and low-dose-rate radiation. Cancer 2002; 94(4 Suppl):1210–4.
161. Carlsson J, Hakansson E, Eriksson V, Grawe J, Wester K, Grusell E, Montelius A, Lundqvist H. Early effects of low dose-rate radiation on cultured tumor cells. Cancer Biotherapy & Radiopharmaceuticals 2003; 18(4):663–70.
162. Iwadate Y, Mizoe J, Osaka Y, Yamaura A, Tsujii H. High linear energy transfer carbon radiation effectively kills cultured glioma cells with either mutant or wild-type p53. International Journal of Radiation Oncology, Biology, Physics 2001; 50(3):803–8.
163. Meijer AE, Ekedahl J, Joseph B, Castro J, Harms-Ringdahl M, Zhivotovsky B, Lewensohn R. High-LET radiation induces apoptosis in lymphoblastoid cell lines derived from atazia-telangiectasia patients. International Journal of Radiation Biology 2001; 77(3):309–17.
164. Takahashi A, Matsumoto H, Furusawa Y, Ohnishi K, Ishioka N, Ohnishi T. Apoptosis induced by high-LET radiations is not affected by cellular p53 gene status. International Journal of Radiation Biology 2005; 81(8):581–6.
165. Takahashi A, Matsumoto H, Yuki K, *et al.* High-LET radiation enhanced apoptosis but not necrosis regardless of p53 status. International journal of radiation oncology, biology, physics 2004;60(2):591–7.

166. Friesen C, Lubatschofski A, Kotzerke J, Buchmann I, Reske SN, Debatin KM. Beta-irradiation used for systemic radioimmunotherapy induces apoptosis and activates apoptosis pathways in leukaemia cells. European Journal of Nuclear Medicine and Molecular Imaging 2003; 30(9):1251–61.
167. Obeid M, Tesniere A, Panaretakis T, et al. Ecto-calreticulin in immunogenic chemotherapy. Immunological Reviews 2007; 220:22–34.
168. Tesniere A, Panaretakis T, Kepp O, Apetoh L, Ghiringhelli F, Zitvogel L, Kroemer G. Molecular characteristics of immunogenic cancer cell death. Cell Death and Differentiation 2008; 15(1):3–12.
169. Colombo A, Repici M, Pesaresi M, Santambrogio S, Forloni G, Borsello T. The TAT-JNK inhibitor peptide interferes with beta amyloid protein stability. Cell Death and Differentiation 2007; 14(10):1845–8.
170. Gisselsson D. Mitotic instability in cancer: is there method in the madness? Cell Cycle (Georgetown, TX) 2005; 4(8):1007–10.
171. Castedo M, Kroemer G. [Mitotic catastrophe: a special case of apoptosis]. Journal de la Societe de biologie 2004; 198(2):97–103.
172. Erenpreisa J, Kalejs M, Ianzini F, et al. Segregation of genomes in polyploid tumour cells following mitotic catastrophe. Cell Biology International 2005; 29(12):1005–11.
173. Mansilla S, Priebe W, Portugal J. Mitotic catastrophe results in cell death by caspase-dependent and caspase-independent mechanisms. Cell Cycle (Georgetown, TX) 2006; 5(1):53–60.
174. Lock RB, Stribinskiene L. Dual modes of death induced by etoposide in human epithelial tumor cells allow Bcl-2 to inhibit apoptosis without affecting clonogenic survival. Cancer Research 1996; 56(17):4006–12.
175. Ruth AC, Roninson IB. Effects of the multidrug transporter P-glycoprotein on cellular responses to ionizing radiation. Cancer Research 2000; 60(10):2576–8.
176. Hall EJ. Radiobiology for the radiologist. Philadelphia, PA: J.B. Lippincott Company, 2000.
177. Bradford CR, Zhu S, Ogawa H, et al. P53 mutation correlates with cisplatin sensitivity in head and neck squamous cell carcinoma lines. Head & Neck 2003; 25(8):654–61.
178. Fan S, Smith ML, Rivet DJ, 2nd, Duba D, Zhan Q, Kohn KW, Fornace AJ, Jr., O'Connor PM. Disruption of p53 function sensitizes breast cancer MCF-7 cells to cisplatin and pentoxifylline. Cancer Research 1995; 55(8):1649–54.
179. Pekkola-Heino K, Servomaa K, Kiuru A, Grenman R. Increased radiosensitivity is associated with p53 mutations in cell lines derived from oral cavity carcinoma. Acta Oto-laryngologica 1996; 116(2):341–4.
180. Servomaa K, Kiuru A, Grenman R, Pekkola-Heino K, Pulkkinen JO, Rytomaa T. p53 mutations associated with increased sensitivity to ionizing radiation in human head and neck cancer cell lines. Cell Proliferation 1996; 29(5):219–30.
181. Brachman DG, Beckett M, Graves D, Haraf D, Vokes E, Weichselbaum RR. p53 mutation does not correlate with radiosensitivity in 24 head and neck cancer cell lines. Cancer Research 1993; 53(16):3667–9.
182. Fan S, el-Deiry WS, Bae I, *et al.* p53 gene mutations are associated with decreased sensitivity of human lymphoma cells to DNA damaging agents. Cancer research 1994;54(22):5824–30.
183. Bhattathiri NV, Bharathykkutty C, Prathapan R, Chirayathmanjiyil DA, Nair KM. Prediction of radiosensitivity of oral cancers by serial cytological assay of nuclear changes. Radiotherapy and Oncology 1998; 49(1):61–5.
184. Bhattathiri NV, Bindu L, Remani P, Chandralekha B, Nair KM. Radiation-induced acute immediate nuclear abnormalities in oral cancer cells: serial cytologic evaluation. Acta Cytologica 1998; 42(5):1084–90.
185. Falkvoll KH. The occurrence of apoptosis, abnormal mitoses, cells dying in mitosis and micronuclei in a human melanoma xenograft exposed to single dose irradiation. Strahlentherapie und Onkologie 1990;166(7):487–92.

186. Ross GM. Induction of cell death by radiotherapy. Endocrine-Related Cancer 1999; 6(1):41–4.
187. Bedford JS, Mitchell JB, Griggs HG, Bender MA. Radiation-induced cellular reproductive death and chromosome aberrations. Radiation Research 1978; 76(3):573–86.
188. Carrano AV. Chromosome aberrations and radiation-induced cell death. II. Predicted and observed cell survival. Mutation Research 1973; 17(3):355–66.
189. Dewey WC, Miller HH, Leeper DB. Chromosomal aberrations and mortality of x-irradiated mammalian cells: emphasis on repair. Proceedings of the National Academy of Sciences of the United States of America 1971; 68(3):667–71.
190. Schneider DO, Whitmore GF. Comparative effects of neutrons and x-rays on mammalian cells. Radiation Research 1963; 18:286–306.
191. Bedford JS, Cornforth MN. Relationship between the recovery from sublethal X-ray damage and the rejoining of chromosome breaks in normal human fibroblasts. Radiation Research 1987; 111(3):406–23.
192. Forrester HB, Albright N, Ling CC, Dewey WC. Computerized video time-lapse analysis of apoptosis of REC:Myc cells X-irradiated in different phases of the cell cycle. Radiation Research 2000; 154(6):625–39.
193. Castedo M, Perfettini JL, Roumier T, Andreau K, Medema R, Kroemer G. Cell death by mitotic catastrophe: a molecular definition. Oncogene 2004; 23(16):2825–37.
194. Vogelstein B, Kinzler KW. Achilles' heel of cancer? Nature 2001; 412(6850):865–6.
195. Taylor WR, Stark GR. Regulation of the G2/M transition by p53. Oncogene 2001; 20(15):1803–15.
196. Stark GR, Taylor WR. Control of the G2/M transition. Molecular Biotechnology 2006; 32(3):227–48.
197. Bourke E, Dodson H, Merdes A, Cuffe L, Zachos G, Walker M, Gillespie D, Morrison CG. DNA damage induces Chk1-dependent centrosome amplification. EMBO Reports 2007; 8(6):603–9.
198. Dodson H, Wheatley SP, Morrison CG. Involvement of centrosome amplification in radiation-induced mitotic catastrophe. Cell Cycle (Georgetown, TX) 2007; 6(3):364–70.
199. Kawamura K, Fujikawa-Yamamoto K, Ozaki M, et al. Centrosome hyperamplification and chromosomal damage after exposure to radiation. Oncology 2004; 67(5–6):460–70.
200. Kawamura K, Morita N, Domiki C, Fujikawa-Yamamoto K, Hashimoto M, Iwabuchi K, Suzuki K. Induction of centrosome amplification in p53 siRNA-treated human fibroblast cells by radiation exposure. Cancer Science 2006; 97(4):252–8.
201. Sato N, Mizumoto K, Nakamura M, Ueno H, Minamishima YA, Farber JL, Tanaka M. A possible role for centrosome overduplication in radiation-induced cell death. Oncogene 2000; 19(46):5281–90.
202. Heald R, Tournebize R, Habermann A, Karsenti E, Hyman A. Spindle assembly in Xenopus egg extracts: respective roles of centrosomes and microtubule self-organization. The Journal of Cell Biology 1997; 138(3):615–28.
203. Loffler H, Lukas J, Bartek J, Kramer A. Structure meets function–centrosomes, genome maintenance and the DNA damage response. Experimental cell research 2006;312(14):2633–40.
204. Stewenius Y, Gorunova L, Jonson T, et al. Structural and numerical chromosome changes in colon cancer develop through telomere-mediated anaphase bridges, not through mitotic multipolarity. Proceedings of the National Academy of Sciences of the United States of America 2005; 102(15):5541–6.
205. Dodson H, Bourke E, Jeffers LJ, et al. Centrosome amplification induced by DNA damage occurs during a prolonged G2 phase and involves ATM. The EMBO Journal 2004; 23(19):3864–73.
206. Blagosklonny MV. Mitotic arrest and cell fate: why and how mitotic inhibition of transcription drives mutually exclusive events. Cell Cycle (Georgetown, TX) 2007; 6(1):70–4.
207. Jallepalli PV, Lengauer C. Chromosome segregation and cancer: cutting through the mystery. Nature Reviews 2001; 1(2):109–17.

208. Zhivotovsky B, Orrenius S. Caspase-2 function in response to DNA damage. Biochemical and Biophysical Research Communications 2005; 331(3):859–67.
209. Weaver BA, Cleveland DW. Decoding the links between mitosis, cancer, and chemotherapy: the mitotic checkpoint, adaptation, and cell death. Cancer Cell 2005; 8(1):7–12.
210. Yamada HY, Gorbsky GJ. Spindle checkpoint function and cellular sensitivity to antimitotic drugs. Molecular Cancer Therapeutics 2006; 5(12):2963–9.
211. Rieder CL, Maiato H. Stuck in division or passing through: what happens when cells cannot satisfy the spindle assembly checkpoint. Developmental Cell 2004; 7(5):637–51.
212. Castedo M, Coquelle A, Vivet S, et al. Apoptosis regulation in tetraploid cancer cells. The EMBO Journal 2006; 25(11):2584–95.
213. Uetake Y, Sluder G. Cell cycle progression after cleavage failure: mammalian somatic cells do not possess a "tetraploidy checkpoint". The Journal of Cell Biology 2004; 165(5):609–15.
214. Blagosklonny MV, Demidenko ZN, Giovino M, Szynal C, Donskoy E, Herrmann RA, Barry JJ, Whalen AM. Cytostatic activity of paclitaxel in coronary artery smooth muscle cells is mediated through transient mitotic arrest followed by permanent post-mitotic arrest: comparison with cancer cells. Cell Cycle (Georgetown, TX) 2006; 5(14):1574–9.
215. Klein LE, Freeze BS, Smith AB, 3rd, Horwitz SB. The microtubule stabilizing agent discodermolide is a potent inducer of accelerated cell senescence. Cell Cycle (Georgetown, TX) 2005; 4(3):501–7.
216. Casenghi M, Mangiacasale R, Tuynder M, et al. p53-independent apoptosis and p53-dependent block of DNA rereplication following mitotic spindle inhibition in human cells. Experimental Cell Research 1999; 250(2):339–50.
217. Stein GH, Dulic V. Origins of G1 arrest in senescent human fibroblasts. Bioessays 1995; 17(6):537–43.
218. Dimri GP, Lee X, Basile G, et al. A biomarker that identifies senescent human cells in culture and in aging skin in vivo. Proceedings of the National Academy of Sciences of the United States of America 1995; 92(20):9363–7.
219. Krishnamurthy J, Torrice C, Ramsey MR, Kovalev GI, Al-Regaiey K, Su L, Sharpless NE. Ink4a/Arf expression is a biomarker of aging. The Journal of Clinical Investigation 2004; 114(9):1299–307.
220. Ben-Porath I, Weinberg RA. The signals and pathways activating cellular senescence. The International Journal of Biochemistry & Cell Biology 2005; 37(5):961–76.
221. van Heemst D, den Reijer PM, Westendorp RG. Ageing or cancer: a review on the role of caretakers and gatekeepers. European Journal of Cancer 2007; 43(15):2144–52.
222. Funk WD, Wang CK, Shelton DN, Harley CB, Pagon GD, Hoeffler WK. Telomerase expression restores dermal integrity to in vitro-aged fibroblasts in a reconstituted skin model. Experimental Cell Research 2000; 258(2):270–8.
223. Yoon IK, Kim HK, Kim YK, et al. Exploration of replicative senescence-associated genes in human dermal fibroblasts by cDNA microarray technology. Experimental Gerontology 2004; 39(9):1369–78.
224. Quick QA, Gewirtz DA. An accelerated senescence response to radiation in wild-type p53 glioblastoma multiforme cells. Journal of Neurosurgery 2006; 105(1):111–8.
225. Igarashi K, Sakimoto I, Kataoka K, Ohta K, Miura M. Radiation-induced senescence-like phenotype in proliferating and plateau-phase vascular endothelial cells. Experimental Cell Research 2007; 313(15):3326–36.
226. Baehrecke EH. How death shapes life during development. Nature Reviews. Molecular Cell Biology 2002; 3(10):779–87.
227. Reggiori F, Klionsky DJ. Autophagosomes: biogenesis from scratch? Current opinion in cell biology 2005;17(4):415–22.
228. Levine B, Yuan J. Autophagy in cell death: an innocent convict? The Journal of Clinical Investigation 2005; 115(10):2679–88.
229. Bursch W, Ellinger A, Gerner C, Frohwein U, Schulte-Hermann R. Programmed cell death (PCD). Apoptosis, autophagic PCD, or others? Annals of the New York Academy of Sciences 2000; 926:1–12.

230. Qu X, Yu J, Bhagat G, et al. Promotion of tumorigenesis by heterozygous disruption of the beclin 1 autophagy gene. The Journal of Clinical Investigation 2003; 112(12):1809–20.
231. Yu L, Alva A, Su H, Dutt P, Freundt E, Welsh S, Baehrecke EH, Lenardo MJ. Regulation of an ATG7-beclin 1 program of autophagic cell death by caspase-8. Science (New York) 2004; 304(5676):1500–2.
232. Yu L, Lenardo MJ, Baehrecke EH. Autophagy and caspases: a new cell death program. Cell Cycle (Georgetown, TX) 2004; 3(9):1124–6.
233. Katayama M, Kawaguchi T, Berger MS, Pieper RO. DNA damaging agent-induced autophagy produces a cytoprotective adenosine triphosphate surge in malignant glioma cells. Cell Death and Differentiation 2007; 14(3):548–58.
234. Kim KW, Mutter RW, Cao C, Albert JM, Freeman M, Hallahan DE, Lu B. Autophagy for cancer therapy through inhibition of pro-apoptotic proteins and mammalian target of rapamycin signaling. The Journal of Biological Chemistry 2006; 281(48):36883–90.
235. Paglin S, Yahalom J. Pathways that regulate autophagy and their role in mediating tumor response to treatment. Autophagy 2006; 2(4):291–3.
236. Ito H, Daido S, Kanzawa T, Kondo S, Kondo Y. Radiation-induced autophagy is associated with LC3 and its inhibition sensitizes malignant glioma cells. International Journal of Oncology 2005; 26(5):1401–10.

Chapter 13
Radiation Induced DNA-Damage/Repair and Associated Signaling Pathways

Bo Stenerlöw[1], Lina Ekerljung[1], Jörgen Carlsson[1], and Johan Lennartsson[2]

Abbreviations ATM, Ataxia telangiectasia mutated; DAG, 1,2-diacylglycerol; DSB, DNA double-strand breaks; DNA-PK, DNA dependent protein kinase; EGF, Epidermal growth factor; EGFR, EGF receptor; Erk, Extracellular regulated kinase; HER, Human epidermal growth factor receptor; HR, Homologous recombination; LET, Linear energy transfer; PI, Phosphatidylinositol; PLC, Phospholipase C; PTEN; Phosphatase and tensin homolog deleted on chromosome 10

Summary Radiation-induced DNA damage and related repair mechanisms are described in this chapter. The emerging connection with growth factor induced signal transduction is described, with important implications for radiotherapy. The prospect of developing targeting agents, which selectively deliver radioactivity to the tumor and at the same time radiosensitize the tumor cells is discussed in some detail.

Introduction

A thorough understanding of the mechanisms for radiation-induced DNA damage and regulation of the DNA repair systems have important implications for radiotherapy. When a cell is exposed to ionizing radiation, or to other DNA damaging agents such as cytotoxic drugs or endogenous free radicals, damage in the chromosomal DNA is critical. Many types of DNA lesions, such as a single strand break or a base damage, can be accurately repaired but it is more difficult for the cell to repair severe damage such as a double-strand break (DSB). Incorrectly repaired or unrepaired DSB:s might lead to chromosomal aberrations that are lethal for the cell.

[1]Department of Oncology, Radiology and Clinical Immunology, Rudbeck Laboratory, Uppsala University, SE-751 85, Uppsala, Sweden

[2]Ludwig Institute for Cancer Research, Uppsala University, Box 595, SE-751 24, Uppsala, Sweden

T. Stigbrand et al. (eds.) *Targeted Radionuclide Tumor Therapy*,

Since more than a decade, it is known that there are at least two important DSB-repair mechanisms in cells. These systems are called non-homologous end joining (NHEJ) and homologous rejoining (HR). The cell use recognition mechanisms (e.g. ATM and related molecules) to sense the DSB:s and initiate and effectuate repair with DNA-PK and related molecules. If the DNA damage is too severe, the repair might fail and the cell can either kill itself through apoptosis (p53 and related molecules are involved), or there will be paralysis of cell division followed by cell death. The signaling system for DNA-repair also induces cell cycle blocks (again with the help of p53 and related molecules), which is essential to gain time for the repair process. (See also chapter 14 in this volume.)

Growth factor receptors are often overexpressed or constitutively activated in many human tumors, which make them suitable as target structures for agents delivering radionuclides. However, many growth factor receptors might emit signals that protect the cell from apoptosis and enhance DNA repair, thereby reducing the therapeutic effect of the radiotherapy. When a growth factor binds to its cognate receptor, intracellular signaling pathways are activated that often lead all the way from the plasma membrane to the nucleus. In many cases the signal is transmitted by a cascade of protein phosphorylation events, i.e. one protein phosphorylates another that becomes activated and phosphorylates another protein and so forth. In the nucleus, these signals are interpreted by the machinery that regulates gene expression, eventually changing the behavior of the cell; promoting cell growth (e.g. via the Ras/Erk-MAPK pathway) or regulate cell death/apoptosis (e.g. via the Akt pathway). Furthermore, cell cycle blocks are also influenced by these signals.

Since apoptosis and cell cycle blocks are regulated via both DSB initiated signaling and growth factor receptor signaling, there is likely to be a connection between these signaling systems. This crosstalk can hopefully be therapeutically exploited by using a receptor-binding agent that both deliver radioactivity to the tumor in order to induce DBS:s, and at the same time modifies both apoptosis capacity and cell cycle blocks to sensitize or protect the cells. In a tumor cell, sensitization is desired, but in a normal cell, protection is of course preferred. However, much is unknown about this and it is a field for intensive research.

In this chapter we describe radiation-induced DNA damage and related repair mechanisms and the emerging connection with growth factor induced signal transduction. We also discuss the prospect of developing targeting agents, which selectively delivers radioactivity to the tumor and at the same time radiosensitizes the tumor cells.

DNA Damage Signaling and Repair

This section is focused on how radiation-induced double-strand breaks (DSB) are handled by the cellular repair processes and we discuss how the formation of DSB triggers signal transduction and cell cycle checkpoints. For further information about the topics in this part we suggest specialized review articles on cell cycle checkpoints [1], cellular stress response [2], apoptosis and DNA repair. (See also chapter 12 in this volume.)

Ionizing Radiation and Induced DNA Damage

The therapy effect by ionizing radiation and many cytotoxic drugs is caused by DSBs in DNA [3]. In addition, radiation induces a wide range of different lesions in the DNA, including numerous base alterations, single-strand breaks and other modifications of the DNA double helix. These DNA damages are also frequently generated by endogenous sources such as free radicals during metabolic processes. In contrast to DSB, such lesions are in general efficiently repaired by the cell. A DSB is formed when two single-strand breaks are spaced less than 14 bases apart [4]. Unrepaired or misrepaired DSB leads to cell death or a surviving cell with altered genome where chromosomal translocations or deletions may affect tumor suppressor genes and oncogenes. About 25–30 DSB are induced in a diploid mammalian cell after irradiation with a dose of 1 Gy low linear energy transfer (LET) radiation [5].

Cellular Response to DNA Damage

The cellular response to DNA damage is complex and relies on several protective responses to counteract the harmful effects of DNA damage. These include DNA damage sensing/recognition, repair, and induction of signaling cascades leading to cell cycle checkpoint activation, apoptosis, and stress related responses [6]. However, it is still not fully understood how the primary DNA damage is detected and how this initiates signal transduction and activates DNA repair proteins. A schematic illustration of the major steps in the DSB response is shown in Fig. 13.1.

Several candidate proteins have been proposed to be involved in the initial sensing of DSB:s [7]. Three proteins of the PI3-kinase-like kinase family, ataxia telangiectasia mutated (ATM), DNA-dependent protein kinase (DNA-PK) and ATM-Rad3-related (ATR) have important roles as initiators of the cellular stress response [8]. The protein kinase ATM, a key protein in this response, is rapidly activated by autophosphorylation after exposure to ionizing radiation. Phosphorylated ATM (p-ATM) then phosphorylates several downstream proteins involved in the repair and damage signaling pathways after exposure to radiation, including 53BP1, NBS1, BRCA1 (Fig. 13.1). Upstream this activation, the MRN complex (MRE11/RAD50/NBS1) may be an important sensor for the ATM pathways [9].

A protein directly affected by the formation of DSB is the histone protein variant H2AX. H2AX constitutes 2–25% of the normal H2A pool in the nucleosomes in a mammalian cell [10] and the H2AX flanking a DSB is rapidly phosphorylated by ATM. The accumulation of phosphorylated H2AX, named γ-H2AX, at a DSB site can be detected as a spot, or a so called focus, in a microscope by applying immunofluorescence techniques (Fig. 13.2).The phosphorylation of H2AX results in extensive chromatin modification around a DSB site and this helps the DNA repair process by recruiting repair proteins to the damaged site. Several proteins involved in DNA repair also accumulate into foci at DSB:s and these foci can contain hundreds of proteins and are believed to represent sites with ongoing repair and/or be an indication of a checkpoint mechanism.

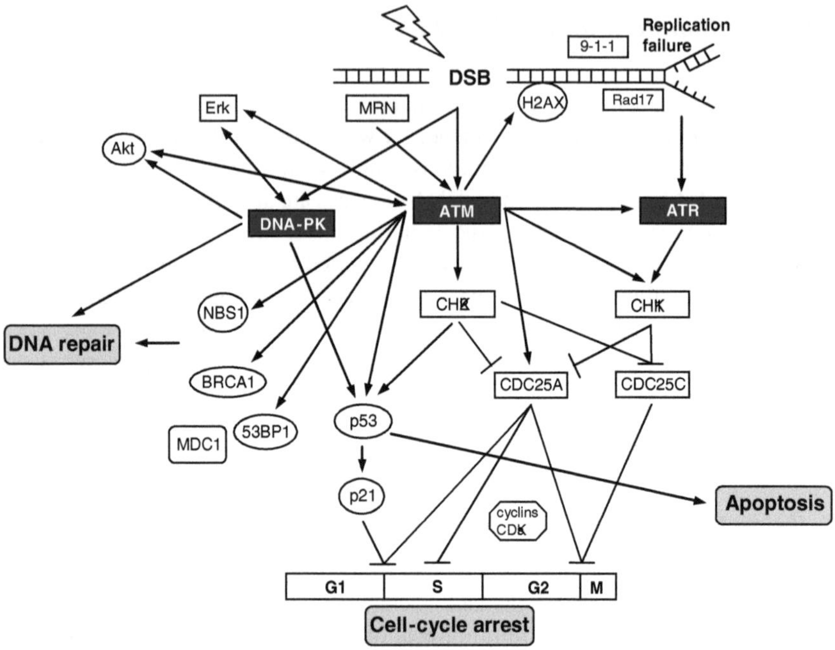

Fig. 13.1 Outline of the major mammalian DNA damage response pathways. Arrowhead indicates activation and a line ending with a bar indicates inhibition. See text for further details (From [80]. With permission)

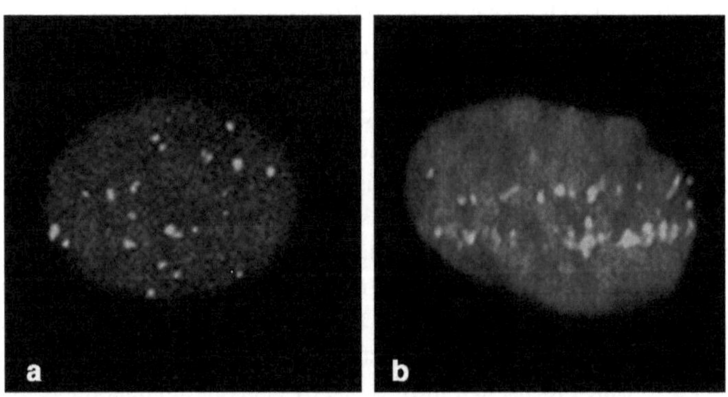

Fig. 13.2 DNA double-strand breaks represented by γ-H2AX foci in a human cell nucleus 30 min after irradiation with 1 Gy. The γ-H2AX (white spots) was visualized by immunofluorescence and grey staining is the DNA in the cell nucleus. (a) Irradiation with gamma radiation (^{137}Cs) gives a random distribution of small γ-H2AX foci. (b) Irradiation with high-LET radiation (160 eV/nm nitrogen ions) gives a few "tracks" with large γ-H2AX foci. See text for details

A number of other proteins have been suggested for proper detection of DNA damage downstream of ATM. The ATR kinase is closely related to ATM and responds to radiation-induced damage and inhibit DNA replication [11]. ATM and ATR further activate substrates, e.g. the protein kinases CHK1 and CHK2, which regulate proteins involved in cell-cycle arrest and DNA repair [12]. CHK1 is predominantly expressed in the S and G_2 phases of the cell cycle and is assumed to be absent in differentiated cells [13]. In contrast, CHK2 is activated by DNA damage throughout the cell cycle and by activating p53, CHK2 indirectly controls G_1 arrest and apoptosis. However, p53 may also be directly activated by ATM (Fig. 13.1) and the p53-dependent apoptosis pathway can be selectively regulated by DNA-PK [8]. Furthermore, recent studies suggest interactions between the Akt and Erk pathways with ATM and DNA-PK (Fig. 13.1) [14–17]. This further accentuates the complexity of the cellular stress response in which nuclear and cytoplasmatic signaling pathways must communicate.

There is a clear link between DNA damage response and genomic instability. Recent findings show that human tumors commonly express markers of activated DNA damage response and that phosphorylated forms of several proteins, e.g. H2AX and ATM, are over-expressed in both early invasive and more advanced carcinomas [18]. The fundamental role of ATM in regulation of the DNA damage response, including activation of proteins involved in apoptosis, repair and cell-cycle arrest, implies that defects in the ATM gene are critical, if the cell is exposed to ionizing radiation. Indeed, ATM defective cells are very radiosensitive and therapeutic strategies that will potentiate the cytotoxicity of ionizing radiation, e.g. via inhibition of ATM, are currently under investigation.

DNA Double-Strand Break Repair

DNA repair is important for preservation of the genomic stability. Double strand breaks can not only be induced by radiation and other exogenous agents, they can also be formed by endogenous processes such as DNA replication, topoisomerase failure, exposure to free radicals or during specialized recombination reactions, e.g. V(D)J recombination [19]. Mammalian cells have evolved highly effective enzyme systems that recognize DSB and co-ordinate its repair to maintain genomic stability.

Two major DSB repair pathways are known in mammalian cells: non-homologous end joining (NHEJ) and homologous recombination (HR). Their conservation in eukaryotes, from yeast to man, demonstrate the importance of efficient DSB repair for survival of organisms. Genetic evidence supports the concept of HR and NHEJ as distinct, but in some cases competing, DSB repair pathways where one pathway directly affects the activity of the other. However, the regulatory interplay between NHEJ and HR is not known.

In mammalian cells, NHEJ is believed to be the major pathway. NHEJ is assumed to be active in all cell-cycle phases and involves key proteins such as DNA-PK, DNA ligase IV and XRCC4 (Fig. 13.3a). DNA-PK consists of a heterodimer composed of KU70 and KU80, and the catalytic subunit DNA-PKcs (also called PRKDC). DNA-PK brings the DNA ends together and activates proteins involved in the NHEJ repair. Before the final rejoining by the DNA Ligase IV/XRCC4 complex, the DNA ends probably need trimming by nucleases, and both Artemis and the MRN complex (MRE11/RAD50/NBS1 complex) could have important roles in this process. Malfunction of DNA-PK makes cells very sensitive to radiation [20].

Homologous recombination (HR) is much less studied in mammals, but appears to play an important role for DSB repair during S- and G_2-phases of the cell cycle due to the availability of sister chromatids as repair templates. The process seems to be initiated by the transfer of DSB ends into 3′-single-stranded DNA (ssDNA) overhangs, possibly by the MRN complex. The replication protein A (RPA) coats the ssDNA and RAD51 then forms nucleoprotein filaments on as outlined in Fig. 13.3b. The binding of the strand-exchange protein RAD51 is facilitated by a number of proteins which then initiate the recombination process.

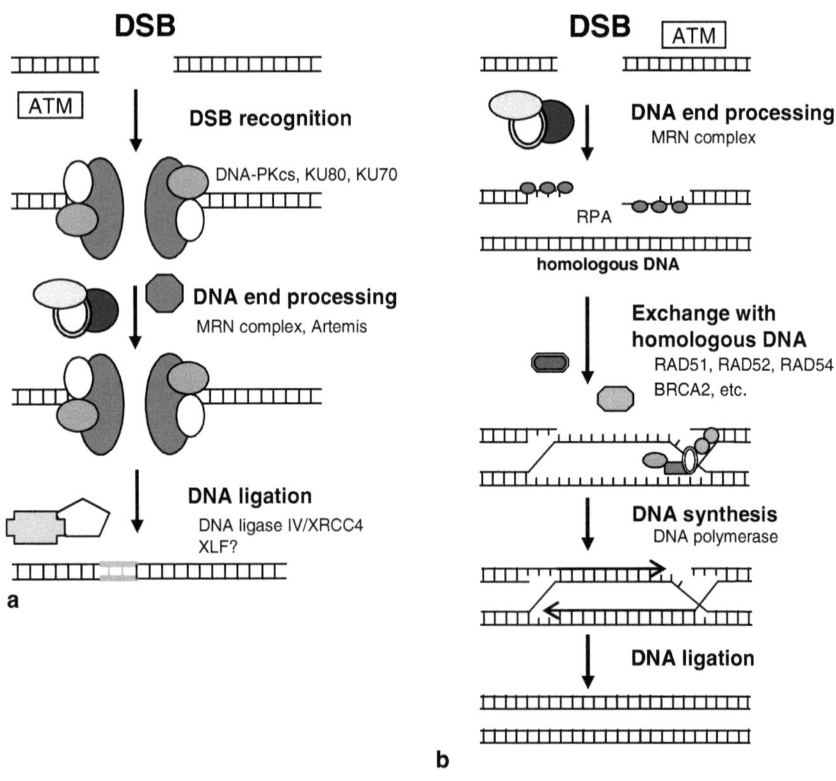

Fig. 13.3 Repair of DNA double-strand breaks by non-homologous end joining, NHEJ (a) and homologous recombination, HR (b) (Modified from [80]. With permission)

It is important to note that the NHEJ repair, in contrast to HR repair, join DNA ends without any template and is therefore unable to restore the original DNA sequence. Still, NHEJ is the major DSB repair pathway, which could be explained by the fact that only a small fraction of the genome is related to gene coding/regulation.

Repair of Radiation-Induced DSB

The NHEJ mechanism accounts for repair of the majority of radiation-induced DSBs. The induction and rejoining of DSB can be measured by pulsed-field gel electrophoresis (PFGE) that enables separation of large DNA fragments. The NHEJ repair is an extremely fast process removing 80% of the radiation-induced DSB within 30 min, although some base pairs of DNA might be deleted. However, radiation-induced DNA lesions are highly heterogeneous and densely ionizing radiation with high-LET (linear energy transfer), e.g. α-particles, delivers a lethal radiation dose by only a few particle hits in the cell nucleus (Fig. 13.2b). This dense deposition of energy results in clustered DNA breaks within 1–2 Mbp of chromatin [21] that heavily affect the repair of DSB [22]. As a consequence, a DSB induced by high-LET radiation is several times more effective than a DSB induced by low-LET radiation in producing lethal or stable genetic rearrangements. Hence, it is clear that clustered lesions are much more difficult to restore, but there is no information about failure in specific steps in the repair process.

Inhibition of DNA-PK activity makes cells very sensitive to radiation [20] and their ability to rejoin DSB is strongly reduced or even absent [5, 23]. Since there is a direct relation between DSB repair capacity and sensitivity to radiation, specific inhibitors to DNA-PK should be developed for use in combination with radiotherapy.

Receptor Mediated Signal Transduction, Cell Survival and Radiation Sensitivity

There are many cell membrane associated tyrosine kinase receptor families that might regulate cell survival and radiation sensitivity, e.g. the EGFR or HER family, the PDGFR family, the FGF family and the IGFR family. Among these the EGFR family is most exploited therapeutically. (See also chapter 3 in this volume.) Cellular signaling is complex and diverse, including issues such as redundancy, cell type specificity etc. Therefore, one must approach the role of a specific signaling molecule in a certain process with great care, and the discussions below only highlight certain aspects of these molecules and are by no means intended to be complete.

Phosphatidylinositol 3′-kinase Signaling

Phosphatidylinositol 3′-kinase (PI3-kinase) is a lipid kinase that phosphorylates the 3′-hydroxyl group of phosphoinositides (PI), particularly phosphatidylinositol-4, 5-biphosphate (PIP_2) generating phosphatidylinositol-3,4,5-triphosphate (PIP_3) [24]. A well characterized protein activated downstream of PI3-kinase is Akt (protein kinase B, PKB), which contains a pleckstrin homology (PH) domain and is predominantly localized to the cytoplasm in resting cells. The PH domain of Akt has high affinity for PIP_3. Consequently, Akt will translocate from the cytoplasm to PIP_3 rich patches in the plasma membrane in response to stimulation of PI3-kinase, where Akt will be activated through PDK-mediated phosphorylation [25]. The active form of Akt may detach from the plasma membrane and can be found both in the cytoplasm and the nucleus [26, 27].

Akt activation promotes cell survival as well as cell cycle progression. The anti-apoptotic effect is mediated through phosphorylation and thereby inactivation of the pro-apoptotic proteins Bad and forkhead transcription factors. In the absence of phosphorylation, Bad sequesters Bcl-2 or Bcl-X_L and prevents their anti-apoptotic activities. However, Akt-mediated phosphorylation of Bad causes the release of Bcl-2 or Bcl-X_L, which enables them to promote cell survival by inhibiting the release of cytochrome c from the mitochondria [28, 29]. Unphosphorylated forkhead transcription factors are located in the nucleus where they induce expression of genes that promote apoptosis and cell cycle arrest, for example the ligand for the death receptor Fas and the cell cycle inhibitor $p27^{Kip1}$ [30]. However, phosphorylation of forkhead transcription factors by Akt causes a relocalization to the cytoplasm where they are unable to induce and activate target genes. In addition, Akt enhances cell cycle progression by phosphorylating and thereby moving pre-existing $p27^{Kip1}$ from the nucleus to the cytoplasm away from the Cdk-cyclin targets [31–33].

The tumor suppressor protein phosphatase and tensin homolog deleted on chromosome 10 (PTEN) is a phosphatase that can dephosphorylate PIP_3 [34] and thus counteract PI3-kinase mediated signal transduction. Thus, loss of PTEN expression, which is observed in several human tumors, causes hyperactivation of proteins that depend on PIP_3 for their function, e.g. Akt. The activity of Akt has important implications for therapy since it has been demonstrated that robust Akt activity protects against radiation-induced apoptosis [35, 36]. Furthermore, in vitro studies have demonstrated that inhibition of the PI3-kinase/Akt pathway results in enhanced radiation-induced apoptosis [37–39]. (A schematic picture of PI3-kinase/Akt signaling is shown in Fig. 13.4a.)

Ras/Erk Signaling

The MAP kinase cascade is evolutionary conserved and eukaryotic cells contain multiple forms (Erk, p38 and Jnk) while more primitive cells have at least one. The Ras/Erk pathway has a central role in regulating cell proliferation and survival and may therefore, if inappropriately activated, contribute to cell transformation [40].

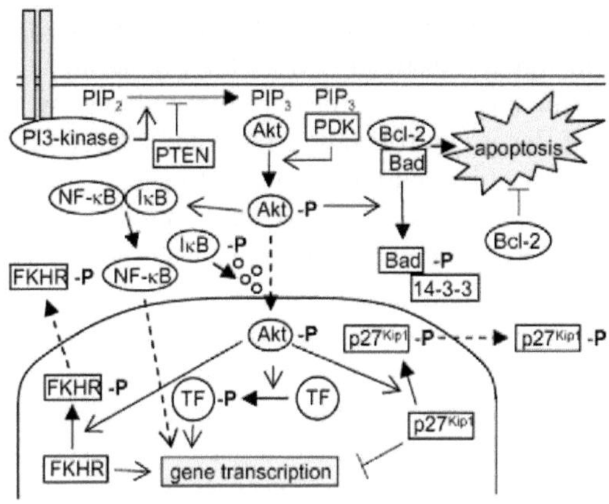

a

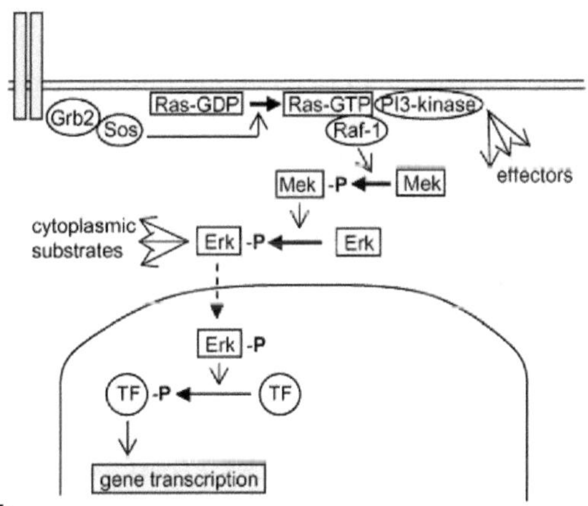

b

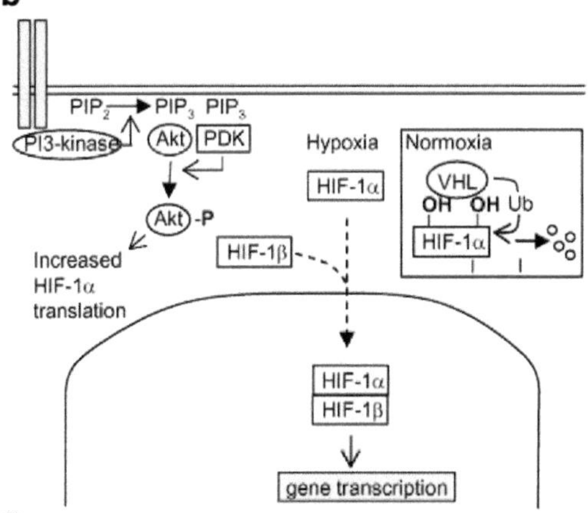

c

Fig. 13.4 Schematic illustration of the major signaling pathways discussed in this article. Solid arrowheads indicate occurrence of a modification, e.g. phosphorylation (**–P**) or degradation (shown as bubbles). Open arrowheads represent the action of an enzyme. A line ending with a bar indicates inhibition and dashed lines translocations. See text for further discussion (From [80]. With permission)

The Ras/Erk pathway is activated by most tyrosine kinase receptors, underscoring its important role in signal transduction from the cell surface to the nucleus. Ras is a small GTPase, which localizes to the plasma membrane by a lipid anchor. The biological activity of Ras is controlled by a regulated GDP/GTP cycle; when GDP is bound to Ras it is inactive and the exchange to GTP causes a conformational change that activates Ras and enables effector proteins to interact. Oncogenic mutations in Ras, which often lock it in an active GTP-bound state, are commonly found in as many as 30% of human tumors [41]. An activating signal is transmitted to Ras through recruitment of nucleotide exchange factors (e.g. Sos) to the cell membrane where they activate Ras by promoting the exchange of GDP for GTP. The active form of Ras interacts with effector proteins such as the serine/threonine kinase Raf-1 and translocates it from the cytoplasm to the cell membrane where it becomes activated. Raf-1 is the first component of a three-tired kinase cascade also containing Mek and Erk. Active Erk localizes both in the cytoplasm and nucleus where it phosphorylates transcription factors and in so doing directly affects gene transcription [42]. In addition to the Erk pathway, Ras may also interact with the catalytic domain of PI3-kinase, establishing crosstalk between the PI3-kinase and Ras/Erk pathways [43]. Consistent with its role in the activation of both Erk and PI3-kinase it has been demonstrated that activated Ras confers radiation resistance to cells [35, 44]. A schematic representation of Ras/Erk pathways is shown in Fig. 13.4b.

Phospholipase Cγ Signaling

Many growth factors activate phospholipase Cγ (PLCγ) which hydrolyses the membrane lipid PIP_2 into the second messengers 1,2-diacylglycerol (DAG) and inositol-1,4,5-triphosphate (IP_3) [45]. Both IP_3, which causes release of Ca^{2+} from intracellular stores, and DAG activate protein kinase C family members, which are involved in a large number of signaling cascades controlling e.g. cell proliferation and migration [46, 47].

The activity of PLCγ has been implicated in radiation and chemotherapy resistance [48, 49]. Furthermore, in A431 human squamous carcinoma cells it has been demonstrated that ionizing radiation can activate PLCγ [50]. However, the molecular mechanism behind these observations has not yet been clarified.

Nuclear Factor–κB Signaling

Nuclear factor-κB (NF-κB) is a transcription factor regulating the expression of a large number of genes, including several involved in protection from apoptosis. In the absence of stimulation NF-κB is localized in the cytoplasm due to binding to inhibitor of κB (IκB) [51]. Activation of cell surface receptors (or cellular stress) causes phosphorylation and ubiquitination of IκB, which targets it for proteasomal degradation. As a consequence, NF-κB is liberated and able to move into the nucleus where it can induce expression of target genes (Fig. 13.4a).

The anti-apoptotic activity of NF-κB probably has a crucial role in the formation of several types of cancers [52]. In fact, it has been demonstrated that radiation activates NF-κB and that down-regulation of NF-κB sensitizes the cells to radiation or DNA damaging chemicals [53, 54].

HIF-1 Signaling

The transcription factor HIF-1, which is a heterodimer consisting of HIF-1α and HIF-1β, accumulates when the cell encounters hypoxia. HIF-1 regulates the expression of a large number of genes, many involved in angiogenesis, e.g. VEGF [55, 56]. At normoxia, two proline residues in HIF-1α are hydroxylated, which enables HIF-1α to bind the von Hippel-Lindau (VHL) tumor suppressor protein that mediates its ubiquitination and degradation (Fig. 13.4c). During hypoxia, the oxygen necessary for the hydroxylation is not available and as a consequence HIF-1α fails to interact with VHL and escapes degradation. Moreover, it has been demonstrated that HIF-1α may be induced by growth factor stimulation [57–61]. Notably, HIF-1 has been suggested to protect tumor cells from radiation-induced apoptosis by increasing the expression of survivin, which is an inhibitor of apoptosis [62].

EGFR Signaling and DNA Repair

The activation of the DNA repair machinery by mitogenic factors might be a way to put the cell in high alert before DNA replication proceeds. For example, Golding et al. demonstrated that Erk MAP kinase can regulate ATM phosphorylation and thereby promote DNA repair [63]. Interestingly, ATM can also influence Erk activity, suggesting the presence of a regulatory feedback loop. Furthermore, interference with PI3-kinase function reduces the ability of radiation to activate ATM [64]. A connection between receptor signaling and DNA repair is thus established by Erk and PI3-kinase since they are proteins activated downstream of the EGFR. This connection is consistent with the fact that many tumor cells become more radiosensitive upon inhibition of EGFR signaling. Treatment with chemotherapeutic drugs or radiation induced EGFR activation as well as translocation to the nucleus [65], resulted in enhanced DNA repair involving activation of DNA-PK as well as other repair protein complexes. The nuclear translocation of the EGFR was inhibited by cetuximab through an unknown mechanism, resulting in slower DSB repair and increased cell death [66]. Additionally, treating cells with the EGFR targeting antibody cetuximab or the low molecular weight EGFR inhibitor gefitinib induced complex formation between the EGFR and the DNA repair protein DNA-PK [67, 68].

Cetuximab treatment leads to translocation of DNA-PK from the nucleus to the cytoplasm [67, 69]. These observations are coherent with the fact that EGFR overexpression confers radioresistance to tumor cells.

In addition to stimulation with ligand, the EGFR also becomes activated in response to radiation or DNA damaging cytotoxic drugs [65]. The mechanism behind the radiation-induced EGFR activation is not fully understood, but probably involves radicals produced by the radiation. In fact, radical scavengers inhibit radiation-induced nuclear import of EGFR [65]. Moreover, exposing cells to hydrogen peroxide or other oxidants lead to ligand-independent signaling [70]. Possible mechanisms include oxidation of the receptor that leads to its activation, or oxidative inactivation of phosphatases that normally keeps the basal activity of the receptor restrained [70–72].

Ideas for Double Action

It is essential to inhibit the cell's defense against apoptosis and DNA damage in order to increase the therapeutical effect of radiation. An ideal situation is to have a tumor-targeting agent that in addition to delivery of radionuclides also modulates intracellular signaling pathways to increase radiosensitivity. Initial studies on combined effects of external radiation and cetuximab indicate this as a possible approach.

We foresee that effective agents for treatment of certain solid tumors can be obtained with radionuclide labeled EGFR and/or HER2 targeting agents (antibodies, antibody fragments, peptides or affibody molecules) that deliver therapeutic radionuclides and also, via binding to EGFR and/or HER2, modify the intracellular signal transduction to give radiosensitization. Thus, the targeted cells will suffer from the direct radiation effect on the cells, i.e. DNA damage and cell death [73–76] and be sensitized via changes in intracellular signal transduction. It is possible that cells from solid tumors, that otherwise would be difficult to treat, might thereby be treatable even with a curative intention.

Akt-Phosphorylation and Apoptosis

The serine/threonine kinase Akt has a central role in protecting the cell from apoptosis and consequently in the sensitivity toward radiation and drugs (Fig. 13.4a). This makes the PI3-kinase/Akt pathway an interesting therapeutic target, and there are currently several inhibitors in preclinical development [77]. It is likely that a targeting agent, recognizing a cell surface structure on the tumor cell, that in addition to selectively deliver a radionuclide or cytotoxic agent to the tumor also enhances the apoptotic response by downregulating Akt will have an enhanced therapeutic effect. Alternatively, a systemic treatment with a low molecular weight inhibitor against Akt may also enhance the therapeutic efficacy of external radiation. In summary, it is possible that a synergistic anti-tumor activity may be achieved by simultaneously exposing the cancer cell to radioactive nuclides and Akt inhibition.

Inhibition of DNA Repair via Inhibition of ATM Phosphorylation

A possible way to increase the response to radiation could be to down-regulate or inhibit phosphorylation of ATM and thereby inhibit DNA repair. Mammalian cells delay their progression through the G_1, S and G_2 phases of the cell cycle in response to radiation damage on DNA and this response is controlled by ATM, ATR and downstream kinases CHK1 and CHK2. Cells with severe DNA damage are forced into replication or to enter mitosis before extensive repair if they are without functional checkpoint regulation. This might be achieved by inhibition of tyrosine kinase receptors, e.g. EGFR. A targeting agent can hopefully be designed to give signal transduction disturbances that give decreased phosphorylation of ATM and at the same time deliver therapeutic radionuclides. Thus, the tumor cell killing effects of radiation might therefore further increase if ATM phosphorylation is inhibited.

Radiosensitization Through Inhibition of DNA-PK

Administration of tyrosine kinase inhibitors such as gefitinib might, via inhibition of EGFR signaling, inhibit DNA-PK activity [78] and thereby inhibit DNA repair. Inhibition of EGFR has been shown to radiosensitize tumor cells [79]. Cetuximab and other macromolecular EGFR inhibiting agents might also be candidates for such radiosensitization. Furthermore, the macromolecules can also be designed to deliver therapeutically active radionuclides.

Tumor Versus Normal Cells

The discussion above is focused on radiation sensitization of tumor cells. In contrast, there is of course an ambition to protect normal cells. Normal tissue toxicity is a major reason why many compounds that are efficient in vitro fail in clinical studies. Thus, for normal cells it is desirable to diminish harmful effects, e.g. by modifying signal pathways to improve DNA-repair. Of course, it will be difficult to obtain differential effects between normal cells and tumor cells but innovative approaches must be tried. The overexpression of for example EGFR and HER2 in many tumor cell types might give one possibility to at least sensitize the tumor cells while induced protection in normal cells probably is difficult. Nevertheless, sensitization of tumor cells will lead to an improved difference in sensitivity between tumor and normal cells and this is a good start.

Conclusions

There exists a connection (crosstalk) between signals emanating from growth factor receptors and the complex DNA repair machinery. Increased knowledge regarding this relation might give new possibilities to modulate radiosensitivity both in tumor cells and normal cells. Development of new targeting agents with double action, i. e. receptor mediated radiosensitization and radiation-induced DNA damage, is an important research direction for many decades ahead. The hope is that agents are developed that can, on a large scale, be successfully used for treatment of malignant tumors while at the same time the damage to normal tissue can be kept on an acceptable level.

Acknowledgements The work was financially supported by the Swedish Cancer Society grants 0980-B06-19XBC and 0540-B05-01XAC, Vinnova 2004-02159, the Ludwig Institute for Cancer Research and the Swedish Research Council (VR). Thanks also to Bentham Science Publishers who permitted us to reproduce three of the figures from our recent review article Lennartsson et al. [80]. Several of the aspects discussed in this chapter were also discussed in that article.

References

1. Niida, H. and Nakanishi, M. (2006) DNA damage checkpoints in mammals. *Mutagenesis*, **21**, 3–9.
2. Bakkenist, C.J. and Kastan, M.B. (2004) Initiating cellular stress responses. *Cell*, **118**, 9–17.
3. Roos, W.P. and Kaina, B. (2006) DNA damage-induced cell death by apoptosis. *Trends Mol Med*, **12**, 440–50.
4. Vispe, S. and Satoh, M.S. (2000) DNA repair patch-mediated double strand DNA break formation in human cells. *J Biol Chem*, **275**, 27386–92.
5. Stenerlöw, B., Karlsson, K.H., Cooper, B. and Rydberg, B. (2003) Measurement of prompt DNA double-strand breaks in mammalian cells without including heat-labile sites: results for cells deficient in nonhomologous end joining. *Radiat Res*, **159**, 502–10.
6. Norbury, C.J. and Zhivotovsky, B. (2004) DNA damage-induced apoptosis. *Oncogene*, **23**, 2797–808.
7. Petrini, J.H. and Stracker, T.H. (2003) The cellular response to DNA double-strand breaks: defining the sensors and mediators. *Trends Cell Biol*, **13**, 458–62.
8. Yang, J., Yu, Y., Hamrick, H.E. and Duerksen-Hughes, P.J. (2003) ATM, ATR and DNA-PK: initiators of the cellular genotoxic stress responses. *Carcinogenesis*, **24**, 1571–80.
9. Lee, J.H. and Paull, T.T. (2005) ATM activation by DNA double-strand breaks through the Mre11-Rad50-Nbs1 complex. *Science*, **308**, 551–4.
10. Rogakou, E.P., Pilch, D.R., Orr, A.H., Ivanova, V.S. and Bonner, W.M. (1998) DNA double-stranded breaks induce histone H2AX phosphorylation on serine **139**. *J Biol Chem*, 273, 5858–68.

11. Jazayeri, A., Falck, J., Lukas, C., Bartek, J., Smith, G.C., Lukas, J. and Jackson, S.P. (2006) ATM- and cell cycle-dependent regulation of ATR in response to DNA double-strand breaks. *Nat Cell Biol*, **8**, 37–45.
12. Bartek, J. and Lukas, J. (2003) Chk1 and Chk2 kinases in checkpoint control and cancer. *Cancer Cell*, **3**, 421–9.
13. Zhou, B.B., Anderson, H.J. and Roberge, M. (2003) Targeting DNA checkpoint kinases in cancer therapy. *Cancer Biol Ther*, **2**, S16–22.
14. Viniegra, J.G., Martinez, N., Modirassari, P., Losa, J.H., Parada Cobo, C., Lobo, V.J., Luquero, C.I., Alvarez-Vallina, L., Ramon y Cajal, S., Rojas, J.M. and Sanchez-Prieto, R. (2005) Full activation of PKB/Akt in response to insulin or ionizing radiation is mediated through ATM. *J Biol Chem*, **280**, 4029–36.
15. Panta, G.R., Kaur, S., Cavin, L.G., Cortes, M.L., Mercurio, F., Lothstein, L., Sweatman, T.W., Israel, M. and Arsura, M. (2004) ATM and the catalytic subunit of DNA-dependent protein kinase activate NF-kappaB through a common MEK/extracellular signal-regulated kinase/p90(rsk) signaling pathway in response to distinct forms of DNA damage. *Mol Cell Biol*, **24**, 1823–35.
16. Dragoi, A.M., Fu, X., Ivanov, S., Zhang, P., Sheng, L., Wu, D., Li, G.C. and Chu, W.M. (2005) DNA-PKcs, but not TLR9, is required for activation of Akt by CpG-DNA. *EMBO J*, **24**, 779–89.
17. Feng, J., Park, J., Cron, P., Hess, D. and Hemmings, B.A. (2004) Identification of a PKB/Akt hydrophobic motif Ser-473 kinase as DNA-dependent protein kinase. *J Biol Chem*, **279**, 41189–96.
18. Bartkova, J., Horejsi, Z., Koed, K., Kramer, A., Tort, F., Zieger, K., Guldberg, P., Sehested, M., Nesland, J.M., Lukas, C., Orntoft, T., Lukas, J. and Bartek, J. (2005) DNA damage response as a candidate anti-cancer barrier in early human tumorigenesis. *Nature*, **434**, 864–70.
19. van Gent, D.C., Hoeijmakers, J.H. and Kanaar, R. (2001) Chromosomal stability and the DNA double-stranded break connection. *Nat Rev Genet*, **2**, 196–206.
20. DiBiase, S.J., Zeng, Z.C., Chen, R., Hyslop, T., Curran, W.J., Jr. and Iliakis, G. (2000) DNA-dependent protein kinase stimulates an independently active, nonhomologous, end-joining apparatus. *Cancer Res*, **60**, 1245–53.
21. Radulescu, I., Elmroth, K. and Stenerlöw, B. (2004) Chromatin organization contributes to non-randomly distributed double-strand breaks after exposure to high-LET radiation. *Radiat Res*, **161**, 1–8.
22. Stenerlöw, B., Höglund, E., Carlsson, J. and Blomquist, E. (2000) Rejoining of DNA fragments produced by radiations of different linear energy transfer. *Int J Radiat Biol*, **76**, 549–57.
23. Karlsson, K.H. and Stenerlöw, B. (2004) Focus formation of DNA repair proteins in normal and repair-deficient cells irradiated with high-LET ions. *Radiat Res*, **161**, 517–27.
24. Foster, F.M., Traer, C.J., Abraham, S.M. and Fry, M.J. (2003) The phosphoinositide (PI) 3-kinase family. *J Cell Sci*, **116**, 3037–40.
25. Coffer, P.J., Jin, J. and Woodgett, J.R. (1998) Protein kinase B (c-Akt): a multifunctional mediator of phosphatidylinositol 3-kinase activation. *Biochem J*, **335 (Pt 1)**, 1–13.
26. Andjelkovic, M., Alessi, D.R., Meier, R., Fernandez, A., Lamb, N.J., Frech, M., Cron, P., Cohen, P., Lucocq, J.M. and Hemmings, B.A. (1997) Role of translocation in the activation and function of protein kinase B. *J Biol Chem*, **272**, 31515–24.
27. Meier, R., Alessi, D.R., Cron, P., Andjelkovic, M. and Hemmings, B.A. (1997) Mitogenic activation, phosphorylation, and nuclear translocation of protein kinase Bbeta. *J Biol Chem*, **272**, 30491–7.
28. Zha, J., Harada, H., Yang, E., Jockel, J. and Korsmeyer, S.J. (1996) Serine phosphorylation of death agonist BAD in response to survival factor results in binding to 14-3-3 not BCL-X(L). *Cell*, **87**, 619–28.
29. Datta, S.R., Dudek, H., Tao, X., Masters, S., Fu, H., Gotoh, Y. and Greenberg, M.E. (1997) Akt phosphorylation of BAD couples survival signals to the cell-intrinsic death machinery. *Cell*, **91**, 231–41.

30. Medema, R.H., Kops, G.J., Bos, J.L. and Burgering, B.M. (2000) AFX-like Forkhead transcription factors mediate cell-cycle regulation by Ras and PKB through p27kip1. *Nature*, **404**, 782–7.
31. Liang, J., Zubovitz, J., Petrocelli, T., Kotchetkov, R., Connor, M.K., Han, K., Lee, J.H., Ciarallo, S., Catzavelos, C., Beniston, R., Franssen, E. and Slingerland, J.M. (2002) PKB/Akt phosphorylates p27, impairs nuclear import of p27 and opposes p27-mediated G1 arrest. *Nat Med*, **8**, 1153–60.
32. Shin, I., Yakes, F.M., Rojo, F., Shin, N.Y., Bakin, A.V., Baselga, J. and Arteaga, C.L. (2002) PKB/Akt mediates cell-cycle progression by phosphorylation of p27(Kip1) at threonine 157 and modulation of its cellular localization. *Nat Med*, **8**, 1145–52.
33. Viglietto, G., Motti, M.L., Bruni, P., Melillo, R.M., D'Alessio, A., Califano, D., Vinci, F., Chiappetta, G., Tsichlis, P., Bellacosa, A., Fusco, A. and Santoro, M. (2002) Cytoplasmic relocalization and inhibition of the cyclin-dependent kinase inhibitor p27(Kip1) by PKB/Akt-mediated phosphorylation in breast cancer. *Nat Med*, **8**, 1136–44.
34. Chu, E.C. and Tarnawski, A.S. (2004) PTEN regulatory functions in tumor suppression and cell biology. *Med Sci Monit*, **10**, RA235–41.
35. Kim, I.A., Bae, S.S., Fernandes, A., Wu, J., Muschel, R.J., McKenna, W.G., Birnbaum, M.J. and Bernhard, E.J. (2005) Selective inhibition of Ras, phosphoinositide 3 kinase, and Akt isoforms increases the radiosensitivity of human carcinoma cell lines. *Cancer Res*, **65**, 7902–10.
36. Tanno, S., Yanagawa, N., Habiro, A., Koizumi, K., Nakano, Y., Osanai, M., Mizukami, Y., Okumura, T., Testa, J.R. and Kohgo, Y. (2004) Serine/threonine kinase AKT is frequently activated in human bile duct cancer and is associated with increased radioresistance. *Cancer Res*, **64**, 3486–90.
37. Lee, C.M., Fuhrman, C.B., Planelles, V., Peltier, M.R., Gaffney, D.K., Soisson, A.P., Dodson, M.K., Tolley, H.D., Green, C.L. and Zempolich, K.A. (2006) Phosphatidylinositol 3-kinase inhibition by LY294002 radiosensitizes human cervical cancer cell lines. *Clin Cancer Res*, **12**, 250–6.
38. Tan, J. and Hallahan, D.E. (2003) Growth factor-independent activation of protein kinase B contributes to the inherent resistance of vascular endothelium to radiation-induced apoptotic response. *Cancer Res*, **63**, 7663–7.
39. Edwards, E., Geng, L., Tan, J., Onishko, H., Donnelly, E. and Hallahan, D.E. (2002) Phosphatidylinositol 3-kinase/Akt signaling in the response of vascular endothelium to ionizing radiation. *Cancer Res*, **62**, 4671–7.
40. Lewis, T.S., Shapiro, P.S. and Ahn, N.G. (1998) Signal transduction through MAP kinase cascades. *Adv Cancer Res*, **74**, 49–139.
41. Thompson, N. and Lyons, J. (2005) Recent progress in targeting the Raf/MEK/ERK pathway with inhibitors in cancer drug discovery. *Curr Opin Pharmacol*, **5**, 350–6.
42. Chen, R.H., Sarnecki, C. and Blenis, J. (1992) Nuclear localization and regulation of erk- and rsk-encoded protein kinases. *Mol Cell Biol*, **12**, 915–27.
43. Rodriguez-Viciana, P., Warne, P.H., Dhand, R., Vanhaesebroeck, B., Gout, I., Fry, M.J., Waterfield, M.D. and Downward, J. (1994) Phosphatidylinositol-3-OH kinase as a direct target of Ras. *Nature*, **370**, 527–32.
44. Kim, I.A., Fernandes, A.T., Gupta, A.K., McKenna, W.G. and Bernhard, E.J. (2004) The influence of Ras pathway signaling on tumor radiosensitivity. *Cancer Metastasis Rev*, **23**, 227–36.
45. Wilde, J.I. and Watson, S.P. (2001) Regulation of phospholipase C gamma isoforms in haematopoietic cells: why one, not the other? *Cell Signal*, **13**, 691–701.
46. Berridge, M.J., Lipp, P. and Bootman, M.D. (2000) The versatility and universality of calcium signalling. *Nat Rev Mol Cell Biol*, **1**, 11–21.
47. Liu, W.S. and Heckman, C.A. (1998) The sevenfold way of PKC regulation. *Cell Signal*, **10**, 529–42.
48. Plo, I., Lautier, D., Casteran, N., Dubreuil, P., Arock, M. and Laurent, G. (2001) Kit signaling and negative regulation of daunorubicin-induced apoptosis: role of phospholipase Cgamma. *Oncogene*, **20**, 6752–63.

49. Maddens, S., Charruyer, A., Plo, I., Dubreuil, P., Berger, S., Salles, B., Laurent, G. and Jaffrezou, J.P. (2002) Kit signaling inhibits the sphingomyelin-ceramide pathway through PLC gamma 1: implication in stem cell factor radioprotective effect. *Blood*, **100**, 1294–301.
50. Todd, D.G., Mikkelsen, R.B., Rorrer, W.K., Valerie, K. and Schmidt-Ullrich, R.K. (1999) Ionizing radiation stimulates existing signal transduction pathways involving the activation of epidermal growth factor receptor and ERBB-3, and changes of intracellular calcium in A431 human squamous carcinoma cells. *J Recept Signal Transduct Res*, **19**, 885–908.
51. Karin, M. (1999) How NF-kappaB is activated: the role of the IkappaB kinase (IKK) complex. *Oncogene*, **18**, 6867–74.
52. Barkett, M. and Gilmore, T.D. (1999) Control of apoptosis by Rel/NF-kappaB transcription factors. *Oncogene*, **18**, 6910–24.
53. Kato, T., Duffey, D.C., Ondrey, F.G., Dong, G., Chen, Z., Cook, J.A., Mitchell, J.B. and Van Waes, C. (2000) Cisplatin and radiation sensitivity in human head and neck squamous carcinomas are independently modulated by glutathione and transcription factor NF-kappaB. *Head Neck*, **22**, 748–59.
54. Miyakoshi, J. and Yagi, K. (2000) Inhibition of I kappaB-alpha phosphorylation at serine and tyrosine acts independently on sensitization to DNA damaging agents in human glioma cells. *Br J Cancer*, **82**, 28–33.
55. Dery, M.A., Michaud, M.D. and Richard, D.E. (2005) Hypoxia-inducible factor 1: regulation by hypoxic and non-hypoxic activators. *Int J Biochem Cell Biol*, **37**, 535–40.
56. Maxwell, P.H. (2005) The HIF pathway in cancer. *Semin Cell Dev Biol*, **16**, 523–30.
57. Zundel, W., Schindler, C., Haas-Kogan, D., Koong, A., Kaper, F., Chen, E., Gottschalk, A.R., Ryan, H.E., Johnson, R.S., Jefferson, A.B., Stokoe, D. and Giaccia, A.J. (2000) Loss of PTEN facilitates HIF-1-mediated gene expression. *Genes Dev*, **14**, 391–6.
58. Fukuda, R., Hirota, K., Fan, F., Jung, Y.D., Ellis, L.M. and Semenza, G.L. (2002) Insulin-like growth factor 1 induces hypoxia-inducible factor 1-mediated vascular endothelial growth factor expression, which is dependent on MAP kinase and phosphatidylinositol 3-kinase signaling in colon cancer cells. *J Biol Chem*, **277**, 38205–11.
59. Jiang, B.H., Jiang, G., Zheng, J.Z., Lu, Z., Hunter, T. and Vogt, P.K. (2001) Phosphatidylinositol 3-kinase signaling controls levels of hypoxia-inducible factor 1. *Cell Growth Differ*, **12**, 363–9.
60. Laughner, E., Taghavi, P., Chiles, K., Mahon, P.C. and Semenza, G.L. (2001) HER2 (neu) signaling increases the rate of hypoxia-inducible factor 1alpha (HIF-1alpha) synthesis: novel mechanism for HIF-1-mediated vascular endothelial growth factor expression. *Mol Cell Biol*, **21**, 3995–4004.
61. Giatromanolaki, A., Koukourakis, M.I., Simopoulos, C., Polychronidis, A., Gatter, K.C., Harris, A.L. and Sivridis, E. (2004) c-erbB-2 related aggressiveness in breast cancer is hypoxia inducible factor-1alpha dependent. *Clin Cancer Res*, **10**, 7972–7.
62. Shi, M., Guo, X.T., Shu, M.G., Chen, F.L. and Li, L.W. (2007) Cell-permeable hypoxia-inducible factor-1 (HIF-1) antagonists function as tumor radiosensitizers. *Med Hypotheses*, **69**, 33–35.
63. Golding, S.E., Rosenberg, E., Neill, S., Dent, P., Povirk, L.F. and Valerie, K. (2007) Extracellular signal-related kinase positively regulates ataxia telangiectasia mutated, homologous recombination repair, and the DNA damage response. *Cancer Res*, **67**, 1046–53.
64. Irarrazabal, C.E., Burg, M.B., Ward, S.G. and Ferraris, J.D. (2006) Phosphatidylinositol 3-kinase mediates activation of ATM by high NaCl and by ionizing radiation: role in osmoprotective transcriptional regulation. *Proc Natl Acad Sci USA*, **103**, 8882–7.
65. Dittmann, K., Mayer, C., Fehrenbacher, B., Schaller, M., Raju, U., Milas, L., Chen, D.J., Kehlbach, R. and Rodemann, H.P. (2005) Radiation-induced epidermal growth factor receptor nuclear import is linked to activation of DNA-dependent protein kinase. *J Biol Chem*, **280**, 31182–9.
66. Dittmann, K., Mayer, C. and Rodemann, H.P. (2005) Inhibition of radiation-induced EGFR nuclear import by C225 (Cetuximab) suppresses DNA-PK activity. *Radiother Oncol*, **76**, 157–61.

67. Bandyopadhyay, D., Mandal, M., Adam, L., Mendelsohn, J. and Kumar, R. (1998) Physical interaction between epidermal growth factor receptor and DNA-dependent protein kinase in mammalian cells. *J Biol Chem*, **273**, 1568–73.
68. Friedmann, B., Caplin, M., Hartley, J.A. and Hochhauser, D. (2004) Modulation of DNA repair in vitro after treatment with chemotherapeutic agents by the epidermal growth factor receptor inhibitor gefitinib (ZD1839). *Clin Cancer Res*, **10**, 6476–86.
69. Huang, S.M. and Harari, P.M. (2000) Modulation of radiation response after epidermal growth factor receptor blockade in squamous cell carcinomas: inhibition of damage repair, cell cycle kinetics, and tumor angiogenesis. *Clin Cancer Res*, **6**, 2166–74.
70. Lucero, H., Gae, D. and Taccioli, G.E. (2003) Novel localization of the DNA-PK complex in lipid rafts: a putative role in the signal transduction pathway of the ionizing radiation response. *J Biol Chem*, **278**, 22136–43.
71. Knebel, A., Rahmsdorf, H.J., Ullrich, A. and Herrlich, P. (1996) Dephosphorylation of receptor tyrosine kinases as target of regulation by radiation, oxidants or alkylating agents. *EMBO J*, **15**, 5314–25.
72. Ostman, A. and Bohmer, F.D. (2001) Regulation of receptor tyrosine kinase signaling by protein tyrosine phosphatases. *Trends Cell Biol*, **11**, 258–66.
73. Ma, B.B., Bristow, R.G., Kim, J. and Siu, L.L. (2003) Combined-modality treatment of solid tumors using radiotherapy and molecular targeted agents. *J Clin Oncol*, **21**, 2760–76.
74. Connell, P.P., Kron, S.J. and Weichselbaum, R.R. (2004) Relevance and irrelevance of DNA damage response to radiotherapy. *DNA Repair (Amst)*, **3**, 1245–51.
75. Pawlik, T.M. and Keyomarsi, K. (2004) Role of cell cycle in mediating sensitivity to radiotherapy. *Int J Radiat Oncol Biol Phys*, **59**, 928–42.
76. Willers, H., Dahm-Daphi, J. and Powell, S.N. (2004) Repair of radiation damage to DNA. *Br J Cancer*, **90**, 1297–301.
77. Hennessy, B.T., Smith, D.L., Ram, P.T., Lu, Y. and Mills, G.B. (2005) Exploiting the PI3K/AKT pathway for cancer drug discovery. *Nat Rev Drug Discov*, **4**, 988–1004.
78. Shintani, S., Li, C., Mihara, M., Terakado, N., Yano, J., Nakashiro, K. and Hamakawa, H. (2003) Enhancement of tumor radioresponse by combined treatment with gefitinib (Iressa, ZD1839), an epidermal growth factor receptor tyrosine kinase inhibitor, is accompanied by inhibition of DNA damage repair and cell growth in oral cancer. *Int J Cancer*, **107**, 1030–7.
79. Sartor, C.I. (2004) Mechanisms of disease: Radiosensitization by epidermal growth factor receptor inhibitors. *Nat Clin Pract Oncol*, **1**, 80–7.
80. Lennartsson, J., Carlsson, J. and Stenerlöw, B. (2006) Targeting the epidermal growth factor receptor family in radionuclide therapy of tumors–signal transduction and DNA repair. *Lett Drug Des Discov*, **3**, 357–368.

Chapter 14
Radiation Induced DNA Damage Checkpoints

David Eriksson, Katrine Riklund, Lennart Johansson, and Torgny Stigbrand

Summary Radiation induced damage to DNA can be limited to exchanges of single DNA bases or extensive double-strand breaks. Nuclear proteins can sense these alterations and are able to cause cell cycle arrests at the G1/S, intra-S or G2/M checkpoints in the cell cycle, until the lesions undergo repair. If the induction of these cell cycle arrests is defective, genomic instability and aberrations in the cell cycle kinetics appear, which may cause cell death. In this chapter radiation induced effects on the cell cycle will be presented.

Introduction

In cells exposed to ionizing radiation, a variety of DNA damages can be induced, including DNA double and single strand breaks (DSBs, SSBs respectively), DNA base and sugar damages and abnormal cross-links within the DNA or between DNA and cellular proteins [1–4]. DNA damage can be lethal to the cell and has to be recognized and repaired in order for the cell to survive, but also to minimize the risk of heritable mutations. To prevent these harmful outcomes, DNA damage checkpoints are activated and interact and operate in concert to recognize these alterations and execute a proper response, thereby controlling and protecting the integrity of the genome [5–7].

The first recognized function of the DNA damage checkpoints was the delayed progression through the cell cycle, which was reported in cells exposed to ionizing radiation more than 50 years ago [5]. Today it is documented that the DNA damage checkpoints respond to damage in a considerably broader way by coordinating DNA reparation with cell cycle progression. This is done by activation of DNA repair pathways and induction of arrests at specific phases of the cell cycle (G1/S, intra S or G2/M-arrests), which provides extra time for DNA reparation.

Departments of Immunology, Diagnostic Radiology and Radiophysics, University of Umeå, SE-90185 Umeå, Sweden

If the reparation process is successful, these cells will survive and can reenter the cell cycle upon termination of checkpoint arrest. When the DNA lesions are extensive, i.e. the damage is beyond repair, cells with activated checkpoints will be eliminated via apoptosis or inactivated by cellular senescence (Fig. 14.1).

Activation of the DNA damage response includes the same central components as other signal transduction pathways, which can be properly divided into sensors, mediators, transducer and effectors [7] (Fig. 14.1). The activating signal is DNA damage and the most crucial DNA lesion following ionizing radiation exposure is DSBs. DSBs are the most dangerous lesions since both DNA strands are broken and consequently the coding sequence lost. If the DSBs are not repaired or repaired incorrectly, they may cause mutations or chromosomal translocations, which may cause cancer [2, 8]. It has been reported that about 40 DSBs are induced per Gy of ionizing radiation in a typical cell [9] and experiments indicate that the DNA damage checkpoints can be very sensitive and can be activated and respond to few or

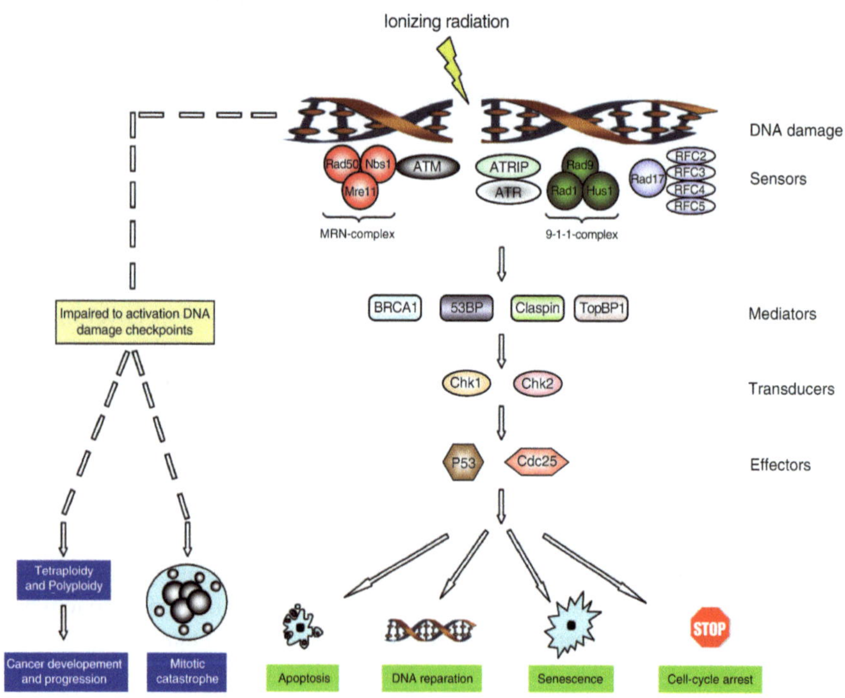

Fig. 14.1 Major components of the DNA damage checkpoints. The DNA damage is recognized by sensors that initiate the signalling. Transduction of the signal to transducers is mediated with the assistance of mediators. The transducers in turn give signals to the effector proteins and depending on the nature of the effector, the cells may initiate cell cycle arrest, DNA repair, senescence or apoptosis. Failure to activate these DNA damage checkpoints can lead to cell death via mitotic catastrophe (chapter 12) or the development of tetraploid/polyploidy and multinucleated giant cells. Abnormal division of tetraploid/polyploid cells then might facilitate genetic changes that contribute to the development and progression of cancer

even one DSB [10, 11]. The sensors constitute the first components of the DNA damage response and they recognise and initiate the response to the DNA damage. Mediators then facilitate signalling by promoting physical interactions between other proteins, whereas signal transducers, typically protein kinases, pass on and amplify the damage signal. Finally, effectors are the ultimate downstream targets that mediate the final response. These effector responses include DNA repair (discussed in chapter 13), apoptosis and senescence (discussed in chapter 12) and cell cycle arrest. This chapter will mainly focus on DNA damage checkpoints for events that arrest cell cycle progression in response to DNA damage. Cells that display an impaired activation of these DNA damage checkpoints will be forced into mitotic catastrophes and die or become tetraploid/polyploid following abnormal divisions (chapter 12). This can facilitate genetic changes that lead to aneuploid cancers and development and progression of cancer (for reviews see [12–14]).

Components of the DNA Damage Checkpoints

The initiating step in activation of the DNA damage checkpoints involves sensors, which recognize DNA damage and initiate a signal, which is transmitted via the central phosphoinositide 3-kinase related kinases (PIKKs, reviewed in [15]) to their downstream substrates that mediate cell cycle arrest in G1, S or G2 phases, DNA repair, and cell death [15–18]. Two important members of the PIKKs, known to be involved in the DNA damage response, are ataxia-telangiectasia mutated (ATM) and ATM and Rad3 related (ATR), which both phosphorylate a large number of substrates. ATM is a serine-threonine kinase and mutations causing a deficiency in functional ATM are responsible for a rare syndrome, ataxia telangiectasia (A-T), characterized by cerebellar neurodegeneration, immunodeficiency, extreme sensitivity to radiation, and increased risk of cancer, attributable largely to insufficient DNA DSB recognition and repair [19]. While cells without active ATM are viable, disruption of ATR causes cell death, which suggests that ATR also is essential in undamaged cells in functions like replication and cellular differentiation [20–23]. This family also includes DNA-dependent protein kinase (DNA-PK), which plays an important role in DNA DSB repair by NHEJ (reviewed in [24, 25] and chapter 13). ATM, ATR, and DNA-PK partially have different substrate specificity and phosphorylate various targets that contribute to the overall DNA damage response.

While the ATM and ATR pathways have some of their downstream functions in common, they are activated by distinct DNA damages. ATM plays a primary role in response to DNA DSBs and appears to be the primary PIKK responding to ionizing irradiation [23, 26, 27]. ATM is mainly found in the nucleus and the level does not change in cells following exposure to irradiation [28–31]. However, the kinase activity of ATM increases rapidly after exposure to irradiation. ATR, conversely, responds broadly to DNA damage, including SSBs, and also to DNA replication stress [32–34]. However, in response to DSBs, ATM is activated immediately as it is responsible for the instantaneous damage response, whereas ATR uses longer time for activation, but joins in later and assists in phosphorylation of specific substrates [6, 15, 34]. These two kinases together strongly promote the activation of downstream substrates in a concerted manner (see below).

ATM and ATR Activation

DSBs initiate the downstream signalling as a consequence of changes in chromatin structure, binding to DNA by the MRN protein complex, and resection of the double strand to expose single stranded DNA, which collectively triggers an increase in ATM and ATR kinase activity. These three modes of activation are described in the following sections.

ATM Activation as a Consequence of Chromatin Conformation Changes

ATM is maintained inactive in unirradiated cells as a dimer or as a multimer of higher-order, which physically blocks the kinase domain. In cells exposed to even very low doses of ionizing radiation a rapid intermolecular autophosphorylation of serine 1981 is triggered, which causes dimer dissociation and initiates chromatin association and kinase activity of ATM [16]. The conformational change that occurs due to this autophosphorylation and causes monomerization and activation of ATM kinase activity is geared by changes in the chromatin structure and does not require binding to the damage site. While autophosphorylation of serine 1981 following irradiation is critical to the activation of ATM, autophosphorylation on other sites of ATM has been recognized, including phosphorylation of serine 367 and serine 1893, which also can be important for the DNA damage response [35].

ATM Activation via MRN-Complex Binding to DSBs and DSB Resection

The other two ways by which ATM activity is regulated depends on a sensor protein complex consisting of Mre11, Rad50, and Nbs1 (MRN-complex). This complex rapidly forms discrete nuclear foci following exposure to DNA DSB inducing agents, including ionizing irradiation. Rad50 forms homodimers which associate with two Mre11 molecules to generate a heterotetramer. Binding of the complex to DNA appears to be achieved through binding motifs of Mre11 tethering together, and therefore contributes to stabilize broken chromosomes, whereas Rad50 mediates unwinding of these DNA ends generating single stranded DNA. Nbs1 binds directly to and recruits ATM to the damage site and serves as a bridge between ATM and the DNA bound hetrotetrameric MR-complex [36, 37]. The MRN-ATM complex subsequently triggers two pathways that culminate in local rearrangements of DNA and neighbouring chromatin (see Fig. 1 in [38]).

The first pathway is very rapid and operates throughout the cell cycle in a CDK-independent manner [38]. In this pathway, ATM phosphorylates downstream substrates including histone H2AX, which localise in the chromatin adjacent to the break and is referred to as γ-H2AX in its phosphorylated state (reviewed in [39]). γ-H2AX, implicated in amplifying the DNA damage signal, can be detected within minutes after irradiation and the fraction of H2AX that becomes phosphorylated is proportional to the dose [40, 41]. These γ-H2AX molecules are not homogeneously distributed within the nucleus but form structures named ionizing radiation induced nuclear foci (IRIF), together with other DNA damage response proteins [42], with each focus corresponding to approximately one DSB [40]. Mdc1, which is a mediator, in turn directly binds to γ-H2AX via its tandem BRCT domains [43] and recruits and retains additional Nbs1 [44]. Accordingly, more molecules of the MRN complex will bind and then bring about the recruitment of further activated ATM molecules to the chromatin regions flanking the lesion. This creates a positive feedback loop that carries DNA damage-induced H2AX phosphorylation over large chromatin regions [44]. Phosphorylated H2AX is initially found close to the site of the break, but the feedback loop leads to growth of the chromatin regions containing γ-H2AX, which facilitate the assembly of other protein complexes [38, 45, 46]. Several other DNA damage response proteins have also been shown to accumulate in IRIF in an H2AX dependent manner including mediators (BRCA1, 53BP1, TopBP1), the MRN-complex, and ATM itself [45, 47–51]. However, as discussed in [44], Mdc1 is probably the pre-dominant γ-H2AX recognition module. Furthermore, despite that γ-H2AX is not required for the initial recruitment of Nbs1, 53BP1 and BRCA1 to DSBs, these DNA damage response proteins subsequently fail to form IRIF as a consequence of inefficient accumulation and a reduced retention within chromatin at the damage site [52]. γ-H2AX seems to work as an amplifier that may be important for maximization of the DNA damage response when the signal is low, as is the case in response to low doses of irradiation, which might otherwise be insufficient to prevent entry of damaged cells into mitosis [53]. γ-H2AX creates large subnuclear domains around the DSBs, which accumulate DNA repair proteins and subsequent chromatin remodelers, which in turn maintain the chromatin domain in a decondensed open configuration [54]. Collectively, this leads to an increased concentration of active ATM, which increases phosphorylation of ATM targets.

Secondly, the MRN-ATM complex is furthermore involved in DSB resection to expose ssDNA, a common intermediate DNA structure that activates the ATR pathway and also is needed for homologous recombination-mediated DSB repair [55–57]. DSB resection is followed by coating of ssDNA with the Replication Protein A (RPA) complex, which display high affinity for single stranded DNA. Single stranded DNA coated with RPA recruits and enriches ATR-ATRIP and facilitate loading of the 9-1-1 complex (Rad9, Rad1, Hus1) by Rad17 to the DNA damage sites. The 9-1-1 complex structurally resembles the proliferating cell nucleus antigen (PCNA)-like sliding clamp, that functions in DNA replication and repair [58]. Rad17 can interact with replication factor c subunits (Rfc2-5) to form a complex, which acts as a DNA damage activated 9-1-1 clamp loading complex [59–61].

ATRIP becomes phosphorylated by ATR and the colocalization of this complex with Rad17 and 9-1-1 complexes at the damage site may upregulate the kinase activity of ATR-ATRIP. This colocalization and the increased kinase activity may lead to phosphorylation of a subset of ATR substrates including Rad17 and Rad9, which then may recruit the downstream mediator proteins Claspin and TopBP1 respectively. Both Claspin and TopBP1 are phosphorylated by ATR, which facilitate TopBP1 to stimulate ATR-ATRIP activity and Claspin to phosphorylate and activate Chk1 via stable protein-protein interactions.

Activation of Transducers and Effectors

The activated kinases (ATM, ATR) cooperate and together strongly promote the activation of downstream substrates in a concerted manner. Following exposure to ionizing radiation ATM substrates include Chk2, p53, NBS1, BRCA1 and itself [16, 28, 29, 62, 63]. ATM and ATR display an overlapping phosphorylation pattern, but substrate specificity also exists [64] including the two important signal transducers for cell cycle regulation, Chk1 and Chk2 [65–67]. Following ionizing radiation, the damage signal that goes via ATM is then transduced by Chk2 [68, 69], whereas UV induced DNA damage or DSB resection signal via ATR and this signal is subsequently transduced by Chk1 [70]. Chk1 and Chk2 (also ATM and ATR themselves) in turn initiate phosphorylation of several effector molecules including p53 and the Cdc25 family of phosphatases, which induce several signalling pathways and activate cell cycle arrest, DNA reparation (chapter 13), and apoptosis (chapter 12).

Irradiation Induced Cell Cycle Checkpoints

In order to provide extra time for DNA reparation to occur, before the DNA damage becomes permanent during replication or mitosis, DNA damage checkpoints are activated following radiation. A range of sensors, mediators and signal transducing molecules involved in activation of the G1/S, intra-S, and G2/M-checkpoints are shared between these checkpoints. However, even though several components might be involved in all three checkpoints they can exert more prominent functions in one compared to another checkpoint (primary role in one, supporting role in another) [32]. Instead it is the effector molecules of the checkpoints that characterize and provide the different checkpoints with their unique identities.

Cyclin dependent kinases (Cdks) and cyclins are two protein families that are critical in the regulation and progression of the cell cycle machinery. Cdks are always present in the cell, but are inactive without cyclin partner. Cyclins are periodically expressed during the cell cycle and associates and activates the Cdks. Specific

Cyclin/Cdk complexes are formed during distinct phases of the cell cycle and coordinate the progression through these different phases by phosphorylation of specific target proteins. Inhibition of these complexes in response to DNA damage is the main strategy that DNA damage checkpoints rely on in order to induce cell cycle arrest in the G1/S, intra-S and G2/M phase of the cell cycle.

The G1/S Checkpoint

The G1/S checkpoint prevents cells with unrepaired DNA damage from entering the S-phase [64]. Following exposure of cells to ionizing radiation, ATM and ATR are activated (as above) and phosphorylates downstream target molecules, especially Chk2/Chk1 and p53, which initiates and maintains the G1/S arrest respectively [64, 71] (Fig. 14.2).

The signalling pathway that involves Chk2 and Chk1 are activated rapidly as they do not require de novo transcription. Chk2 and Chk1 phosphorylates Cdc25a, which leads to its inactivation by ubiquitination and rapid degradation by the proteasome as well as its exclusion from the nucleus [72–74]. Cdc25a is a phosphatase responsible for removing inhibitory phosphatases on Cdk2 and inactivation of Cdc25a consequently leads to accumulation of inactive Cdk2 [64]. Cdk2 is a cyclin dependent kinase and its activation is essential for S-phase entry and progression as the inactive form is unable to phosphorylate Cdc45 to initiate replication [64, 71, 75, 76].

This immediate arrest is followed by a transcription dependent, p53-mediated continuation of the G1/S arrest [75, 76, 80]. P53 participates in multiple cell cycle checkpoints (for review see [81]). Expression of p53 following DNA damage maintains the arrests at the G1/S transition [82, 83]. This pathway is mediated via activation of ATM (or ATR), which phosphorylates p53 on Ser15, or indirectly via Chk2 or Chk1 phosphorylation of p53 on Ser20 [28, 29, 80, 84]. These phosphorylations lead to an accumulation as well as an increased activity of p53 (for a more detailed description see chapter 12). Following activation, p53 mainly work as a transcription factor with transcriptional control over target genes, including p21, which is an inhibitor of cyclin-dependent kinases and a critical regulator of the G1/S arrest [75, 76, 80, 85, 86]. P21 binds and inhibits S-phase promoting Cdk/cyclin complexes including Cdk2-cyclin A, Cdk2-cyclin E, Cdk4-cyclin D and Cdk6-cyclin D [71]. Inhibition of these complexes prevents them from phosphorylating Rb, which inhibits the release of the transcription factor E2F. E2F is responsible for transcription of genes needed for S-phase entry including DNA polymerase, cyclin A and cyclin E (reviewed in [87]). P21 can also interact with PCNA, which prevents, or displaces subsequent binding of DNA polymerase delta to PCNA and replication [88]. Furthermore, ionizing radiation cause a rapid p53-independent arrest as a consequence of proteolysis of cyclin D1, which leads to a release of p21 from Cdk4 to inhibit Cdk2 [89].

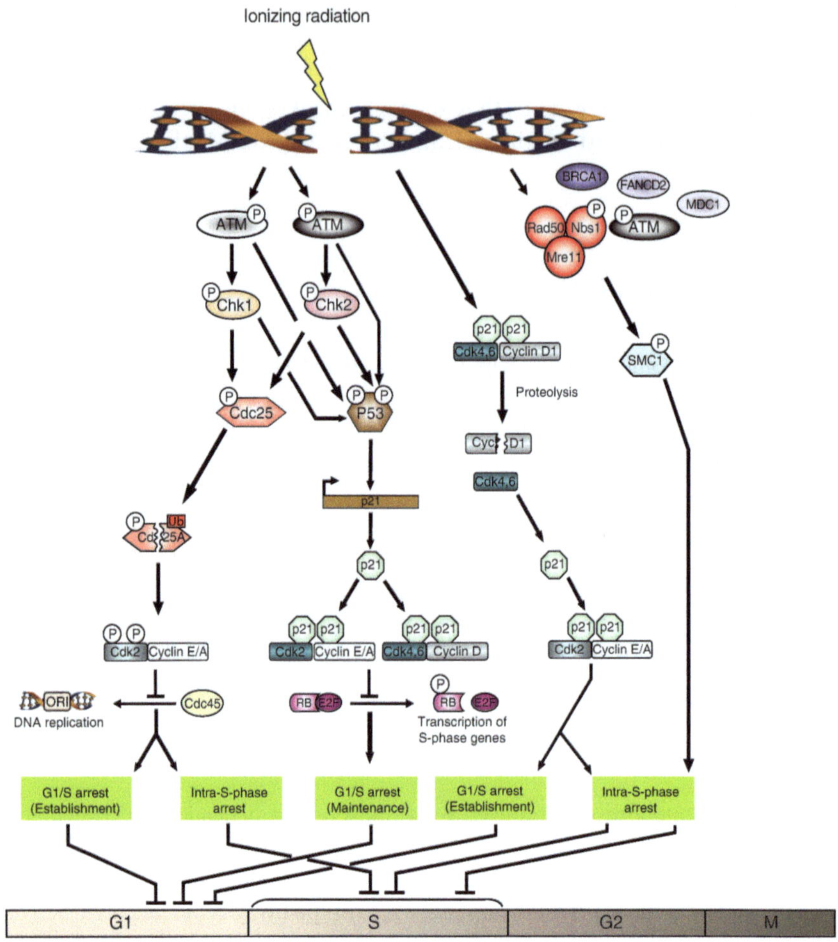

Fig. 14.2 A schematic overview of the multiple molecular pathways involved in the establishment and maintenance of the G1/S-phase arrest and the transient intra-S-phase arrest following exposure to ionizing radiation. See text for more details

The Intra-S-Phase Checkpoint

The intra-S-phase checkpoint is activated in response to DNA damage encountered during DNA replication. The S-phase DNA damage checkpoint inhibits DNA replication either by suppressing new replication origin firing or replication fork progression [90, 91]. The intra-S-phase checkpoint delays the progression through the S-phase in a transient manner and lacks the sustained maintenance phase of the cell cycle arrest, as compared to the G1/S and G2/M checkpoints. Consequently, if the damage is not repaired during this delay the cells enter G2 and in turn arrest at the G2/M checkpoint [92].

There is a significant overlap between components of G1/S and the intra-S-phase checkpoint. For instance, activation of the intra-S-phase checkpoints involves the ATM/ATR-Chk2/Chk1-Cdc25A-Cdk2/cyclin E(A)-Cdc45 cascade, which is also important for the rapid establishment of the G1-arrest [17, 72, 93–95] (Described more in detail in the previous section). Furthermore, also in S-phase cells, ionizing radiation cause a rapid p53-independent arrest as a consequence of proteolysis of cyclin D1, which leads to a release of p21 from Cdk4 to inhibit Cdk2 and later to an intra-S-phase arrest (Fig. 14.2).

Another parallel activation route that is crucial for the intra-S-phase checkpoint involves the ATM-mediated phosphorylation of Nbs1, one of the proteins in the MRN-complex [94]. The importance of the MRN-complex for intra-S-phase activation was first acknowledged when studies on NBS and ATLD cells demonstrated that these cells, unlike normal cells, continue DNA replication after treatment with ionizing radiation [72]. This phenomenon is known as radioresistant DNA synthesis (RDS) [96] and the cells appear to go through S-phase without any delay, which indicates an inability to activate the intra-S-phase checkpoint efficiently [97–99].

SMC1, a component of a protein-complex (cohesion) that is essential for the establishment of sister-chromatid cohesion during S-phase [100] is in turn phosphorylated in response to ionizing radiation in an ATM-Nbs1 dependent manner [101, 102]. Phosphorylation of Nbs1 and SMC1 following irradiation are important as interference with either of these two phosphorylations impairs the intra-S-phase checkpoint. Additionally, efficient phosphorylation of SMC1 also requires the presence of BRCA1 [92]. However, the details of the downstream mechanism that lead to inhibition of DNA synthesis are still not clear. Furthermore, in a recent study a new mechanism of the ATM-Nbs1 pathway to mediate the S-phase checkpoint in response to ionizing radiation was described [103]. This study suggested that the recruitment of MRN by RPA to replication-proximal sites is a major mechanism in the ATM-Nbs1 pathway to regulate the S-phase checkpoint.

Also MDC1, 53BP1 and FANCD2 seem to be involved in this pathway, as cells where these proteins are impaired was reported to have a defective intra-S-phase checkpoint [50, 104, 105].

Until recently it was generally believed that activation of the intra-S-phase checkpoint was independent of p53 [15, 32, 72, 75, 106]. However, these studies were performed using doses higher than 5 Gy and recently a novel low-dose-specific (below 2.5 Gy) p53-dependent but p21-independent S-phase DNA damage checkpoint was reported [107].

The G2/M Checkpoint

The G2/M checkpoint is activated in cells that have either acquired DNA damage in the G2-phase of the cell cycle, or retain DNA damage, inflicted in previous cell cycle phases, when they enter G2. This checkpoint is induced to prevent cells from entering mitosis with damaged DNA. Like with the G1/S arrest, the G2/M arrest is the result of mechanisms that rapidly initiate the arrest and those that maintain it. The immediate response operates via post-translational modifications, mainly phosphorylations of effector proteins, whereas the more delayed but sustained maintenance of the G2/M arrest also requires changes in transcription [17].

The main strategy for activation of the G2/M-arrest involves silencing of the critical mitosis-promoting Cdk1-Cyclin B complex. The first mechanism exploited for this purpose prevents activation of the Cdk1-Cyclin B complex by inactivating the Cdc25 family of proteins (Cdc25A, Cdc25B, Cdc25C) (reviewed in [108, 109]). Initially, Cdc25C was considered to be the most important member of the Cdc25 family for the G2/M DNA damage arrest [110]. However, Cdc25C and Cdc25B deficient cells display a normal G2/M checkpoint [110–112], implying that Cdc25A is also the most important Cdc25 family member for activation of the G2/M arrest. The Cdc25 family at normal conditions cooperates as positive regulators of the Cdk1-Cyclin B complex by removing inhibitory phosphatases on Cdk1, thereby promoting mitosis during normal division [109, 113]. Following exposure to ionizing radiation, Chk1 and Chk2 are phosphorylated and in turn phosphorylate several substrates including Cdc25 family members [109, 110]. Consequently, Cdc25A is degraded, by the same mechanism employed by the G1/S and intra-S-phase checkpoints [17, 74, 95, 113, 114]. Furthermore, hyperphosphorylation of Cdc25A by both Chk1 and Chk2 following exposure to ionizing radiation promotes an accelerated turnover via ubiquitin-mediated proteolysis of Cdc25A [115], which is mediated by β-TrCP [116]. Additionally, Chk1 phosphorylates Cdc25A at an extra C-terminal site, which directly inhibits the phosphatase activity [117]. Cdc25C is also phosphorylated by Chk1 and Chk2 in response to ionizing radiation, which promotes binding of 14-3-3 proteins and subsequent sequestration of Cdc25 in the cytoplasm and degradation via the ubiquitin-proteasome pathway [118–120].

One of the most important components for the maintenance of the G2/M arrest is p53. As with the G1/S checkpoint, the ATM/ATR-CHK2/CHK1 pathway becomes activated, which leads to phosphorylation and stabilization of p53. P53 in turn upregulates transcription of p21, 14-3-3, and Gadd45, which collectively inhibit Cdk1 and activation of the G2/M arrest (reviewed in [121]). 14-3-3 binds to the Cdk1-cyclinB complex and sequesters it in the cytoplasm where it cannot induce mitosis [121, 122]. P21 can inhibit the Cdk1-cyclin B complex directly [123–125] but can also inhibit Cdk2-cyclin A, Cdk2-cyclin E, Cdk4-cyclin D and Cdk6-cyclin D complexes and consequently phosphorylation of Rb, which inhibits the E2F-dependent transcription [71, 126]. Genome-wide analysis of E2F transcriptional regulation using a microarray imply that multiple genes important in mitosis are regulated by the RB-E2F pathway [127, 128]. E2F target genes, which are important in the G2/M regulation include Cdk1, cyclin A, and cyclin B1,2 [129]. Gadd45 inhibits the Cdk1-cyclinB complex activity by dissociating Cdk1 from cyclin B [121]. However, GADD45 may only be important for the activation of G2/M arrest following exposure to UV, but not ionizing radiation [130] (Fig. 14.3).

Finally, also the checkpoint mediators, including 53BP1, BRCA1 and MDC1 have been reported to contribute to the G2/M checkpoint response [50, 53, 105, 131, 132].

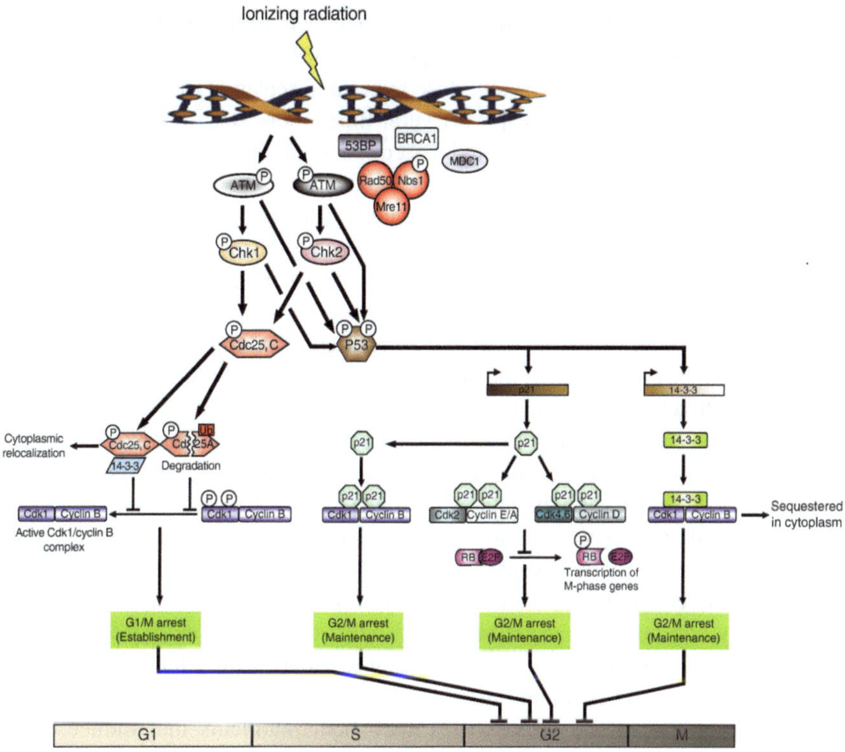

Fig. 14.3 A schematic overview of the multiple molecular pathways involved in the establishment and maintenance of the G2/M-phase arrest following exposure to ionizing radiation. See text for more details

Conclusions

A strict and highly coordinated activation of DNA damage checkpoints, including cell cycle arrest, DNA repair and proliferative cell death (apoptosis, senescence), in response to ionizing radiation is important to protect the integrity of the genome and prevent oncogenesis. As a consequence, alterations in these pathways increase the risk for cancer development and are frequently observed in malignancies (reviewed in [80, 133, 134]). The regulatory mechanisms in the G1/S checkpoint, including those governed by p53 and pRB, are major targets for tumor development [85, 86, 133, 135, 136]. Genetic analysis of human tumors has demonstrated that gene deletion, overexpression or point mutations that impair gene function of important G1/S checkpoint genes can be found in the major part of the cases, whereas such alterations are rarer for the G2/M checkpoint. Consequently, many tumors lose the ability to activate the G1/S checkpoint although they undergo G2/M arrest. One explanation for this, reported recently [137], may be that the G2/M checkpoint has a defined threshold of ~10–20 DSBs both for activation and maintenance and that due to this inefficiency it may not be necessary to abrogate the G2/M checkpoint for tumorigenesis [138]. Furthermore, this threshold has been implied as a reason for low-dose hyperradiosensitivity [139, 140], which is a phenomenon where cells display several times more sensitivity to low doses of radiation (~0.2 Gy) than expected based on data obtained at higher doses (chapter 19).

New molecular radiosensitizers targeting cell cycle checkpoint controls and taking advantage of differences in genotype between malignant and normal cells are currently being evaluated [141]. These radiosensitizers include inhibitors of ATM, of Chk1, of CDKs, and of p53 [141, 142].

As the G1/S-checkpoint is frequently impaired in malignancies, the G2/M-checkpoint can be considered as the key guardian of the cancer cell genome and has become an attractive therapeutic target for cancer therapy (reviewed in [143]). Following exposure to ionizing radiation, G2/M checkpoint abrogation prevents the cancer cells from DNA reparation and also induces a premature mitosis. This promotes cell cycle progression, which results in the induction of cell death via mitotic catastrophe and apoptosis. Currently, several Chk1 inhibitors are in advanced preclinical and/or early clinical development [143].

A better understanding of how the genotype predisposes a cell to respond in a specific way and how this gears malignant cells and normal cells into different fates, following exposure to ionizing radiation can help us design better therapies. Furthermore, using specific inhibitors that take advantage of cell cycle defects in cancer cells and combine them with established treatments that induce DNA damage, including ionizing radiation, can prove to be efficient for eradicating tumors.

Acknowledgements Financial support from the Swedish Cancer Society, the County of Västerbotten and the Medical Faculty at Umeå University for research related to the content of this chapter is acknowledged.

References

1. Hoeijmakers JH. Genome maintenance mechanisms for preventing cancer. Nature 2001; 411(6835):366–74.
2. Khanna KK, Jackson SP. DNA double-strand breaks: signaling, repair and the cancer connection. Nature Genetics 2001; 27(3):247–54.
3. Nias AHW. Radiobiology. New York: Wiley, 1998.
4. Ward JF. Biochemistry of DNA lesions. Radiation Research 1985; 8(Suppl):S103–11.
5. Iliakis G, Wang Y, Guan J, Wang H. DNA damage checkpoint control in cells exposed to ionizing radiation. Oncogene 2003; 22(37):5834–47.
6. Nyberg KA, Michelson RJ, Putnam CW, Weinert TA. Toward maintaining the genome: DNA damage and replication checkpoints. Annual Review of Genetics 2002; 36:617–56.
7. Zhou BB, Elledge SJ. The DNA damage response: putting checkpoints in perspective. Nature 2000; 408(6811):433–9.
8. Tsukamoto Y, Ikeda H. Double-strand break repair mediated by DNA end-joining. Genes Cells 1998; 3(3):135–44.

9. Prise KM, Schettino G, Folkard M, Held KD. New insights on cell death from radiation exposure. The Lancet Oncology 2005; 6(7):520–8.
10. Huang LC, Clarkin KC, Wahl GM. Sensitivity and selectivity of the DNA damage sensor responsible for activating p53-dependent G1 arrest. Proceedings of the National Academy of Sciences of the United States of America 1996; 93(10):4827–32.
11. Rich T, Allen RL, Wyllie AH. Defying death after DNA damage. Nature 2000; 407(6805):777–83.
12. Erenpreisa J, Cragg MS. Cancer: a matter of life cycle? Cell Biology International 2007; 31(12):1507–10.
13. Ganem NJ, Storchova Z, Pellman D. Tetraploidy, aneuploidy and cancer. Current Opinion in Genetics & Development 2007; 17(2):157–62.
14. Storchova Z, Pellman D. From polyploidy to aneuploidy, genome instability and cancer. Nature Reviews. Molecular Cell Biology 2004; 5(1):45–54.
15. Shiloh Y. ATM and related protein kinases: safeguarding genome integrity. Nature Reviews 2003; 3(3):155–68.
16. Bakkenist CJ, Kastan MB. DNA damage activates ATM through intermolecular autophosphorylation and dimer dissociation. Nature 2003; 421(6922):499–506.
17. Lukas J, Lukas C, Bartek J. Mammalian cell cycle checkpoints: signalling pathways and their organization in space and time. DNA Repair 2004; 3(8–9):997–1007.
18. Su TT. Cellular responses to DNA damage: one signal, multiple choices. Annual Review of Genetics 2006; 40:187–208.
19. Lavin MF, Shiloh Y. The genetic defect in ataxia-telangiectasia. Annual Review of Immunology 1997; 15:177–202.
20. Brown EJ, Baltimore D. ATR disruption leads to chromosomal fragmentation and early embryonic lethality. Genes & Development 2000; 14(4):397–402.
21. Brown EJ, Baltimore D. Essential and dispensable roles of ATR in cell cycle arrest and genome maintenance. Genes & Development 2003; 17(5):615–28.
22. Cortez D, Guntuku S, Qin J, Elledge SJ. ATR and ATRIP: partners in checkpoint signaling. Science (New York) 2001; 294(5547):1713–6.
23. Houtgraaf JH, Versmissen J, van der Giessen WJ. A concise review of DNA damage checkpoints and repair in mammalian cells. Cardiovascular Revascularization Medicine 2006; 7(3):165–72.
24. Collis SJ, DeWeese TL, Jeggo PA, Parker AR. The life and death of DNA-PK. Oncogene 2005; 24(6):949–61.
25. Sakata K, Someya M, Matsumoto Y, Hareyama M. Ability to repair DNA double-strand breaks related to cancer susceptibility and radiosensitivity. Radiation Medicine 2007; 25(9):433–8.
26. Bakkenist CJ, Kastan MB. Initiating cellular stress responses. Cell 2004; 118(1):9–17.
27. Kastan MB, Lim DS, Kim ST, Yang D. ATM–a key determinant of multiple cellular responses to irradiation. Acta Oncologica (Stockholm, Sweden) 2001; 40(6):686–8.
28. Banin S, Moyal L, Shieh S, et al. Enhanced phosphorylation of p53 by ATM in response to DNA damage. Science (New York) 1998; 281(5383):1674–7.
29. Canman CE, Lim DS, Cimprich KA, et al. Activation of the ATM kinase by ionizing radiation and phosphorylation of p53. Science (New York) 1998; 281(5383):1677–9.
30. Chan DW, Gately DP, Urban S, Galloway AM, Lees-Miller SP, Yen T, Allalunis-Turner J. Lack of correlation between ATM protein expression and tumour cell radiosensitivity. International Journal of Radiation Biology 1998; 74(2):217–24.
31. Lakin ND, Weber P, Stankovic T, Rottinghaus ST, Taylor AM, Jackson SP. Analysis of the ATM protein in wild-type and ataxia telangiectasia cells. Oncogene 1996; 13(12):2707–16.
32. Abraham RT. Cell cycle checkpoint signaling through the ATM and ATR kinases. Genes & Development 2001; 15(17):2177–96.
33. Paulsen RD, Cimprich KA. The ATR pathway: fine-tuning the fork. DNA Repair 2007; 6(7):953–66.

34. Zou L. Single- and double-stranded DNA: building a trigger of ATR-mediated DNA damage response. Genes & Development 2007; 21(8):879–85.
35. Kozlov SV, Graham ME, Peng C, Chen P, Robinson PJ, Lavin MF. Involvement of novel autophosphorylation sites in ATM activation. The EMBO Journal 2006; 25(15):3504–14.
36. Falck J, Coates J, Jackson SP. Conserved modes of recruitment of ATM, ATR and DNA-PKcs to sites of DNA damage. Nature 2005; 434(7033):605–11.
37. You Z, Chahwan C, Bailis J, Hunter T, Russell P. ATM activation and its recruitment to damaged DNA require binding to the C terminus of Nbs1. Molecular and Cellular Biology 2005; 25(13):5363–79.
38. Bartek J, Lukas J. DNA damage checkpoints: from initiation to recovery or adaptation. Current Opinion in Cell Biology 2007; 19(2):238–45.
39. Pilch DR, Sedelnikova OA, Redon C, Celeste A, Nussenzweig A, Bonner WM. Characteristics of gamma-H2AX foci at DNA double-strand breaks sites. Biochemistry and Cell Biology = Biochimie et biologie cellulaire 2003; 81(3):123–9.
40. Rogakou EP, Boon C, Redon C, Bonner WM. Megabase chromatin domains involved in DNA double-strand breaks in vivo. The Journal of Cell Biology 1999; 146(5):905–16.
41. Rogakou EP, Pilch DR, Orr AH, Ivanova VS, Bonner WM. DNA double-stranded breaks induce histone H2AX phosphorylation on serine 139. The Journal of Biological Chemistry 1998; 273(10):5858–68.
42. Fernandez-Capetillo O, Celeste A, Nussenzweig A. Focusing on foci: H2AX and the recruitment of DNA-damage response factors. Cell Cycle (Georgetown, TX) 2003; 2(5):426–7.
43. Stucki M, Clapperton JA, Mohammad D, Yaffe MB, Smerdon SJ, Jackson SP. MDC1 directly binds phosphorylated histone H2AX to regulate cellular responses to DNA double-strand breaks. Cell 2005; 123(7):1213–26.
44. Stucki M, Jackson SP. GammaH2AX and MDC1: anchoring the DNA-damage-response machinery to broken chromosomes. DNA Repair 2006; 5(5):534–43.
45. Bekker-Jensen S, Lukas C, Kitagawa R, Melander F, Kastan MB, Bartek J, Lukas J. Spatial organization of the mammalian genome surveillance machinery in response to DNA strand breaks. The Journal of Cell Biology 2006; 173(2):195–206.
46. Lukas C, Melander F, Stucki M, et al. Mdc1 couples DNA double-strand break recognition by Nbs1 with its H2AX-dependent chromatin retention. The EMBO Journal 2004; 23(13):2674–83.
47. Carney JP, Maser RS, Olivares H, et al. The hMre11/hRad50 protein complex and Nijmegen breakage syndrome: linkage of double-strand break repair to the cellular DNA damage response. Cell 1998; 93(3):477–86.
48. Schultz LB, Chehab NH, Malikzay A, Halazonetis TD. p53 binding protein 1 (53BP1) is an early participant in the cellular response to DNA double-strand breaks. The Journal of Cell Biology 2000; 151(7):1381–90.
49. Scully R, Chen J, Ochs RL, Keegan K, Hoekstra M, Feunteun J, Livingston DM. Dynamic changes of BRCA1 subnuclear location and phosphorylation state are initiated by DNA damage. Cell 1997; 90(3):425–35.
50. Stewart GS, Wang B, Bignell CR, Taylor AM, Elledge SJ. MDC1 is a mediator of the mammalian DNA damage checkpoint. Nature 2003; 421(6926):961–6.
51. Yamane K, Wu X, Chen J. A DNA damage-regulated BRCT-containing protein, TopBP1, is required for cell survival. Molecular and Cellular Biology 2002; 22(2):555–66.
52. Celeste A, Fernandez-Capetillo O, Kruhlak MJ, et al. Histone H2AX phosphorylation is dispensable for the initial recognition of DNA breaks. Nature Cell Biology 2003; 5(7):675–9.
53. Fernandez-Capetillo O, Chen HT, Celeste A, et al. DNA damage-induced G2-M checkpoint activation by histone H2AX and 53BP1. Nature Cell Biology 2002; 4(12):993–7.
54. Kruhlak MJ, Celeste A, Nussenzweig A. Spatio-temporal dynamics of chromatin containing DNA breaks. Cell Cycle (Georgetown, TX) 2006; 5(17):1910–2.
55. Adams KE, Medhurst AL, Dart DA, Lakin ND. Recruitment of ATR to sites of ionising radiation-induced DNA damage requires ATM and components of the MRN protein complex. Oncogene 2006; 25(28):3894–904.

56. Chen L, Nievera C, Lee AY, Wu X. Cell cycle-dependent complex formation of BRCA1/CtIP/MRN is important for DNA double-strand break repair. The Journal of Biological Chemistry 2008; 283(12):7713–20.
57. Myers JS, Cortez D. Rapid activation of ATR by ionizing radiation requires ATM and Mre11. The Journal of Biological Chemistry 2006; 281(14):9346–50.
58. Venclovas C, Thelen MP. Structure-based predictions of Rad1, Rad9, Hus1 and Rad17 participation in sliding clamp and clamp-loading complexes. Nucleic Acids Research 2000; 28(13):2481–93.
59. Bermudez VP, Lindsey-Boltz LA, Cesare AJ, Maniwa Y, Griffith JD, Hurwitz J, Sancar A. Loading of the human 9-1-1 checkpoint complex onto DNA by the checkpoint clamp loader hRad17-replication factor C complex in vitro. Proceedings of the National Academy of Sciences of the United States of America 2003; 100(4):1633–8.
60. Ellison V, Stillman B. Biochemical characterization of DNA damage checkpoint complexes: clamp loader and clamp complexes with specificity for 5 recessed DNA. PLoS Biology 2003; 1(2):E33.
61. Majka J, Chung BY, Burgers PM. Requirement for ATP by the DNA damage checkpoint clamp loader. The Journal of Biological Chemistry 2004; 279(20):20921–6.
62. Cortez D, Wang Y, Qin J, Elledge SJ. Requirement of ATM-dependent phosphorylation of brca1 in the DNA damage response to double-strand breaks. Science (New York) 1999; 286(5442):1162–6.
63. Lim DS, Kim ST, Xu B, Maser RS, Lin J, Petrini JH, Kastan MB. ATM phosphorylates p95/nbs1 in an S-phase checkpoint pathway. Nature 2000; 404(6778):613–7.
64. Sancar A, Lindsey-Boltz LA, Unsal Kacmaz K, Linn S. Molecular mechanisms of mammalian DNA repair and the DNA damage checkpoints. Annual Review of Biochemistry 2004; 73:39–85.
65. McGowan CH. Checking in on Cds1 (Chk2): a checkpoint kinase and tumor suppressor. Bioessays 2002; 24(6):502–11.
66. Melo J, Toczyski D. A unified view of the DNA-damage checkpoint. Current Opinion in Cell Biology 2002; 14(2):237–45.
67. Rhind N, Russell P. Chk1 and Cds1: linchpins of the DNA damage and replication checkpoint pathways. Journal of Cell Science 2000; 113(Pt 22):3889–96.
68. Hirao A, Kong YY, Matsuoka S, et al. DNA damage-induced activation of p53 by the checkpoint kinase Chk2. Science (New York) 2000; 287(5459):1824–7.
69. Matsuoka S, Rotman G, Ogawa A, Shiloh Y, Tamai K, Elledge SJ. Ataxia telangiectasia-mutated phosphorylates Chk2 in vivo and in vitro. Proceedings of the National Academy of Sciences of the United States of America 2000; 97(19):10389–94.
70. Zhao H, Piwnica-Worms H. ATR-mediated checkpoint pathways regulate phosphorylation and activation of human Chk1. Molecular and Cellular Biology 2001; 21(13):4129–39.
71. Cann KL, Hicks GG. Regulation of the cellular DNA double-strand break response. Biochemistry and Cell Biology = Biochimie et biologie cellulaire 2007; 85(6):663–74.
72. Falck J, Mailand N, Syljuasen RG, Bartek J, Lukas J. The ATM-Chk2-Cdc25A checkpoint pathway guards against radioresistant DNA synthesis. Nature 2001; 410(6830):842–7.
73. Molinari M, Mercurio C, Dominguez J, Goubin F, Draetta GF. Human Cdc25 A inactivation in response to S phase inhibition and its role in preventing premature mitosis. EMBO Reports 2000; 1(1):71–9.
74. Zhao H, Watkins JL, Piwnica-Worms H. Disruption of the checkpoint kinase 1/cell division cycle 25A pathway abrogates ionizing radiation-induced S and G2 checkpoints. Proceedings of the National Academy of Sciences of the United States of America 2002; 99(23):14795–800.
75. Bartek J, Lukas J. Mammalian G1- and S-phase checkpoints in response to DNA damage. Current Opinion in Cell Biology 2001; 13(6):738–47.
76. Bartek J, Lukas J. Pathways governing G1/S transition and their response to DNA damage. FEBS Letters 2001; 490(3):117–22.
77. Chen Y, Sanchez Y. Chk1 in the DNA damage response: conserved roles from yeasts to mammals. DNA Repair 2004; 3(8–9):1025–32.

78. Cuadrado M, Martinez-Pastor B, Murga M, Toledo LI, Gutierrez-Martinez P, Lopez E, Fernandez-Capetillo O. ATM regulates ATR chromatin loading in response to DNA double-strand breaks. The Journal of Experimental Medicine 2006; 203(2):297–303.
79. Jazayeri A, Falck J, Lukas C, Bartek J, Smith GC, Lukas J, Jackson SP. ATM- and cell cycle-dependent regulation of ATR in response to DNA double-strand breaks. Nature Cell Biology 2006; 8(1):37–45.
80. Kastan MB, Bartek J. Cell-cycle checkpoints and cancer. Nature 2004; 432(7015):316–23.
81. Giono LE, Manfredi JJ. The p53 tumor suppressor participates in multiple cell cycle checkpoints. Journal of Cellular Physiology 2006; 209(1):13–20.
82. Kastan MB, Onyekwere O, Sidransky D, Vogelstein B, Craig RW. Participation of p53 protein in the cellular response to DNA damage. Cancer Research 1991; 51(23 Pt 1):6304–11.
83. Lin D, Shields MT, Ullrich SJ, Appella E, Mercer WE. Growth arrest induced by wild-type p53 protein blocks cells prior to or near the restriction point in late G1 phase. Proceedings of the National Academy of Sciences of the United States of America 1992; 89(19):9210–4.
84. Chehab NH, Malikzay A, Stavridi ES, Halazonetis TD. Phosphorylation of Ser-20 mediates stabilization of human p53 in response to DNA damage. Proceedings of the National Academy of Sciences of the United States of America 1999; 96(24):13777–82.
85. Kastan MB, Lim DS. The many substrates and functions of ATM. Nature Reviews. Molecular Cell Biology 2000; 1(3):179–86.
86. Wahl GM, Carr AM. The evolution of diverse biological responses to DNA damage: insights from yeast and p53. Nature Cell Biology 2001; 3(12):E277–86.
87. Sun A, Bagella L, Tutton S, Romano G, Giordano A. From G0 to S phase: a view of the roles played by the retinoblastoma (Rb) family members in the Rb-E2F pathway. Journal of Cellular Biochemistry 2007; 102(6):1400–4.
88. Cazzalini O, Perucca P, Riva F, Stivala LA, Bianchi L, Vannini V, Ducommun B, Prosperi E. p21CDKN1A does not interfere with loading of PCNA at DNA replication sites, but inhibits subsequent binding of DNA polymerase delta at the G1/S phase transition. Cell Cycle (Georgetown, TX) 2003; 2(6):596–603.
89. Agami R, Bernards R. Distinct initiation and maintenance mechanisms cooperate to induce G1 cell cycle arrest in response to DNA damage. Cell 2000; 102(1):55–66.
90. Boddy MN, Russell P. DNA replication checkpoint. Current Biology 2001; 11(23):R953–6.
91. Osborn AJ, Elledge SJ, Zou L. Checking on the fork: the DNA-replication stress-response pathway. Trends in Cell Biology 2002; 12(11):509–16.
92. Bartek J, Lukas C, Lukas J. Checking on DNA damage in S phase. Nature Reviews. Molecular Cell Biology 2004; 5(10):792–804.
93. Costanzo V, Robertson K, Ying CY, Kim E, Avvedimento E, Gottesman M, Grieco D, Gautier J. Reconstitution of an ATM-dependent checkpoint that inhibits chromosomal DNA replication following DNA damage. Molecular Cell 2000; 6(3):649–59.
94. Falck J, Petrini JH, Williams BR, Lukas J, Bartek J. The DNA damage-dependent intra-S phase checkpoint is regulated by parallel pathways. Nature Genetics 2002; 30(3):290–4.
95. Mailand N, Falck J, Lukas C, Syljuasen RG, Welcker M, Bartek J, Lukas J. Rapid destruction of human Cdc25A in response to DNA damage. Science (New York) 2000; 288(5470):1425–9.
96. Painter RB, Young BR. Radiosensitivity in ataxia-telangiectasia: a new explanation. Proceedings of the National Academy of Sciences of the United States of America 1980; 77(12):7315–7.
97. Shiloh Y. Ataxia-telangiectasia and the Nijmegen breakage syndrome: related disorders but genes apart. Annual Review of Genetics 1997; 31:635–62.
98. Stewart GS, Maser RS, Stankovic T, et al. The DNA double-strand break repair gene hMRE11 is mutated in individuals with an ataxia-telangiectasia-like disorder. Cell 1999; 99(6):577–87.
99. Taalman RD, Jaspers NG, Scheres JM, de Wit J, Hustinx TW. Hypersensitivity to ionizing radiation, in vitro, in a new chromosomal breakage disorder, the Nijmegen Breakage Syndrome. Mutation Research 1983; 112(1):23–32.

100. Hirano T. The ABCs of SMC proteins: two-armed ATPases for chromosome condensation, cohesion, and repair. Genes & Development 2002; 16(4):399–414.
101. Kim ST, Xu B, Kastan MB. Involvement of the cohesin protein, Smc1, in Atm-dependent and independent responses to DNA damage. Genes & Development 2002; 16(5):560–70.
102. Yazdi PT, Wang Y, Zhao S, Patel N, Lee EY, Qin J. SMC1 is a downstream effector in the ATM/NBS1 branch of the human S-phase checkpoint. Genes & Development 2002; 16(5):571–82.
103. Olson E, Nievera CJ, Liu E, Lee AY, Chen L, Wu X. The Mre11 complex mediates the S-phase checkpoint through an interaction with replication protein A. Molecular and Cellular Biology 2007; 27(17):6053–67.
104. Nakanishi K, Taniguchi T, Ranganathan V, et al. Interaction of FANCD2 and NBS1 in the DNA damage response. Nature Cell Biology 2002; 4(12):913–20.
105. Wang B, Matsuoka S, Carpenter PB, Elledge SJ. 53BP1, a mediator of the DNA damage checkpoint. Science (New York) 2002; 298(5597):1435–8.
106. Merrick CJ, Jackson D, Diffley JF. Visualization of altered replication dynamics after DNA damage in human cells. Journal of Biological Chemistry 2004; 279(19):20067–75.
107. Shimura T, Toyoshima M, Adiga SK, Kunoh T, Nagai H, Shimizu N, Inoue M, Niwa O. Suppression of replication fork progression in low-dose-specific p53-dependent S-phase DNA damage checkpoint. Oncogene 2006; 25(44):5921–32.
108. Boutros R, Lobjois V, Ducommun B. CDC25 phosphatases in cancer cells: key players? Good targets? Nature Reviews 2007; 7(7):495–507.
109. Donzelli M, Draetta GF. Regulating mammalian checkpoints through Cdc25 inactivation. EMBO Reports 2003; 4(7):671–7.
110. Niida H, Nakanishi M. DNA damage checkpoints in mammals. Mutagenesis 2006; 21(1):3–9.
111. Chen MS, Hurov J, White LS, Woodford-Thomas T, Piwnica-Worms H. Absence of apparent phenotype in mice lacking Cdc25C protein phosphatase. Molecular and Cellular Biology 2001; 21(12):3853–61.
112. Lincoln AJ, Wickramasinghe D, Stein P, Schultz RM, Palko ME, De Miguel MP, Tessarollo L, Donovan PJ. Cdc25b phosphatase is required for resumption of meiosis during oocyte maturation. Nature Genetics 2002; 30(4):446–9.
113. Mailand N, Podtelejnikov AV, Groth A, Mann M, Bartek J, Lukas J. Regulation of G(2)/M events by Cdc25A through phosphorylation-dependent modulation of its stability. The EMBO Journal 2002; 21(21):5911–20.
114. Xiao Z, Chen Z, Gunasekera AH, Sowin TJ, Rosenberg SH, Fesik S, Zhang H. Chk1 mediates S and G2 arrests through Cdc25A degradation in response to DNA-damaging agents. Journal of Biological Chemistry 2003; 278(24):21767–73.
115. Sorensen CS, Syljuasen RG, Falck J, et al. Chk1 regulates the S phase checkpoint by coupling the physiological turnover and ionizing radiation-induced accelerated proteolysis of Cdc25A. Cancer Cell 2003; 3(3):247–58.
116. Busino L, Donzelli M, Chiesa M, et al. Degradation of Cdc25A by beta-TrCP during S phase and in response to DNA damage. Nature 2003; 426(6962):87–91.
117. Uto K, Inoue D, Shimuta K, Nakajo N, Sagata N. Chk1, but not Chk2, inhibits Cdc25 phosphatases by a novel common mechanism. The EMBO Journal 2004; 23(16):3386–96.
118. Matsuoka S, Huang M, Elledge SJ. Linkage of ATM to cell cycle regulation by the Chk2 protein kinase. Science (New York) 1998; 282(5395):1893–7.
119. Peng CY, Graves PR, Thoma RS, Wu Z, Shaw AS, Piwnica-Worms H. Mitotic and G2 checkpoint control: regulation of 14-3-3 protein binding by phosphorylation of Cdc25C on serine-216. Science (New York) 1997; 277(5331):1501–5.
120. Sanchez Y, Wong C, Thoma RS, Richman R, Wu Z, Piwnica-Worms H, Elledge SJ. Conservation of the Chk1 checkpoint pathway in mammals: linkage of DNA damage to Cdk regulation through Cdc25. Science (New York) 1997; 277(5331):1497–501.
121. Taylor WR, Stark GR. Regulation of the G2/M transition by p53. Oncogene 2001; 20(15):1803–15.

122. Chan TA, Hermeking H, Lengauer C, Kinzler KW, Vogelstein B. 14-3-3Sigma is required to prevent mitotic catastrophe after DNA damage. Nature 1999; 401(6753):616–20.
123. Baus F, Gire V, Fisher D, Piette J, Dulic V. Permanent cell cycle exit in G2 phase after DNA damage in normal human fibroblasts. The EMBO Journal 2003; 22(15):3992–4002.
124. Obaya AJ, Sedivy JM. Regulation of cyclin-Cdk activity in mammalian cells. Cellular and Molecular Life Sciences 2002; 59(1):126–42.
125. Xiong Y, Hannon GJ, Zhang H, Casso D, Kobayashi R, Beach D. p21 is a universal inhibitor of cyclin kinases. Nature 1993; 366(6456):701–4.
126. Stark GR, Taylor WR. Analyzing the G2/M checkpoint. Methods in Molecular Biology (Clifton, NJ) 2004; 280:51–82.
127. Ishida S, Huang E, Zuzan H, Spang R, Leone G, West M, Nevins JR. Role for E2F in control of both DNA replication and mitotic functions as revealed from DNA microarray analysis. Molecular and Cellular Biology 2001; 21(14):4684–99.
128. Ren B, Cam H, Takahashi Y, Volkert T, Terragni J, Young RA, Dynlacht BD. E2F integrates cell cycle progression with DNA repair, replication, and G(2)/M checkpoints. Genes & Development 2002; 16(2):245–56.
129. DeGregori J. The genetics of the E2F family of transcription factors: shared functions and unique roles. Biochimica et biophysica acta 2002; 1602(2):131–50.
130. Wang XW, Zhan Q, Coursen JD, et al. GADD45 induction of a G2/M cell cycle checkpoint. Proceedings of the National Academy of Sciences of the United States of America 1999; 96(7):3706–11.
131. DiTullio RA, Jr., Mochan TA, Venere M, Bartkova J, Sehested M, Bartek J, Halazonetis TD. 53BP1 functions in an ATM-dependent checkpoint pathway that is constitutively activated in human cancer. Nature Cell Biology 2002; 4(12):998–1002.
132. Xu B, Kim S, Kastan MB. Involvement of Brca1 in S-phase and G(2)-phase checkpoints after ionizing irradiation. Molecular and Cellular Biology 2001; 21(10):3445–50.
133. Molinari M. Cell cycle checkpoints and their inactivation in human cancer. Cell Proliferation 2000; 33(5):261–74.
134. Shimada M, Nakanishi M. DNA damage checkpoints and cancer. Journal of Molecular Histology 2006; 37(5–7):253–60.
135. Bartek J, Bartkova J, Lukas J. The retinoblastoma protein pathway in cell cycle control and cancer. Experimental Cell Research 1997; 237(1):1–6.
136. Sherr CJ, McCormick F. The RB and p53 pathways in cancer. Cancer Cell 2002; 2(2):103–12.
137. Deckbar D, Birraux J, Krempler A, et al. Chromosome breakage after G2 checkpoint release. The Journal of Cell Biology 2007; 176(6):749–55.
138. Lobrich M, Jeggo PA. The impact of a negligent G2/M checkpoint on genomic instability and cancer induction. Nature Reviews 2007; 7(11):861–9.
139. Marples B, Wouters BG, Collis SJ, Chalmers AJ, Joiner MC. Low-dose hyper-radiosensitivity: a consequence of ineffective cell cycle arrest of radiation-damaged G2-phase cells. Radiation Research 2004; 161(3):247–55.
140. Short SC, Woodcock M, Marples B, Joiner MC. Effects of cell cycle phase on low-dose hyper-radiosensitivity. International Journal of Radiation Biology 2003; 79(2):99–105.
141. Choudhury A, Cuddihy A, Bristow RG. Radiation and new molecular agents part I: targeting ATM-ATR checkpoints, DNA repair, and the proteasome. Seminars in Radiation Oncology 2006; 16(1):51–8.
142. Gasser S. DNA damage response and development of targeted cancer treatments. Annals of Medicine 2007; 39(6):457–64.
143. Bucher N, Britten CD. G2 checkpoint abrogation and checkpoint kinase-1 targeting in the treatment of cancer. British Journal of Cancer 2008; 98(3):523–8.

Chapter 15
Cancer Stem Cells and Radiation

David Eriksson, Katrine Riklund, Lennart Johansson, and Torgny Stigbrand

Summary Cancer stem cells have recently been proposed to play a significant role in the initiation and propagation of tumor cells. They display indefinite self-renewal capacity and multilineage potential as well as an excessive proliferation capacity. Cancer stem cells are quiescent with low mitotic frequencies. They seem to be relatively radioresistant and have been demonstrated to increase in relative amount following radiotherapy. The stem cells express a number of marker molecules, which hopefully can be used for therapeutic purposes. These possibilities will be discussed in this chapter.

The Cancer Stem Cell Hypothesis

All malignant cells within the same tumor have been considered able to generate new tumors by clonal expansion of the transformed cells (stochastic model). The heterogeneity of cells displaying different stages of development (with divergent nuclear morphologies and differentiation features) often seen within a tumor has been explained by microenvironmental influence and genomic instability. However, new findings demonstrate that not all cells within a tumor are equally able to initiate new tumors. Only small subsets of cells have been proposed to be able to do so at a high incidence (hierarchic theory). This theory has been important for establishing the cancer stem cell model. This model was envisioned already in 1855 by Rudolph Virchow, when he proposed that tumor cells arise from embryonic-like cells [1]. Today, with new technologies and techniques for the identification, isolation and characterization of subpopulations of cells within a tumor, renewed and increased interest has been focused on this research.

The existence of cancer stem cells is today generally accepted, but still discussed [2–4]. Growing evidence for the importance of cancer stem cells (CSCs), also referred to as tumor-initiating cells (TICs) (for reviews see [5–7]), for tumor

Departments of Immunology, Diagnostic Radiology and Radiophysics, University of Umeå, SE-90185 Umeå, Sweden

T. Stigbrand et al. (eds.) *Targeted Radionuclide Tumor Therapy*,

development and progression, is today supported by reports for several malignant diseases including leukemia and solid tumors from breast, colon, brain and prostate [5, 8]. The cancer stem cell model furthermore is a complementary concept that helps explaining the heterogenous cell populations in a tumor as a consequence of a continuously operating differentiation route.

The term cancer stem cells have generated some misunderstandings since it can be interpreted that such cells are derived from the stem cells of the corresponding normal tissue. Whether cancer stem cells develop from normal tissue stem cells, which have acquired genetic and epigenetic changes to acquire tumorigenicity or whether tumor stem cells are derived from differentiated cells, which have reacquired stem cell characteristics, is not established and both mechanisms may occur [9–11] and may depend on organ of origin [12]. However, considering the low mutation rate of somatic cells and that tumorigenesis requires multiple mutations, it is conceivable that cancer stem cells are more likely to be derived from adult stem cells, which have higher capacity to proliferate and are long-lived [13, 14]. Repeated cell divisions allow accumulation of mutations during their lifespan.

The consensus definition of a cancer stem cell has been proposed to be a cell within a tumor that possess the capacity to self-renew and to cause the heterogeneous lineages of cancer cells that comprise the tumor [12].

Analogous to adult stem cells found in normal tissues, cancer stem cells are undifferentiated and have indefinite self-renewal capacity and multilineage potential as well as an excessive proliferation capacity [12, 15, 16]. A self renewing cell division produces two identical daughter cells, which retain the stem cell potential of the parental cell (symmetric division) or one daughter stem cell and one more differentiated progenitor cell (asymmetric division), consequently generating a heterogeneous cell population [17, 18]. As a result, cancer stem cells will drive and maintain tumor progression [19, 20] as they have the potential to generate tumor cells without self-renewing capacity, which are responsible for generating the main tumor mass and the heterogenous cell population found within the tumor. Recently, the potential role of cancer stem cells as key players in the metastatic process has been reviewed and metastatic cells were found to share many similarities with normal stem cells [21]. This include an unlimited capacity for self-renewal, requirements for specific niches or microenvironment to grow, use of the SDF-1/CXCR4 axis for migration, enhanced resistance to apoptosis and increased capacity for drug resistance [21].

Cancer Stem Cell Identification

Evidences for the cancer stem cell hypothesis (self-renewal and lineage capacity) are mainly obtained from studies in which the enriched cancer stem cell subgroup, isolated by use of specific stem cell markers, was able to form new tumors when transplanted into immunodeficient mice. Typically, isolated tumor cells are transplanted into an orthotopic site in a NOD/SCID mouse, which is analysed over time for tumor formation. To assay for self-renewal capacity, cells are subsequently isolated from the tumors that are formed and grafted into another immunocompromised mouse.

The range of cancer stem cell markers are rapidly increasing and differ between cancer forms and so far none of the markers used is exclusively expressed by stem cells (Table 15.1).

The first distinct evidence for the cancer stem cell hypothesis was provided by Lapidot et al. in 1994, when they observed that AML cells, fractionated into subgroups based on their cell surface markers, displayed different abilities to engraft SCID mice and to produce large numbers of colony-forming progenitor cells [22]. The subgroup of cells that displayed stem-like properties was characterised by their cell surface phenotype, which was CD34+ CD38-, similar to that typical of normal human primitive hematopoietic progenitors [22, 23].

Lately, the initial findings of cancer stem cells in leukemia got support from the existence of cancer stem cells also present in increasing numbers of solid tumors [24–37]. Extensive efforts have been directed towards identifying stem cell markers also for solid tumors, but this challenge has been considerable, since cells within solid tumors are less accessible and little is known about their normal tissue developmental hierarchies compared to those of the hematopoietic system. Furthermore, properties that are useful for identification, isolation and characterisation of cancer stem cells from one form of solid malignancy are often individual and not the same for cancer stem cells from different tumor types. The first solid cancer stem-like cells were identified and isolated from primary breast cancer tumors based upon their CD44+ CD24-/low cell surface phenotype [24]. Recent evidence also suggests that CD44+ CD24- prostate cells are stem-like cells responsible for tumor initiation [38]. In order to induce a tumor in an animal, hundreds of thousands of cancer cells generally need to be transplanted. When CD44+ CD24- breast cancer cells were transplanted into immunocompromised mice, as few as one hundred of these cells were sufficient to form tumors. In contrast, when mice where transplanted with breast cancer cells not expressing the CD44+ CD24- phenotype, even tens of thousands of cells failed to form tumors. Furthermore, these cells expressed genes known to be important for stem cell maintenance, such as BMI-1, Oct-3/4, β-catenin

Table 15.1 Cell surface phenotypes of cancer stem cells in human malignancies

Tumor type	CSC phenotype	Reference
Acute myeloid leukemia	CD34+, CD38-; CD90-	[23, 43]
Breast cancer	CD44+, CD24-/low	[24]
Brain tumor	CD133+	[35, 36]
Multiple myeloma	CD138-	[44]
Prostate cancer	CD44+, $\alpha 2\beta 1$+, CD133+; CD44+, CD24-	[25, 38]
Melanoma	CD20+; CD133+, ABCG2+; ABCB5+	[28, 31, 34]
Head and neck squamous cell carcinoma	CD44+	[33]
Pancreatic cancer	CD44+, ESA+, CD24+	[29]
Lung cancer	CD133+	[27]
Colon cancer	CD44+, EpCAM+, CD166+; CD133+	[26, 32]
Liver cancer	CD133+; CD90+	[37]

and SMO [38, 39]. Additionally, CD44+ prostate cancer cells can generate CD44- cells in vitro and in vivo [39]. CD44+ normal and breast cancer cells have also been shown to have an upregulated expression of Notch 3, which has been observed to play a role in stem cell renewal, cell fate, apoptosis and proliferation [40].

CD133 has recently been described as "the molecule of the moment" [41] and was originally classified as a marker for hematopoietic and neural stem cells, but has lately been identified as a marker often expressed in combination with other markers of cancer stem cells. This includes several solid malignancies such as brain, prostate, pancreatic and colon tumors (reviewed in [42]). Again, as few as one hundred CD133+ stem like cells have been shown to be sufficient to form tumors when injected into immunocompromised mice, whereas injections with the negative population consistently failed to form tumors.

Although the in vivo reconstitution ability, following isolation based on stem cell markers, is the most established and best method used for identification of cancer stem cells, assays which measure functional characteristics of normal stem cells may be an additional and complementary way to identify cancer stem cells. One example of these functional assays is side-population (SP) analysis, which identifies a fraction of cells within a population that express high levels of various members from the family of ABC transporters. These ABC transporters include MDR1 and BCRP, which may be responsible for drug resistance as they promote a more efficient efflux of drugs or dyes [45, 46]. Normal stem cells [45] as well a small SP in primary tumors and several cancer cell lines [46] have been shown to effectively efflux Hoechst 33342 dye. The SP phenotype, defined as the reserpine-blockable ability to efflux the nucleic acid dye Hoechst 33342, may therefore be useful for the identification and isolation of cancer stem cells. However the concept of the SP phenotype as a universal marker for stem cells does not apply to gastrointestinal cancer cells [47].

Cancer Stem Cell Therapy and Radiation Resistance

When a wider panorama of these specific markers has been established, characterization of the molecular and biological properties of the cancer stem cells will be the next step. This can be done using global gene expression profiling, which enables comparisons of the cancer stem cell profile to that of non stem cancer cells, or to profiles from the corresponding normal tissue, with expectations to identify ways to specifically target and eradicate these cells [5]. An extensive review of seven of the major molecular signalling pathways in cancer and embryonic stem cells, which have been elucidated in the past decade, was recently published by Dreesen and Brivanlou and included JAK/STAT, Notch, MAPK/ERK, PI3K/AKT, NF-κB, Wnt and the TGF-β pathway [13]. These pathways were evaluated for their role in stem cell renewal and development and key molecules whose aberrant expression has been associated with malignant phenotypes were identified. Furthermore, Sell recently presented a guide to preventive and therapeutic strategies for cancer stem cells, based upon identification of transactivating pathways that are over-expressed in cancer stem cells compared to normal stem cells [48]. Blocking or modifying these pathways will potentially allow for a selective cancer stem cell therapy.

Solid malignancies are therapeutic challenges for all treatment modalities including radioimmunotherapy. Today all established non-surgical treatments for solid malignancies are directed against non-stem cancer cells with instant kill (radiation and chemotherapy), limitation of their blood supply (anti-angiogenic therapy) or induction of apoptosis or terminal differentiation. Following treatment, an initial favourable therapeutic result may be obtained, which reduces the tumor burden significantly, but tumor recurrence usually occurs and may be followed by resistance to radiation and chemotherapy. Cancer stem cells are quiescent or slow cycling and also express drug membrane transporters. As a result they are resistant to conventional therapies, which mainly target proliferating cells [49]. Cancer stem cell radiotherapy and their proposed intrinsic radioresistance has recently been reviewed [50]. In a study by Bao et al. glioma stem cells (CD133+) were shown to be resistant to radiation as a result of preferential activation of the DNA damage checkpoint response and an increase in DNA repair capacity (Fig. 15.1A) [51]. Consequently, CD133+ cells accumulated after irradiation both in vitro and in vivo, which has therapeutic implications as they found that a slight increase in the CD133+ fraction of cells used to initiate tumors significantly increased their growth rate. Furthermore, also breast cancer and mammary progenitor cells have been reported to be radioresistant [52–54]. Philips et al. reported that when CD44+ CD24-/low cells were isolated from breast cancer cell lines and exposed to 2 Gy of radiation (^{137}Cs) they were more radioresistant, with a difference in mean surviving fraction of approximately 20%, when compared to the remaining breast cancer cell population [53]. Consistent with the increased radioresistance, radiation treatment caused comparatively lower levels of reactive oxygen species, followed by decreased double-strand break formation in cancer initiating cells (CD44+ CD24-/low). The breast cancer initiating cells increased in numbers after short courses of fractionated irradiation, which suggest a possible mechanism for an accelerated repopulation of tumor cells observed during gaps in radiotherapy. According to the cancer stem cell hypothesis, the initial effect from radiation treatment will debulk the tumor burden, killing proliferating cells that are more responsive to this treatment, whereas cancer stem cells will be spared and highly enriched [51], which may cause a subsequent relapse (Fig. 15.1B). Consequently, research on novel treatment modalities that target not only the proliferating cells but also the cancer stem cells may be required.

Future Directions

Developing novel antibodies that specifically target and deliver radionuclides to cancer stem cells is an attractive approach that depends on the precise identification of cancer stem cell markers, distinguishing them both from their non-tumorigenic

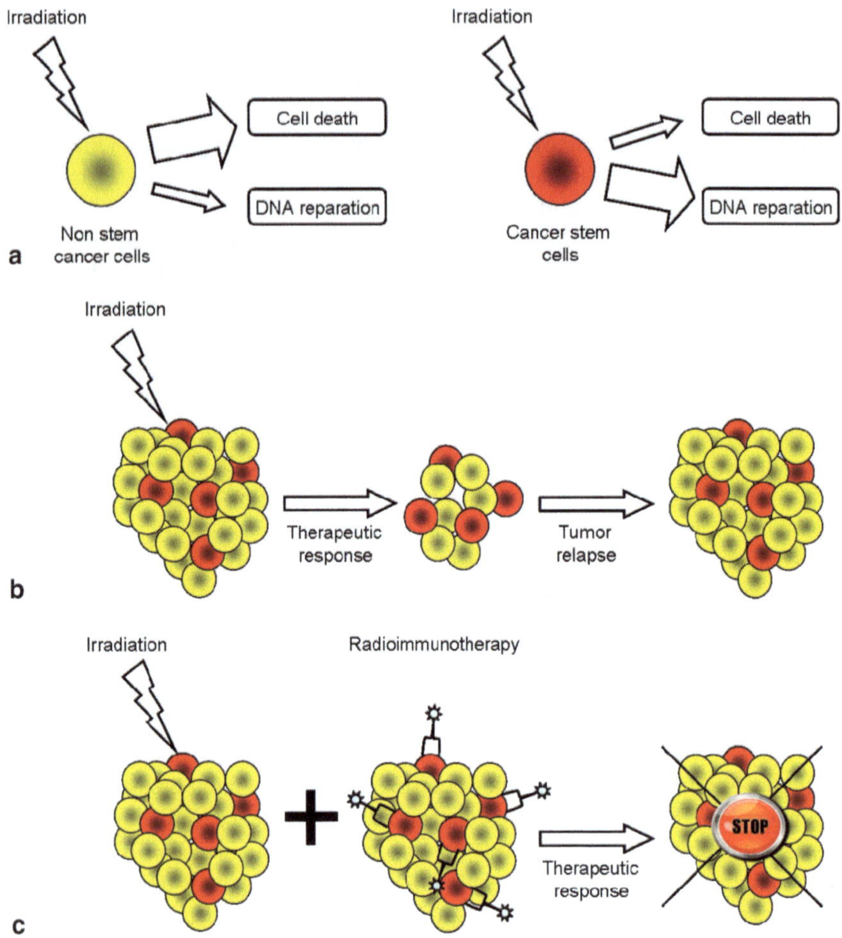

Fig. 15.1 Cancer stem cells demonstrate enhanced resistance to radiation. Cancer stem cells activate the DNA damage checkpoints and DNA repair more and cell death less following irradiation when compared to non stem cancer cells (A). This imply that cancer stem cells are more likely to survive irradiation and as a consequence will be enriched, which can lead to tumor relapse (B). A combination of conventional cancer therapies with targeted cancer stem cell therapies may improve the treatment response (C) (Modified from [55])

progeny and from normal adult stem cells. Once potential functional targets and epitopes have been found, antibodies can be used to target and destroy these cancer stem cells while sparing normal stem cells. As an example, hematopoietic stem cells were shown to express THY-1 and c-kit, whereas leukemic stem cells strongly expressed the alpha subunit of the interleukin-3 receptor (IL-3Rα, CD123) [56]. Such markers may be the key to antibody targeted therapies. Recently, a study was published in which an immunotoxin targeting CD123 was constructed for treatment of acute myeloid leukemia and other CD123 expressing malignancies [57].

A combination of conventional cancer therapies with targeted cancer stem cell therapies might be effective and may extend the durability of the tumor response (Fig. 15.1C).

Acknowledgements Financial support from the Swedish Cancer Society, the County of Västerbotten and the Medical Faculty at Umeå University is acknowledged.

References

1. Virchow R. Editorial Archiv für pathologische Anatomie und Physiologie und für klinische Medizin 1855; 8:23.
2. Hill RP. Identifying cancer stem cells in solid tumors: case not proven. Cancer Research 2006; 66(4):1891–5; discussion 0.
3. Kelly PN, Dakic A, Adams JM, Nutt SL, Strasser A. Tumor growth need not be driven by rare cancer stem cells. Science (New York) 2007; 317(5836):337.
4. Kern SE, Shibata D. The fuzzy math of solid tumor stem cells: a perspective. Cancer Research 2007; 67(19):8985–8.
5. Ailles LE, Weissman IL. Cancer stem cells in solid tumors. Current Opinion in Biotechnology 2007; 18(5):460–6.
6. Alison MR, Murphy G, Leedham S. Stem cells and cancer: a deadly mix. Cell and Tissue Research 2008; 331(1):109–24.
7. Burkert J, Wright NA, Alison MR. Stem cells and cancer: an intimate relationship. The Journal of Pathology 2006; 209(3):287–97.
8. Sanchez-Garcia I, Vicente-Duenas C, Cobaleda C. The theoretical basis of cancer-stem-cell-based therapeutics of cancer: can it be put into practice? Bioessays 2007; 29(12):1269–80.
9. Cozzio A, Passegue E, Ayton PM, Karsunky H, Cleary ML, Weissman IL. Similar MLL-associated leukemias arising from self-renewing stem cells and short-lived myeloid progenitors. Genes & Development 2003; 17(24):3029–35.
10. Jamieson CH, Ailles LE, Dylla SJ, et al. Granulocyte-macrophage progenitors as candidate leukemic stem cells in blast-crisis CML. The New England Journal of Medicine 2004; 351(7):657–67.
11. Weissman IL. Normal and neoplastic stem cells. Novartis Foundation symposium 2005; 265:35–50; discussion -4, 92–7.
12. Clarke MF, Dick JE, Dirks PB, et al. Cancer stem cells–perspectives on current status and future directions: AACR Workshop on cancer stem cells. Cancer Research 2006; 66(19):9339–44.
13. Dreesen O, Brivanlou AH. Signaling pathways in cancer and embryonic stem cells. Stem Cell Reviews 2007; 3(1):7–17.
14. Wang TL, Rago C, Silliman N, et al. Prevalence of somatic alterations in the colorectal cancer cell genome. Proceedings of the National Academy of Sciences of the United States of America 2002; 99(5):3076–80.
15. Jordan CT, Guzman ML, Noble M. Cancer stem cells. The New England Journal of Medicine 2006; 355(12):1253–61.
16. Wicha MS, Liu S, Dontu G. Cancer stem cells: an old idea–a paradigm shift. Cancer Research 2006; 66(4):1883–90; discussion 95–6.
17. Al-Hajj M, Clarke MF. Self-renewal and solid tumor stem cells. Oncogene 2004; 23(43):7274–82.
18. Sell S. Stem cell origin of cancer and differentiation therapy. Critical Reviews in Oncology/Hematology 2004; 51(1):1–28.

19. Dalerba P, Cho RW, Clarke MF. Cancer stem cells: models and concepts. Annual review of Medicine 2007; 58:267–84.
20. Reya T, Morrison SJ, Clarke MF, Weissman IL. Stem cells, cancer, and cancer stem cells. Nature 2001; 414(6859):105–11.
21. Croker AK, Allan AL. Cancer stem cells: implications for the progression and treatment of metastatic disease. Journal of Cellular and Molecular Medicine 2008; 12(2):374–90.
22. Lapidot T, Sirard C, Vormoor J, et al. A cell initiating human acute myeloid leukaemia after transplantation into SCID mice. Nature 1994; 367(6464):645–8.
23. Bonnet D, Dick JE. Human acute myeloid leukemia is organized as a hierarchy that originates from a primitive hematopoietic cell. Nature Medicine 1997; 3(7):730–7.
24. Al-Hajj M, Wicha MS, Benito-Hernandez A, Morrison SJ, Clarke MF. Prospective identification of tumorigenic breast cancer cells. Proceedings of the National Academy of Sciences of the United States of America 2003; 100(7):3983–8.
25. Collins AT, Berry PA, Hyde C, Stower MJ, Maitland NJ. Prospective identification of tumorigenic prostate cancer stem cells. Cancer Research 2005; 65(23):10946–51.
26. Dalerba P, Dylla SJ, Park IK, et al. Phenotypic characterization of human colorectal cancer stem cells. Proceedings of the National Academy of Sciences of the United States of America 2007; 104(24):10158–63.
27. Eramo A, Lotti F, Sette G, et al. Identification and expansion of the tumorigenic lung cancer stem cell population. Cell Death and Differentiation 2008; 15(3):504–14.
28. Fang D, Nguyen TK, Leishear K, et al. A tumorigenic subpopulation with stem cell properties in melanomas. Cancer Research 2005; 65(20):9328–37.
29. Li C, Heidt DG, Dalerba P, et al. Identification of pancreatic cancer stem cells. Cancer Research 2007; 67(3):1030–7.
30. Ma S, Chan KW, Hu L, Lee TK, Wo JY, Ng IO, Zheng BJ, Guan XY. Identification and characterization of tumorigenic liver cancer stem/progenitor cells. Gastroenterology 2007; 132(7):2542–56.
31. Monzani E, Facchetti F, Galmozzi E, et al. Melanoma contains CD133 and ABCG2 positive cells with enhanced tumourigenic potential. European Journal of Cancer 2007; 43(5):935–46.
32. O'Brien CA, Pollett A, Gallinger S, Dick JE. A human colon cancer cell capable of initiating tumour growth in immunodeficient mice. Nature 2007; 445(7123):106–10.
33. Prince ME, Sivanandan R, Kaczorowski A, et al. Identification of a subpopulation of cells with cancer stem cell properties in head and neck squamous cell carcinoma. Proceedings of the National Academy of Sciences of the United States of America 2007; 104(3):973–8.
34. Schatton T, Murphy GF, Frank NY, et al. Identification of cells initiating human melanomas. Nature 2008; 451(7176):345–9.
35. Singh SK, Clarke ID, Terasaki M, Bonn VE, Hawkins C, Squire J, Dirks PB. Identification of a cancer stem cell in human brain tumors. Cancer Research 2003; 63(18):5821–8.
36. Singh SK, Hawkins C, Clarke ID, et al. Identification of human brain tumour initiating cells. Nature 2004; 432(7015):396–401.
37. Yang ZF, Ho DW, Ng MN, et al. Significance of CD90(+) Cancer stem cells in human liver cancer. Cancer Cell 2008; 13(2):153–66.
38. Hurt EM, Kawasaki BT, Klarmann GJ, Thomas SB, Farrar WL. CD44(+)CD24(-) prostate cells are early cancer progenitor/stem cells that provide a model for patients with poor prognosis. British Journal of Cancer 2008; 98(4):756–65.
39. Patrawala L, Calhoun T, Schneider-Broussard R, et al. Highly purified CD44 + prostate cancer cells from xenograft human tumors are enriched in tumorigenic and metastatic progenitor cells. Oncogene 2006; 25(12):1696–708.
40. Farnie G, Clarke RB. Mammary stem cells and breast cancer–role of Notch signalling. Stem Cell Reviews 2007; 3(2):169–75.
41. Mizrak D, Brittan M, Alison MR. CD133: molecule of the moment. The Journal of Pathology 2008; 214(1):3–9.

42. Neuzil J, Stantic M, Zobalova R, et al. Tumour-initiating cells vs. cancer 'stem' cells and CD133: what's in the name? Biochemical and Biophysical Research Communications 2007; 355(4):855–9.
43. Blair A, Hogge DE, Ailles LE, Lansdorp PM, Sutherland HJ. Lack of expression of Thy-1 (CD90) on acute myeloid leukemia cells with long-term proliferative ability in vitro and in vivo. Blood 1997; 89(9):3104–12.
44. Matsui W, Huff CA, Wang Q, et al. Characterization of clonogenic multiple myeloma cells. Blood 2004; 103(6):2332–6.
45. Hadnagy A, Gaboury L, Beaulieu R, Balicki D. SP analysis may be used to identify cancer stem cell populations. Experimental Cell Research 2006; 312(19):3701–10.
46. Hirschmann-Jax C, Foster AE, Wulf GG, Nuchtern JG, Jax TW, Gobel U, Goodell MA, Brenner MK. A distinct "side population" of cells with high drug efflux capacity in human tumor cells. Proceedings of the National Academy of Sciences of the United States of America 2004; 101(39):14228–33.
47. Burkert J, Otto W, Wright N. Side populations of gastrointestinal cancers are not enriched in stem cells. The Journal of Pathology 2008; 214(5):564–73.
48. Sell S. Cancer and stem cell signaling: a guide to preventive and therapeutic strategies for cancer stem cells. Stem Cell Reviews 2007; 3(1):1–6.
49. Dean M, Fojo T, Bates S. Tumour stem cells and drug resistance. Nature Reviews 2005; 5(4):275–84.
50. Diehn M, Clarke MF. Cancer stem cells and radiotherapy: new insights into tumor radioresistance. Journal of the National Cancer Institute 2006; 98(24):1755–7.
51. Bao S, Wu Q, McLendon RE, et al. Glioma stem cells promote radioresistance by preferential activation of the DNA damage response. Nature 2006; 444(7120):756–60.
52. Chen MS, Woodward WA, Behbod F, Peddibhotla S, Alfaro MP, Buchholz TA, Rosen JM. Wnt/beta-catenin mediates radiation resistance of Sca1 + progenitors in an immortalized mammary gland cell line. Journal of Cell Science 2007; 120(Pt 3):468–77.
53. Phillips TM, McBride WH, Pajonk F. The response of CD24(-/low)/CD44 + breast cancer-initiating cells to radiation. Journal of the National Cancer Institute 2006; 98(24):1777–85.
54. Woodward WA, Chen MS, Behbod F, Alfaro MP, Buchholz TA, Rosen JM. WNT/beta-catenin mediates radiation resistance of mouse mammary progenitor cells. Proceedings of the National Academy of Sciences of the United States of America 2007; 104(2):618–23.
55. Rich JN. Cancer stem cells in radiation resistance. Cancer Research 2007; 67(19):8980–4.
56. Testa U, Riccioni R, Diverio D, Rossini A, Lo Coco F, Peschle C. Interleukin-3 receptor in acute leukemia. Leukemia 2004; 18(2):219–26.
57. Du X, Ho M, Pastan I. New immunotoxins targeting CD123, a stem cell antigen on acute myeloid leukemia cells. Journal of Immunotherapy (1997) 2007; 30(6):607–13.

Chapter 16
Effects of Low Dose-Rate Radiation on Cellular Survival

Jörgen Carlsson

Abbreviations LDR, Low dose-rate; CAF, Cross-fire amplifying factor; LET, Linear energy transfer; HRS, Hyperradiosensitivity

Summary The experience of external radiotherapy can only to a limited extent be used to understand therapeutic effects of radionuclide therapy. A major difference is that the dose-rate at radionuclide therapy is at least two orders of magnitude lower. Part of this chapter deals with estimates of the necessary dose-rate and exposure time in combination in order to deliver therapeutic effects to tumour cells. It is proposed that combinations of about 0.1–0.2 Gy/h for several days or about 1 Gy/h for at least 1 day is necessary. Such dose-rates can be achieved with the help of cross fire radiation. Effects of radionuclide therapy in terms of apoptosis, cell-cycle blocks and hyperradiosensitivity are also discussed.

Introduction

The cell killing capacity of low LET radiation, i.e. photons (x-rays and gammas) and electrons (beta-particles and shell-electrons), is well known at high dose-rates, typically 0.5–2.0 Gy/min, as often applied with photons at external radiotherapy [1–3]. However, the extensive experimental and clinical knowledge on effects of external radiotherapy can only be used to a limited extent for understanding effects of radionuclide therapy. A major difference is that the dose-rate in radionuclide therapy can be at least two orders of magnitude lower than in external radiotherapy. The dose-rates in low LET targeted radionuclide therapy can typically be in the order of 0.01–1.0 Gy/h [3–9].

The dose-rate effects discussed in this chapter are only valid for low-LET radiation. The properties of the low-LET emitters most often applied in radionuclide

Unit of Biomedical Radiation Sciences, Department of Oncology, Radiology and Clinical Immunology, Rudbeck Laboratory, Uppsala University, SE-751 85, Uppsala, Sweden

T. Stigbrand et al. (eds.) *Targeted Radionuclide Tumor Therapy*,

therapy (e.g. ^{67}Cu, ^{90}Y, ^{131}I, ^{177}Lu, ^{186}Re and ^{188}Re) are described elsewhere and discussed in this book (e.g. chapter 8). Effects of high-LET radiation (such as alpha-particles from ^{211}At, ^{212}Bi and ^{213}Bi) and of Auger emitters (e.g. ^{111}In and ^{125}I) are described and discussed in chapters 9–11.

Low DoseRate

Exposure to low dose-rate radiation permits DNA repair and repopulation during the radiation exposure, which is not the case during high dose-rate exposure. Basic radiobiological studies have demonstrated that low dose-rates, in the range of 0.1–1.0 Gy/h, give a much lower biological effect per dose unit than high dose-rates in the range 0.5–2.0 Gy/min [2, 10] as shown in Fig. 16.1a. It is also known that an inverse dose-rate effect exists with dose-rates of 0.2–0.4 Gy/h, which can give more cell kill than dose-rates within the range 0.7–1.0 Gy/h [2, 11] as indicated in Fig. 16.1a. Figure 16.1 also points at the problem of extrapolation. If a survival level of 10^{-5} is necessary to achieve, then it is uncertain which radiation dose to apply since experimental data in a survival curve are not valid for low survival levels and high radiation doses. There can also be a significant cell type dependent variation in cell kill following low dose-rate exposure depending on the shape of the "conventional" high dose-rate survival curves in the low dose region as indicated in Fig. 16.1b. The reason is that the initial low dose part of the conventional high dose-rate survival curves varies in slope between different cell types and this slope will determine the dose-effect relation when low dose-rate effects are evaluated [2, 3, 9].

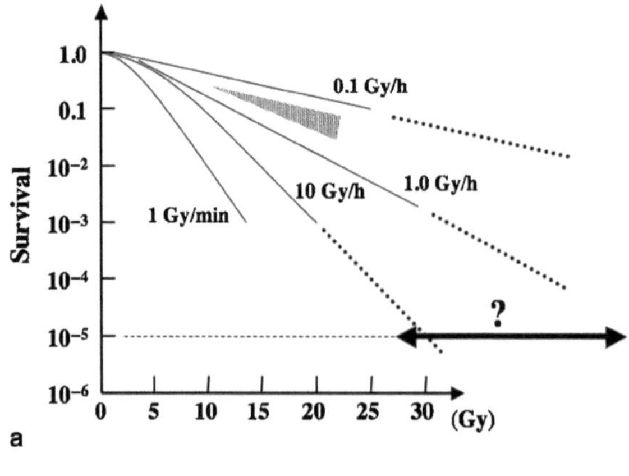

Fig. 16.1 Relative reduction in cellular survival is schematically drawn as a function of radiation dose. (1a) Dose-rates in the interval 1–10 Gy/h gives smaller survival reductions than 1 Gy/min due to DNA-repair during the radiation exposures. Dose rates in the interval 0.1–1.0 Gy/h gives even smaller survival reductions but there can be inverted dose-rate effects (shaded area) due to redistributions between sensitive and resistant cell cycle phases. Dose-rates below 0.1 Gy/h gives real small survival reductions due to cell proliferation during the radiation exposures

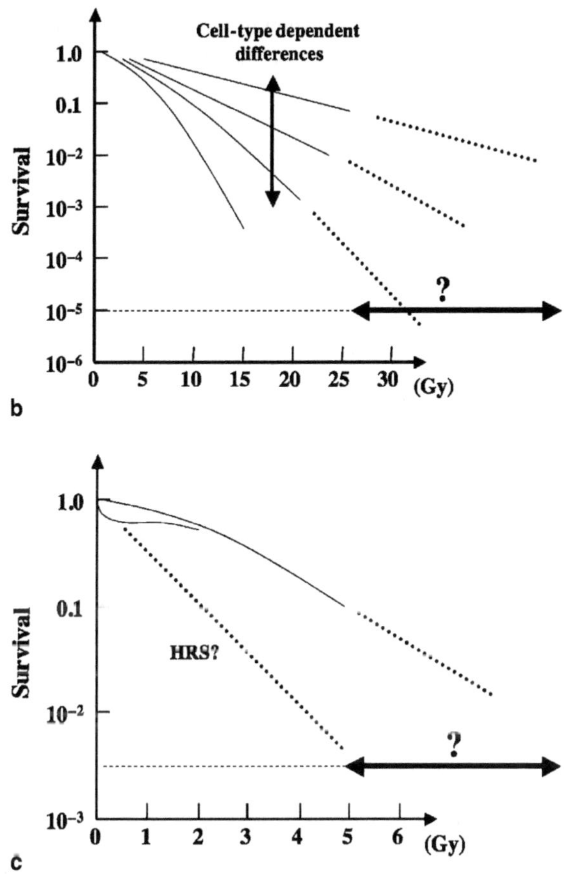

Fig. 16.1 (continued) (1b) Different types of cells can display different radiosensitivity, especially in the low dose shoulder region of the survival curves. This can give appreciable variations in the effects of low dose-rate radiation since the initial low dose part of the survival curve to a large extent determines the dose-effect relation when low dose-rate is applied. (1c) If hyperradiosensitivity, HRS, can be kept during prolonged radionuclide therapy (lower dotted line), there will be an appreciable sensitization, nearly equal to effects of high-LET radiation. An estimate of the necessary radiation dose to reach survival levels down to e.g. 10^{-5} is uncertain due to the obvious uncertainties in the shapes of all these survival curves

The survival at the dose 2 Gy, S_{2Gy}, following exposure to high dose-rate (most often 0.5–2.0 Gy/min) photons is assumed to reflect intrinsic radiosensitivity. There is a published review on such intrinsic radiosensitivity for 694 human cell lines, of which 271 were from tumours [12]. However, it has in one recent study, Carlsson et al. [13], been claimed that there is no obvious relation between S_{2Gy} and the obtained cell killing after low dose-rate irradiation. This is a controversial statement since the general view is that such a relation should exist [2, 3]. The conclusions drawn by Carlsson et al. [13] were made from only a limited number of cell-types.

It was found that the cells most radioresistant to low dose-rate irradiation (U-118MG cells) had about the same S_{2Gy} value as the cell lines more sensitive to low dose-rate.

One possible explanation to the lack of agreement between intrinsic radiosensitivity, measured as S_{2Gy} and low dose-rate effects, is that cell type dependent differences in repopulation during low dose-rate irradiations occur. Such differences can possibly "overshadow" the differences in intrinsic radiosensitivity. Another possible explanation might be cell type dependent differences in the capacity for low dose-rate induced apoptosis. The latter hypothesis is supported by a study demonstrating that low dose-rate induced apoptosis was more frequent in low dose-rate sensitive cells than in low dose-rate resistant cells [14]. More information on apoptosis is given in chapter 12.

It has also been assumed that the radiosensitive state called hyperradiosensitivity, HRS (see also chapter 19), at high dose-rate, low doses, <0.5 Gy [15], can be maintained during a prolonged radionuclide therapy with low dose-rate [16] as indicated by the lower dotted line in Fig. 16.1c. A prolonged state of hyperradiosensitivity has so far, to the knowledge of the author, not been generally proven to exist. Actually, it seems as if differences in HRS are, at least in some cases, not of great importance since cells reported to have HRS (e.g. U-118MG and HT-29 cells) can be rather resistant to low dose-rate exposure while low dose-rate sensitive cells (e.g. U-373MG) can be without HRS [14, 15].

It is difficult to foresee which combinations of low dose-rate and exposure time that can completely eliminate a metastasis containing e.g. 10^5 cells. It is likely, considering data in earlier publications, that doses in the order of at least 30–50 Gy, given with low dose-rate with 0.1–1.0 Gy/h, are necessary to decrease the single cell survival probability to 10^{-5} [17, 18], and as a consequence give a reasonable chance to kill 10^5 tumour cells. Note that such doses given with low dose-rate require continuous irradiation for at least some days.

Furthermore, dosimetry for targeted radionuclide therapy is complicated, since it is not enough only to consider the macroscopic dose concept; different cellular and intracellular distributions of radionuclides may give different biological effects although the macroscopic dose is the same [19, 20].

The LDR-Model

Information on low dose-rate and exposure time combinations that most likely give a curative treatment can be obtained both experimentally and by clinical trials. The author use the name "LDR-model" (low dose-rate model) for an experimental design applied in a recently published in vitro study [13]. The model specifies that low dose-rate radiation has to kill all 10^5 tumour cells in a culture dish for simulating a successful ("curative") treatment of the same number of disseminated tumour cells or the same number of cells in a small metastasis. The follow up time after treatment has so far been 3 months when applying this model.

The choice of 10^5 tumour cells is somewhat arbitrary and based on two reasons. The first is that this number represents a small tumour cell cluster normally not identifiable by diagnostic routine procedures such as CT or MRI [21] unless the tumour cells cause macroscopic changes in the surrounding normal tissues. Furthermore, this number of tumour cells does not in most cases give clinical symptoms. Thus, a cluster of 10^5 tumour cells in a patient can be considered an "occult" or "subclinical" tumour or metastasis. The second argument is more practical; 10^5 tumour cells in a normal cell culture dish or flask provide enough space to allow exponential growth and, at the same time, frequent cell-cell contacts.

The use of the LDR-model is not primarily for simulation of the dose-rate variations in time and space that occur at radionuclide therapy. Instead, it allows the choice of various combinations of dose-rates and exposure times in a reproducible way. In the clinical setting, the dose-rate varies with time, not only as a consequence of the physical half life of the radionuclides, but also due to time dependent changes in the spatial distribution of the radionuclides [4, 5, 18, 20] (Fig. 16.2). These time dependent changes are difficult to simulate in an experimental model. Factors that

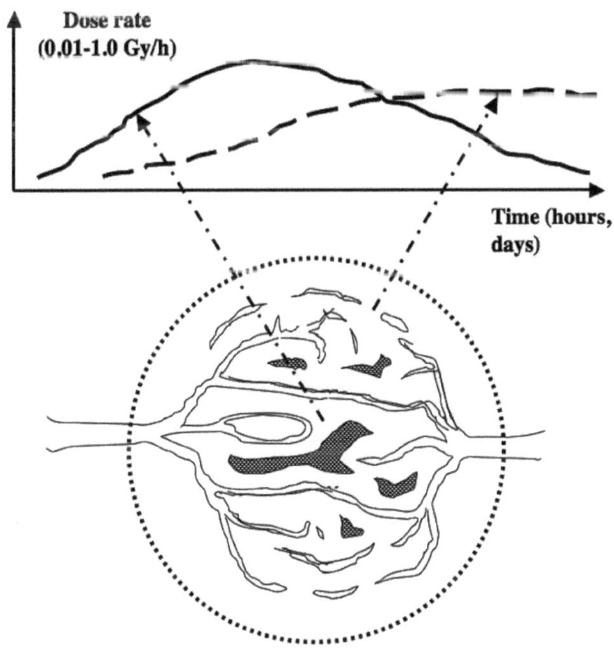

Fig. 16.2 Schematic illustration of the time- and position dependent variations in dose-rate in a tumour nodule. There are variations in vascularisation, vessel wall leakage, changes in blood flow and in diffusion and convection conditions for the radiolabelled targeting agents. There might also be time dependent variations in the expression of target structures on the tumour cells. These factors make it difficult to establish basic and reproducible dose-rate response relations in a tumour. This is illustrated by the schematic curves presenting different dose-rate patterns in two different positions in the tumour. Shaded areas indicate necrosis

determine the dose-rate in solid tumours and metastases are, except for the injected amount of radioactivity, ongoing vascularisation processes, variations in vessel wall leakage and changes in blood flow. Probably also differences in diffusion and convection conditions appear in different areas of the tumour causing variation in penetration properties of the radiolabelled targeting agent. In addition, there might be time dependent variations in the expression of target structures on the tumour cells. All these time dependent factors make it difficult to establish basic and reproducible dose-rate response relations.

The experimental LDR-model was designed to give reproducible and valid irradiation conditions, and has so far been applied for external beta particle irradiation from a ^{32}P-source ($T_{1/2}$ = 14.3 days) giving only a slow decrease in dose-rate during the exposures. The maximal range of the emitted beta particles is about 8 mm in plastic, water or tissue (mean range about 2.7 mm). The beta particles had to pass through totally 1.5 mm plastic before reaching the monolayer of growing tumour cells. Relevant dose-rates were selected through the amount of radionuclide placed in the irradiation chambers. The exposure times were selected to correspond to assumed effective half lives of the radionuclides, delivered by targeting agents of different types.

Hyperradiosensitivity [15, 16] at low doses, bystander effects [22–24] and low dose-rate induced apoptosis [25, 26] are all extensively studied processes and the LDR-model allows these processes to work together. The overall goal with the model is to find "dose-rate – exposure time" relations that can kill all of the exposed 10^5 tumour cells, with no remaining cells observed after at least 3 months. The initial dose-rates were, in the study by Carlsson et al. [13], in the interval 0.1–0.8 Gy/h and the cells were continuously exposed for 1, 3 or 7 days. These combinations covered dose-rates and doses achievable in targeted radionuclide therapy. Five tumour cell lines, gliomas U-373MG and U-118MG, colon carcinoma HT-29, cervix squamous carcinoma A-431 and breast cancer SKBR-3 cells were used.

Dose-Rate and Exposure Time, Using the LDR-Model

The results of the first LDR-model experiments was that mean dose-rates of 0.2–0.3 and 0.4–0.6 Gy/h for 7 and 3 days, respectively, could kill all tumour cells in each "10^5-sample". These treatments gave total radiation doses of 30–40 Gy. However, when exposed for only 24 h with about 0.8 Gy/h, only the comparatively radiosensitive SKBR-3 cells were successfully treated, all the other cell-types recovered [13]. Lower dose-rates than 0.1 Gy/h will probably, in most cases, not lead to curative treatments when beta particles are applied. The results are shown in Fig. 16.3.

The U-118MG cells were most resistant and U-373MG and SKBR-3 cells most sensitive to treatment while the HT-29 and A-431 cells behaved in between. The shift from recovery to "cure" fell within a rather narrow range of dose-rate and exposure time combinations.

There were variations in the growth delay patterns for the cells that recovered. For example, when the cells were exposed to 0.8 Gy/h for 24 h, the HT-29 cells recovered to the control growth rate after a growth delay, the U-118MG cells recovered after a growth delay but continued to grow at a slower rate than the controls and the

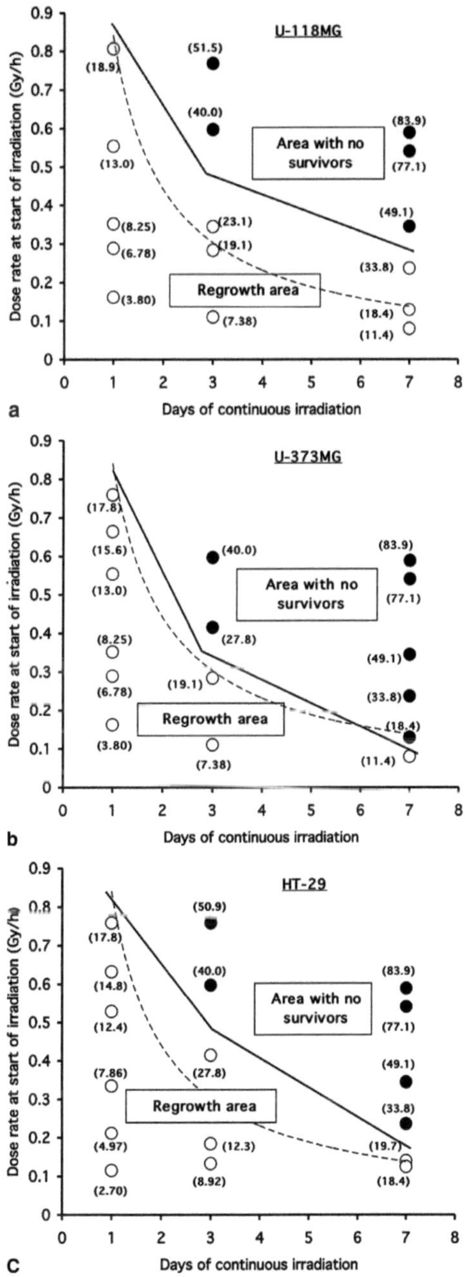

Fig. 16.3 Summary of low dose-rate experiments carried out for (a) U-118MG, (b) U-373MG, (c) HT-29, (d) A-431 cells and (c) SKBR-3 cells. The cells were irradiated with different initial dose rates and exposed for 1, 3 or 7 days. The figures (a)–(e) show at which combinations of dose rate and exposure time all cells were killed (area with no survivors), and at which at least some cells survived and displayed regrowth (the regrowth area). The separation between the two areas is indicated by bold solid lines. The total delivered radiation dose (Gy) is given in parentheses near each point. The 20 Gy isodose curve is indicated by a dashed line (Reproduced from [13] with kind permission from Springer Science and Business Media)

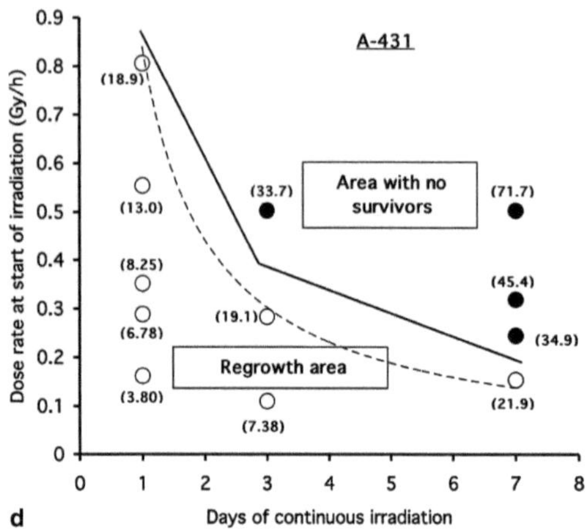

d

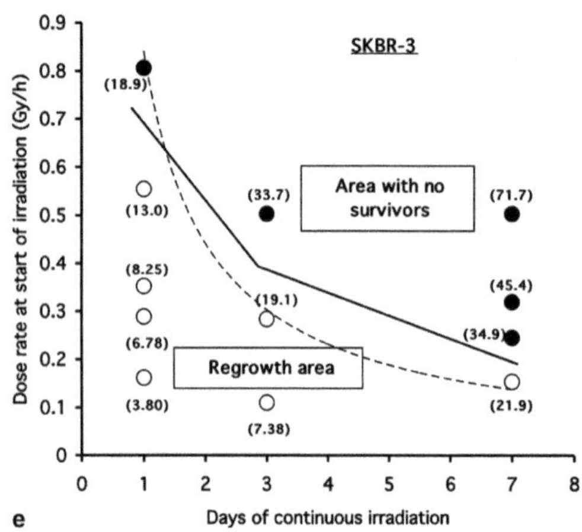

e

Fig. 16.3 (continued)

A-431 cells continued to grow without delay but with a slower rate than the controls. The reasons for these differences in the regrowth patterns are not known.

The highest studied dose-rates, about 0.8 Gy/h, are probably near the highest values that can be achieved in targeted radionuclide therapy [4–7]. The total doses achieved after 1, 3 or 7 days exposure (see parentheses in Fig. 16.3) probably also correspond to the highest achievable doses in targeted radionuclide therapy [4], and most often total doses of not more than 10–20 Gy are obtained in targeting of B-cell lymphomas [8]. However, there are indications from preclinical studies that dramatic "killing effect amplification" per receptor interaction can be achieved by using effective residualising agents [27].

There might be cases when only a fraction of the tumour cells have to be killed directly by radiation, since the remaining tumour cells might be killed through bystander effects [22–24] or other factors (e.g. limited nutrition supply, immune response, adjuvant chemo- or immunotherapy). Considering the LDR-model the assumption was made that 10^5 tumour cells have to be killed by radiation, even if there are other tumour cells killed by other reasons.

Apoptosis and Cell Cycle Blocks

We have in the previous study [14] published data on low dose-rate acute effects, using three of the cells that were later used in the LDR-model study. These were the cell-lines U-118MG, U-373MG and HT-29. In the study from 2003, the initial dose-rate was only 0.05–0.09 Gy/h and the exposure time 7 days. As expected, all cultures did regrow after such treatments. It was shown that the U-373MG cells had, at day 7, the strongest cell number reduction due to a combination of a G_2 block and radiation induced apoptosis. The U-118MG and HT29 cells had surprisingly low cell number reductions. U-118MG had only a G_2 block but no radiation induced apoptosis. HT29 presented both a G_2 block and some radiation induced apoptosis, but the amount of apoptosis was smaller than for the U-373MG cells. Thus, the results from that study indicate that the U-373MG cells were more sensitive than the other two cell lines due to a higher degree of apoptosis. The achieved sensitivity differences are in agreement with the cell killing results from the experimental LDR-model study. Thus, apoptosis seems, from these results, to be an important factor for cell kill when low dose-rate is applied. This is in agreement with several other research reports; see review by Murray and McEwan [9]. Further information on the role of apoptosis and other cell deaths during and after low dose-rate radiation exposure is given in chapter 12 in this book.

Cross Fire and Dose-Rate

The obtained dose-rates in beta particle based radionuclide therapy are to a large extent a consequence, not only of the amount of radionuclides associated to each tumour cell, but also to the cross-fire effect. The dose-rate will be low for a single isolated tumour cell considering only the radionuclides bound to that cell [19]. Beta particles with long range will enable rather uniform dose-distributions and hopefully give therapeutic relevant radiation doses also to non-targeted tumour cells. Thus, radionuclides associated to one cell can also irradiate cells close by due to the long range of the radiation [28, 29]. This can increase the dose rate 10–100-fold as shown in Table 16.1. The irradiation doses applied in the LDR-model experiments (see above) can be considered to be either from direct irradiation of the targeted cell, from cross-fire radiation or, most likely, due to the combination. Actually, the doses achieved through cross fire irradiation makes it reasonable that dose-rates in the range used in the LDR-model experiments also can be achieved when treating patients.

Essand et al. [29] studied the effects of targeting antibodies binding to the E4-antigen in prostate cancer spheroids. The antibodies were labelled with ^{131}I and bound only to the outer 0–120 µm cell layers in the spheroids, but significant amounts of radiation dose were given to the inner 120–200 µm cell layers due to the cross fire radiation. For example, a total dose of about 8 Gy was given during 2 days to the cell layer positioned 160–200 µm inside the spheroids. The average dose-rate, due to the cross fire irradiation, was then in the order of 0.1–0.2 Gy/h. The outer cell layers received about 13 Gy and the dose-rate was 0.2–0.3 Gy/h in those layers. The therapy effects were, after the exposure to the radiolabelled antibodies, studied using sequential trypsinisation thereby "piling off" layer by layer from the spheroids followed by cloning of these cell fractions. The exposure to the inner layers gave a survival of about 20% of the survival within the same region of non-exposed spheroids.

The study by Essand et al. [29] is old but, to the knowledge of the author, so far the most reproducible and detailed experimental demonstration of the cross fire effect. Furthermore, the results showed that only a fraction of the tumour cells were killed when the overall dose-rate was in the order of 0.1–0.3 Gy/h and the exposure time was 2 days. This is in accordance with more recent results applying the LDR-model.

In a theoretical study by Hartman et al. [19] applying homogeneous ^{131}I-antibody uptake in spherical metastases, it was shown that the cross-fire effect gives high dose contributions when the metastases grow real big. It was assumed that 10^5 ^{131}I atoms were bound to each cell, independent of position within the metastases, and that the efficient half life (biological and physical half lives weighted) was 24 h. The dose-rates achieved in the study by Hartman et al. [19] are given in Table 16.1.

When the micrometastases contained ten cells, the dose to all cells was more than doubled in comparison to the dose given to each cell by the "self dose" (i.e. the dose delivered by the antibodies that bound to that cell) (Table 16.1).

Table 16.1 Number of cells in metastases, radiation dose, CAF (cross-fire amplifying factor), dose-rates as function of time and mean dose-rates

			Dose-rates as a function of time (Gy/h)				
Number of cells	Dose (Gy)	CAF	Day 1	Day 2	Day 3	Day 4	Mean dose Rate (Gy/h)
1	3	1	0.06	0.03	0.015	0.008	0.03–0.04
10	7.3	2.4	0.15	0.075	0.038	0.019	0.07–0.10
100	50	17	1.0	0.50	0.25	0.13	0.50–0.70
10^6	330	110	6.9	3.5	1.75	0.86	3.2–4.5
10^9	570	190	12	6.0	3.0	1.5	5.6–8.0

The values were calculated with the help of the results reported by Hartman et al. [19]. They were calculated assuming that 10^5 ^{131}I atoms, via the antibodies, were bound to each cell and that the effective half life (biological and physical half lives weighted) was 24 h.

The dose increase, due to the cross fire effect, is here called the "cross-fire amplification factor", CAF. When the metastases contained 100 cells the CAF-value was about 17 but when the metastases reached 1 mg (about 10^6 cells) and 1 g (about 10^9 cells) the CAF-values were as high as about 110 and 190, respectively. The latter two CAF values were obtained irrespectively if the calculations were made via direct integration or using the MIRDOSE 3 program [19]. The dose to the nucleus of a single isolated cell (no cross fire irradiation) was for simplicity set to the typical value 3 Gy although this dose can be both lower and higher depending on the subcellular localisation of the radioactivity and on the size of the cells [19].

The doses above 100 Gy in Table 16.1 are unrealistic since in a real metastasis it is unlikely that approximately 10^5 radioactive atoms can be bound to all the tumour cells in the metastasis. It is more reasonable with a heterogeneous distribution of nuclide uptake as demonstrated in Fig. 16.4. It is probably neither possible that 10^5 radioactive atoms can bind to a tumour cell even if the number of binding sites per cell can be in the order of 10^6 as is the case for the EGFR and HER2 receptors in certain types of tumour cells (see chapter 3 in this book).

However, if a mean dose-rate of at least 0.5 Gy/h can be achieved during a 3 days exposure, or a mean dose-rate of 1 Gy/h can be achieved during only 1 day exposure, then complete kill of a small metastasis containing 10^5 cells might be possible as indicated in the LDR model study.

Inhomogeneous Uptake of Radionuclides

An example of inhomogeneous radionuclide uptake in a tumour is presented here. The ovarian cancer cells, SKOV-3, expressing about 10^6 HER2-receptors per cell, were allowed to generate xenotransplant tumours at the right hind leg of nude mice. The mice were injected with $^{125}I\text{-}(Z_{HER2:4})_2$ (MW ≈ 15 kDa) into the tail vein. The mice were anesthetised and euthanised by heart puncture various times after the injection of the radiolabelled affibody molecule. The tumours were dissected and fixed in formaldehyde and then sectioned and processed for immunohistochemical HER-2 staining and autoradiography as described by Steffen et al [30]. An example is shown in Fig 16.4. The immunohistochemistry confirmed uniform HER-2 expression in the tumour, with typical membrane staining (Fig 16.4b). The autoradiography (Fig 16.4c) demonstrated a granular distribution of the radioactivity within the tumours. There were no grains in the HER-2 negative normal tissues surrounding the tumour (not shown). As indicated in Fig. 16.4c, the radioactivity was, 6 h after injection, perivascular and visualized close to blood vessels, confirming an inhomogeneous uptake of the radionuclide.

Information on the intratumoural uptake pattern of radionuclides is unfortunately most often not given in tumour targeting studies. It is possible that there is a "binding site barrier" in the tumour [31, 32], that delays penetration of macromolecular ligands to regions far from the blood vessels, as a result of successful binding to their target receptors. It has actually been shown, in tumour spheroid

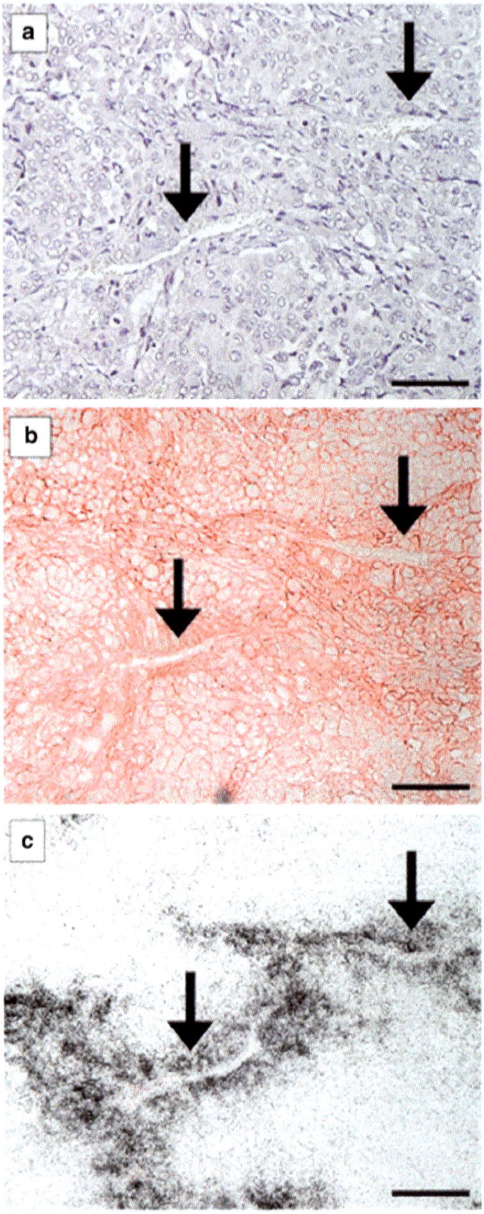

Fig. 16.4 Illustration of heterogeneous radionuclide uptake in a transplanted tumour. The diameter of the transplanted tumour was 3 mm, which is of the same size as a typical micrometastases in a patient. Serial tumour sections were made 6 h post injection of a ^{125}I-labelled anti-HER2 affibody molecule (MW ≈ 15 kDa). (A) Demonstrates a section with conventional haematoxylin blue staining. (B) A neighbour section with immunohistochemical red staining of the HER2 expression. (C) The intratumoural ^{125}I distribution with the help of autoradiography. Note that (C) only shows the distribution of the radiation source in the 4 μm thin section. The radiation dose distribution in the tumour is expected to be more homogeneous due to cross-fire irradiation from surrounding cells in the three-dimensional tumour mass if a suitable beta-emitter (e.g. ^{177}Lu, ^{131}I or ^{90}Y) is applied. The arrows indicate blood vessels. The bar is 100 μm (Reproduced from [30] with kind permission from Springer Science and Business Media)

models, that blockage of receptors with unlabelled ligand, leads to an increased penetration depth of a subsequent incubation of radiolabelled ligand [33, 34]. A better tumour penetration could possibly be achieved by using fractionated therapy, or by blocking readily accessible antigen with unlabeled targeting agents to overcome the binding site barrier. It has also been described that the affinity coefficient of the binders influence penetration and that the optimal affinity seems to be around 10^{-9} M [35].

It is important to observe that the radionuclide distribution as observed in Fig. 16.4c not represents the radiation dose distribution in the tumour. The autoradiograph only presents the distribution of radioactive decays in the 4 μm thin section, i.e. the position of the radiation source in the investigated section [30]. The radiation dose distribution in the tumour is expected to be much more homogenous due to cross-fire irradiation from other areas of the tumour. Thus, also areas around vessels not positioned in the section will contribute to the dose distribution. This is important to consider when beta emitters, giving extensive cross-fire irradiation, such as ^{177}Lu, ^{131}I and ^{90}Y, are used. Actually, also alpha emitters, having a range of only a few cell diameters, give some cross-fire irradiation.

Normal Tissues

It is of course important to consider unwanted effects in normal cells and tissues. The tolerance doses for most normal tissues are, unfortunately, not known in much detail when exposed to low dose-rate irradiation. The major exception seems to be the bone marrow, i.e. effects on the stem cells, as experienced from lymphoma treatments [36, 37]. However, targeted radionuclide therapy is generally expected to give high tumour specific uptake of the therapeutic radionuclides and acceptable doses to normal tissues. It is important to evaluate which targeting agent that is suitable for each type of tumour and, most important, if the required tumour dose-rates and exposure times can be achieved without too severe side effects on normal tissues [9, 38].

Molecular Mechanisms

The molecular mechanisms determining if a low dose-rate exposed cell will be killed or not are essentially the same as those determining the effects after exposure to high dose-rate irradiation. The function of the DNA damage sensing proteins like ATM (ataxia telangiectasia mutated) and DNA repair complexes like DNA-PK (DNA-dependent protein kinase) are most likely similar independent of dose-rate, see chapter 13 in this book for more details on these mechanisms. The significance of non-repaired DNA double-strand breaks seems to be similar irrespective if the cells are irradiated with high or low dose-rate [39]. The major differences that possibly exist between exposures to high and low dose-rate radiation have recently been discussed in the article by Murray and McEwan [9]. Apoptosis could probably be the major mechanism for cell death following low dose-rate exposures, while necrosis, mitotic catastrophes and possibly also premature senescence can be more important for cell death following exposure to high dose-rate. Further details about apoptosis and low dose-rate are given in chapter 12 in this book.

The molecular mechanisms of the reversed dose-rate effect is possibly due the action of molecules regulating growth arrest and activating cell cycle check-points [2], see also chapters 13 and 14 in this volume. This might cause, during exposure to low dose-rate irradiation, an accumulation of cells in radiosensitive phases, e.g. late G_2.

The molecular mechanisms behind HRS are probably to be found in a suboptimal triggering (phosphorylation) of DNA damage sensing or DNA repair complexes. Suboptimal triggering means most likely that the cells are sensitized. Full triggering of DNA repair can, in such cases, be achieved after radiation doses ≥1 Gy given at high dose-rate. A clue to the molecular factors involved in that were indicated in a recent report, demonstrating that activation or inhibition of the DNA-damage sensor ATM is of importance [40]. It was found that DNA damages inflicted at low dose-rate did fail to activate ATM. However, if ATM was activated by chloroquine the cells survived the low dose-rate better.

Furthermore, it has been suggested that variations in radiosensitivty at low dose-rates are related to the compactness of chromatin [41] but this has, to the knowledge of the author, not been confirmed by further studies. In another recent experimental study, favourable outcome by low dose-rate treatment was reported and the effect was, if the totally delivered dose was in the range 1–2 Gy, as good for low dose-rate as for high dose-rate, although the difference in dose-rate was nearly three orders of magnitude [42]. This indicates that there are basic biological aspects of low dose-rate radiation, which have to be analyzed in more detail.

Conclusions

Several factors in tumours and metastases such as vascularisation, variations in vessel wall leakage and changes in blood flow affect the dose and dose-rate. The diffusion and convection conditions in different areas of tumours and metastases affect the penetration of the radiolabelled targeting agents. In addition, there might be variations in the expression of target structures on the tumour cells. It is likely that the uptake of radioactivity is inhomogeneous and that most of the radionuclides will be situated close to blood vessels and capillaries, which makes the effect of cross-fire irradiation important.

We conclude that mean dose-rates in the range 0.2–0.3 Gy/h are necessary in order to kill 10^5 tumour cells in a metastasis during 1 week exposure. Higher dose-rates, such as 0.4–0.6 Gy/h and >0.8 Gy/h, are necessary if the exposure times are only 3 days or 1 day, respectively. Dose-rates of that magnitude are possible to achieve when there is cross fire irradiation from long range beta emitters.

Acknowledgements Financial support from the Swedish Cancer Society, grant 0980-B06–19XBC, and Vinnova, grant 2004–02159, is acknowledged. Thanks also to the journals that allowed the author to reproduce, and in some cases slightly modify, figures from previously published articles (see figure texts).

References

1. Steel GG (2002) Basic clinical radiobiology. Hodder Education. London (ISBN 9780340807835).
2. Hall EJ, Giaccia AJ (2006) Radiobiology for the radiologist. Chapter 5. Lippincott, Williams & Wilkins. Philadelphia, PA (ISBN 0-7817-4151-3).
3. Dale R, Jones B (2007) Radiobiological modelling in radiation oncology. BIR, the British Institute of radiology, London (ISBN 13978-0-905749-60-0).
4. Dillehay LE, Williams JR (1990) Radiobiology of dose-rate patterns achievable in radioimmuno globulin therapy. Front Radiat Ther Oncol 24:96–103.
5. Dale RG (1996) Dose-rate effects in targeted radiotherapy. Phys Med Biol 41(10):1871–1884.
6. Murtha AD (2000) Radiobiology of low-dose-rate radiation relevant to radioimmunotherapy. Cancer Biother Radiopharm 15(1):7–14.
7. Carlsson J, Forssell Aronsson E, Hietala SO, Stigbrand T, Tennvall J (2003) Tumour therapy with radionuclides: assessment of progress and problems. Radiother Oncol 66(2):107–117.
8. Hernandez MC, Knox SJ (2004) Radiobiology of radioimmunotherapy: targeting CD20 B-cell antigen in non-Hodgkin's lymphoma. Int J Radiat Oncol Biol Phys 59(5):1274–1287.
9. Murray D, McEwan AJ (2007) Radiobiology of systemic radiation therapy. Cancer Biother Radiopharm 22(1):1–23.
10. Bedford JS, Mitchell JB (1973) Dose-rate effects in synchronous mammalian cells in culture. Radiat Res 54(2):316–327.
11. Mitchell JB, Bedford JS, Bailey S (1979) Dose-rate effects in mammalian cells in culture III. Comparison of cell killing and cell proliferation during continuous irradiation for six different cell lines. Radiat Res 79(3):537–551.
12. Deschavanne PJ, Fertil B (1996) A review of human cell radiosensitivity in vitro. Int J Radiat Oncol Biol Phys 34(1):251–266.
13. Carlsson J, Eriksson V, Stenerlow B, Lundqvist H (2006) Requirements regarding dose rate and exposure time for killing of tumour cells in beta particle radionuclide therapy. Eur J Nucl Med Mol Imaging 33(10):1185–1195.
14. Carlsson J, Hakansson E, Eriksson V, Grawe J, Wester K, Grusell E, Montelius A, Lundqvist H (2003) Early effects of low dose-rate radiation on cultured tumor cells. Cancer Biother Radiopharm 18(4):663–670.
15. Joiner MC, Marples B, Lambin P, Short SC, Turesson I (2001) Low-dose hypersensitivity: current status and possible mechanisms. Int J Radiat Oncol Biol Phys 49(2):379–389.
16. Mitchell CR, Folkard M, Joiner MC (2002) Effects of exposure to low-dose-rate 60Co gamma rays on human tumor cells in vitro. Radiat Res 158(3):311–318.
17. Dillehay LE (1990) A model of cell killing by low-dose-rate radiation including repair of sublethal damage, G2 block, and cell division. Radiat Res 124(2):201–207.
18. Wong JY, Williams LE, Demidecki AJ, Wessels BW, Yan XW (1991) Radiobiologic studies comparing Yttrium-90 irradiation and external beam irradiation in vitro. Int J Radiat Oncol Biol Phys 20(4):715–722.
19. Hartman T, Lundqvist H, Westlin JE, Carlsson J (2000) Radiation doses to the cell nucleus in single cells and cells in micrometastases in targeted therapy with 131I labelled ligands or antibodies. Int J Radiat Oncol Biol Phys 46(4):1025–1036.
20. Howell RW, Neti PV (2005) Modeling multicellular response to nonuniform distributions of radioactivity: differences in cellular response to self-dose and cross-dose. Radiat Res 163(2):216–221.
21. Saha GB (2006) Physics and radiobiology of nuclear medicine. Springer. New York (ISBN 9780387307541).
22. Prise KM, Folkard M, Michael BD (2003) A review of the bystander effect and its implications for low-dose exposure. Radiat Prot Dosimetry 104(4):347–355.
23. Hall EJ (2003) The bystander effect. Health Phys 85(1): 31–35.
24. Mothersill C, Seymour CB (2004) Radiation-induced bystander effects–implications for cancer. Nat Rev Cancer 4(2):158–164.

25. Mirzaie-Joniani H, Eriksson D, Johansson A, Lofroth PO, Johansson L, Ahlstrom KR, Stigbrand T (2002) Apoptosis in HeLa Hep2 cells is induced by low-dose, low-dose-rate radiation. Radiat Res 158(5):634–640.
26. Mirzaie-Joniani H, Eriksson D, Sheikholvaezin A, Johansson A, Lofroth PO, Johansson L, Stigbrand T (2002) Apoptosis induced by low-dose and low-dose-rate radiation. Cancer 94 (4 Suppl):1210–1214.
27. Sundberg AL, Blomquist E, Carlsson J, Steffen AC, Gedda L (2003) Cellular retention of radioactivity and increased radiation dose. Model experiments with EGF-dextran. Nucl Med Biol 30(3):303–315.
28. O'Donoghue JA, Bardies M, Wheldon TE (1995) Relationships between tumor size and curability for uniformly targeted therapy with beta-emitting radionuclides. J Nucl Med 36(10):1902–1909.
29. Essand M, Gronvik C, Hartman T, Carlsson J (1995) Radioimmunotherapy of prostatic adenocarcinomas: effects of 131I-labelled E4 antibodies on cells at different depth in DU 145 spheroids. Int J Cancer 63(3):387–394.
30. Steffen AC, Orlova A, Wikman M, Nilsson FY, Stahl S, Adams GP, Tolmachev V, Carlsson J (2006) Affibody-mediated tumour targeting of HER-2 expressing xenografts in mice. Eur J Nucl Med Mol Imaging 33(6):631–638.
31. Weinstein JN, Eger RR, Covell DG, Black CD, Mulshine J, Carrasquillo JA (1987) The pharmacology of monoclonal antibodies. Ann N Y Acad Sci 507:199–210.
32. Fujimori K, Covell DG, Fletcher JE, Weinstein JN (1989) Modeling analysis of the global and microscopic distribution of immunoglobulin G, F(ab')2, and Fab in tumors. Cancer Res 49:5656–5663.
33. Lindstrom A, Carlsson J (1993) Penetration and binding of epidermal growth factor-dextran conjugates in spheroids of human glioma origin. Cancer Biother 8:145–158.
34. Carlsson J, Gedda L (2006) Penetration of tumor therapy interesting substances in non-vasularized metastases: review of studies in multicellular spheroids. Curr Cancer Ther Rev 2:293–304.
35. Adams GP, Schier R, McCall AM, Simmons HH, Horak EM, Alpaugh RK, Marks JD, Weiner LM (2001) High affinity restricts the localization and tumor penetration of single-chain fv antibody molecules. Cancer Res June 15; 61(12):4750–4755.
36. DeNardo SJ, Williams LE, Leigh BR, Wahl RL (2002) Choosing an optimal radioimmunotherapy dose for clinical response. Cancer 94(4 Suppl):1275–1286.
37. Witzig TE (2006) Radioimmunotherapy for B-cell non-Hodgkin lymphoma. Best Pract Res Clin Haematol 19(4):655–668.
38. Larson SM, Krenning EP (2005) A pragmatic perspective on molecular targeted radionuclide therapy. J Nucl Med 46(Suppl 1):1S–3S.
39. Dikomey E, Brammer I (2000) Relationship between cellular radiosensitivity and non-repaired double-strand breaks studied for different growth states, dose-rates and plating conditions in a normal human fibroblast line. Int J Radiat Biol 76(6):773–781
40. Collis SJ, Schwaninger JM, Ntambi AJ, Keller TW, Nelson WG, Dillehay LE, Deweese TL (2004) Evasion of early cellular response mechanisms following low level radiation-induced DNA damage. J Biol Chem 279 (48):49624–49632.
41. Chapman JD (2003) Single-hit mechanism of tumour cell killing by radiation. Int J Radiat Biol 79(2):71–81.
42. Verwijnen S, Capello A, Bernard B, van den Aardweg G, Konijnenberg M, Breeman W, Krenning E, de Jong M (2004) Low-dose-rate irradiation by ^{131}I versus high-dose-rate external beam irradiation in the rat pancreatic tumor cell line CA20948. Cancer Biother Radiopharm 19(3):285–292.

Chapter 17
Bystander Effects and Radionuclide Therapy

Kevin M. Prise

Summary The standard paradigm for radiation effects in biological systems is that direct DNA damage within the nucleus of a cell is required to trigger the downstream biological consequences. However, significant evidence has been obtained for the presence of bystander effects where cells respond to the fact that their neighbours have been irradiated. As well as extensive evidence from external beam exposures, several studies have reported bystander responses after radionuclide incorporation. These have included the use of ^{3}H, ^{121}I, ^{123}I, ^{131}I and ^{211}At-labelled targets. Responses have been reported both *in vitro* and *in vivo* and are distinct from physical cross-fire effects. For the development of new targeted therapies involving radionuclides, it is clear that bystander responses have the potential to significantly enhance the effectiveness of these approaches if the underlying mechanisms can be fully elucidated.

Introduction

The longstanding paradigm for the effects of radiation exposure in biological systems has been that energy deposition in nuclear DNA and the direct production of DNA damage drives the downstream biological consequences. Some of the key early studies promoting this model used radioisotopes localized to different cellular regions to determine locations of radiosensitive targets. In a series of defining papers, Warters and colleagues compared the effects of ^{125}I incorporated into cellular DNA versus ^{125}I tagged onto the cell membrane bound protein Concanavalin A [1, 2]. Significant cell killing was observed when radioactivity was incorporated directly into the nuclear DNA but not when associated with cell membranes. These studies were done using synchronized cells incubated at 37 °C for accumulation of ^{125}I-UdR into nuclear DNA or 4 °C for ^{125}I-Concanavalin A labeling. Further studies confirmed that it was dose to the cell nucleus which determined the level of cell

Professor of Radiation Biology, Centre for Cancer Research and Cell Biology,
Queen's University Belfast, 97 Lisburn Road, Belfast, BT9 7BL, UK

killing rather than dose to the cytoplasm or cell membranes. Along with other studies, using microbeam approaches to localise dose [3–5], this has consolidated the DNA damage model of direct radiation effects. Central to the role of DNA damage has been the involvement of DNA double-strand breaks as critical lesions the repair of which determines whether cells can survive radiation exposure or if misrepaired accrue potentially harmful mutations [6]. Despite this longstanding evidence however, the universality of the direct DNA damage paradigm has recently been questioned. A range of responses have been reported where cells do not respond in direct proportion to energy deposited in their nuclear DNA. These have been classified as non-targeted or more accurately non-(DNA)-targeted responses [7]. Archetypal of these is the radiation-induced bystander response where cells respond to the fact that their neighbours have been irradiated (for reviews see [8, 9]). Other non-(DNA)-targeted responses include adaptive responses [10], genomic instability [11], low-dose hypersensitivity [12] and the inverse dose-rate effect [13].

Evidence for Radiation-Induced Bystander Responses

Evidence for bystander responses has been know for many years. In the early 1960s it was shown that blood samples from irradiated individuals could lead to the production of chromosome aberrations in freshly isolated lymphocytes [14]. A range of studies followed from this to characterize these "clastogenic factors", These clastogenic factors have been postulated to be between 1,000 and 10,000 daltons in size and include lipid peroxide products [15], ionisine nucleotides [16] and cytokines such as TNF-α [17], but underlying their actions is the involvement of reactive oxygen species (ROS) such as superoxide radicals.

In the early 1990s a classical experiment was performed by Jack Little and colleagues defining the presence of bystander responses. Using a low fluence α-particle exposure of confluent CHO cells they showed that under conditions where less than 1% of the population was exposed to α-particle traversals, 30% of the population showed chromosomal changes in the form of sister chromatid exchanges [18]. Since then a range of studies have shown bystander response for endpoints including cell killing, mutation, chromosomal damage, apoptosis and transformation. Two main modes of action appear to be involved. One involves release of cell signaling molecules into the cell culture medium [19] and the second involves direct cell-cell communication via gap-junctional intercellular communication (GJIC) [20]. Several key pathways and species have been implicated in bystander signaling. These include a range of studies showing evidence for the involvement of cytokines, reactive oxygen (ROS) and nitrogen species (RNS) along with calcium and other species. More recently it has also been shown that bystander responses can be induced even if radiation is not deposited in the nucleus of a cell. Localised irradiation of the cytoplasm only using the current generation of microbeams, has confirmed that cellular responses can occur in the absence of direct nuclear irradiation despite the earlier studies suggesting that this was not significant [21–23].

Also, bystander signaling has been observed in more complex cell tissue models. For example, localized irradiation of 3-D human skin reconstructs has reported transmission of bystander responses up to 1 mm away from the irradiated region [24]. Further studies have repeated these findings in lung tissue [25].

Several studies have also shown evidence for the production of radiation-induced bystander studies *in vivo*. In studies where rats with partially shielded lungs were irradiated, damaged cells were observed in the shielded regions, with cytokine signaling known to play a role [26]. Other studies have shown *in vivo* bystander responses in shielded spleen and in transplanted tumors after irradiation of normal tissues [27]. The anecdotal evidence of abscopal or out-of-field effects at a clinical level have been postulated to be evidence for long-range bystander responses in humans (see [28] for a review).

Bystander Studies with Radionuclides

Significant evidence is now emerging for bystander responses in studies where the effects of radionuclides have been studied rather than external beam exposures. A range of studies using different radionuclides have been reported (see Table 17.1). Testing for bystander responses with radionuclides is technically much more challenging than the approaches taken with external beam irradiation. For the assessment of bystander responses from external beam radiation exposure several experimental approaches are used. In the early studies, low fluence delivery of charged particles was used which restricted the fraction of cells randomly irradiated within a population to, for example, less than 1% [18]. More sophisticated approaches using microbeams have also been extensively used. Microbeams enable radiation to be specifically targeted to individual cells within a population and more specifically to sub-cellular locations [29]. For conventional X-ray or γ-ray studies of bystander responses two approaches have been used. Firstly, cell culture medium from irradiated cells is simply transferred to non-irradiated cells [19]. Secondly, an insert system is used where two populations are physically separated from each other [30]. All of these approaches can rely on the fact that the bystander populations have not received any direct radiation exposure. For studies with radionuclides testing for bystander responses, important challenges exist to ensure no radioactivity is incorporated into cells which would otherwise be defined as

Table 17.1 Properties of radionuclides used in bystander studies

Isotope	Decay	Energy (mean)	Half-life $T_{1/2}$	Range (mean)	Compounds labelled
^{3}H (tritium)	β-particles	5.67 keV	12.32 years	1.0 μm	Thymidine
^{123}Iodine	Auger	1.234 MeV	13.2 hours	<0.5 μm	MIBG/IUdR
^{125}Iodine	Auger	179 keV	60.1 days	<0.5 μm	IUdR
^{131}Iodine	β-particles	606 keV	8.04 days	0.36 mm	MIBG/IUdR
^{211}Astatine	α-particles	5.98 MeV	7.2 hours	50–70 μm	MIBG

bystander cells. Extensive washing to remove excess non-incorporated radionuclide and careful assessment of the effects of radionuclide efflux are required. This is especially critical, given the evidence from external radiation studies showing bystander responses are essentially a low dose response.

The earliest studies on radionuclide induced bystander responses have been using ^{3}H (tritium) and specifically labeling the DNA of cells using ^{3}H-TdR (thymidine). The mean energy of the β-rays is 5.67 keV with a mean range of 1 μm. Bishayee and colleagues compared the effectiveness of radiolabelled cells at being inactivated in small multicellular spheroids typically of 1.6 mm diameter consisting of 4×10^{6} V79 cells. Cells were allowed to accumulate various levels of ^{3}H at 4 °C over 36 hours. They compared the effectiveness of 100% of the cells within the small cell clusters being labeled versus 50% labeled. They saw an increased effectiveness, measured as loss of clonogenic survival, under the 50% conditions over that predicted from irradiation of the labeled cells only which they concluded was a bystander response. They also tested for a role for GJIC using the inhibitor lindane and found evidence for direct cell-cell communication in this model [31, 32].

In further studies, the group compared the effects of mixing ^{3}H-TdR rat liver epithelial cells (WB-F344) cells in monolayer in co-culture with non-labelled cells. Using a fluorescent staining approach, where one of the populations was stained with the membrane permeant reactive tracer, carboxyfluorescein diacetate succinimidyl ester (CFDA SE), the two cell populations could be discriminated using flow cytometry. Co-culturing of cells lead to an increase in the proliferation of bystander cells, which was dependent on the fraction of labeled cells present [33, 34].

In another similar study, Persaud and colleagues studied the effectiveness of ^{3}H-TdR-labelled CHO cells grown in multicellular spheroid with unlabelled hamster A_L cells in the ratio of 1:5 to produce a bystander response. After incubation, the A_L cells were separated by magnetic CD59 antibody technique and mutation analysis in these cells performed. Significant bystander mediated mutations were produced which contained a higher than expected frequency of deletion mutations. They similarly showed evidence for a role for reactive oxygen species and GJIC [35, 36].

Bystander responses after radionuclide incorporation have also been reported *in vivo*. In a highly sophisticated protocol, human colon LS174T adenocarcinoma tumour cells were prelabelled with ^{125}I-UdR and injected subcutaneously into nude mice with a mixture of non-labelled cells and dead cells. The labeled cells were loaded with the equivalent of a lethal dose of ^{125}I-UdR so were destined to die. The dead cells produced by freeze thawing cycles were included as "cell spacers" to ensure a consistent spacing of labeled and unlabelled cells in the exposed tumours. As the range of the auger electrons is in the order of <0.5 μm the authors estimated that bystander cells received no more than 10 cGy. Under these conditions with 1:1 and 1:5 ratio of labeled to unlabelled cells, significant tumour regression derived from the unlabelled cells was observed [37]. In further studies they compared the effects of ^{125}I with ^{123}I-labelling strategies in the same *in vivo* tumour model. They reported both an inhibitory bystander response for ^{125}I but for ^{123}I-labelled studies a stimulatory bystander response was observed which was confirmed from *in vitro* studies. The reasons for these differences are unclear as both radionuclides produced short range auger electron cascades. Interestingly, however there are significant differences in dose-rate due to the differences in half-life (^{123}I $t_{1/2}$ = 13.3 hours and ^{125}I $t_{1/2}$ = 60.5 days) with over a 100-fold difference.

These discrepancies in effect for different radionuclides in the same biological model are indicative of the need to more carefully compare different radionuclide mediated bystander responses in comparison to external beam exposure. In a recent important study, Boyd and colleagues [38] have compared the effect of an external radiation-mediated bystander response with different radionuclide approaches. In particular, they compared three different halogenated analogues of metaiodobenzylguanidine (MIBG). MIBG is selectively taken up into cells containing the noradrenaline transporter gene (NAT). The authors compared the effectiveness of the β-emitter ^{131}I-MIBG with the auger electron emitter ^{123}I-MIBG and the α emitter ^{211}At-astatobenzylguanidine (^{211}At-MABG) in two tumour lines transfected with NAT. For external beam irradiation followed by medium transfer onto non-irradiated cells a significant bystander response measured as a loss of clonogenic survival was observed. As found for other studies with external radiation approaches, the degree of bystander response increased at low dose and then saturated at ~60–70% survival in the two cell lines. This was in contrast to the studies with radionuclides where, although bystander responses were detected, no saturation was observed. For ^{131}I-MIBG, a significant bystander response was detected which increased in proportion to the activity added to the directly exposed cells, leading to killing of 70–80% of the bystander cells. In contrast treatment of cells with either ^{123}I-MIBG or ^{211}At-MABG led to an increased cell kill in recipient bystander cells upto a maximum of 35–70% but with increasing activity, the effect decreased again, leading to U-shaped response curves (see Fig. 17.1 for a schematic representation of these data). These studies suggest there may be important LET differences in the response of cells to bystander factors produced in response to radionuclide incorporation and that the types of bystander responses induced may be distinct from those observed after external radiation studies. One possibility is that the design of these studies may also be highlighting important dose-rate dependencies of bystander responses which have to date not been explored with external radiation approaches.

Impact on Radionuclide Therapy

It is important to speculate on what are the consequences of the observation of bystander responses after radionuclide treatments for therapy. Significant advances are being made on the use of targeted radionuclides in therapy. These include, for example, the ability to target small metastatic regions which are not accessible with conventional external beam approaches and the development of good biological targeting strategies to give tumour cell specificity [39, 40].

Earlier studies have predicted that the use of radionuclides which produce electrons with relatively long regions interacting with multiple cells would give benefits due to the observation of radiological cross-fire (see Fig. 17.2). For example, studies

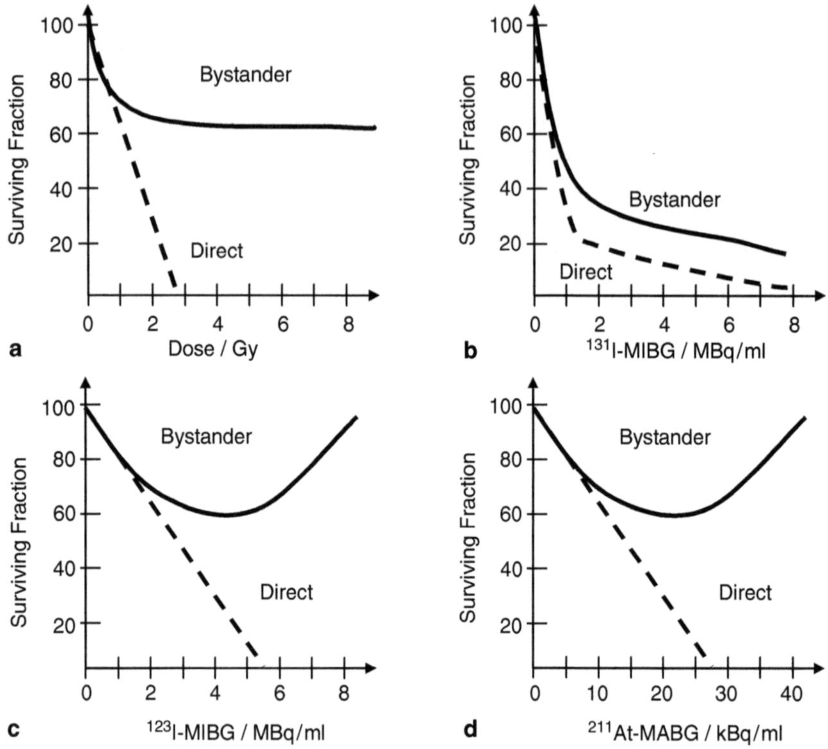

Fig. 17.1 Comparison of bystander responses for external beam irradiation versus radionuclide incorporation (Schematic summary of survival curves adapted from [38]). Panel A represents a typical bystander response after external γ-ray exposure, Panel B after ^{131}I-MIBG labeling, Panel C is for ^{123}I-MIBG labeling and Panel D for ^{211}At-MABG

in multicellular spheroids have shown that the effectiveness of ^{131}I-MIBG is twice that observed in cell monolayer studies due to significant cross-fire from the long range of the β-rays [41]. If recent experimental studies are extrapolated into a tumour killing situation it is clear that a radiobiological bystander response as well as cross-fire effects could be highly significant in producing additional cell kill. Future therapies involving radionuclides need, *a priori*, to consider the impact of bystander responses in overall outcome. The suggestion that dose-rate may be important needs to be further defined for both external beam and radionuclide exposures, as this may even impact on our use and development of brachytherapy approaches. To date we have bystander information on a very limited range of radionuclides despite the large range of potential candidates for therapy [42].

Finally, another consequence of the dose-effect relationships that have been reported for bystander responses in the literature is that they are predominantly low-dose effects. This has lead to considerable debate as to their relevance to radiation-risk at low doses with some authors suggesting that they impact on the current use of the LNT hypothesis for risk estimation [43]. This has lead to discussion that

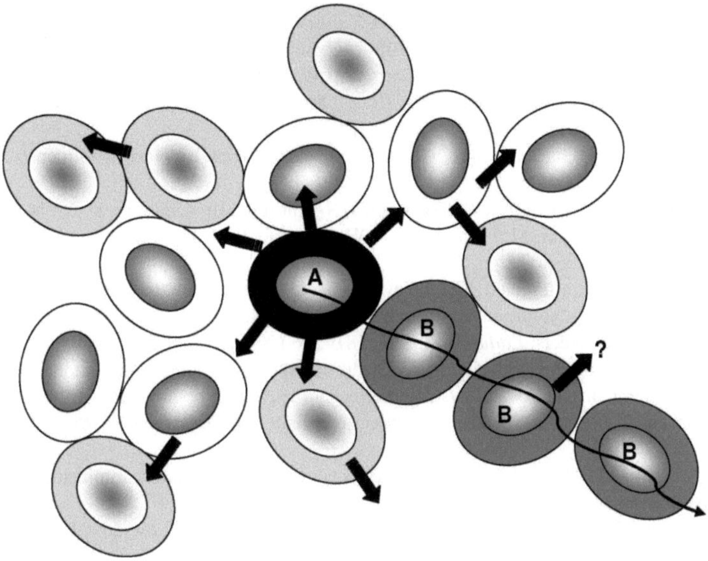

Fig. 17.2 Cross-fire versus bystander response. Cell A has a radionuclide incorporated into its nucleus which produces a long range electron track which interacts with cells B via a cross-fire response. Other cells can also respond due to the release of bystander signals from cell A and possibly from cells B also

low dose exposures may be considerably more "active" than previously thought and could for example impact on secondary cancer rates after external beam therapies [44]. A similar argument could also apply for radionuclide exposures if the robust bystander responses reported *in vitro* translate to *in vivo*. This could impact on the use of radionuclides for therapeutic and imaging approaches in the longer term. Clearly, however much more study of the role of cell-cell communication in a range of biological contexts is required for this to be fully elucidated.

Acknowledgements The author acknowledges the support of Cancer Research UK [CUK] grant number C1513/A7047, the European NOTE project (FI6R 036465) and the US National Institutes of Health (5P01CA095227-02).

References

1. R. L. Warters, K. G. Hofer, C. R. Harris and J. M. Smith, Radionuclide toxicity in cultured mammalian cells: elucidation of the primary site of radiation damage. *Curr. Top. Radiat. Res. Q.* **12**, 389–407 (1977).
2. R. L. Warters and K. G. Hofer, Radionuclide toxicity in cultured mammalian cells. Elucidation of the primary site for radiation-induced division delay. *Radiat. Res.* **69**, 348–358 (1977).
3. T. R. Munro, The relative radiosensitivity of the nucleus and cytoplasm of Chinese hamster fibroblasts. *Radiat. Res.* **42**, 451–470 (1970).

4. R. E. Zirkle, Partial-cell irradiation. In *Advances in Biology and Medical Physics* (J. H. Lawrence and C. A. Tobias, Eds.), pp. 103–146. Academic, New York, 1957.
5. A. Cole, R. E. Meyn, R. Chen, P. M. Corry and W. Hittelman, Mechanisms of cell injury. In *Radiation Biology in Cancer Research* (R. E. Meyn and H. R. Withers, Eds.), pp. 33–58. Raven Press, New York, 1980.
6. E. J. Hall and A. J. Giaccia, *Radiobiology for the Radiologist*. Lippincott William & Wilkins, Philadelphia, PA, 2006.
7. J. F. Ward, Non-DNA targeted effects and DNA models. In *Radiat. Res.* (M. Moriarty, C. Mothersill, C. Seymour, M. Edington, J. F. Ward and R. J. M. Fry, Eds.), pp. 379–402. Allen Press, Lawrence, KS, 2000.
8. W. F. Morgan, Non-targeted and delayed effects of exposure to ionizing radiation: II. Radiation-induced genomic instability and bystander effects in vivo, clastogenic factors and transgenerational effects. *Radiat. Res.* **159**, 581–596 (2003).
9. W. F. Morgan, Non-targeted and delayed effects of exposure to ionizing radiation: I. Radiation-induced genomic instability and bystander effects in vitro. *Radiat. Res.* **159**, 567–580 (2003).
10. S. Tapio and V. Jacob, Radioadaptive response revisited. *Radiat. Environ. Biophys.* **46**, 1–12 (2006).
11. E. G. Wright and P. J. Coates, Untargeted effects of ionizing radiation: implications for radiation pathology. *Mutat. Res.* **597**, 119–132 (2006).
12. M. C. Joiner, B. Marples, P. Lambin, S. C. Short and I. Turesson, Low-dose hypersensitivity: current status and possible mechanisms. *Int. J. Radiat. Oncol. Biol. Phys.* **49**, 379–389 (2001).
13. C. R. Mitchell, M. Folkard and M. C. Joiner, Effects of exposure to low-dose-rate (60)co gamma rays on human tumor cells in vitro. *Radiat. Res.* **158**, 311–318 (2002).
14. J. G. Hollowell and G. Littlefield, Chromosome damage induced by plasma of x-rayed patients: an indirect effect of x-ray. *Proc. Soc. Exp. Biol. Med.* **129**, 240–244 (1968).
15. I. Emerit, S. H. Khan and H. Esterbauer, Hydroxynonenal, a component of clastogenic factors? *Free Radic. Biol. Med.* **10**, 371–377 (1991).
16. C. Auclair, A. Gouyette, A. Levy and I. Emerit, Clastogenic inosine nucleotide as components of the chromosome breakage factor in scleroderma patients. *Arch. Biochem. Biophys.* **278**, 238–244 (1990).
17. I. Emerit, F. Garban, J. Vassy, A. Levy, P. Filipe and J. Freitas, Superoxide-mediated clastogenesis and anticlastogenic effects of exogenous superoxide dismutase. *Proc. Natl. Acad. Sci. USA* **93**, 12799–12804 (1996).
18. H. Nagasawa and J. B. Little, induction of sister chromatid exchanges by extremely low doses of α-particles. *Cancer Res.* **52**, 6394–6396 (1992).
19. C. Mothersill and C. Seymour, Medium from irradiated human epithelial cells but not human fibroblasts reduces the clonogenic survival of irradiated cells. *Int. J. Radiat. Biol.* **71**, 421–427 (1997).
20. E. I. Azzam, S. M. de Toledo, T. Gooding and J. B. Little, Intercellular communication is involved in the bystander regulation of gene expression in human cells exposed to very low fluences of alpha particles. *Radiat. Res.* **150**, 497–504 (1998).
21. C. Shao, M. Folkard, B. D. Michael and K. M. Prise, Targeted cytoplasmic irradiation induces bystander responses. *Proc. Natl. Acad. Sci. USA* **101**, 13495–13500 (2004).
22. L. Tartier, S. Gilchrist, S. Burdak-Rothkamm, M. Folkard and K. M. Prise, Cytoplasmic irradiation induces mitochondrial-dependent 53BP1 protein relocalization in irradiated and bystander cells. *Cancer Res.* **67**, 5872–5879 (2007).
23. L. J. Wu, G. Randers-Pehrson, A. Xu, C. A. Waldren, C. R. Geard, Z. Yu and T. K. Hei, Targeted cytoplasmic irradiation with alpha particles induces mutations in mammalian cells. *Proc. Natl. Acad. Sci. USA* **96**, 4959–4964 (1999).
24. O. V. Belyakov, S. A. Mitchell, D. Parikh, G. Randers-Pehrson, S. A. Marino, S. A. Amundson, C. R. Geard and D. J. Brenner, Biological effects in unirradiated human tissue induced by radiation damage up to 1 mm away. *Proc. Natl. Acad. Sci. USA* **102**, 14203–14208 (2005).

25. O. A. Sedelnikova, A. Nakamura, O. Kovalchuk, I. Koturbash, S. A. Mitchell, S. A. Marino, D. J. Brenner and W. M. Bonner, DNA double-strand breaks form in bystander cells after microbeam irradiation of three-dimensional human tissue models. *Cancer Res.* **67**, 4295–4302 (2007).
26. M. A. Khan, R. P. Hill and J. Van Dyk, Partial volume rat lung irradiation: an evaluation of early DNA damage. *Int. J. Radiat. Oncol. Biol. Phys.* **40**, 467–476 (1998).
27. I. Koturbash, R. E. Rugo, C. A. Hendricks, J. Loree, B. Thibault, K. Kutanzi, I. Pogribny, J. C. Yanch, B. P. Engelward and O. Kovalchuk, Irradiation induces DNA damage and modulates epigenetic effectors in distant bystander tissue in vivo. *Oncogene* **25**, 4267–4275 (2006).
28. J. M. Kaminski, E. Shinohara, J. B. Summers, K. J. Niermann, A. Morimoto and J. Brousal, The controversial abscopal effect. *Cancer Treat. Rev.* **31**, 159–172 (2005).
29. K. M. Prise, O. V. Belyakov, M. Folkard and B. D. Michael, Studies of bystander effects in human fibroblasts using a charged particle microbeam. *Int. J. Radiat. Biol.* **74**, 793–798 (1998).
30. H. Yang, N. Asaad and K. D. Held, Medium-mediated intercellular communication is involved in bystander responses of X-ray-irradiated normal human fibroblasts. *Oncogene* (2005).
31. A. Bishayee, D. V. Rao and R. W. Howell, Evidence for pronounced bystander effects caused by nonuniform distributions of radioactivity using a novel three-dimensional tissue culture model. *Radiat. Res.* **152**, 88–97 (1999).
32. A. Bishayee, H. Z. Hill, D. Stein, D. V. Rao and R. W. Howell, Free radical-initiated and gap junction-mediated bystander effect due to nonuniform distribution of incorporated radioactivity in a three-dimensional tissue culture model. *Radiat. Res.* **155**, 1–10 (2000).
33. B. I. Gerashchenko and R. W. Howell, Bystander cell proliferation is modulated by the number of adjacent cells that were exposed to ionizing radiation. *Cytometry A* **66**, 62–70 (2005).
34. B. I. Gerashchenko and R. W. Howell, Proliferative response of bystander cells adjacent to cells with incorporated radioactivity. *Cytometry A* **60**, 155–164 (2004).
35. R. Persaud, H. Zhou, S. E. Baker, T. K. Hei and E. J. Hall, Assessment of low linear energy transfer radiation-induced bystander mutagenesis in a three-dimensional culture model. *Cancer Res.* **65**, 9876–9882 (2005).
36. R. Persaud, H. Zhou, T. K. Hei and E. J. Hall, Demonstration of a radiation-induced bystander effect for low dose low LET beta-particles. *Radiat. Environ. Biophys.* **46**, 395–400 (2007).
37. L. Y. Xue, N. J. Butler, G. M. Makrigiorgos, S. J. Adelstein and A. I. Kassis, Bystander effect produced by radiolabeled tumor cells in vivo. *Proc. Natl. Acad. Sci. USA* **99**, 13765–13770 (2002).
38. M. Boyd, S. C. Ross, J. Dorrens, N. E. Fullerton, K. W. Tan, M. R. Zalutsky and R. J. Mairs, Radiation-induced biologic bystander effect elicited in vitro by targeted radiopharmaceuticals labeled with alpha-, beta-, and auger electron-emitting radionuclides. *J. Nucl. Med.* **47**, 1007–1015 (2006).
39. J. L. Dearling and R. B. Pedley, Technological advances in radioimmunotherapy. *Clin. Oncol. (Royal College of Radiologists (Great Britain))* **19**, 457–469 (2007).
40. S. J. DeNardo and G. L. Denardo, Targeted radionuclide therapy for solid tumors: an overview. *Int. J. Radiat. Oncol., Biol., Phys.* **66**, S89–95 (2006).
41. M. Boyd, S. H. Cunningham, M. M. Brown, R. J. Mairs and T. E. Wheldon, Noradrenaline transporter gene transfer for radiation cell kill by 131I meta-iodobenzylguanidine. *Gene Ther.* **6**, 1147–1152 (1999).
42. C. A. Boswell and M. W. Brechbiel, Development of radioimmunotherapeutic and diagnostic antibodies: an inside-out view. *Nucl. Med. Biol.* **34**, 757–778 (2007).
43. D. J. Brenner, R. Doll, D. T. Goodhead, E. J. Hall, C. E. Land, J. B. Little, J. H. Lubin, D. L. Preston, R. J. Preston, et al., Cancer risks attributable to low doses of ionizing radiation: assessing what we really know. *Proc. Natl. Acad. Sci. USA* **100**, 13761–13766 (2003).
44. E. J. Hall, Intensity-modulated radiation therapy, protons, and the risk of second cancers. *Int. J. Radiat. Oncol. Biol. Phys.* **65**, 1–7 (2006).

Chapter 18
Enhancing the Efficiency of Targeted Radionuclide Therapy

Gregory P. Adams

Summary While radionuclide therapy has been effective using radiolabeled antibodies in the treatment of solid tumors in animal models and in the clinical treatment of diffuse (liquid) malignancies, similar successes are rarely seen in the treatment solid tumors in the clinical setting. Alternate strategies are needed to improve the clinical efficacy. There is an emerging body of evidence that this could be accomplished through a number of means including; the use of radiation sensitizers, the normalization of tumor vasculature, the selectively enhancement of tumor vascular permeability or the use of combination therapy with agents that have complementary therapeutic effects.

Radiation Sensitizers

Radiation sensitizers function by increasing the sensitivity of tissues to the effects of radioactive emissions, often by decreasing DNA repair, increasing double stranded DNA breaks, overcoming the hypoxia problem or inducing apoptosis. By far the majority of the clinical experience with radiation sensitizers comes from their use with external beam radiation therapy (XRT), however, in many cases there is potential for these same agents to enhance the efficacy of targeted radionuclide therapy. Most of the commonly employed agents are chemotherapy drugs, such as 5-fluorouracil (5-FU) and cisplatin (reviewed in [23]), however, more recently new classes of molecularly targeted agents such as monoclonal antibodies and small molecule tyrosine kinase inhibitors have emerged as potential sensitizers for XRT (reviewed in [30]). While the former class of agents are not themselves targeted to the site of tumor, combining them with targeted radionuclide therapy can focus their effects.

Department of Medical Oncology, Fox Chase Cancer Center, Philadelphia, PA 19111, USA

T. Stigbrand et al. (eds.) *Targeted Radionuclide Tumor Therapy*,

Autosensitization

In general, using an antibody-based molecule strictly as a delivery vehicle for therapeutic radionuclides seems in many cases to be insufficient. The most effective radioimmunotherapy, RAIT, agents are those in which the naked antibody itself has an anti-tumor effect, which is further amplified by the addition of the radionuclide that it is delivering. An example is the effective use of Ibritumomab tiuxetan (Zevalin) for the treatment of non-Hodgkins lymphomas, NHL. Zevalin is composed of Ibritumomab, the murine parent antibody of rituximab (Rituxan), combined with ^{90}Y. While treatment with rituximab is associated with true clinical responses, the addition of the beta-emitting radionuclide ^{90}Y significantly enhances therapeutic outcome (reviewed in [18]). In fact, the ideal antibody and radionuclide pair for RAIT would be one in which the binding of the antibody to its target receptor directly leads to a signaling event that results in the radiosensitization of the cell.

A number of antibodies have been shown to possess radiosensitization properties when used in combination with XRT (reviewed in [30]). For example, antibodies that target EGFR enhance XRT efficacy both in the preclinical and clinical setting [4, 20]. However, the most impressive report was that of Bonner et al in which the addition of treatment with the anti-EGFR MAb cetuximab to XRT significantly prolonged both survival (49 months vs. 29 months for XRT alone) and the duration of locoregional control of tumor growth (24 months vs. 15 months for XRT alone) [1]. Antibodies against HER2 (erbB-2), another member of the epidermal growth factor receptor family, have been found to sensitize HER2 overexpressing tumor cells *in vitro* [17, 28] and preliminary clinical trial results suggest that a similar effect may be possible in the clinical setting [27].

These effects are likely due to the alteration of downstream signal transduction of the RAF and PI3 kinase signaling pathways that normalize the enhanced radiation resistance often associated with overexpression of these growth factor receptors (see also chapter 13). A rigorous examination of the role of autosensitization in RAIT by antibodies that effect of down stream signaling pathways associated with radiation sensitivity has yet to be performed, and in fact could be difficult to establish due to a number of issues with targeting efficiency, receptor expression levels, etc. However, the observations from the XRT studies described above strongly suggest that autosensitization is potentially a factor in the efficacy of RAIT targeted against growth factor receptors.

Sensitizing Agents

Significantly more evidence is available supporting use of "secondary" radiosensitizing agents to enhance the efficacy of targeted radionuclide therapy. The most compelling reports are from studies combining chemotherapeutic agents and RAIT.

Chemotherapy commonly causes delays in the growth of cancer cells, often arresting them in a radiation sensitive phase of the cell cycle [15, 19, 29]. Examples of effective combinations of chemotherapy and RAIT are provided below.

Gemcitabine. Gemcitabine is a commonly employed chemotherapeutic agent that functions as a nucleoside analog and arrests cells during DNA replication. In preclinical studies, Milenic et al. demonstrated that pretreatment of athymic mice with gemcitabine (50 mg/kg) 24–30 hours prior to RAIT significantly enhanced the efficacy of therapy with the alpha emitter ^{212}Pb-trastuzumab immunoconjugate (5–10 μCi) of i.p. disseminated LS-174T human colon adenocarcinoma tumor cells [21]. In these studies mice without treatment exhibited a median survival of 16 days, treatment with 5 μCi ^{212}Pb-trastuzumab without gemcitabine improved the mean survival to 31 days and pretreatment with gemcitabine prior to RAIT extended the mean survival to 51 days. The 10 μCi dose group exhibited further improvements with survivals of 45 and 70 days, respectively for RAIT alone and gemcitabine plus RAIT. Interestingly, the effect was further enhanced when the mice were given three doses of gemcitabine, one prior to RAIT and two afterwards.

Systemic low dose RAIT with beta emitting radionuclide conjugates has also been shown to benefit from the addition of gemcitabine. Gold et al reported that athymic nude mice bearing large s.c. human CaPan1 pancreatic cancer xenografts exhibited significantly enhanced reductions in tumor growth rate and prolonged survival when treated with the combination of RAIT with ^{90}Y-labeled anti-MUC-1 PAM4 MAb and gemcitabine [7]. In these studies, three week cycles of gemcitabine (1,000 mg/m^2/week) and ^{90}Y-labeled PAM4 (25 μCi; 10% of the single agent MTD) resulted in a median survival of 24 weeks, treatment with only ^{90}Y-labeled PAM4 yielded a median survival of 16 weeks and treatment with gemcitabine alone resulted in a median survival of 10 weeks. As the administered doses of radioimmunoconjugate were well below what would be required for single-agent antitumor effects, this combination therapy was associated with minimal toxicity to normal tissues.

The same group reported similar responses to combinations of gemcitabine and the same antibody conjugated to another beta emitting radioisotope, ^{131}I [3]. The timing of the administration of RAIT and gemcitabine is likely critical in the initiation of a radiosensitizing effect. While pre-administration of gemcitabine, as described above, led to radiosensitization, co-administration of ^{131}I-MN-14, an anti-CEA Mab did not enhance the efficacy as compared to ^{131}I-MAb alone [13].

Taxanes. Paclitaxel is another commonly employed chemotherapeutic agent that has shown promise as a radiosensitizer for RAIT applications. The efficacy as a radiosensitizer stems from its ability to stabilize microtubules, thereby preventing the separation of chromosomes and arresting cells in the G_2/M phase of the cell cycle. O'Donnell et al effectively used paclitaxel (Taxol) to enhance the efficacy of ^{90}Y-DOTA-chimeric L6 (ChL6) MAb therapy in mice bearing human PC3 prostate cancer xenografts [22]. Paclitaxel (600 μg) plus RAIT (75 μCi) resulted in a 100% response rate with 20% cures as compared to the RAIT alone or paclitaxel alone groups, which exhibited no cures. Overall, the average tumor size in the groups that received combination treatment was reduced compared to the control groups and the anti-tumor responses that were achieved were durable. Significantly, the degree of myelotoxicity was similar in the combined modality groups and the groups receiving the same dose of RAIT alone. The combination of paclitaxel and RAIT with a ^{90}Y-conjugated MAb (m170) was tolerated with toxicities limited to bone marrow suppression in a small pilot phase I clinical trial [26], suggesting that the clinical use of this combination of agents is reasonable.

Paclitaxel has also been reported to enhance the effects of alpha particle RAIT on newly formed tumors, suggesting that the combination may be effective in the setting of minimum residual disease. Kelly et al. found that increasing doses (15–60 μCuries) of ^{213}Bi-hu3S193 anti-LewisY immunoconjugate was significantly more effective at reducing the growth rate of two days old MCF-7 tumors when the animals were given a subtherapeutic dose of 300 μg of Paclitaxel 24 hours after RAIT [8].

Engineered bispecific antibodies (bsAb) have also been successfully used in combination with paclitaxel to increase the therapeutic efficacy of pretargeted radionuclide therapy. Kraeber-Bodéré found that paclitaxel, but not doxorubicin, improved the anti-tumor response of thyroid cancer xenografts to an anti-CEA/anti-indium-DTPA bsAb followed by ^{131}I-labeled bivalent hapten and the chemotherapeutic drugs [14]. As in the studies described above, there were no increases in toxicity associated with the addition of paclitaxel to RAIT.

A second taxane, docetaxel (Taxotere), has also demonstrated efficacy in *in vivo* models. In mice, combined treatments of docetaxel (300 μg) plus RAIT with ^{90}Y-DOTA-ChL6 MAb (75 μCi) resulted in a 67% cure rate of human PC3 prostate tumor xenografts, whereas no response was observed in mice treated with RAIT or chemotherapy alone [22].

Small molecule inhibitors. Small molecule tyrosine kinase inhibitors (TKI) are playing an increasingly important role in tumor therapy. These agents work by interfering with the mitogenic/anti-apoptotic signaling cascade that results from the presence of either constitutively activated overexpressed members of the EGFR family of receptor tyrosine kinases or ligand induced signaling through these receptors. TKIs have been effectively combined with RAIT in preclinical studies. Lee et al recently reported that administration of sub-therapeutic doses of the EGFR inhibitor, AG1478, to BALB/c nude mice bearing A431squamous carcinoma tumors improved the outcome of RAIT [16]. In this study treatment with a single 25 μCi dose of ^{90}Y-CHX-″A-DTPA-hu3S193, a humanized anti-Lewis Y antibody led to a small, but significant reduction in tumor growth rate.

A second small molecule TKI, imatinib (Glivec or Gleevec), was also recently employed in combination with RAIT in preclinical studies. The potent PDGFRbeta inhibitor imatinib, when combined with ^{131}I-CC49 MAb, also resulted in small, but significant, reduction in tumor growth rate of PC-3 prostate cancer xenografts as compared with RAIT alone [9]. As above with AG1478, treatment with imatinib alone had no effect on tumor growth.

While the overall outcome of the studies reported above were rather modest, their major significance is that they represent the vanguard of a new class of potentially potent combination therapy strategies. As the signaling networks impacted by these small molecule TKIs are complex and often redundant, it is possible that signaling through other members of the network was not sufficiently blocked, thereby attenuating the effect of these combination therapy strategies. This suggests that combinations of RAIT with small molecule TKIs with a broader specificity profiles or cocktails of TKIs may lead to enhanced results. This is supported by the observation by Fukutome et al. that combinations of gefitinib (ZD1839) and trastuzumab additively increased the *in vitro* radiosensitivity of A431 cells [6].

Anti-angiogenics. Another method to augment the effects of RAIT is through the addition of anti-angiogenic agents. As radiolabeled antibodies are often found to be limited in their ability to penetrate into solid tumors, the cancer cells directly affected by RAIT are typically closer to the well-vascularized regions of the tumor. This limits the ability of RAIT to successfully treat the viable cells residing in the hypoxic areas of the tumor. The combination of RAIT and anti-vascular agents in theory should be complementary as the former focuses on the perivascular regions and the latter shuts down the blood flow to the deeper regions of the tumor.

Burke et al. examined the effect of combinations of the anti-alpha$_v$beta$_3$ integrin receptor cyclic Arg-Gly-Asp peptide, Cilengitide (EMD 121974), which targets neovasculature, and ^{90}Y-ChL6 on HBT 3477 human breast tumor xenografts growing in nude mice [2]. Cilengitide alone had no effect on tumor growth. RAIT with ^{90}Y-ChL6 resulted in a 15% cure rate and the addition of Cilengitide increased the cure rate to 53%. Interestingly, post-treatment analysis of the tumors from the mice that received both RAIT and Cilengitide revealed significantly increased apoptosis of both endothelial and tumor cells at five days post treatment as compared to mice that only received RAIT.

Another effective combination of RAIT and the anti-vascular therapy was reported by Pedley et al. [24]. Combretastatin A-4 3-O-phosphate (CA4-P) P and RAIT with^{131}I conjugated anti-CEA MAb produced complete cures in five of six mice bearing colorectal xenografts. In contrast, mice treated with RAIT alone exhibited a median survival of 60 days while those treated with CA4-P or left untreated had a median survival of 20 days. Macroscopic examination of the tumors following treatment with RAIT or CA4-P alone revealed the expected complementary cytotoxicity patterns. Other angiogenesis inhibitors, such as thalidomide, have been effective in animal models in combination with RAIT using murine MAbs [12].

Enhanced vascular permeability. Increased efficacy of RAIT can also be achieved by enhancing the localization of the radioimmunoconjugate in the tumor. Systemic administration of angiotensin II (ATII) mediates arteriolar constriction throughout the body, leading to widespread hypertension. In contrast to the vaculature of normal tissues, the vessels located in tumors lack smooth muscles and are therefore not constricted [10]. This leads to increased blood flow to solid tumors and enhanced, selective uptake of systemically administered radiolabeled antibody. However, for this application, ATII exposure must only occur for a limited time as infusions beyond 72 hours in duration lead to increased normal tissue uptake.

Combinations of ATII and enalapril, a kinase inhibitor, can also be used to mediate both improved tumor blood flow and increased vascular permeability, leading to further enhancement of tumor uptake of radiolabeled antibodies and improved efficacy in preclinical RAIT studies. Kinuya et al. reported that administration of ATII and enalapril to immunodeficient mice bearing human colon cancer xenografts one hour prior to RAIT with ^{131}I-A7 Mab, increased the tumor absorbed dose 1.5-fold without altering the absorbed doses in normal tissues. This led to a significant reduction in tumor growth rate [11]. The A7 Mab is specific for a 45-kDa glycoprotein expressed on colorectal cancer.

Normalization of tumor vasculature. Tumor vasculature is characteristically abnormal, exhibiting significant twists and fenestrations. This can lead to elevated interstitial pressure and non-uniform tumor perfusion of therapeutic agents such as radiolabeled MAbs (reviewed in [5]). As one of the effects resulting from treatment with the anti-VEGF MAb bevacizumab is the normalization of tumor blood flow, anti-VEGF therapy is emerging as a method of enhancing delivery of a variety of anti-cancer agents, including those linked to antibodies, to tumors [31].

The normalization of tumor blood flow with anti-VEGF agents also leads to reduced tumor hypoxia, thereby making the targeted tissues more sensitive to the effects of ionizing radiation. Winkler et al reported that the use of the anti-VEGF-2 receptor MAb DC101 enhanced the efficacy of radiation therapy in mice bearing human glioblastoma xenografts [32]. Combinations of bevacizumab and trastuzumab have also been found to be safe in a phase I clinical trial and were associated with therapeutic responses [25]. This suggests that a similar approach would be feasible, combining anti-VEGF and RAIT agents.

Conclusions

While targeted radionuclide therapy as a monotherapy has been severely limited in its ability to mediate meaningful clinical anti-tumor effects in the setting of solid malignancies, numerous strategies are available to enhancement of both the localization and efficacy of such therapy. A variety of agents ranging from antibodies and TKIs to chemotherapeutic drugs have been effective at enhancing the efficacy of targeted radionuclide therapy in the preclinical setting, assessment of their utility in the clinical setting should be a high priority for our field.

References

1. Bonner JA, Harari PM, Giralt J, et al. Radiotherapy plus Cetuximab for Squamous-Cell Carcinoma of the Head and Neck. NEJM, 354:567–578, 2006.
2. Burke PA, DeNardo SJ, Miers LA, Lamborn KR, Matzku S, DeNardo GL. Cilengitide targeting of alpha(v)beta(3) integrin receptor synergizes with radioimmunotherapy to increase efficacy and apoptosis in breast cancer xenografts. Cancer Res. 62:4263–4272, 2002.
3. Cardillo TM, Blumenthal R, Ying Z, Gold DV. Combined gemcitabine and radioimmunotherapy for the treatment of pancreatic cancer. Int. J. Cancer 97:386–392, 2002.

4. Curran D, Giralt J, Harari PM, et al. Quality of life in head and neck cancer patients after treatment with high-dose radiotherapy alone or in combination with cetuximab. J. Clin. Oncol. 25:2191–2197, 2007.
5. Ellis LM. Mechanisms of action of bevacizumab as a component of therapy for metastatic colorectal cancer. Semin. Oncol. 33(5 Suppl 10):S1–7, 2006.
6. Fukutome M, Maebayashi K, Nasu S, Seki K, Mitsuhashi N. Enhancement of radiosensitivity by dual inhibition of the HER family with ZD1839 ("Iressa") and trastuzumab ("Herceptin"). Int. J. Radiat. Oncol. Biol. Phys. 66:528–536, 2006.
7. Gold DV, Schutsky K, Modrak D, Cardillo TM. Low-dose radioimmunotherapy (90Y-PAM4) combined with gemcitabine for the treatment of experimental pancreatic cancer. Clin. Cancer Res. 9(Suppl):3929s–3937s, September 1, 2003.
8. Kelly MP, Lee FT, Tahtis K, Smyth FE, Brechbiel MW, Scott AM. Radioimmunotherapy with alpha-particle emitting 213Bi-C-functionalized trans-cyclohexyl-diethylenetriaminepentaacetic acid-humanized 3S193 is enhanced by combination with paclitaxel chemotherapy. Clin. Cancer Res. 13:5604s–5612s, 2007.
9. Kimura Y, Inoue K, Abe M, Nearman J, Baranowska-Kortylewicz J. PDGFRbeta and HIF-1alpha inhibition with imatinib and radioimmunotherapy of experimental prostate cancer. Cancer Biol. Ther. 6(11):1763–1772, 2007 [Epub].
10. Kinuya S, Yokoyama K, Yamamoto W, et al. Short-period-induced hypertension could improve tumor-to-nontumor ratios of radiolabeled monoclonal antibody. Nucl. Med. Biol. 24:547–551, 1997.
11. Kinuya S, Yokoyama K, Kawashima A, et al. Pharmacologic intervention with angiotensin II and kininase inhibitor enhanced efficacy of radioimmunotherapy in human colon cancer xenografts. J. Nucl. Med. 41:1244–1249, 2000.
12. Kinuya S, Kawashima A, Yokoyama K, et al. Cooperative effect of radioimmunotherapy and antiangiogenic therapy with thalidomide in human cancer xenografts. J. Nucl. Med. 43:1084–1089, 2002.
13. Koppe MJ, Oyen WJ, Bleichrodt RP, Verhofstad AA, Goldenberg DM, Boerman OC. Combination therapy using gemcitabine and radioimmunotherapy in nude mice with small peritoneal metastases of colonic origin. Cancer Biother. Radiopharm. 21:506–514, 2006.
14. Kraeber-Bodéré F, Saï-Maurel C, Campion L, et al. Enhanced antitumor activity of combined pretargeted radioimmunotherapy and paclitaxel in medullary thyroid cancer xenograft. Mol. Cancer Ther. 1:267–274, 2002.
15. Lawrence TS, Eisbruch, A, Shewach DS. Gemcitabine mediated radiosensitization. Semin. Oncol. 24: S7–24, 1997.
16. Lee FT, Mountain AJ, Kelly MP, et al. Enhanced efficacy of radioimmunotherapy with 90Y-CHX-A″-DTPA-hu3S193 by inhibition of epidermal growth factor receptor (EGFR) signaling with EGFR tyrosine kinase inhibitor AG1478. Clin Cancer Res. 11:7080s–7086s, 2005.
17. Liang K, Lu Y, Jin W, Ang KK, Milas L, Fan Z. Sensitization of breast cancer cells to radiation by trastuzumab. Mol. Cancer Ther. 2:1113–1120, 2003.
18. Macklis RM. Radioimmunotherapy as a therapeutic option for non-Hodgkin's lymphoma. Semin. Radiat. Oncol. 17:176–183, 2007.
19. McGinn CJ, Shewach DS, Lawrence TS. Radiosensitizing nucleosides. J. Nat. Cancer. Inst. (Bethesda) 88:1193–1203, 1996.
20. Milas L, Fang FM, Mason KA, et al. Importance of maintenance therapy in C225-induced enhancement of tumor control by fractionated radiation. Int. J. Radiat. Oncol. Biol. Phys. 67:568–572, 2007.
21. Milenic DE, Garmestani K, Brady ED, et al. Potentiation of high-LET radiation by gemcitabine: targeting HER2 with trastuzumab to treat disseminated peritoneal disease. Clin. Cancer Res. 13:1926–1935, 2007.
22. O'Donnell RT, DeNardo SJ, Miers LA, et al. Combined modality radioimmunotherapy for human prostate cancer xenografts with taxanes and ^{90}yttrium-DOTA-peptide-ChL6. Prostate 50:27–37, 2002.

23. Oehler C, Dickinson DJ, Broggini-Tenzer A, et al. Current concepts for the combined treatment modality of ionizing radiation with anticancer agents. Curr. Pharm. Des. 13:519–535, 2007.
24. Pedley RB, El-Emir E, Flynn AA, et al. Synergy between vascular targeting agents and antibody-directed therapy. Int. J. Radiat. Oncol. Biol. Phys. 54:1524–1531, 2002.
25. Pegram M, Chan D, Dichmann RA, et al. Phase II combined biological therapy targeting the HER2 proto-oncogene and the vascular endothelial growth factor using trastuzumab (T) and bevacizumab (B) as first line treatment of HER2-amplified breast cancer. Breast Cancer Res. Treat. 100(Suppl 1):S28 (abstract 301).
26. Richman CM, Denardo SJ, O'Donnell RT, et al. High-dose radioimmunotherapy combined with fixed, low-dose paclitaxel in metastatic prostate and breast cancer by using a MUC-1 monoclonal antibody, m170, linked to indium-111/yttrium-90 via a cathepsin cleavable linker wit cyclosporine to prevent human anti-mouse antibody. Clin. Cancer Res. 11:5920–5927, 2005.
27. Sartor, CG, Carey, L, Dees, EC, Ollila, D, Sherron, R, et al. Radiosensitization of locally advanced breast cancer with Herceptin – initial toxicity results of a phase II trial. In: San Antonio Breast Cancer Meeting, 2003.
28. Sato S, Kajiyama Y, Sugano M, et al. Monoclonal antibody to HER-2/neu receptor enhances radiosensitivity of esophagealcancer cell lines expressing HER-2/neu oncoprotein. Int. J. Radiat. Oncol. Biol. Phys. 61:203–211, 2005.
29. Shewach DS, Hahn TM, Chang E., Hertel LW, Lawrence TS. Metabolism of 2_,2_-Difluoro-2_-deoxycytidine and radiation sensitization of human colon carcinoma cells. Cancer Res, 54:3218–3223, 1994.
30. Spalding AC, Lawrence TS. New and emerging radiosensitizers and radioprotectors. Cancer Invest 24:444–546, 2006.
31. Tong RT, BoucherY, Kozin SV,Winkler F, Hicklin DJ, Jain RK. Vascular normalization by vascular endothelial growth factor receptor 2 blockade induces a pressure gradient across the vasculature and improves drug penetration in tumors. Cancer Res. 64:3731–3736, 2004.
32. Winkler F, Kozin SV,Tong RT, et al. Kinetics of vascular normalization byVEGFR2 blockade governs brain tumor response to radiation: role of oxygenation, angiopoietin-1, and matrix metalloproteinases. Cancer Cell. 6:553–563, 2004.

Chapter 19
Low Dose Hyper-Radiosensitivity: A Historical Perspective

Brian Marples[1], Sarah A. Krueger[1], Spencer J. Collis[2], and Michael C. Joiner[3]

Summary This chapter discusses the biology of low-dose hyper-radiosensitivity (HRS) with reference to radiation-induced DNA damage and cellular repair processes. Particular attention is paid to the significance of G2-phase cell cycle checkpoints in overcoming low-dose hyper-radiosensitivity and the impact of HRS on low-dose rate radiobiology. The history of HRS from the original *in vivo* discovery to the most recent *in vitro* and clinical data are examined to present a unifying hypothesis concerning the molecular control and regulation of this important low-dose radiation response. Finally, pre-clinical and clinical data are discussed, from a molecular viewpoint, to provide theoretical approaches to exploit HRS biology for clinical gain.

Introduction

The past two decades have seen the discovery and characterization of several low-dose radiobiological phenomena. These include genomic instability [1], the adaptive responses [2, 3], bystander effects [4] and cell survival as characterized by low-dose hyper-radiosensitivity (HRS) [5]. These responses exhibit some similar biological traits but each shows individual distinguishing characteristics [6]. The purpose of this chapter is to describe the molecular developments of HRS biology within the context of DNA repair processes, and explain how utilization of this knowledge could impact clinical practice.

[1]Department of Radiation Oncology, William Beaumont Hospital, 3811 W. Thirteen Mile Road, 105-RI, Royal Oak, MI 48073-0213, USA

[2]DNA Damage Response Laboratory, Cancer Research UK, Clare Hall Laboratories, Blanche Lane, South Mimms, EN6 3LD, UK

[3]Department of Radiation Oncology, Wayne State University, Gershenson Radiation Oncology Center, 4100 John R, Detroit, MI 48201-2013, USA

T. Stigbrand et al. (eds.) *Targeted Radionuclide Tumor Therapy*,

Background

The Measurement of Low-Dose Cell Survival

The association between cell survival and radiation dose was originally described in prokaryotes. Some 80 years later, techniques were developed for the extended culturing of eukaryotic cells [7], which allowed production of the first radiation cell survival measurements using mammalian cells [8]. The clonogenic survival assay, pioneered by Puck and Marcus, quickly became the standard technique for measuring cellular radiosensitivity [8]. However, the assay lacked the necessary resolution to accurately define radiosensitivity after low clinically-relevant radiation doses (<1 Gy), since it relied on the serial dilution of cells during plating [9]. Consequently, the survival response of cells following low radiation doses could only be estimated by back-extrapolating clonogenic data obtained from high doses using biomathematical models. Bedford and Griggs [10] overcame this low-dose limitation by accurately counting the number of cells plated at each dose point, and in doing so improved the statistical confidence of the assay. This experimental approach was later refined by Durand [11], who applied flow cytometry to plate a precise number of cells. Around the same time, a group lead by Palcic devised an entirely different approach that used an automated scanning microscope to locate and track individual cells after plating [12]. Importantly, low-dose hyper-radiosensitivity (HRS) was first identified *in vitro* by Marples and Joiner, using this location technique [13]. More recently, Weinfeld and colleagues have described an additional high-precision cell plating system called the gel microdrop (GMD) protocol [14] which has been successfully applied to define HRS. Despite these alternative techniques, the most widely applied methodology used routinely is the flow cytometric protocol of Durand [11], since this assay can be readily adapted to study cells in specific cell cycle phases [15, 16]. This latter advantage subsequently became pivotal in further understanding the cellular mechanisms underlying HRS biology.

Low Dose Cell Survival: The HRS/IRR Transition

Mammalian cells exhibit enhanced radiosensitivity to radiation doses below ~0.2 Gy when given at acute dose rates; the so-called low-dose hyper-radiosensitivity (HRS) response (See Fig. 19.1) [13]. Whereas, over the ~0.3–0.6 Gy dose range, a more radioresistant response per unit dose builds up as illustrated by the shallower slope of the radiation dose-response curve. The transition towards this radiation resistance associated with overcoming HRS is generically described by the term "increased radioresistance" (IRR). Then, above 1 Gy a more conventional downward-bending survival curve is seen that is well-described by a linear-quadratic relationship between –log(surviving fraction) and dose. Data from several laboratories have now unambiguously verified the existence of HRS and demonstrated that low-dose radiation effects (<0.3 Gy) cannot reliably be predicted by back-extrapolating from measurements made at high doses for the majority of cell lines.

The presence of HRS can be confirmed by fitting cell survival data with Joiner's Induced Repair model [13, 17] (Equation 1); and demonstrating that the low-dose value of α describing the HRS region (α_s) is higher than that of the conventional high dose response (α_r), combined with a value of d_c (the transition point indicating the change from low (HRS) to high dose (IRR) survival response) that is significantly greater than zero. The validation of HRS using this model necessitates that multiple measurements of low-dose cell survival are made, with several measurements below 1 Gy including values below 0.3 Gy.

$$s = \exp\left\{-\alpha_r\left(1+\left(\alpha_s/\alpha_r - 1\right)e^{-d/d_c}\right)d - \beta d^2\right\} \tag{1}$$

Where d is dose, and α_s represents the low-dose value of α (derived from the response at very low doses), α_r is the value extrapolated from the conventional high-dose response, d_c is the 'transition' dose point at which the change from the very low-dose HRS to the IRR response occurs (i.e. when α_s to α_r is 63% complete) and α is a constant as in the high-dose LQ equation.

Two recent molecular studies [18, 19] have also reported non-linear dose-dependent radiation responses over the 0–1 Gy dose range, the most notable of these being the activation of ataxia telangiectasia mutated (ATM) activity [19]. These reports are consistent with the concept that repair systems respond to

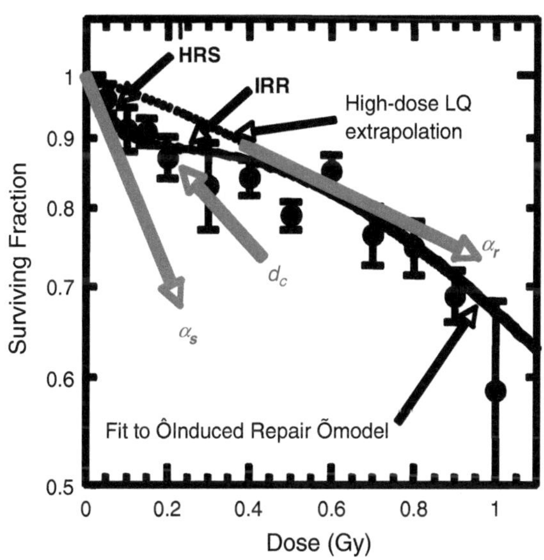

Fig. 19.1 Low dose survival of mammalian cell line measured by Flow cytometry plating assay. The broken line shows low-dose extrapolation from the linear quadratic model applied to the high dose survival data. The solid line shows the Induced Repair fit which describes the data well at all doses. The derivation of the α_s, α_r and d_c parameters are shown. To accurately define the HRS response several measurements below 0.3 Gy are needed

changing levels of radiation-induced DNA damage produced by increasing radiation exposures. The cell survival consequent of a dose-dependent activation pattern for the ATM protein would be expected to produce a changeover point in the low-dose survival region, which has been already demonstrated with the HRS to IRR transition. An expanded discussion of the link between molecular activation of repair processes and the HRS/IRR transition can be found later in this chapter.

Transitional Low-Dose Radiation Responses in Lower Organisms

Transitional or bi-phasic cell survival responses are not a new concept in radiobiology. In 1963, experiments on irradiated maize plants described both enhanced mutation induction and lethality in pollen grains after acute low-dose gamma-ray exposures [20]. Dose-response reports from Chadwick and Leenhouts [21] indicated a degree of low-dose hypersensitivity which was analogous to earlier reports in budding yeast [22], algae [23] and a lepidopteron TN-368 cell line [24]. The biphasic cell-survival pattern seen in the insect cells was explained by invoking a dose-dependent-radiosensitivity hypothesis, implying transitional radioresistance with increasing dose [25]. This interpretation of the data was reasonable given the earlier evidence for adaptive responses seen in the green unicellular alga Chlamydomonas [26] and the fern Osmunda [27] and in yeast by Boreham and Mitchel [28].

Transitional Low-Dose Radiation Responses in Mammalian and Human Cell Systems

As previously outlined, improvements in the methodology of clonogenic assays made it possible to resolve changes in radiosensitivity at doses where cell survival approached 100%, leading to the discovery of HRS and the transitional HRS/IRR survival response in mammalian cells [13, 29]. As with non-mammalian systems, HRS in mammalian cells could not be explained by any differential passive sensitivity of cells in specific phases of the cell cycle [13] but instead reflected the initiation of dynamic damage response pathways [5, 15, 30] and activation of checkpoints that control the progression of cells through the cell cycle [5, 30].

HRS and IRR responses have been characterized in many mammalian tumor and normal cell lines using different radiation qualities and biological endpoints [14, 31–45]. The HRS/IRR pattern of survival response has also been detected after acute dose-rate proton and pi-meson irradiation [46–48] and after high-linear energy transfer (LET) neutrons given at a low dose rate [49], albeit that the HRS/IRR transition point occurred at a different dose level. More recently, HRS was reported after proton irradiation using a charged particle microbeam targeted directly at the nuclei of individual cells [38]. Taken together, these data demonstrate that HRS is a response universal to low levels of radiation injury irrespective of incident radiation LET, whereas the IRR response is only evident in repair competent cell lines after low-LET irradiation [46]. The association between incident radiation LET and presence of IRR provides anecdotal evidence for the involvement of repair processes in both overcoming HRS and triggering the development of the IRR response, an observation that is discussed in more detail later in this chapter.

The existence of HRS has been questioned by some research groups. For example, the Columbia laboratory have published data showing evidence of a transitional HRS-type response to multiple low radiation doses [50] but chose to read the data differently. Although their data were well described by Joiner's low-dose Induced Repair model [13], the authors chose to interpret the data as representing cell-cycle redistribution. While this explanation may be appropriate for the fractionated exposures in the Columbia study, it cannot explain the transitional low-dose radiation responses seen after a single 0.3 Gy dose and therefore this explanation remains hypothetical. These single-dose data are consistent with the majority of studies reporting that HRS is the default survival response of mammalian cells to low-dose radiation exposure.

Transitional Low-Dose Radiation Responses In Vivo

Joiner and colleagues working at the Gray Laboratory were the first to report that very small radiation doses were more effective at causing injury than predicted by conventional radiobiological modeling [17, 51]. When the dose per fraction was reduced below 1 Gy, the total dose needed to produce damage was found to *decrease* in mouse skin and kidney. Similar conclusions were reported by Parkins and Fowler for murine lung [52]. This 'reverse' fractionation effect is precisely that expected from the transitional low-dose radiation response following low doses in cell lines. Importantly for radioprotection, these *in vivo* data demonstrate that cell lethality is enhanced following low-dose radiation exposure in normal tissues and that successive exposures may also elicit the enhanced lethality and hence augment residual genetic perturbations. This hypothesis is consistent with theoretical arguments made by Brenner and colleagues [53], but appears contradictory to measurements of a reduction in transformation frequency following low dose irradiation recently described by Redpath [32]. Clinical data obtained so far are also consistent with the concept of transitional low-dose radiation responses (*i.e.* differential effectiveness of radiation killing *per unit dose*) in normal human epidermis [34, 54–56] and tumor nodules derived from solid tumors [56] exposed to successive very low doses, although an alternate explanation of cell proliferation has been invoked to explain some of these clinical data.

How Does It Work?

Transitional Low-Dose Radiation Responses and Cell-Cycle Checkpoints

To ensure the faithful repair of radiation-induced DNA lesions, DNA repair is coordinated with the function of cell-cycle checkpoints. (See also chapter 14 in this volume.) Radiation-responsive checkpoints have been described in each cell-cycle phase and they operate to arrest normal cell-cycle progression to provide time for repair to occur [57]. Utilizing the flow-cytometry cell sorting technique of Durand [11], exaggerated HRS survival responses were found for enriched populations of G2-phase cells [16, 30], indicating that the mechanism regulating the HRS/IRR transition was likely to involve checkpoint events in the G2-phase of the cell cycle. Two distinct radiation-inducible cell-cycle checkpoints have been described for G2-phase cells. The first checkpoint has been known for many decades and operates in a dose-dependent manner to arrest the progression of radiation-damaged G1- or S-phase cells in the G2 phase [58] (hereafter referred to as the 'Sinclair' checkpoint). The second G2 checkpoint has only been described recently, and is detected rapidly after radiation exposure [18]. This aptly named 'early' checkpoint is believed to protect radiation-damaged G2-phase cells from progressing through G2 and prematurely entering mitosis with unrepaired radiation-induced DNA damage [18]. In contrast to the 'Sinclair' checkpoint, the 'early' checkpoint is ATM-dependent and functions in a dose *independent* manner over the range 1–10 Gy, but exhibits a distinct threshold for activation at around 0.4 Gy [59]. Therefore, only radiation doses above ~0.4 Gy produce sufficient damage to fully activate this damage response pathway. Moreover, the G2 specificity of this early checkpoint would imply an exaggerated transitional low-dose radiation response for G2-phase enriched cell populations, as has been demonstrated [16, 30].

Recently, this novel 'early' G2-phase cell-cycle checkpoint [18] was proposed as a critical event controlling the transitional low-dose radiation response [15, 30]. Supporting this hypothesis, Krueger et al. [60] demonstrated a strong association between the HRS/IRR transition and induction of the 'early' G2 checkpoint. Using a dual labeling flow cytometry method to distinguish between G2-phase and mitotic cells, Krueger and colleagues demonstrated for the first time that radiation doses below 0.2 Gy did not activate the early G2-checkpoint, and this was commensurate with HRS. The checkpoint was seen only to function in response to radiation doses above the HRS dose region. Presumably therefore, acute G2-phase arrest allows time for DNA repair to occur in radiation-damaged G2-phase cells prior to mitosis, thereby permitting an increase in cell survival and the overcoming of HRS transitioning into IRR. It will be interesting to see if future studies determine at the molecular level whether the 'early' G2/M checkpoint is defective in cell lines that fail to exhibit HRS and if the precise location of the checkpoint in the G2-phase of the cell cycle can be established. A clue to these mechanisms may be provided by data which has shown that G2-phase cells arrested immediately before mitosis using nocodazole show a complete absence of an IRR response, which demonstrates the need for progression through the early part of the G2-phase for IRR to develop [60]. Also, because the signaling cascade regulating this G2/M checkpoint is initiated through ATM activity and maintained by several key kinases and phosphorylation events, determination of how these activities relate to HRS could yield potential therapeutic targets to improve the cytotoxicity of low radiation doses, which could be useful in the treatment of conventionally radioresistant cancers.

Transitional Low-Dose Radiation Responses Are a Measure of Damage Repair Pathways

HRS is abrogated by pre-treatment with DNA damaging agents [61], and the extent of the protective effect induced is dependent on the amount of DNA damage produced. X-ray pre-treatments of 0.2 Gy or higher eliminated HRS, unlike smaller doses (0.05 Gy), which is consistent with the activation of the ‘early’ G2 checkpoint. A comparable dose-dependent abrogation was also seen after pre-treatment with various concentrations of hydrogen peroxide [61]. These cell-survival data indicate that priming or activating the DNA repair machinery with sufficient damage renders the cell resistant to HRS-type killing in subsequent irradiation. Conversely, inhibiting DNA repair processes with chemical agents eliminates the IRR response and extends HRS to higher doses, above which cell survival then proceeds according to the traditional LQ model [62]. The association between HRS killing and radiation-induced DNA strand breaks has been demonstrated by the hyper-radiosensitivity pattern for micronucleus induction [40, 63] and chromatid aberrations [64]. Similarly, the role of DNA strand-break repair in overcoming HRS was established by the extension of the HRS response (*ergo* lack of an IRR response) in repair deficient cell lines [65], which is the same response that is seen with repair competent cells after treatment with DNA repair modifiers [62]. Together, these data demonstrate that the HRS/IRR transition is a dynamic process that responds to changes in DNA damage and the functionality of DNA repair processes.

Radiation-induced DNA double-strand breaks (DSBs) trigger the activation of highly-conserved damage response processes to preserve genome integrity (see Fig. 19.2 and [66–72] for comprehensive reviews). If unrepaired, DNA DSBs can lead to chromosomal aberrations, genetic instability, permanent cell-cycle arrest, and cell death. Therefore, within minutes of radiation exposure, damage response proteins initiate repair by localizing to sites of DNA DSBs. The exact sequence of events involved with the initial molecular recognition of radiation-induced DSBs is still not fully clear, but recent reports have established a vital role for the Mre11-Rad50-Nbs1 (MRN) complex [73, 74] and ATM kinase [72, 75] in the early cellular response to such lesions [72, 76–78]. Current evidence is that the production of DSBs alters the local chromatin architecture [19], which then promotes both NBS1

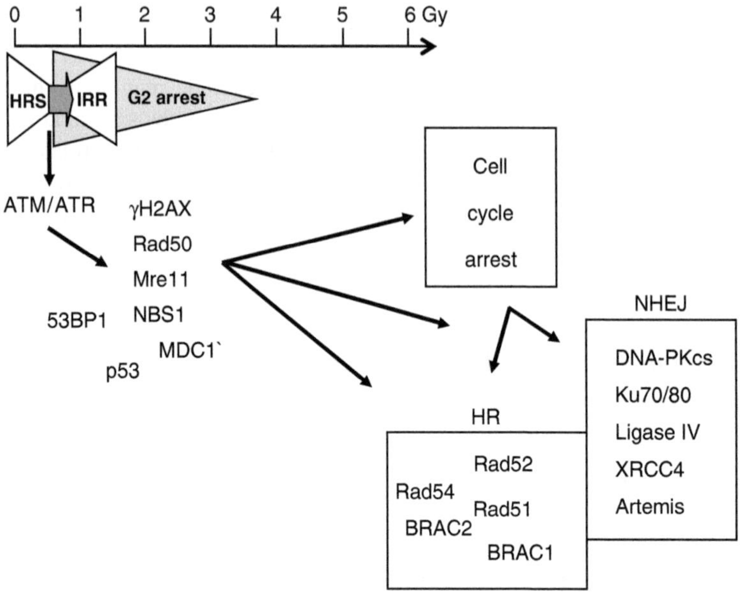

Fig. 19.2 A simplified view of the DNA damage response. Low levels of radiation-induced DNA damage lead to the activation of the ATM/ATR signaling cascades which, via mediator proteins, lead to the arrest of cell cycle progression. Halting cell cycle progression is important to allow sufficient time for DSBs to be repaired by the non-homologous end joining (NHEJ) and homologous recombination (HR) repair mechanisms, thereby preventing potentially pro-mutagenic lesions from being passed on to progeny cells

and ATM activity [79]. Once active, ATM, together with its substrates, regulates downstream cell-cycle checkpoints to avoid the replication of damaged DNA or prevent aberrant mitotic events [75, 80–82].

It has been established that radiation-induced activation of ATM, by phosphorylation at the ser1981 residue, does not directly regulate the transition in survival from HRS to IRR [60]. Rather, the balance of evidence indicates that the downstream ATM-dependent 'early' G2/M checkpoint plays a more important role (see above). Therefore, since the recruitment of ATM to DSBs and its activation is mediated by the MRN complex it is probable that the MRN complex is also not a key regulator of HRS/IRR transition, despite the fact that mutations in the NBS1 and MRE11 genes are associated with radiation sensitivity [74]. However, this speculation needs to be experimentally confirmed and may be complicated by the direct role that the MRE11 component plays in the processing of DSBs [74]. Another important issue to be addressed when evaluating the role of the MRN complex in HRS activation is the "cross-talk" between the ATM and ATR pathways, where downstream targets can be sufficiently activated by one kinase in the absence of the other [76, 83–88]. With specific regard to the rejoining of radiation-induced DNA DSBs, roles for poly(ADP-ribose) polymerase-1 (PARP) activation [62, 89] and functional DNA-PK (DNA dependent protein kinase) activity [90, 91] have also been demonstrated for overcoming HRS and instigating the IRR response. These proteins are involved in the major pathways important in the repair of radiation-induced DNA double-strand break damage in G2-phase cells; namely homologous recombination (HR) and nonhomologous end-joining (NHEJ) (see for example [66, 69–72, 92, 93]). However, what is less well understood both for HRS and the repair of DNA DSBs is the initial sensing event of radiation-induced DNA damage, and how the initial detection of damage is signaled to initiate DNA repair. The central transducers of the DNA damage responses are the phosphatidylinositol 3-kinase protein kinase-like (PIKK) family members: ATM, ATR (ATM and rad3-related) and DNA-PK (see for example [72, 75, 81, 82, 94–96]). Defects in PIKK activity are associated with hypersensitivity to radiation injury, impairment in cell-cycle checkpoints and cancer susceptibility [71, 95, 97]. Once activated, these PIKK kinases activate a plethora of downstream factors including the key kinases Chk1 and Chk2, which in turn orchestrate cell-cycle arrest and DNA repair activities. Given the dose- and ATM-dependence of the early G2 checkpoint in the context of HRS biology, it was important to assess if similar low-dose responses were evident in other factors associated with the DNA damage/repair pathways. Recent work by Short et al. [98] has suggested a molecular activation threshold *per se* does not exist for many factors that they tested as cells transition from HRS to IRR. Interestingly, there is a change in the balance between DNA repair enzyme activity with increasing radiation dose, which was demonstrated to be particularly true for RAD51, the key recombinase involved in the repair of DSBs breaks through homologous recombination events. Such recombination events predominate at the G2/M checkpoint, where homologous chromosomes are readily available to provide error-free repair of DSBs, and therefore fit well with the importance of early phase G2 cells in HRS responses (see above).

DNA Repair Foci Data and Damage Recognition

The initiation and repair of radiation-induced DNA DSBs can be measured by agarose-based assays [99, 100]. However, these traditional methods lack the resolution needed in order to examine DNA DSBs in the HRS dose region. In contrast, the γ-H2AX assay is capable of measuring single DSBs following X-irradiation ([101, 102], and references therein). One of the earliest cellular responses to radiation-induced DNA damage is the phosphorylation of the variant of histone H2A known as H2AX [103], facilitating the spatio-temporal assembly of multi-protein complexes around the region of damaged DNA [68]. Even though cells respond to very low doses of radiation by the phosphorylation of H2AX [101], work by Wykes et al. [104] with cell lines in culture has shown that there is no relationship between the initial numbers of DNA DSBs assessed by γ-H2AX foci with either low- or high-dose cell survival, indicating that the prevalence of HRS is not related to the initial event of DNA DSB recognition. However, data presented at the 13th

ICRR meeting in San Francisco 2007 by Simonsson, Qvarmström and colleagues (Uppsala Universitet, Sweden) showed a hypersensitive dose response for the persistence of γ-H2AX in epidermal skin cells receiving 0.3 Gy in biopsies taken from patients 30 minutes after radiation treatment, indicating a tentative relationship with DNA DSB repair, albeit from a small number of samples. The role of other DNA binding proteins in the HRS/IRR transition could be investigated using DNA foci techniques together with time-course studies. Such work is likely to provide further molecular insight into the control of the HRS/IRR transition process.

P53 and Low Dose Survival: The Role of Apoptosis in HRS

As well as initiation of downstream kinases to co-ordinate checkpoint activation with the repair of DNA damage, the ATM/ATR signaling cascades are also responsible for eliciting an apoptotic response as a last resort to prevent potential pro-mutagenic lesions from being passed on to daughter cells, thereby promoting genomic integrity. Recent work initially by Enns et al. [14] and later by Krueger et al. [105] has determined a role for apoptotic processes in HRS. Interestingly, it was demonstrated that such responses were mediated through the p53-dependent activation of Caspase-3, which forms part of the signaling cascade downstream of ATM activation [78, 106]. Although it appears that ATM activation alone is not the key determinant for overcoming HRS [105], given the importance of ATM-mediated apoptosis in removal of cells during HRS it appears that HRS might be a default mechanism to prevent potentially mutagenic G2 cells from entering mitosis. Consistent with this view, recent data from Iliakis and colleagues demonstrates that G2-phase AT cells (from patients mutated in ATM) are particularly prone to radiation-induced chromosome breaks due to a failure of the early G2 checkpoint [107]. One potential caveat with these findings with regards to clinical applications of HRS biology is that if apoptosis of early G2 cells during HRS is fully dependent on active p53, then this may somewhat limit the potential exploitation of HRS biology for improved killing of cancer cells within the clinical setting, given the high frequency of p53 mutations during cancer progression.

HRS and the Inverse Dose-Rate Effect

As discussed earlier, there are other cellular responses to low levels of radiation exposure that cannot be extrapolated from clonogenic survival data obtained using higher doses [108]. An example is the inverse dose-rate effect, where equivalent radiation doses delivered at lower amounts of dose per unit time lead to enhanced cell killing compared with equivalent doses delivered at higher dose-rates [109, 110]. As with the transition from HRS to IRR, there appears to be a 'threshold' dose-rate for a particular cell type below which inverse effects on cell killing are observed. Consistent with this notion are the findings that exposures to low dose-rates prior to low doses of radiation, can abrogate HRS responses [110]. Furthermore, prior activation of ATM can abrogate the molecular defects observed following low dose-rate exposures and prevent inverse dose-rate effects [31]. Thus, as is true for HRS responses, certain cellular processes that rely upon ATM activity may be responsible for inverse dose-rate effects.

Early studies attributed inverse dose-rate effects to changes in cell-cycle kinetics, *e.g.* accumulation of cells within the G2 phase during protracted radiation exposure, which resulted in unexpected enhanced cell killing effects [111, 112]. However, other studies suggested that such G2 accumulation could not explain the inverse dose-rate effect [110, 113, 114]. Perhaps more importantly, a detailed molecular understanding to the phenomenon remained to be determined. The first study to address this problem demonstrated that at certain low dose-rates, activation of the ATM signaling cascade does not occur [31]. At the molecular level, this is manifest as a failure to sufficiently activate NBS1 via phosphorylation of serine 343. Failure to activate the MRN complex means that ATM autophosphorylation at serine 1981 is also abrogated at low dose-rates, leading to an ineffective activation of H2AX [31]. With regards to the initiating event that triggers activation of the ATM pathway in response to DNA damage, these abrogated responses to low dose-rates could be overturned simply by the addition of agents that modify chromatin structure, consistent with the notion that some level of higher order chromatin modifications are required to elicit an efficient ATM-mediated damage response. More recent studies have also implicated ATM activation as an important factor in the cellular response to radiation exposures delivered at a reduced dose-rate [115–117]. Following acute dose exposures, ATM activation alone was not sufficient to overcome HRS, but activation of the ATM-dependent early G2 checkpoint was shown to be the key event in HRS/IRR biology [60]. Therefore, it is possible that the same is also true for inverse dose-rate effects; that a failure to activate the ATM pathway at the early G2 phase of the cell cycle, leads to an increased sensitivity to such low exposures to radiation. This finding regarding the importance of ATM activation within the context of cell-cycle phase may explain the conflict in the past literature regarding cell-cycle distributions and cellular responses to low dose-rate radiation, as described above.

Potential Clinical Implications of HRS

Although the complete mechanism of HRS is not yet understood, the potential clinical implications of HRS is an area of considerable debate [35, 118, 119]. This discussion has initially focused on how HRS may affect treatment planning for intensity modulated radiotherapy (IMRT). Honoré and Bentzen [118] argue that in some situations, HRS will tend to increase the effect of low doses in normal tissues and this could negate the benefits of IMRT over conventional treatment plans, and that the importance of HRS would be potentially larger in tissues with a pronounced volume effect. A similar concern was highlighted by Lin and Wu [120] when modeling the effects of partial fractions of different dose sizes less than 2 Gy [120]. Another consideration is that since HRS has been strongly linked with G2-phase cells, this may imply that HRS is not important in slowly proliferating normal tissues with a small growth fraction; such tissues are typically characterized as late-responding tissues to radiation injury. HRS is more likely to affect early-responding proliferating tissues, such as skin. Indeed, Harney et al. [56] have demonstrated a response consistent with HRS in human skin. Clearly, more molecular-based experiments are needed using whole animal models to characterize the mechanisms of HRS in normal tissue radiation damage, to complement the earlier functional data [17, 51, 52]. The role of cell-to-cell contact should also be considered in the clinical situation since this has been suggested to lessen the effect of HRS [45], which therefore may serve to negate any potential clinical complications that arise from HRS killing in normal tissues outside the clinical target volume.

The large HRS effects observed in many malignant cell lines imply that there may also be a positive effect on radiotherapy treatment planning, by increasing the biologically-effective dose beyond the margins expected from a purely physical dose distribution. Figure 19.3 shows hypothetically how this could work in a tumor, based on the radiation sensitivity and HRS parameters of the T98G cell line. In the field edges, the increase in biologically effective dose due to HRS, over and above with the actual physical dose delivered, might be worth as much as 33% of the target dose. This biologically-effective dose spreading might be particularly important in situations where tumor margins are ill-defined. Glioblastoma is an example, and

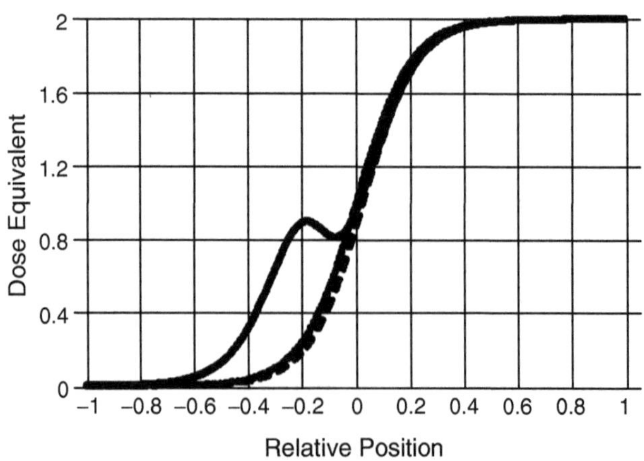

Fig. 19.3 Physical dose (dotted line) is plotted against the relative position across the boundary of a tumor target volume prescribed a dose of 2 Gy. The dashed line shows the biological effect of that dose expressed as the equivalent dose that would need to be given in 2-Gy fractions, calculated according to the Linear-Quadratic model. The solid line shows the biologically effective equivalent dose that would need to be given in 2-Gy fractions calculated according to the Induced-Repair model and assuming the presence of low-dose hyper-radiosensitivity in the tumor cells. Parameters in the models are those from the study on T98G human glioblastoma cells [16]

is also expected to benefit particularly from this "HRS dose spreading" effect as particularly large HRS effects have been seen in glioblastoma cell lines. Given that this effect is already "built in" to conventional radiotherapy, the cautionary note here is that this benefit might be lost when adopting more highly conformal treatment plans, especially using protons or carbon ions which can deliver exceptionally sharp dose transitions.

The therapeutic benefits of HRS for tumor cell killing have been more extensively considered, but more pre-clinical studies are still needed. Spring and colleagues [33, 35] combined low dose fractionated irradiation with cell synchronization using taxanes to radiosensitize SCCHN (squamous cell carcinoma of head and neck) tumor xenografts in nude mice. The taxanes were suggested to increase the proportion of G2-phase cells in the tumor xenograft thereby enhancing the HRS response of the tumor. The experimental success of this treatment strategy has prompted a clinical trial of bi-weekly combined gemcitabine and paclitaxel with 50–80 cGy twice daily (ClinincalTrials.gov NCT 00176241), the results of which are on-going. By contrast, ultrafractionation using 0.4 Gy per fraction, three fractions per day at 7 days per week, did not improve the results of radiotherapy in radioresistant murine DDL1 Lymphoma compared with conventional fractionation with 1.68 Gy per fraction, one fraction per day at 5 days per week [121]. A similar disappointing outcome was also seen with human T98G and HGL21 glioblastoma xenograft models [122]. These radiotherapy alone experiments therefore do not support the hypothesis that HRS *in vitro* translates into improved outcome of full-course ultrafractionated irradiation *in vivo*. The failure of ultrafractionation to produce HRS killing in the tumor could reflect one of many possibilities inherit in the experimental design. The turnover of cells within the xenograft may promote the continual activation of damage response kinases that operate to constantly prime the tumor cell population to repair DNA damage, thereby abrogating any potential benefit of HRS. If this explanation proves correct, the same mechanism may also occur in a clinical setting. Or, it is possible that the prolonged treatment times associated with such long ultrafractionation schedules lead to the eventual accumulation of sufficient damage to trigger the IRR response, such that an enhanced HRS response is not detectable. This accumulation hypothesis is based on the fact that low levels of radiation damage are known to go undetected by repair systems [101], therefore in the ultrafractionation setting time would be needed for sufficient amounts of damage to occur to induce repair and radioresistance. In contrast, a combined chemo-radiotherapy approach to enrich the G2-phase fraction prior to radiotherapy as demonstrated by Spring [35], shows considerable promise at improving tumor curability. Moreover, if the *in vitro* studies translate clinically, then increasing the proportional of G2-phase cells in the target population would extend the HRS response to high doses. This would therefore permit larger fraction sizes to be used clinically, with fewer numbers of fractions. Indeed, extrapolating from the animal data, a combination of taxanes could be used with a 0.8 Gy dose b.i.d., to achieve HRS-type killing to improve tumor curability. Finally, given that previous studies have suggested a role for ATM, DNA-PK and PARP-1 in overcoming HRS [60, 89–91], potent and specific inhibitors of these enzymes could potentially be useful adjuvant agents to extend HRS in tumor cells. Indeed, several biotechnology companies are currently developing improved inhibitors of ATM, DNA-PK, Chk1 and Chk1 which should be studied both *in vitro* and *in vivo* in the context of HRS biology. With regard to PARP-1, several inhibitors are currently being assessed within the clinical setting ([123] and references therein) and these should be considered in future studies designed to exploit HRS biology to improve the therapeutic index of current radiotherapy regimes.

Conclusion

The past decade has seen great progress in delineating the molecular mechanism of HRS. Together, the data support a hypothesis that cell killing in the HRS region reflects the apoptotic death of cells that fail to undergo an ATM-dependent early G2-phase cell cycle arrest, while the transition in the survival response to IRR reflects a change in the balance of G2-phase checkpoint induction, allowing time for repair and increased cell survival. Therefore, tumor-targeted strategies that combine an element of cell-cycle manipulation with low dose radiotherapy have a theoretical basis for improving therapeutic outcomes, particularly in the relative absence of proliferation in the surrounding normal tissue.

Acknowledgements We would like to thank Dr. George D. Wilson (William Beaumont Hospital, Royal Oak) and Dr. Theodore L. DeWeese (Johns Hopkins University, Baltimore) for helpful discussions and for their support of this work.

References

1. Huang L, Kim PM, Nickoloff JA, et al. Targeted and nontargeted effects of low-dose ionizing radiation on delayed genomic instability in human cells. *Cancer Res* 2007; 67:1099–1104.
2. Day TK, Zeng G, Hooker AM, et al. Adaptive response for chromosomal inversions in pKZ1 mouse prostate induced by low doses of X radiation delivered after a high dose. *Radiat Res* 2007; 167:682–692.
3. Matsumoto H, Hamada N, Takahashi A, et al. Vanguards of paradigm shift in radiation biology: radiation-induced adaptive and bystander responses. *J Radiat Res (Tokyo)* 2007; 48:97–106.
4. Mothersill C, Seymour CB. Radiation-induced bystander effects and the DNA paradigm: an "out of field" perspective. *Mutat Res* 2006; 597:5–10.
5. Marples B. Is low-dose hyper-radiosensitivity a measure of G2-phase cell radiosensitivity? *Can Met Reviews* 2004; 23:197–207.
6. Schwartz JL. Variability: the common factor linking low dose-induced genomic instability, adaptation and bystander effects. *Mutat Res* 2007; 616:196–200.
7. Puck TT, Marcus PI, Cieciura SJ. Clonal growth of mammalian cells in vitro; growth characteristics of colonies from single HeLa cells with and without a feeder layer. *J Exp Med* 1956; 103:273–283.
8. Puck TT, Marcus PI. Action of x-rays on mammalian cells. *J Exp Med* 1956; 103:653–666.
9. Boag JW. The statistical treatment of cell survival data. In: Alper T, editor. Cell Survival After Low Doses of Radiation: Theoretical and Clinical Implications. London: Institute of Physics/Wiley; 1975. pp. 40–53.

10. Bedford JS, Griggs HG. The estimation of survival at low doses and the limits of resolution of the single-cell-plating technique. In: Alper T, editor. Cell Survival After Low Doses of Radiation: Theoretical and Clinical Implications. London: Wiley; 1975. pp. 34–39.
11. Durand RE. Use of a cell sorter for assays of cell clonogenicity. *Cancer Res* 1986; 46:2775–2778.
12. Spadinger I, Poon SS, Palcic B. Automated detection and recognition of live cells in tissue culture using image cytometry. *Cytometry* 1989; 10:375–381.
13. Marples B, Joiner MC. The response of Chinese hamster V79 cells to low radiation doses: evidence of enhanced sensitivity of the whole cell population. *Radiat Res* 1993; 133:41–51.
14. Enns L, Bogen KT, Wizniak J, et al. Low-dose radiation hypersensitivity is associated with p53-dependent apoptosis. *Mol Cancer Res* 2004; 2:557–566.
15. Marples B, Wouters BG, Collis SJ, et al. Low-dose hyper-radiosensitivity: a consequence of ineffective cell cycle arrest of radiation-damaged G(2)-phase cells. *Radiat Res* 2004; 161:247–255.
16. Short SC, Woodcock M, Marples B, et al. The effects of cell cycle phase on low dose hyper-radiosensitivity. *Int J Radiat Biol* 2003; 79:99–105.
17. Joiner MC, Johns H. Renal damage in the mouse: the response to very small doses per fraction. *Radiat Res* 1988; 114:385–398.
18. Xu B, Kim ST, Lim DS, et al. Two molecularly distinct G(2)/M checkpoints are induced by ionizing irradiation. *Mol Cell Biol* 2002; 22:1049–1059.
19. Bakkenist CJ, Kastan MB. DNA damage activates ATM through intermolecular autophosphorylation and dimer dissociation. *Nature* 2003; 421:499–506.
20. Eriksson G. Induction of waxy mutants in maize by acute and chronic gamma irradiation. *Hereditas* 1963; 50:161–178.
21. Chadwick KH, Leenhouts HP. The effect of an asynchronous population of cells on the initial slope of dose-effect curves. In: Alper T, editor. Cell Survival After Low Doses of Radiation: Theoretical and Clinical Implications. London: Institute of Physics/Wiley; 1975. pp. 57–63.
22. Beam CA, Mortimer RK, Wolfe RG, et al. The relation of radioresistance to budding in Saccharomyces cerevisiae. *Arch Biochem Biophys* 1954; 49:110–122.
23. Horsley RJ, Pujara CM. Study of the inflexion of X-radiation survival curves for synchronized cell populations of the green alga (*Oedogonium cardiacum*). *Radiat Res* 1969; 40:440–449.
24. Koval TM. Multiphasic survival response of a radioresistant lepidopteran insect cell line. *Radiat Res* 1984; 98:642–648.
25. Koval TM. Inducible repair of ionizing radiation damage in higher eukaryotic cells. *Mutat Res* 1986; 173:291–293.
26. Hillova J, Drasil V. The inhibitory effect of iodoacetamide on recovery from sub-lethal damage in Chlamydomonas reinhardti. *Int J Radiat Biol* 1967; 12:201–208.
27. Hendry JH. Radioresistance induced in fern spores by prior irradiation. *Radiat Res* 1986; 106:396–400.
28. Boreham DR, Mitchel RE. DNA lesions that signal the induction of radioresistance and DNA repair in yeast. *Radiat Res* 1991; 128:19–28.
29. Marples B, Joiner MC, Skov KA. An X-ray inducible repair response: evidence from high resolution survival measurements in air and hypoxia. In: Sugahara T, Sagan LA, Aoyama T, editors. Low Dose Irradiation and Biological Defense Mechanisms. Amsterdam: Elsevier; 1992. pp. 295–298.
30. Marples B, Wouters BG, Joiner MC. An association between the radiation-induced arrest of G2 phase cells and low-dose hyper-radiosensitivity: A plausible underlying mechanism? *Radiat Res* 2003; 160:38–45.
31. Collis SJ, Schwaninger JM, Ntambi AJ, et al. Evasion of early cellular response mechanisms following low level radiation-induced DNA damage. *J Biol Chem* 2004; 279:49624–49632.
32. Redpath JL, Short SC, Woodcock M, et al. Low-dose reduction in transformation frequency compared to unirradiated controls: the role of hyper-radiosensitivity to cell death. *Radiat Res* 2003; 159:433–436.
33. Dey S, Spring PM, Arnold S, et al. Low-dose fractionated radiation potentiates the effects of Paclitaxel in wild-type and mutant p53 head and neck tumor cell lines. *Clin Cancer Res* 2003; 9:1557–1565.

34. Arnold SM, Regine WF, Ahmed MM, et al. Low-dose fractionated radiation as a chemopotentiator of neoadjuvant paclitaxel and carboplatin for locally advanced squamous cell carcinoma of the head and neck: results of a new treatment paradigm. *Int J Radiat Oncol Biol Phys* 2004; 58:1411–1417.
35. Spring PM, Arnold SM, Shajahan S, et al. Low dose fractionated radiation potentiates the effects of taxotere in nude mice xenografts of squamous cell carcinoma of head and neck. *Cell Cycle* 2004; 3:479–485.
36. Caney C, Singh G, Lukka H, et al. Combined gamma-irradiation and subsequent cisplatin treatment in human squamous carcinoma cell lines sensitive and resistant to cisplatin. *Int J Radiat Biol* 2004; 80:291–299.
37. Prise KM, Belyakov OV, Newman HC, et al. Non-targeted effects of radiation: bystander responses in cell and tissue models. *Radiat Prot Dosimetry* 2002; 99:223–226.
38. Schettino G, Folkard M, Prise KM, et al. Low-dose hypersensitivity in Chinese hamster V79 cells targeted with counted protons using a charged-particle microbeam. *Radiat Res* 2001; 156:526–534.
39. Schettino G, Folkard M, Prise KM, et al. Low-dose studies of bystander cell killing with targeted soft X rays. *Radiat Res* 2003; 160:505–511.
40. Vral A, Louagie H, Thierens H, et al. Micronucleus frequencies in cytokinesis-blocked human B lymphocytes after low dose gamma-irradiation. *Int J Radiat Biol* 1998; 73:549–555.
41. Tsoulou E, Baggio L, Cherubini R, et al. Radiosensitivity of V79 cells after alpha particle radiation at low doses. *Radiat Prot Dosimetry* 2002; 99:237–240.
42. Tsoulou E, Baggio L, Cherubini R, et al. Low-dose hypersensitivity of V79 cells under exposure to gamma-rays and 4He ions of different energies: survival and chromosome aberrations. *Int J Radiat Biol* 2001; 77:1133–1139.
43. Bartkowiak D, Hogner S, Nothdurft W, et al. Cell cycle and growth response of CHO cells to X-irradiation: threshold-free repair at low doses. *Int J Radiat Oncol Biol Phys* 2001; 50:221–227.
44. Carlsson J, Hakansson E, Eriksson V, et al. Early effects of low dose-rate radiation on cultured tumor cells. *Cancer Biother Radiopharm* 2003; 18:663–670.
45. Chandna S, Dwarakanath BS, Khaitan D, et al. Low-dose radiation hypersensitivity in human tumor cell lines: effects of cell-cell contact and nutritional deprivation. *Radiat Res* 2002; 157:516–525.
46. Marples B, Lam GK, Zhou H, et al. The response of Chinese hamster V79-379A cells exposed to negative pi-mesons: evidence that increased radioresistance is dependent on linear energy transfer. *Radiat Res* 1994; 138:S81–S84.
47. Marples B, Skov KA. Small doses of high-linear energy transfer radiation increase the radioresistance of Chinese hamster V79 cells to subsequent X irradiation. *Radiat Res* 1996; 146:382–387.
48. Marples B, Adomat H, Koch CJ, et al. Response of V79 cells to low doses of X-rays and negative pi-mesons: clonogenic survival and DNA strand breaks. *Int J Radiat Biol* 1996; 70:429–436.
49. Dionet C, Tchirkov A, Alard JP, et al. Effects of low-dose neutrons applied at reduced dose rate on human melanoma cells. *Radiat Res* 2000; 154:406–411.
50. Smith LG, Miller RC, Richards M, et al. Investigation of hypersensitivity to fractionated low-dose radiation exposure. *Int J Radiat Oncol Biol Phys* 1999; 45:187–191.
51. Joiner MC, Denekamp J, Maughan RL. The use of 'top-up' experiments to investigate the effect of very small doses per fraction in mouse skin. *Int J Radiat Biol* 1986; 49:565–580.
52. Parkins CS, Fowler JF. The linear quadratic fit for lung function after irradiation with X-rays at smaller doses per fraction than 2 Gy. *Br J Cancer Suppl* 1986; 7:320–323.
53. Brenner DJ, Doll R, Goodhead DT, et al. Cancer risks attributable to low doses of ionizing radiation: assessing what we really know. *Proc Natl Acad Sci USA* 2003; 100:13761–13766.
54. Turesson I, Joiner MC. Clinical evidence of hypersensitivity to low doses in radiotherapy. *Radiother Oncol* 1996; 40:1–3.

55. Hamilton CS, Denham JW, O'Brien M, et al. Underprediction of human skin erythema at low doses per fraction by the linear quadratic model. *Radiother Oncol* 1996; 40:23–30.
56. Harney J, Shah N, Short S, et al. The evaluation of low dose hyper-radiosensitivity in normal human skin. *Radiother Oncol* 2004; 70:319–329.
57. Wilson GD. Radiation and the cell cycle, revisited. *Cancer Metastasis Rev* 2004; 23:209–225.
58. Sinclair WK. Cyclic X ray responses in mammalian cells in vitro. *Radiat Res* 1968; 33:620–643.
59. Krempler A, Deckbar D, Jeggo PA, et al. An imperfect G2M checkpoint contributes to chromosome instability following irradiation of S and G2 phase cells. *Cell Cycle* 2007; 6:1682–1686.
60. Krueger SA, Collis SJ, Joiner MC, et al. Transition in survival from Low-dose hyper-radiosensitivity to increased radioresistance is independent of activation of ATM Ser1981 activity. *Int J Radiat Oncol Biol Phys* 2007; 69:1262–1271.
61. Marples B, Joiner MC. The elimination of low-dose hypersensitivity in Chinese hamster V79–379A cells by pretreatment with X rays or hydrogen peroxide. *Radiat Res* 1995; 141:160–169.
62. Marples B, Joiner MC. Modification of survival by DNA repair modifiers: a probable explanation for the phenomenon of increased radioresistance. *Int J Radiat Biol* 2000; 76:305–312.
63. Slonina D, Biesaga B, Urbanski K, et al. Evidence of low-dose hyper-radiosensitivity in normal cells of cervix cancer patients? *Radiat Prot Dosimetry* 2006; 122:282–284.
64. Nasonova EA, Shmakova NL, Komova OV, et al. Cytogenetic effects of low-dose radiation with different LET in human peripheral blood lymphocytes. *Radiat Environ Biophys* 2006; 45:307–312.
65. Skov KA. Radioresponsiveness at low doses: hyper-radiosensitivity and increased radioresistance in mammalian cells. *Mutat Res* 1999; 430:241–253.
66. Jackson SP. Sensing and repairing DNA double-strand breaks. *Carcinogenesis* 2002; 23:687–696.
67. Petrini JH, Stracker TH. The cellular response to DNA double-strand breaks: defining the sensors and mediators. *Trends Cell Biol* 2003; 13:458–462.
68. Bekker-Jensen S, Lukas C, Kitagawa R, et al. Spatial organization of the mammalian genome surveillance machinery in response to DNA strand breaks. *J Cell Biol* 2006; 173:195–206.
69. Harrison JC, Haber JE. Surviving the breakup: the DNA damage checkpoint. *Annu Rev Genet* 2006; 40:209–235.
70. Hoeijmakers JH. Genome maintenance mechanisms for preventing cancer. *Nature* 2001; 411:366–374.
71. O'Driscoll M, Jeggo PA. The role of double-strand break repair - insights from human genetics. *Nat Rev Genet* 2006; 7:45–54.
72. Shiloh Y. ATM and related protein kinases: safeguarding genome integrity. *Nat Rev Cancer* 2003; 3:155–168.
73. Lee JH, Paull TT. ATM activation by DNA double-strand breaks through the Mre11-Rad50-Nbs1 complex. *Science* 2005; 308:551–554.
74. Williams RS, Williams JS, Tainer JA. Mre11-Rad50-Nbs1 is a keystone complex connecting DNA repair machinery, double-strand break signaling, and the chromatin template. *Biochem Cell Biol* 2007; 85:509–520.
75. Lavin MF, Kozlov S. DNA damage-induced signalling in ataxia-telangiectasia and related syndromes. *Radiother Oncol* 2007; 83:231–237.
76. Hirano Y, Sugimoto K. ATR homolog Mec1 controls association of DNA polymerase zeta-Rev1 complex with regions near a double-strand break. *Curr Biol* 2006; 16:586–590.
77. Horejsi Z, Falck J, Bakkenist CJ, et al. Distinct functional domains of Nbs1 modulate the timing and magnitude of ATM activation after low doses of ionizing radiation. *Oncogene* 2004; 23:3122–3127.
78. Lavin MF, Kozlov S. ATM activation and DNA damage response. *Cell Cycle* 2007; 6:931–942.

79. Berkovich E, Monnat RJ, Jr., Kastan MB. Roles of ATM and NBS1 in chromatin structure modulation and DNA double-strand break repair. *Nat Cell Biol* 2007; 9:683–690.
80. Abraham RT. Cell cycle checkpoint signaling through the ATM and ATR kinases. *Genes Dev* 2001; 15:2177–2196.
81. Shiloh Y. ATM: ready, set, go. *Cell Cycle* 2003; 2:116–117.
82. Bartek J, Lukas J. DNA damage checkpoints: from initiation to recovery or adaptation. *Curr Opin Cell Biol* 2007; 19:238–245.
83. Cuadrado M, Martinez-Pastor B, Murga M, et al. ATM regulates ATR chromatin loading in response to DNA double-strand breaks. *J Exp Med* 2006; 203:297–303.
84. Garcia-Muse T, Boulton SJ. Distinct modes of ATR activation after replication stress and DNA double-strand breaks in Caenorhabditis elegans. *EMBO J* 2005; 24:4345–4355.
85. Hurley PJ, Wilsker D, Bunz F. Human cancer cells require ATR for cell cycle progression following exposure to ionizing radiation. *Oncogene* 2007; 26:2535–2542.
86. Jazayeri A, Falck J, Lukas C, et al. ATM- and cell cycle-dependent regulation of ATR in response to DNA double-strand breaks. *Nat Cell Biol* 2006; 8:37–45.
87. Larocque JR, Jaklevic BR, Su TT, et al. Drosophila ATR in double-strand break repair. *Genetics* 2007; 175:1023–1033.
88. Myers JS, Cortez D. Rapid activation of ATR by ionizing radiation requires ATM and Mre11. *J Biol Chem* 2006; 281:9346–9350.
89. Chalmers A, Johnston P, Woodcock M, et al. PARP-1, PARP-2, and the cellular response to low doses of ionizing radiation. *Int J Radiat Oncol Biol Phys* 2004; 58:410–419.
90. Vaganay-Juery S, Muller C, Marangoni E, et al. Decreased DNA-PK activity in human cancer cells exhibiting hypersensitivity to low-dose irradiation. *Br J Cancer* 2000; 83:514–518.
91. Marples B, Cann NE, Mitchell CR, et al. Evidence for the involvement of DNA-dependent protein kinase in the phenomena of low dose hyper-radiosensitivity and increased radioresistance. *Radiat Res* 2002; 78:1151–1159.
92. Featherstone C, Jackson SP. DNA double-strand break repair. *Curr Biol* 1999; 9:759–761.
93. Jeggo PA, Taccioli GE, Jackson SP. Menage a trois: double strand break repair, V(D)J recombination and DNA-PK. *Bioessays* 1995; 17:949–957.
94. Rouse J, Jackson SP. Interfaces between the detection, signaling, and repair of DNA damage. *Science* 2002; 297:547–551.
95. Zhou BB, Elledge SJ. The DNA damage response: putting checkpoints in perspective. *Nature* 2000; 408:433–439.
96. Collis SJ, DeWeese TL, Jeggo PA, et al. The life and death of DNA-PK. *Oncogene* 2005; 24:949–961.
97. Kastan MB, Bartek J. Cell-cycle checkpoints and cancer. *Nature* 2004; 432:316–323.
98. Short SC, Bourne S, Martindale C, et al. DNA damage responses at low radiation doses. *Radiat Res* 2005; 164:292–302.
99. Olive PL. The comet assay. An overview of techniques. *Methods Mol Biol* 2002; 203:179–194.
100. Whitaker SJ, Powell SN, McMillan TJ. Molecular assays of radiation-induced DNA damage. *Eur J Cancer* 1991; 27:922–928.
101. Rothkamm K, Lobrich M. Evidence for a lack of DNA double-strand break repair in human cells exposed to very low x-ray doses. *Proc Natl Acad Sci USA* 2003; 100:5057–5062.
102. Olive PL. Detection of DNA damage in individual cells by analysis of histone H2AX phosphorylation. *Methods Cell Biol* 2004;75:355–373.
103. Burma S, Chen BP, Murphy M, et al. ATM phosphorylates histone H2AX in response to DNA double-strand breaks. *J Biol Chem* 2001; 276:42462–42467.
104. Wykes SM, Piasentin E, Joiner MC, et al. Low-dose hyper-radiosensitivity is not caused by a failure to recognize DNA double-strand breaks. *Radiat Res* 2006; 165:516–524.
105. Krueger SA, Joiner MC, Weinfeld M, et al. Role of apoptosis in low-dose hyper-radiosensitivity. *Radiat Res* 2007; 167:260–267.
106. Roos WP, Kaina B. DNA damage-induced cell death by apoptosis. *Trends Mol Med* 2006; 12:440–450.

107. Terzoudi GI, Manola KN, Pantelias GE, et al. Checkpoint abrogation in G2 compromises repair of chromosomal breaks in ataxia telangiectasia cells. *Cancer Res* 2005; 65:11292–11296.
108. Leonard BE. Thresholds and transitions for activation of cellular radioprotective mechanisms - correlations between HRS/IRR and the 'inverse' dose-rate effect. *Int J Radiat Biol* 2007; 83:479–489.
109. Marin LA, Smith CE, Langston MY, et al. Response of glioblastoma cell lines to low dose rate irradiation. *Int J Radiat Oncol Biol Phys* 1991; 21:397–402.
110. Mitchell CR, Folkard M, Joiner MC. Effects of exposure to low-dose-rate (60)co gamma rays on human tumor cells in vitro. *Radiat Res* 2002; 158:311–318.
111. Knox SJ, Sutherland W, Goris ML. Correlation of tumor sensitivity to low-dose-rate irradiation with G2/M-phase block and other radiobiological parameters. *Radiat Res* 1993; 135:24–31.
112. Mitchell JB, Bedord JS, Bailey SM. Dose-rate effects on the cell cycle and survival of S3 HeLa and V79 cells. *Radiat Res* 1979; 79:520–536.
113. DeWeese TL, Shipman JM, Dillehay LE, et al. Sensitivity of human prostatic carcinoma cell lines to low dose rate radiation exposure. *J Urol* 1998; 159:591–598.
114. DeWeese TL, Walsh JC, Dillehay LE, et al. Human papillomavirus E6 and E7 oncoproteins alter cell cycle progression but not radiosensitivity of carcinoma cells treated with low-dose-rate radiation. *Int J Radiat Oncol Biol Phys* 1997; 37:145–154.
115. Kato TA, Nagasawa H, Weil MM, et al. gamma-H2AX foci after low-dose-rate irradiation reveal atm haploinsufficiency in mice. *Radiat Res* 2006; 166:47–54.
116. Kato TA, Nagasawa H, Weil MM, et al. Levels of gamma-H2AX Foci after low-dose-rate irradiation reveal a DNA DSB rejoining defect in cells from human ATM heterozygotes in two at families and in another apparently normal individual. *Radiat Res* 2006; 166:443–453.
117. Nakamura H, Yasui Y, Saito N, et al. DNA repair defect in AT cells and their hypersensitivity to low-dose-rate radiation. *Radiat Res* 2006; 165:277–282.
118. Honore HB, Bentzen SM. A modelling study of the potential influence of low dose hypersensitivity on radiation treatment planning. *Radiother Oncol* 2006; 79:115–121.
119. Tome WA, Howard SP. On the possible increase in local tumour control probability for gliomas exhibiting low dose hyper-radiosensitivity using a pulsed schedule. *Br J Radiol* 2007; 80:32–37.
120. Lin PS, Wu A. Not all 2 Gray radiation prescriptions are equivalent: Cytotoxic effect depends on delivery sequences of partial fractionated doses. *Int J Radiat Oncol Biol Phys* 2005; 63:536–544.
121. Krause M, Prager J, Wohlfarth J, et al. Ultrafractionation does not improve the results of radiotherapy in radioresistant murine DDL1 lymphoma. *Strahlenther Onkol* 2005; 181:540–544.
122. Krause M, Hessel F, Wohlfarth J, et al. Ultrafractionation in A7 human malignant glioma in nude mice. *Int J Radiat Biol* 2003; 79:377–383.
123. Ratnam K, Low JA. Current development of clinical inhibitors of poly(ADP-ribose) polymerase in oncology. *Clin Cancer Res* 2007; 13:1383–1388.

Chapter 20
Clinical Radionuclide Therapy

Andrew M. Scott[1,2,3] and Sze-Ting Lee[1,2,3]

Summary Clinical applications of targeted radionuclide treatment have evolved considerably over the last 10–20 years, principally as a result of an improved understanding of tumour biology, and the identification of biochemical pathways and protein targets expressed preferentially on tumours compared to normal tissue. As a result, targeted therapy of cancer with radionuclides has evolved to include a number of therapies that have achieved success in the clinic, and a broad range of strategies that are being actively pursued in laboratory studies and clinical trials.

Radioiodine Therapy

Radioiodine had been the most common and widely used radionuclide therapy for more than half a century. The first reported use of radioiodine for treatment of differentiated thyroid cancer (DTC) was in the 1940s. ^{131}I concentrates in DTC due to the expression of sodium-iodine symporter (NIS) on the thyroid cells, which is the key feature of the cells allowing specific uptake of radioactive iodine [58]. This results in the achievement of therapeutic effects due to emission of charged particles, which irradiate the cellular structures. Therefore, the use of radioiodine therapy in DTC results in selective irradiation of iodine avid thyroid tissue and thyroid carcinoma cells, and is the mainstay of successful therapy of this disease [136].

Radioiodine ablation treatment is usually given 4–8 weeks after total thyroidectomy, as there is usually some residual thyroid tissue remaining in the thyroid bed. The aims of this initial treatment are to destroy residual thyroid tissue in order to facilitate long term surveillance with serum thyroglobulin levels and increasing the sensitivity of detection of recurrent or metastatic disease on whole body diagnostic scans, and decreasing the rate of recurrence and increasing survival by removing

[1]Department of Nuclear Medicine and Centre for PET, Austin Health, Melbourne, Australia

[2]Department of Medicine, University of Melbourne, Parkville, Australia

[3]Ludwig Institute for Cancer Research, Austin Hospital, Heidelberg, Victoria, 3084, Australia

T. Stigbrand et al. (eds.) *Targeted Radionuclide Tumor Therapy*,

microscopic tumour postoperatively. Post-ablation ^{131}I scans have a higher sensitivity for detection of metastatic disease than diagnostic scans [214].

The final dose to the target tissue is the main determinant for successful therapy. Individual doses of radioiodine can be given using 'standard' doses, which generally range from 1.1–3.7 GBq (30–100 mCi) [19]. The major disadvantage of this empirical treatment is the failure to determine whether the treatment dose may have a therapeutic effect or exceed a predetermined maximum radiation absorbed dose to a critical organ, which is an important factor to consider in radionuclide therapy. An alternative approach is based on using individual dosimetry based on quantitative dosimetry on individual patients to calculate the dose required to administer an effective radiation dose to the thyroid tissue, whilst minimising unacceptable results [135]. This can be based on either lesional or whole body dosimetry, and requires the uptake of a small tracer dose of radioiodine prior to treatment, as seen in Fig. 20.1. The major advantage of this method is that treatment outcome is improved by selecting and administering higher treatment doses in order to achieve a tumoricidal effect whilst reducing side effects, and potentially avoiding unnecessary costs and untoward effects in some patients. In addition, the administration of multiple empiric doses fractionated over time may not be equivalent to the same total radiation absorbed dose to the target organ administered as a single dosimetric determined dose because the dose rate is lower, and previous dosages would have destroyed some of the target lesion, therefore reducing the uptake of subsequent doses. The major disadvantages of dosimetry-based administration are the increased inconvenience and the potential for stunning from the tracer doses of ^{131}I. This concept of stunning is the rationale that administration of a small pre-ablation (diagnostic) dose of ^{131}I may reduce the trapping of subsequent radiotracer by normal thyroid remnant, therefore reducing the efficacy of ablation treatment [44, 120]. There have been studies which showed the superiority of ^{123}I over ^{131}I for scanning of thyroid remnant, therefore reducing the possibility of stunning, but these studies have used ^{131}I doses up to 185 MBq (5 mCi) of ^{131}I [5, 120, 130] (Fig. 20.2). However, a recent study comparing the ablation rate in patients who received a dose of 74 MBq (2 mCi) of ^{131}I vs. 14.8 MBq (0.4 mCi) of ^{123}I found that the ablation rate, as assessed by follow-up whole body scintigraphy 6–8 months later and stimulated thyroglobulin assessment, was similar for both radiotracers [193].

The effectiveness of radioiodine treatment is inversely correlated with tumour mass and extent. The prognosis is dependent on features such as the presence of metastases, age of diagnosis, completeness of resection, invasion and tumour size [214]. The current international consensus is that patients with high risk disease should have radioiodine ablation treatment, with high dose ^{131}I, following an appropriate period of thyroid hormone withdrawal to stimulate thyroid stimulating hormone (TSH) levels [46, 153]. Patients with very low risk disease, defined as unifocal microcarcinoma (<1 cm) without extracapsular extension or lymph node involvement, or generally low risk disease, do not necessarily have to receive radioiodine ablation treatment, but this may be given to facilitate long term follow up with serum thyroglobulin assessment.

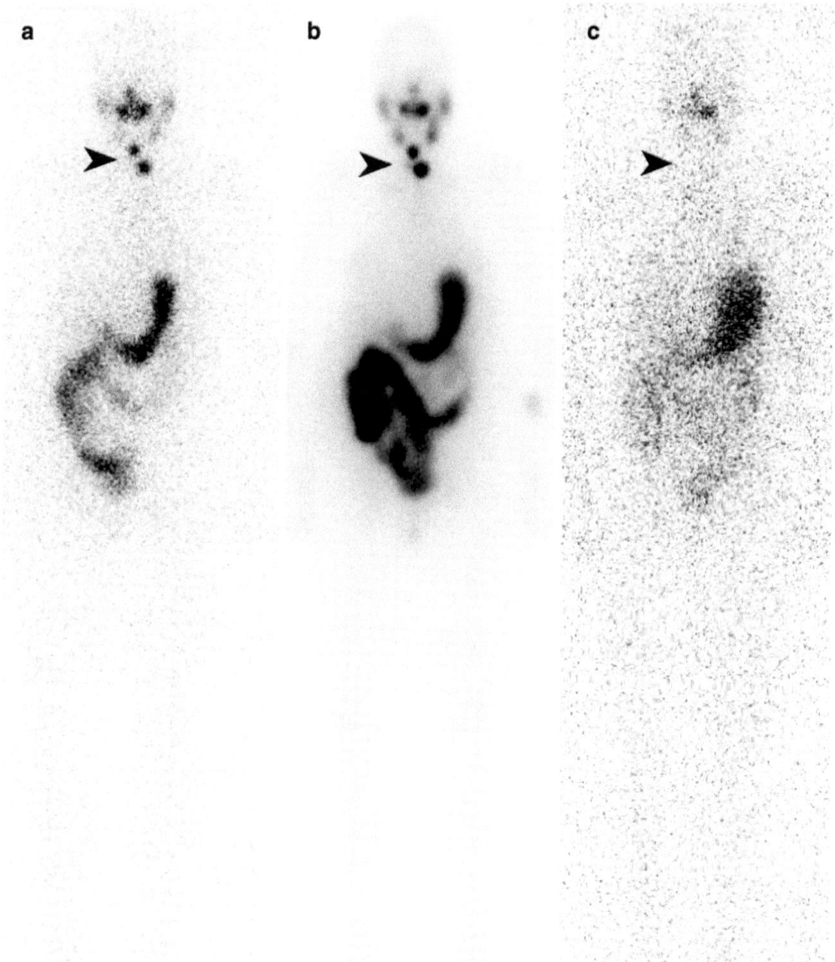

Fig. 20.1 The use of ^{131}I as a diagnostic scan to determine the ablation dose. (A) Diagnostic 75 MBq (2 mCi) ^{131}I whole body scan. (B) The post-ablation scan shows remnant uptake with local lymph node disease. Physiologic activity is seen in the nasopharynx, salivary glands, stomach, bowel and urinary bladder. (C) A follow-up scan 1 year later demonstrates successful remnant and local lymph node ablation

Thyroid hormone remnant ablation requires elevated levels of TSH to allow selective uptake of radioiodine in the thyroid tissue. Serum TSH must be measured prior to ^{131}I administration, and should be >30 mU/l. Traditionally, this has been achieved by withdrawing thyroid hormone (THW) for 4–5 weeks. This will increase endogenous release of TSH and promote radioiodine uptake in the remaining cells. More recently, the advent of recombinant human TSH (rhTSH) has allowed the TSH rise to be achieved without undergoing thyroid hormone withdrawal.

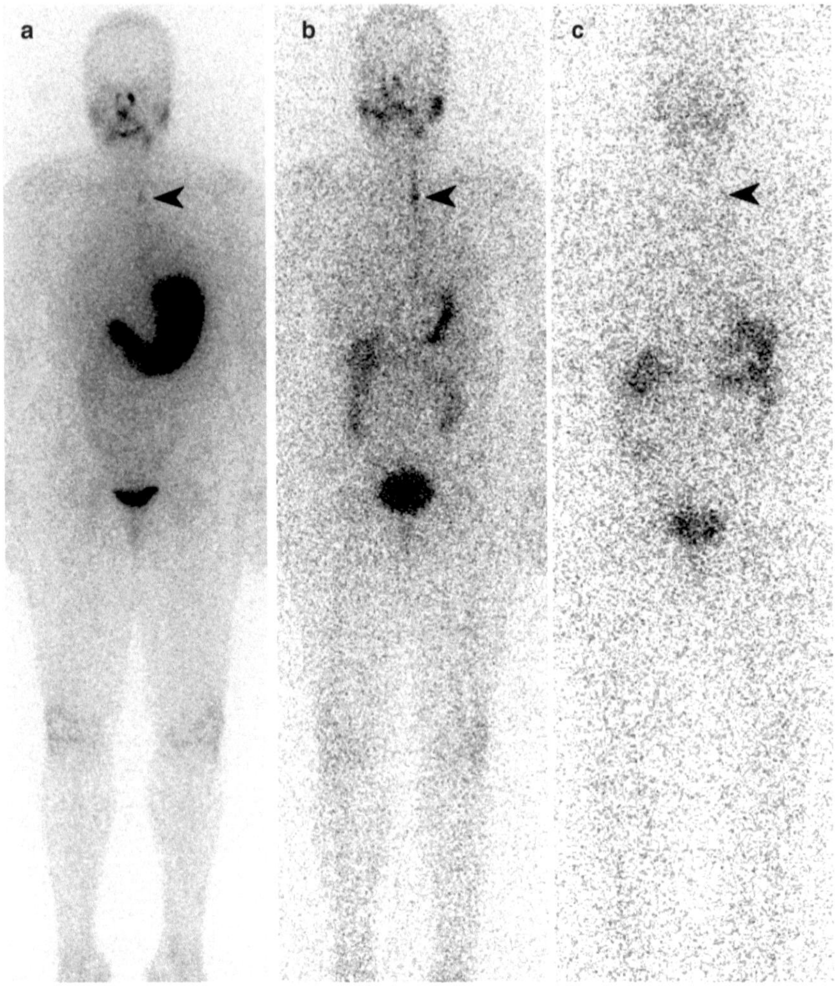

Fig. 20.2 The use of ^{123}I for diagnostic purposes compared to ^{131}I. (A) ^{123}I images obtained at 4 hours showed faint activity in the left of the midline in the upper mediastinum, which becomes more evident on (B) delayed 24 hour images. This appeared to be along the esophagus, and not seen on (C) the 75 MBq (2 mCi) diagnostic ^{131}I whole body scan, and was associated with a negative thyroglobulin level. Physiologic activity in the nasopharynx, salivary glands, stomach, bowel and urinary bladder is evident

The main indications for the use of rhTSH are insufficient TSH production despite adequate thyroid hormone withdrawal, significant comorbidities with thyroid hormone withdrawal. Initial pilot studies of rhTSH with radioiodine ablation did not demonstrate promising results, but these were with low doses of ^{131}I (30 mCi/ 1.1 BGq) or were combined with a shorter duration of THW [12, 154]. A subsequent international, prospective randomised controlled study of 63 patients demonstrated comparable thyroid remnant ablation rates with 100 mCi (3.7 GBq) of ^{131}I in patients prepared with rhTSH or with THW [156]. A review of the use of rhTSH in the preparation of patients for treatment with ^{131}I has validated the safety and efficacy of rhTSh for this purpose [126].

Recombinant human TSH is more commonly used in the follow-up of patients with diagnostic ^{131}I scan and stimulated thyroglobulin assessment. Previous studies have shown that the results of ^{131}I whole body scans and thyroglobulin levels obtained after rhTSH was not significantly different from those obtained after THW [83, 114, 155]. The main advantage of using rhTSH is the avoidance of the physical and psychological effects of hypothyroidism, which can have a significant impact on the patient's quality of life [60, 184]. The fractional remnant uptake is higher in patients who had rhTSH but the difference in residence times and mean whole body ^{131}I uptake at 48 hours are not significant [81], and the ablation rates are also not significantly different [156]. In addition, the radiation dose to the blood (a surrogate marker for bone marrow exposure) is 35% lower in the patients prepared with rhTSH compared to THW group, which may have implications on the potential risk of radiation-induced malignancies [81].

Patients with elevated stimulated thyroglobulin levels or rising thyroglobulin levels after radioiodine ablation treatment should have a whole body diagnostic radioiodine scan with an appropriately elevated TSH level. This scan may reveal a focus of neoplastic activity which needs to have the appropriate treatment. However, in the event of a negative scan, radioiodine ablation treatment should only be given if the Tg level is on an increasing trend. If the post-ablation scan is negative, high dose ^{131}I should not be administered again, as this may indicate the presence of de-differentiated thyroid cancer, which have lost the ability to concentrate iodine. In these cases, consideration should be given to other imaging modalities such as ^{18}F-FDG PET scan [124], as shown in Fig. 20.3. Multiple studies have shown the superiority of FDG-PET in the detection of recurrent or metastatic disease [7, 45, 76, 157, 182, 189]. The sensitivity if FDG-PET is also higher in patients with elevated TSH levels, with statistically significant improvement in tumour-to-background ratio [124, 144].

The short term side effects of ^{131}I treatment include nausea, gastric discomfort, salivary gland pain, taste disturbance and ocular dryness. However, these are usually transient and rarely progress to chronic ailments. There is some evidence that manoeuvres such as lemon juice or chewing gum will reduce the incidence or severity of salivary gland symptoms, but subsequent obstruction of the salivary gland ducts have been reported weeks to years after radioiodine treatment [175]. Permanent side effects have not been consistently demonstrated by large follow-up studies and are most likely to be dependent on other co-existing factors [151].

Although several studies have not found an increased risk of second malignancies related to radioiodine therapy, a linear dose-response relationship between the cumulative ^{131}I dosage and the risk of secondary malignancies, including leukaemia, bone, soft tissue, colorectal and salivary gland tumours [177] has been noted. This incidence is also thought to be dependent on genetic disposition and other environmental factors [200]. The incidence of leukaemia has been reported to be

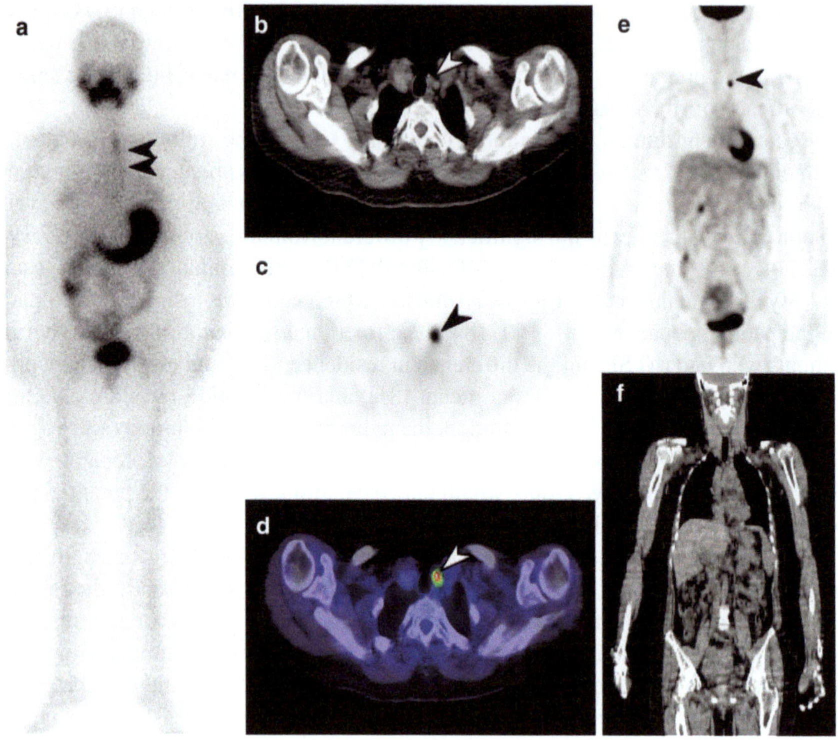

Fig. 20.3 The use of ^{18}F-FDG PET/CT to investigate a thyroglobulin positive, iodine scan negative patient. (A) Post-ablation scan after 5.5 GBq (150 mCi) ^{131}I show physiologic activity in the nasopharynx, esophagus (double arrows), breast, stomach, bowel and bladder. ^{18}F-FDG PET/CT scan shows a discrete focal lesion in the lower left neck adjacent to the trachea (single arrow) on (B) axial CT, (C) axial PET, (D) fusion PET/CT, (E) coronal PET and (F) coronal CT images

higher after >37 GBq (1 Ci) of ^{131}I [80], or >18.5 GBq (500 mCi) when associated with external beam radiotherapy [175].

The absolute contraindication to radioiodine therapy is pregnancy and lactating females. The effective dose to the gonads are in the same order of magnitude to the doses delivered by a pelvic radiograph. Two studies of large patient cohorts treated with ^{131}I did not show a significant difference in female fertility rate, birth weight, prematurity, congenital malformations, death in the first year of life, thyroid diseases or non-thyroid malignancies in the offspring [59, 175]. The prevalence of miscarriages in 290 pregnancies has not been shown to vary with cumulative exposure to ^{131}I, but was maximal in women who became pregnant within 1 year of treatment with ^{131}I [175]. Therefore, delay in conception is recommended 1 year after therapeutic administration of ^{131}I and control of thyroid status has been achieved. Thyroid hormone status should also be monitored every 2–3 months during pregnancy, as pregnancy often requires increases in thyroid hormone doses [129, 181].

The de-differentiation of thyroid cancer cells has been implicated in the lack of radioiodine uptake, resulting in poor response to treatment. Several strategies have been trialed in an attempt to increase intracellular occupancy time of radioiodine. It has been observed that high levels of exogenous iodine can block radioiodine uptake, and exogenous iodine (such as iodinated contrast agents for CT scans and multivitamins) should be avoided prior to treatment with radioiodine [175]. Lithium has also been shown to reduce the exit of iodine from normal thyroid cells, and therefore increase retention in thyroid remnant. The half-life of radioiodine has resulted in the doubling of radiation to the lesions in one study, but no long term outcomes are available [106]. The re-differentiation of thyroid cancer cells with retinoic acid derivatives has been reported to enhance radioiodine uptake [105], but these findings are being further validated [82, 183].

Radiolabelled Antibody Therapy

The development of monoclonal antibody-based therapeutics for cancer patients has been highly successful over the last 10 years [217]. A number of these new treatments have been based on the ability of monoclonal antibodies to modulate receptor-based intracellular signalling (such as trastuzumab, rituximab, cetuximab and bevacizumab), as well as tumour cell cytotoxicity mediated by immune effector function initiated by the Fc portions of these antibodies. The combination of monoclonal antibodies with other therapies, including chemotherapy and other biologics, and using monoclonal antibodies to deliver toxins and radioisotopes to tumour sites, have also emerged as mechanisms of increasing response rates and duration of response.

Antigen Targets

The selection of suitable antigens on the surface of cancer cells for targeting with monoclonal antibodies (mAbs) [187, 210] and the biology of cellular function related to cognate antigens, remain critical factors in the success of this type of therapy, as well as in identifying new strategies for antibody-based treatment. (See also chapter 2 in this volume). Different categories of tumour antigens have been identified in a variety of malignancies, and include: (1) hematopoietic differentiation antigens: glycoproteins usually associated with cluster differentiation (CD) groupings (e.g. CD5, CD19, CD20, CD33, CD45, CD52); (2) cell surface differentiation antigens, including glycoproteins [such as carcinoembryonic antigen (CEA), sialyl Tn antigen (TAG-72), polymorphic epithelial mucin (PEM), epithelial cell adhesion molecule (Ep-CAM), A33, G250, prostate-specific membrane antigen (PSMA) and prostate-specific antigen (PSA)], glycolipids (such as gangliosides, e.g. GD2, GD3, GM2) and carbohydrates (such as blood group-related antigens, e.g. Le^y and Le^b); (3) growth factor receptors, including epidermal growth factor receptor (EGFR) and its mutant form EGFRvIII, HER-2/neu and IL-2 receptor (See also chapter 3 in this volume); and (4) angiogenesis and stromal antigens, including fibroblast activation protein (FAP), vascular endothelial growth factor receptor (VEGFR), tenascin and integrin $\alpha_v\beta_3$.

Radioisotopes can be chemically linked to anti-tumour mAbs and administered to patients to deliver radiation selectively to tumour sites. Radioimmunoconjugates are constructed either by covalently binding the radioisotope directly to the antibody, or by crosslinking through a chelating agent or chemical linker. The selection of radionuclide is particularly important for cell surface targets that are internalised through intracellular trafficking pathways, resulting in dehalogenation of radioiodine and justifying the use of radiometals for this type of antigen based approach. The cytotoxic efficacy of a given radioimmunoconjugate also depends on the kinetics of antibody localisation and retention of the radionuclide, as well as the radiosensitivity of the target cell. For example, lymphoma cells are particularly sensitive to radiation, and ^{90}Y-CD20 mAb (Zevalin®) has been shown to increase delivery of radiation to neoplastic versus normal tissue by nearly 1,000-fold [223].

Radioimmunotherapy of Haematologic Malignancies

Radioimmunotherapy of lymphomas has shown impressive clinical results, which is in part related to the effects of the immune effector function of antibodies used (particularly anti-CD20), as well as the intrinsic radiosensitivity of lymphomas [86]. This is particularly relevant in view of the fact that uptake of radiolabelled antibodies in lymphoma is often lower than in solid tumours, and responses may be seen even when uptake is not visualised in a lymphoma lesion [99, 190, 191].

There have been many radioimmunotherapy studies reported in lymphoma, mainly against differentiation antigen targets including CD19, CD20, CD21, CD22, CD37 and CD45, and HLA-DR [39]. The development of two FDA approved antibodies, ^{131}I-tositumomab (Bexxar®) and ^{90}Y-ibritumomab tiuxetan (Zevalin®) are highlights of the successful application of radiolabelled antibodies in cancer patients. These therapies are approved for the treatment of non-Hodgkin's lymphoma patients either relapsed or refractory to chemotherapy and rituximab (chimeric anti-CD20 antibody). For both, a trace labelled infusion is used prior to therapy to assess biodistribution, and in the case of ^{131}I-tositumomab to calculate the appropriate therapy dose by dosimetry calculations [55]. In the European Union, however, a tracer dose is not required for therapeutic use of ^{90}Y-ibritumomab tiuxetan.

Initial Phase I/II trials of ^{90}Y-ibritumomab tiuxetan showed an overall response rate of 82% in patients with follicular lymphoma, with 26% complete responses [225]. Patients with bulky disease were shown to have a reduced response rate. The maximum tolerated dose in patients with normal blood counts prior to treatment was 0.4 mCi/kg, and 0.3 mCi/kg in patients with platelet counts <150,000. This latter group was shown to have a response rate of 83%, and complete response rate of 47% [180]. In a pivotal randomised trial comparing ^{90}Y-ibritumomab tiuxetan with rituximab in 143 patients with relapsed or refractory follicular low grade non-Hodgkin's lymphoma that were rituximab naive, ^{90}Y-ibritumomab tiuxetan demonstrated responses in 80% of patients compared to 56% with rituximab ($p = 0.002$) [226]. Reponses to ^{90}Y-ibritumomab tiuxetan have also been shown in patients who are refractory to rituximab [224].

The initial Phase I trials of ^{131}I-tositumomab showed that an initial imaging infusion allowed optimal selection of therapy dose of 75 cGy to whole body [99, 101]. The subsequent Phase I/II trial demonstrated a response rate of 71% including 34% complete responders, with responders more common in the low grade or transformed non-Hodgkin's lymphoma group (83%) [102]. A subsequent multicenter trial of ^{131}I-tositumomab in patients with low grade or transformed non-Hodgkin's lymphoma who were resistant to or had relapsed following therapy showed a response rate of 81% in patients with low grade histology, including 20% complete responses [103]. ^{131}I-tositumomab was also shown in a randomised study to be superior to antibody alone, with an overall response rate of 68% vs 16% ($p = 0.002$) [48].

The practical issues surrounding radioimmunotherapy with ^{131}I-tositumomab and ^{90}Y-ibritumomab tiuxetan principally relate to the imaging studies that may be required, and the radiation safety issues for patients and the community following treatment, which vary according to local guidelines and radiation policies. In addition, myelosuppression remains a predictable but usually manageable toxicity following treatment. A principle concern is the incidence of acute myeloid leukaemia (AML) or myelodysplastic syndrome following treatment, although long term follow-up studies have found the incidence to be no greater than that seen with chemotherapy alone [39].

The potential for using radioimmunotherapy in early stage treatment of lymphomas is also being explored. A recent Phase II study of first line ^{131}I-tositumomab in stage III and IV follicular lymphoma showed a complete response rate of 75%, and an overall objective response rate of 95% [100]. Additional trials exploring ^{131}I-tositumomab with chemotherapy [121], and with rituximab, are ongoing in order to define the utility of this therapy in combination treatment settings. High dose ^{131}I-tositumomab therapy with stem cell support has shown high response rates and long term durable responses [161]. Trials with repeat treatments with ^{90}Y-ibritumomab tiuxetan, and including stem cell support, are also being actively pursed.

Radioimmunotherapy of lymphoma is also being explored with other antibodies, including the humanised anti-CD22 antibody epratuzumab labelled with ^{90}Y and ^{186}Re [160, 191], and ^{131}I- labelled rituximab [119].

Radioimmunotherapy of leukemias has focused on differentiation antigen targets expressed on malignant B and T cells [96, 134, 222]. Encouraging results of trials in acute leukemias have been reported with anti-CD33 M195, which has been humanised and studied in patients with AML [97]. ^{131}I-M195 has been used in conjunction with busulphan and cyclophosphamide for cytoreduction prior to bone marrow transplantation in patients with relapsed or refractory AML and blastic or accelerated chronic myeloid leukemia (CML). The use of radiolabelled antibodies directed against leukemic cells as part of a bone marrow transplant protocol has also been evaluated with a ^{131}I anti-CD45 antibody in patients with AML or acute lymphocytic leukemia (ALL) [134]. Minimal non-hematologic toxicity has been seen with both approaches, and comparable results to conventional BMT protocols with total body irradiation has been observed. Overall, the results of radioimmunotherapy in leukemia suggest the ability to reduce the risk of relapse in high-risk AML patients transplanted early in the course of their disease (<15% blasts) to 20–30%, and to safely intensify reduced-intensity conditioning regimens (non-relapse mortality of 25% compared to relapse rate of 55% within 2 years). The optimal therapeutic approach has extended to the use of alpha-labelled antibodies (e.g. ^{213}Bi-M195) in patients with refractory AML [107], and trials with ^{225}Ac-M195 are ongoing. The role of radioimmunotherapy of leukemias is continuing to evolve and will require further trials to establish its place in this disease.

Radioimmunotherapy of Solid Tumours

While radioimmunotherapy has shown success in hematologic malignancy (such as ^{131}I-tositumomab and ^{90}Y-ibritumomab tiuxetan in non-Hodgkin's lymphoma), responses in solid tumours have been infrequent. This is due in part to the inability to deliver sufficient radiation dose to tumour cells, the relative lack of sensitivity of solid tumours to radiation compared to lymphoma, and the size of metastatic lesions combined with physiologic barriers to uniform tumour penetrance by antibodies [42, 188]. Studies of antibody penetration into solid tumours have shown variable uptake in epithelial tumours due to tumour size, histological type, vascularity, degree of necrosis, antigen expression, and poor or non-uniform penetration into the tumour [29, 65, 91, 199]. The physical properties of isotopes, particularly the path length and energy of emission, and physical half-life, need to be selected based on the size of lesion and the targeting and internalisation properties of the antibody. For solid tumours, β-emitters remain the principal choice for effective therapy for lesions greater than 2–3 mm in size, while α-emitters may be best suited to micrometastatic disease [148]. ^{90}Y has a higher beta particle energy and longer range compared to ^{177}Lu; however, this does increase potential normal tissue toxicity. Both ^{90}Y and ^{177}Lu are well-suited to internalising antigens like PSMA compared to radiohalides (such as ^{131}I), due to superior tumor retention. ^{177}Lu radioimmunotherapy has also been demonstrated in computational models and animal experiments to be more effective in treating small lesions compared to ^{90}Y radioimmunotherapy [11, 32, 197].

The short range of α-particle emitters (50–80 μm) is more suited to the treatment of small volume disease, as the high energy (4–9 MeV) emissions are deposited directly over two to four cell diameters, resulting in a high absorbed dose and Linear Energy Transfer (LET) [141]. The high LET of α emitters in part contributes to their high relative biological effectiveness (RBE), with the cytotoxicity of α-emitters 5–100 times that of an equivalent dose of β-emitter [229]. Recent studies of α-emitters labelled to monoclonal antibodies have shown promising efficacy in a range of preclinical models including acute myeloid leukemia, metastatic melanoma, and solid tumour including prostate, breast and gastric cancer [6, 22, 98, 104, 137, 194, 196].

The use of radiolabelled antibodies in a loco-regional infusion setting in solid tumours has shown some promise. The selective targeting of tumour, particularly in ovarian cancer and glioma, has been demonstrated following intraperitoneal infusion, or direct intralesional infusion, of ^{131}I, ^{177}Lu and ^{90}Y-labelled antibodies, with improvements in response and progression free survival observed [8, 9, 68, 128, 139, 165, 174]. A recent large Phase III trial of ^{90}Y-anti-MUC1 antibody in ovarian cancer did not, however, show an improvement in response rate or progression free survival [152]. It is likely that larger Phase II trials in glioma, which are ongoing, may show more promising results and a possible clinical indication for this approach.

In view of the immunogenicity of murine antibodies, chimeric and humanised antibodies have emerged as the optimal constructs for radioimmunotherapy of solid tumours. A recent important development is the treatment of non-small cell lung cancer with ^{131}I-chTNT, which showed an objective response rate of 33% in 97 non-small-cell lung cancer patients [38]. ^{131}I-chTNT has subsequently been approved for the treatment of non-small cell lung cancer in China, and additional clinical indications are being explored.

Other ^{131}I labelled humanised mAbs have also shown responses in humans with solid tumours. hMN-14 is a humanised mAb targeting CEA [18, 78] and phase II radioimmunotherapy trials utilising ^{131}I-hMN-14 have been performed in patients with metastatic colorectal cancer, and in patients with resected colorectal liver metastases. In the latter group, encouraging progression free survival data has been shown compared to historical controls [123], and larger randomised trials are underway. Trials with ^{131}I-huA33, targeting the A33 antigen, have been performed in patients with advanced or metastatic colorectal cancer, with a unique finding of prolonged retention of ^{131}I-huA33 in tumour (at least 6 weeks) observed due to the cellular location of the A33 antigen in tumour cells and lack of trafficking of A33 antigen/antibody complex to intracellular lysosomes [40, 188] (Fig. 20.4). In renal cell carcinoma, ^{131}I-cG250 has demonstrated excellent targeting of primary and metastatic lesions, and in radioimmunotherapy studies of ^{131}I-cG250 some objective responses (partial response and stabilisation of disease) has been observed [32, 199]. Additional trials with ^{177}Lu and ^{90}Y labelled cG250 have also been initiated.

To exploit internalising antigens, radioimmunotherapy studies with ^{90}Y and ^{177}Lu with humanised antibodies have been performed. In a Phase I trial of ^{90}Y-J591 (anti-PSMA) in prostate cancer patients, treatment was found to be well tolerated, and with some biologic activity seen including objective responses and reduction in PSA [142]. In a subsequent trial of ^{177}Lu-J591, 4/35 (11%) patients had a decrease in PSA following treatment and 16/35 (46%) had stabilization of PSA [11]. These studies suggest that ^{177}Lu-J591 may be better suited to small volume disease, and ^{90}Y-J591 to larger (ie >1 cm) volume disease, although this requires confirmation in

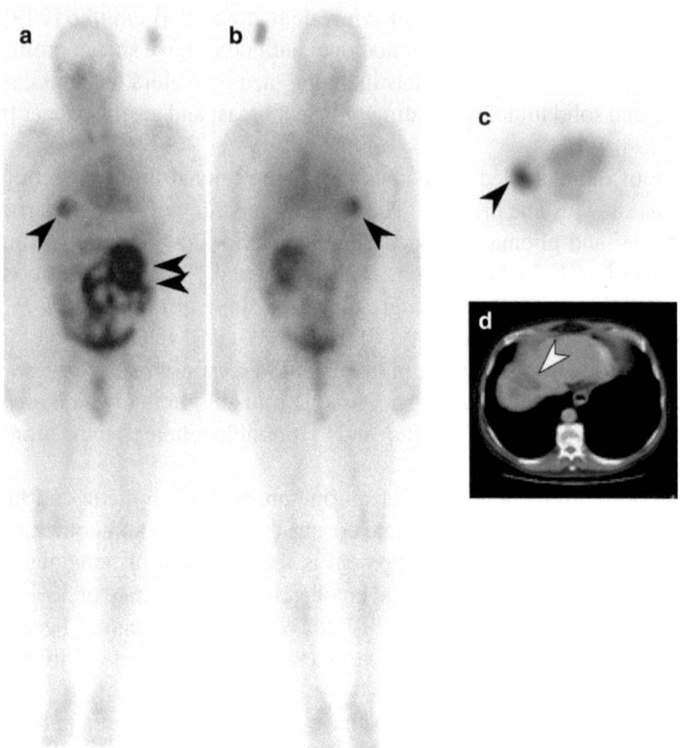

Fig. 20.4 ^{131}I-humanised huA33 monoclonal antibody biodistribution study. (A) Anterior and (B) posterior whole body planar images show uptake in the metastatic liver lesion in the right upper quadrant (arrow), which localises to the liver lesion seen on (C) axial SPECT and (D) CT images. Normal bowel uptake is also seen (double arrows)

larger Phase II trials. In a phase I trial of ^{90}Y-MX-DTPA-hBrE-2 was conducted in patients with breast cancer with stem cell support, two patients showed partial responses and three patients showed stabilization of previously progressive disease [172]. ^{90}Y-cT84.66 has been studied in a dose escalation trial in patients with CEA positive malignancies, with stable disease in three and mixed responses in two patients [227].

In many radioimmunotherapy trials, no clinical or diagnostic parameter (including past therapy, and marrow involvement by tumour) can easily predict red marrow toxicity in individual patients, which is the commonest dose limiting toxicity seen. The need for patient specific dosimetry, which has been successfully utilized for anti-CD20 radioimmunotherapy (such as ^{131}I-tositumomab) [86, 219], has not shown encouraging results in solid tumour radioimmunotherapy trials. Serum levels of FLT-3 ligand as a biomarker of red marrow functional reserve have been shown to assist in predicting hematologic toxicity following radioimmunotherapy [192], however, this has not been reproduced in other trials.

The actual radiation dose delivered to tumour remains the principal factor affecting efficacy of radioimmunotherapy. To address this issue, clinical trials have been conducted where multiple treatments have been performed, with dose and scheduling predicated on red marrow toxicity and recovery [54]. This has been explored with repeat infusion studies [11, 32], however, the toxicity of this approach has been high, and larger trials are required to define the benefits of this approach. The theoretical advantages of such fractionated radioimmunotherapy have been demonstrated in animal model studies, although recent human trials have not confirmed these results [57]. Pretargeting of antibodies may also improve tumour to normal tissue ratios and possible therapeutic efficacy [26, 70]. This approach involves the pretargeting of an antibody-avidin (or streptavidin) conjugate to tumour, clearance of the conjugate from blood, followed by a biotin-radioisotope step, or the use of bispecific antibodies [70]. Trials with pretargeted antibodies have shown acceptable toxicity and some indications of anti-tumour response [37, 108, 218], and this is an area of ongoing clinical investigation.

Radioimmunotherapy in Combination with Other Treatment Modalities

The combination of monoclonal antibody therapy with other treatments, particularly chemotherapy and radiotherapy, has been shown in *in vivo* models and in clinical trials to have potential additive or synergistic effects. The mechanisms of this effect are complex, and related to the interactions between conventional therapy mechanisms of action, and the effect of Fc function or signalling inhibition on tumour cell proliferation and repair mechanisms. The majority of data exists from combining mAb based therapy with chemotherapy [14]. Preclinical data have shown enhanced radiation sensitivity of tumour cells pretreated with cytotoxics such as paclitaxel [122]. As a result, the combination of chemotherapy and radiotherapy has become standard treatment for a number of epithelial tumours over the last 10 years. Animal model studies have shown the combination of radioimmunotherapy with chemotherapy results in enhanced therapeutic effect, with the timing of chemotherapy often playing an important role in improved response [34, 43, 56, 104, 205]. Clinical trials combining chemotherapy and radioimmunotherapy have also shown encouraging results. In a trial of ^{90}Y-anti-CEA chimeric T84.66 with 5-FU, the tolerability of this approach was demonstrated [227]. Additional trials have explored the use of radioimmunotherapy and chemotherapy [66, 172] including the use of peripheral stem cell support for haematologic toxicity [190]. A recently completed trial of ^{131}I-huA33 with capecitabine (an orally bioavailable 5-FU prodrug) has also demonstrated the feasibility of this approach, with measurable responses and prolonged progression free survival in some patients observed [85]. This approach of combination therapy will have increasing importance in the development of radiolabelled mAbs as therapeutics, particularly in solid tumours.

Radiolabelled Peptide Therapy

The labelling of peptides with radiotracers enable the specific treatment of tumours which express peptide receptors, and can overcome the usual resistance to conventional chemotherapy agents. (See also chapter 7 in this volume.) The emission of particles during radionuclide decay can result in cell death of adjacent cells depending on the energy of the emitted particles. The optimal characteristics for systemic radionuclide therapy include emissions, half-life, maximum tumour uptake and retention with minimal non-tumour tissue uptake. These characteristics will depend on the type of tumour and radionuclide used [158].

Small radiolabelled peptide derivatives (1.5 kDa) were developed more than 15 years ago, as an alternative to radiolabelled antibodies [158]. These are normal regulatory peptides found *in vivo*, therefore have a natural high affinity to receptors which are selectively expressed on cell membranes. This resulted in the development of peptide receptor radionuclide therapy (PRRT). PRRT achieves volume reduction by delivering radiation doses to tumours. The biological basis of this treatment is receptor-mediated internalisation and intracellular retention of the radiopeptide, with the key to successful treatment being a residence time in the tumour cell which is appropriate for the physical half-life of the radionuclide [151]. Most regulatory peptides undergo receptor-mediated endocytosis enabling internalisation of the attached radiometal within the targeted cell [195, 230].

Small radiopeptides have an advantage by having rapid tissue penetration (due to their hydrophilic properties), fast clearance, and low antigenicity, and can be produced easily and inexpensively [147]. Peptides do not cross intact blood brain barriers which is obviously an advantage when the targets are in the peripheral organs, but not if central nervous system receptors are the targets. However, peptides may be able to penetrate disturbed blood brain barrier which is seen in undifferentiated glioblastomas [116]. Subtle changes in the placement of the radiolabel on the peptides can produce significant changes in the biodistribution of the radiopeptide [67]. The natural structure of the peptides also render them sensitive to peptidases and catabolism in the body, which can potentially reduce the effective doses delivered to the tumour [131]. Peptides are excreted from the body either via renal and/or hepatobiliary excretion. The rapid and prolonged accumulation of radiopeptides in the kidneys is a recognised issue for PRRT, which needs to be considered prior to treatment, as further described below.

There are two main criteria for the eligibility of PRRT, which are based on clinical and biologic features of the tumour [169]. The clinical criteria are that patients must have cancer with multiple inoperable metastases, and the tumour must express the corresponding peptide receptor, with a receptor density which is sufficiently high to allow delivery of the required absorbed dose [169]. This is where pretherapy imaging with a radiopeptide (preferably with the same targeting agent used for radiopeptide therapy) will play a crucial part in identifying patients who will gain sufficient benefit from radiopeptide therapy. It should be noted that although tumour size was shown to play a role in the efficacy of PRRT in animal tumour models, this was not seen in similar human studies [51].

Table 20.1 Physical properties of common radionuclides used for imaging and therapy ^{18}F, ^{111}In, and ^{123}I are in most cases only used for imaging

Radionuclide	Gamma emission (keV)	Half-life
^{111}In	171	2.8 days
^{90}Y	–	2.7 days
^{177}Lu	497	6.7 days
^{68}Ga	511	68 minutes
^{18}F	511	110 minutes
^{131}I	284/364/637	8.0 days
^{123}I	159	13.2 hours
^{186}Re	137	90 hours
^{188}Re	155	16.9 hours

There is a range of radionuclides which can be used either as an imaging agent, therapeutic agent, or a combination of both. Table 20.1 lists the various radionuclides which can be used for this purpose.

Somatostatin Receptor Therapy

The most widely used radiopeptide therapy is the radiolabelling of somatostatin analogues in the treatment of neuroendocrine tumours, see also chapter 7 in this book. Somatostatin is a cyclic 14 amino acid which acts as a neurotransmitter in the central nervous system [72]. There are five subtypes of human somatostatin receptors (SSTR), somatostatin receptors 1–5, and natural somatostatin has a high affinity for all of these receptors [159].

Neuroendocrine tumours such as carcinoid tumours and pancreatic islet cell tumours overexpress somatostatin receptors. The expression profile of different tumours have been described [170], and the differences in somatostatin receptor expression may account for differences in treatment efficacy [203]. A predominance of SSTR1 or SSTR2 in gastropancreatic tumours has been noted [170], whilst *in vitro* studies of thyroid cancer cells show a predominant expression of SSTR3 and SSTR5 [3]. The overexpression of different somatostatin receptors in different tumour types can be exploited to enable treatment of primary and metastatic lesions due to postreceptor signalling, which is triggered by receptor-ligand internalisation [109, 115, 170].

The labelling of somatostatin analogues with radiotracers such as ^{111}Indium [^{111}In-diethylenetriaminepentaacetic acid (DTPA)^{0}-octreotide] (Octreoscan®; Mallinckrodt Medical), have not only allowed the *in vivo* visualisation of the presence of somatostatin receptors with imaging techniques, but the administration of radiolabel somatostatin analogues at higher doses can also be used [113] (Fig. 20.5). There have been different radiopeptides used for treatment of neuroendocrine tumours, which is summarised in Table 20.2.

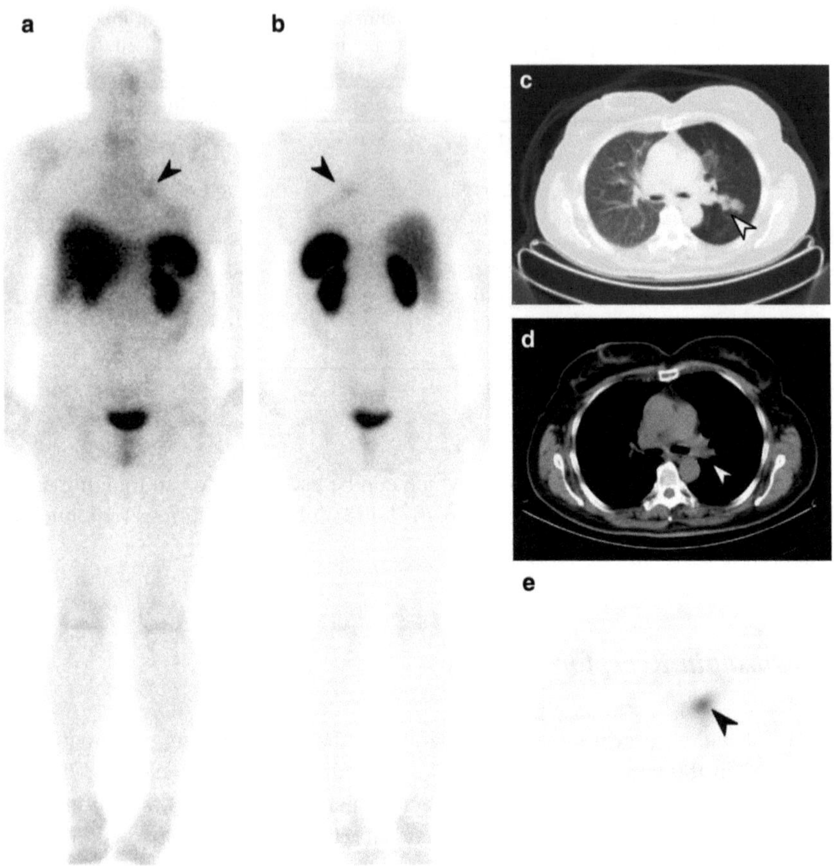

Fig. 20.5 ^{111}In-Octreotide study to assess the presence of somatostatin receptors. Bronchial carcinoid disease in the left hilum and left lung (arrows) are seen on: (A) anterior and (B) posterior whole body images. Correlative CT images in (C) lung and (D) mediastinal windows localises the lesion on (E) axial SPECT image

Table 20.2 Radiopeptides used in clinical somatostatin receptor radionuclide therapy

Radiopeptide	Reference
^{111}In-diethylenetriaminepentaacetic acid (DTPA)-octreotide	[10, 208]
^{90}Y-dodecanetetraacetic acid (DOTA),Tyr3-octreotide	[23, 25, 220, 221]
^{90}Y-DOTA-lantreotide	[150, 215]
^{177}Lu-DOTA-octreotate	[110–112]

Initial peptide receptor radiotherapy, with ^{111}In-labelled peptides did not demonstrate significant objective responses on CT or MR imaging, although favourable symptomatic relief was observed [10, 208]. This finding may be explained by the lower tissue penetration range of this particular radiotracer, which cannot kill adjacent receptor-negative tumour cells which may have heterogeneous receptor expression. Toxicities observed with this agent generally consisted of mild bone marrow toxicity, but myelodysplastic syndrome or leukaemia was observed in patients who received >100 GBq of ^{111}In-DTPA-octreotide [208].

More recently, another radiolabelled somatostatin analogue is being used for PRRT with more promising results. This is [^{90}Y-1,4,7,10-tetraazacyclododecane-N,N',N'',N'''-tetraacetic acid (DOTA)^{0},Tyr^{3}]octreotide [113]. There have been a number of phase I and II studies performed in patients with neuroendocrine tumours, and despite differences in protocols the complete and partial remission rates in these studies were between 10–30%, which is higher than those obtained with [^{111}In-DTPA^{0}]octreotide [24, 206, 220, 221].

The replacement of threoninol in the C-terminal of [DTPA^{0}Tyr^{3}]octreotide with threonine in [DTPA^{0}Tyr^{3}]octreotate shows improved binding to somatostatin receptor-positive tissues in preclinical experiments [52, 113]. The use of this agent in humans shows comparable radiotracer uptake in the kidneys, spleen and liver as [DTPA^{0}Tyr^{3}]octreotide, but up to nine-fold higher affinity for the somatostatin receptor subtype 2 in 80% of tumours [171]. Therefore, there is higher absorbed doses in the tumour with similar doses to potentially dose-limiting organs [110, 171]. This particular somatostatin analogue is labelled with ^{177}Lu, which has a lower tissue penetration range, and may be relevant in small tumours [113]. Clinical use of this radiopeptide in neuroendocrine tumours has shown a 30% complete and partial remission rate, with tumour regression positively correlated with a high level of uptake on OctreoScan® imaging, limited hepatic tumour mass, and a high Karnofsky performance score [113]. The side effects of treatment with this agent were few and mostly transient, with mild bone marrow suppression being the commonest side effect [112, 113]. ^{111}In-Lantreotide is a radiolabelled somatostatin analogue which has been reported to have a higher affinity for subtype 3 somatostatin receptor [150], and has been used as an alternative to cold octreotide. However, there is no clear advantage of using lantreotide over octreotide, apart from a lower tumour-to background ratio for lantreotide due to its lipophilic properties [73].

The most critical organ in PRRT are the kidneys, due to their radiosensitivity and high renal retention of the radiopeptides. The loss of renal function may occur years after PRRT, and is primarily due to the reabsorption of radiopeptide in the proximal tubules and retention in the interstitium resulting in renal irradiation [50, 151]. The use of positively charged molecules such as L-lysine and/or L-arginine, have been used to competitively inhibit the proximal tubular absorption of the radiopeptide [21, 23, 92]. A median decline of creatinine clearance was 7.3%/year with [^{90}Y-DOTA^{0},Tyr^{3}]octreotide compared to 3.8%/year in patients treated with [^{177}Lu-DOTA^{0}Tyr^{3}]octreotate [207]. The risk factors to the decline of renal function after PRRT include age, hypertension, diabetes and cumulative and per-cycle renal absorbed dose [151].

Preclinical experiments have suggested that the use of ^{90}Y labelled somatostatin analogues may be more effective for larger tumours, whilst ^{177}Lu-labelled somatostatin analogues may be more effective for smaller tumours [148]. However, the combination of these analogues labelled with various radionuclides may improve objective outcomes, and should be evaluated with randomised clinical trials.

Other Peptide Targets

Although the current use of radiopeptide therapy has been with somatostatin receptors in neuroendocrine tumours, there are other less commonly used peptide radioligands which have been developed. The rationale for utilising peptides against other receptor targets is due to these receptors being overexpressed in more common human cancers. For example, breast, prostate, pancreas and brain tumours have been shown to overexpress several other peptide receptors, such as cholecystokinin-2 (CCK2) [16, 17], gastrin releasing peptide (GRP), neurotensin [84], substance P[211], glucagon-like peptide 1, neuropeptide Y, or corticotropin-releasing-factor-receptors [169]. The functional expression of GRP receptors (GRP-R) demonstrated in prostate [1, 94, 95], breast [27, 143, 146, 228], colon [27, 143, 146, 228], and lung cancer [4, 35, 47] make it a very attractive target for development of new radiopeptides [93].

GRP consists of 27 amino acids, and is the human counterpart to bombesin (BBN), which is a 14 amino-acid peptide found in amphibian tissues [166]. GRP results in a broad spectrum of biological responses, which include gastric acid secretion and secretion of adrenal, pituitary and gastrointestinal hormones, which act on the central and enteric nervous systems to regulate normal biological systems. GRP and BBN have different subtypes which mediate their actions through membrane-bound G protein coupled receptors characterised by seven transmembrane domains which cluster to form the ligand-binding pocket. GRP-R expression in cancer cells is either due to the malignant expansion of cells which normally express this receptor, or to receptor upregulation in cells which do not normally express GRP-R [93]. This is because GRP-R is not normally expressed in normal epithelial cells in the lung, prostate and colon [13, 36, 63, 162], but are present in the non-cancerous, non-neuroendocrine tissue of the pancreas and breast [77, 79, 179]. However, GRP-R is expressed in the majority of neuroendocrine cells present in the lung, prostate and gastrointestinal tract [198, 201, 202]. GRP-R is abnormally expressed in cancer, and often mutated in cancers of the stomach and colon. This results in the variability of these cancers and also explains the reason why a higher percentage of cancers express GRP-R mRNA than functional protein [93]. Immunohistochemical analysis of human colon cancer specimens demonstrated that 84% of cancers expressed GRP or GRP-R, but although these tissues were more likely to express proliferating cell nuclear antigen, the presence of this expression was found equally in stage A and stage D cancers, and did not affect survival either. These features suggest that although GRP is only a modest mitogen in malignancy, and is not a clinically significant growth factor in human colon cancers [36]. There have been other studies evaluating the use of ^{68}Ga-labelled GRP-R in prostate cancer, but a radiopharmaceutical with optimal characteristics for PRRT with this peptide is yet to emerge [127, 185, 186, 209].

CCK2 receptors are found in abundance in >90% of medullary thyroid carcinoma (MTC) [167, 168]. A radiolabelled radiopharmaceutical – ^{111}In-DTPA-D-Glu-Minigastrin [15] – binds to the CCK2 receptors, and has been able to demonstrate in clinical studies metastatic MTC with a higher sensitivity than PET, CT and somatostatin receptor scanning [74]. Vasoactive intestinal peptide (VIP) is overexpressed in adenocarcinoma of the gastroenteropancreatic system. The use of ^{123}I-labelled VIP has been used to detect metastatic pancreatic cancer. There have been two conflicting reports on the diagnostic ability of this radiopeptide. The initial study showed an advantage for ^{123}I-labelled over CT for detection of metastatic disease [216]. In the second study however, VIP-receptor expression was found to be higher in normal tissue than malignant tissue, therefore ^{123}I-VIP was not found to have a good sensitivity or specificity for detection of metastatic disease [87]. However, given that radiolabelled somatostatin analogues are able to diagnose and treat many neuroendocrine tumours, the use of radiolabelled VIP has not been actively pursued clinically.

Radiolabelled MIBG Therapy

Meta-iodobenzylguanidine (MIBG) is a norepinephrine analogue which is taken up by organs rich in adrenergic innervation and/or catecholamine excretion. Therefore, radiolabelled MIBG allows successful imaging of these systems and neuroectodermally derived tumours, such as neuroblastomas, pheochromocytomas, paragangliomas, medullary thyroid carcinoma, carcinoid tumours and Merkel cell skin tumours. The use of radiolabelled MIBG to treat neuroectodermally derived tumours have arisen from the high sensitivity and specificity of *in vivo* MIBG imaging for detection of primary and metastatic tumours [151] (Fig. 20.6). MIBG is most commonly labelled with either ^{123}I or ^{131}I, therefore requires thyroid protection to be administered in the form of potassium iodine drops prior to administration of the radiolabelled MIBG.

Radiolabelled MIBG therapy is most commonly used in the treatment of neuroblastoma, which is a high grade malignancy of childhood [151]. Although this tumour is chemo- and radio-sensitive, it is prone to relapse after initial induction of remission. Stage 1 and 2 tumours can be cured with surgery alone, whilst stage 3 tumours require preoperative chemotherapy. Sixty percent of neuroblastomas in children are diagnosed in stage 4, of whom many have biological markers of poor prognosis, such as MYCN amplification or 1p deletion [149]. ^{131}I –MIBG was initially reserved for palliation of patients with recurrent disease. However, clinical trials evaluating the role of ^{131}I-MIBG as a first line drug, either as a single agent, or in combination with chemotherapy or myeloablation treatment, or in consolidation treatment has been performed with mixed results and significant potential side effects. The response rates varied between 20% and 60% in newly diagnosed and relapsed or refractory patients [53, 69, 89, 90, 138, 140].

The most important considerations in radiolabelled MIBG therapy are the antitumour efficacy and the toxicity of treatment [132]. Phase I and II studies of ^{131}I-MIBG treatment in neuroblastoma have shown limited non-specific organ toxicity [117, 133], and haematological toxicity is the main side effect which needs to be taken into consideration [132]. The most significant hematotoxicity is severe

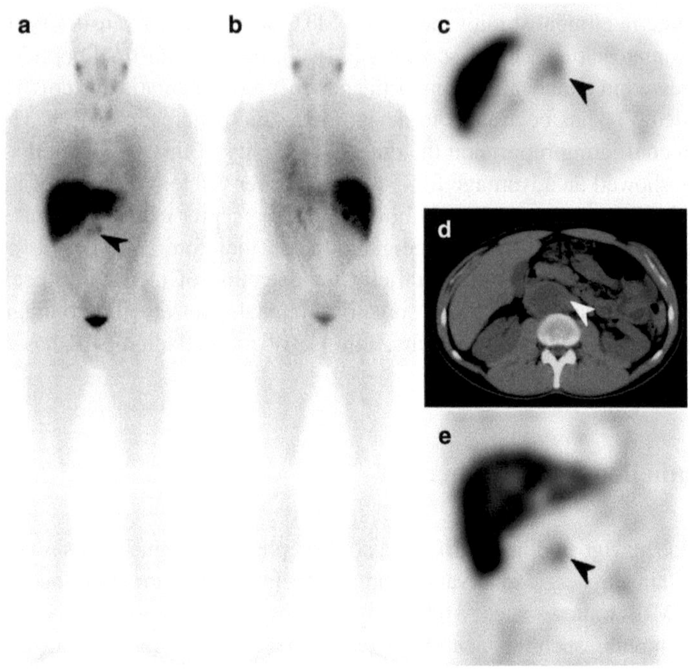

Fig. 20.6 ^{123}I-MIBG study for a neuroectoderm-derived tumour in the right paraaortic mass in the upper abdomen (arrow) seen on: (A) anterior, (B) posterior whole body images, and (C) axial SPECT, (D) axial CT and (E) coronal SPECT images. No distant metastatic disease was identified

thrombocytopenia found in most patients receiving high dose ^{131}I-MIBG therapy [61]. The toxicity-dose relationship for bone marrow toxicity can be determined with pretherapy dosimetry evaluation to predict the individual degree of bone marrow toxicity [132].

Pheochromocytomas are tumours which arise from chromaffin tissue of the adrenal medulla, whilst paragangliomas are chromaffin-cell tumours located distant to the adrenals, along the sympathetic/parasympathetic chain [41]. The mainstay of treatment is surgical resection of macroscopic disease, and debulking prior to adjuvant chemotherapy/radiotherapy [62]. Preoperative scintigraphy with ^{123}I scan is beneficial to identify distant metastatic disease, of which approximately 60% are ^{131}I-MIBG avid [33, 64]. The rationale for using radiolabelled MIBG for treatment of these tumours is based on its ability to enter the cell membrane and be stored in cytoplasmic granules via the VMA transporters (VMAT) [2, 41]. Patients must have significant radiotracer uptake on diagnostic radiolabelled-MIBG scan (>1% uptake of the injected dose), and the only limitation being the total radiation dose to the bone marrow, which is the critical organ in this scenario [2, 28]. There has been a wide range of doses administered, which range from 100 mCi to >500 mCi for treatment. "Low dose" treatment has doses ranging between 100–300 mCi, but objective tumour response have been seen in 30% of patients, disease stabilisation in 57% and hormonal responses range between 15% and 45% [125]. Hormonal and symptomatic responses are more frequently noted than anatomical response [145, 204]. However, the initial radiolabelled MIBG dose can be an important determination of patient's response and survival, because patients who receive a high dose (>500 mCi) of ^{131}I had been shown to have longer survival rates [178]. More recently, higher single doses of ^{131}I-MIBG (386–866 mCi) in a study of 12 patients resulted in a complete response in patients with skeletal and soft tissue metastasis [176]. The high-dose regimen did induce bone marrow toxicity, which required stem cell rescue [2]. Therefore, high dose ^{131}I-MIBG treatment should be customised to be based on dose limiting toxicity to the bone marrow. As patient outcome is highly dependent on the extent of disease at the time of treatment, ^{131}I-MIBG is a useful therapy to consider in an adjuvant setting after surgery.

Radiolabelled Nanoparticles

A nanoparticle is a small particle with a typical dimension less than 100 nm, and this technology is being increasingly used as pharmaceutical delivery systems for drugs, DNA and imaging agents. The use of nanoparticles to enhance the *in vivo* efficiency of anti-cancer drugs has expanded considerably over the last decade, both in the research and clinical setting. The rationale for using these particles to deliver the therapy drug is based on minimising drug degradation and inactivation upon administration, prevent unwanted side effects, and increase the drug bioavailability to the affected area. The ideal features of such particles include its biodegradability, cost and ease of preparation, small particle size with high loading capacity, and demonstrable prolonged circulation and accumulation in specific target sites in the body. The most extensively studied nanoparticles are liposomes (for delivery of water-soluble drugs), micelles (for delivery of poorly soluble drugs), and polymeric nanoparticles. They can be modified to impart specific properties and functionalities as required.

The principal use of nanoparticles for targeted radionuclide therapy has been in locoregional hepatic radionuclide treatment of hepatocellular carcinoma and metastatic liver disease (Fig. 20.7). The main advantage of locoregional administration of radiotherapeutic agents is that a much higher dose delivery to the tumour can be achieved in a single treatment, whilst minimising systemic side effects. The earliest reports of local hepatic tumour treatment date back to the 1970s when albumin colloids labelled with ^{32}Phosphorus were first used [151]. Due to the fact that the liver has a dual blood supply, whereby liver tumours are predominantly perfused by the hepatic artery, whist normal liver parenchyma is perfused by the portal vein, there is preferential flow of injected radioparticles to the liver tumour if injected into the hepatic artery. When these particles are lodged in the small arterioles and capillary sinusoids, they internally irradiate the local tumour tissue. There are two commercially available agents for this purpose, which are resin microspheres (SIR-spheres®,

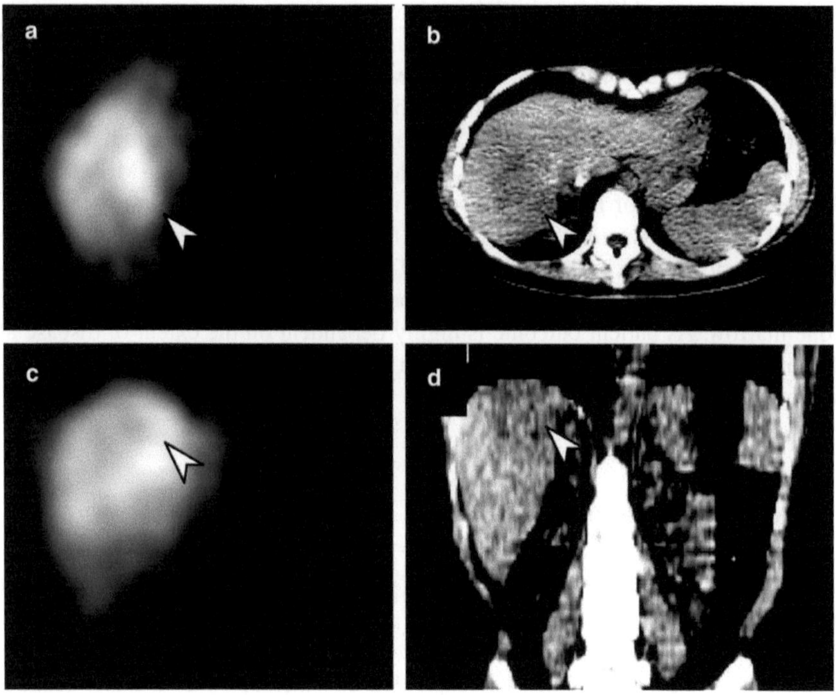

Fig. 20.7 ^{90}Y-microsphere treatment of metastatic liver disease in colorectal carcinoma. Bremsstrahlung imaging performed post-treatment to demonstrate delivery of microspheres to the large metastatic lesion in the dome of the liver seen on: (A) axial SPECT and (C) coronal SPECT, which correlates with the anatomical liver lesion on (B) axial CT and (D) coronal CT images (liver window)

Sirtex, Bonn, Germany) and glass spheres (Theraspheres®, Nordion, Felurus, Belgium), both of which are labelled with ^{90}Y [151].

SIR-spheres therapy (SIRT) has been shown to have promising results in the treatment of liver metastases from colorectal carcinoma, with a reported benefit in objective response and improved survival in patients treated with hepatic artery chemoembolisation (HAC) plus SIRT compared to HAC alone [75]. An objective response was noted in 44% versus 17% of patients, with a median time to progression of 15.9 months in patients receiving both treatments versus 9.7 months for patients receiving HAC alone. This prompted the addition of SIRT to systemic chemotherapeutic regimens which also showed an improvement in response and survival in patients with combination treatment. A randomised Phase II study of patients receiving 5-FU and leucovorin with one cycle of SIRT showed an objective response of 73% in patients receiving chemotherapy with SIRT vs. 0% in patients receiving chemotherapy alone. The time to progression was 18.6 months in the dual treatment group versus 3.6 months in the chemotherapy alone group. There were no significant differences in the grade 3 or 4 toxicity or quality of life, although grade 3 and 4 toxicity was noted in 7% (23/336) of patients [151, 212]. Combination of SIRT with chemotherapeutic regimen consisting of irinotecan or FOLFOX showed similar preliminary results [71, 213]. SIRT was also used before or after surgical resection. An analysis of 226 tumours showed a decrease in median tumour of 60%, irrespective of tumour size, whilst 20% clinically disappeared (<10 cm). The downstaging of tumour was found in 20% of patients, which allowed tumours to be surgically resected [151]. Consideration should be given to incorporating this treatment more readily in the management of liver tumours.

^{131}I-lipiodol is a commercially available agent (Lipiocis® Schering S.A., Berlin, Germany) which is trapped in tortuous tumour blood vessels, and taken up in tumour cells by endocytosis. Lipiodol is a fatty acid ester derivative of naturally occurring iodine-rich seed oil, which was previously widely used as a contrast agent in computed tomography. ^{131}I-lipiodol has been most extensively used in hepatocellular carcinoma (HCC) as a single agent in palliative treatment of inoperable cases. The overall objective response on radiological evaluation has been shown to be 28% with an average 1 year survival of 31% [31, 49, 88, 173]. A large randomised study which compared ^{131}I-lipiodol with transarterial chemoembolisation (TACE) showed similar response rates and survival, but far better tolerability compared to TACE. Serious side effects with ^{131}I-lipiodol was seen in 3% compared to 29% after TACE, with no treatment related deaths with ^{131}I-lipiodol [164]. A pilot study evaluating the use of ^{131}I-lipiodol post-resection reported recurrences in 28.5% in the treated group versus 59% in the untreated group, with a 3 year survival of 86% and 46% respectively ($p = 0.04$) [118]. In two studies evaluating the use of ^{131}I-lipiodol therapy, the radiological response rate was 50% with reported 1- and 3-year recurrence-free survival rate of 91% and 83% respectively, although these patients had limited disease [30, 163]. Therefore, the role of ^{131}I-lipiodol in these cases may be to keep the disease under control whilst waiting for surgery. A more recent development in this field has been the use of ^{188}Re instead of ^{131}I. This radiotracer is readily available via a generator, and does not require hospitalisation or isolation due to its favourable physical properties. An international phase II trial evaluated the efficacy of ^{188}Re-Lipiodol in 185 patients with HCC in developing countries, with safety and feasibility of this therapy demonstrated [20]. Further trials are required to fully evaluate the utility of this therapeutic approach.

Conclusions

Targeted radionuclide therapy has an increasingly important role in treating cancer patients. The range of treatment strategies continues to expand, and based on a sophisticated understanding tumour biology, targeting techniques and radiobiology, there will be further new clinical indications for this approach to cancer therapy in the future.

References

1. Abrahamsson PA (1999) Neuroendocrine cells in tumour growth of the prostate. Endocr Relat Cancer 6:503–19
2. Ahlman H (2006) Malignant pheochromocytoma: state of the field with future projections. Ann N Y Acad Sci 1073:449–64
3. Ain KB, Taylor KD, Tofiq S, Venkataraman G (1997) Somatostatin receptor subtype expression in human thyroid and thyroid carcinoma cell lines. J Clin Endocrinol Metab 82:1857–62
4. Alexander RW, Upp JR, Jr., Poston GJ, Gupta V, Townsend CM, Jr., Thompson JC (1988) Effects of bombesin on growth of human small cell lung carcinoma in vivo. Cancer Res 48:1439–41
5. Ali N, Sebastian C, Foley RR, Murray I, Canizales AL, Jenkins PJ, Drake WM, Plowman PN, Besser GM, Chew SL, Grossman AB, Monson JP, Britton KE (2006) The management of differentiated thyroid cancer using 123I for imaging to assess the need for 131I therapy. Nucl Med Commun 27:165–9
6. Allen BJ, Raja C, Rizvi S, Li Y, Tsui W, Graham P, Thompson JF, Reisfeld RA, Kearsley J (2005) Intralesional targeted alpha therapy for metastatic melanoma. Cancer Biol Ther 4:1318–24
7. Altenvoerde G, Lerch H, Kuwert T, Matheja P, Schafers M, Schober O (1998) Positron emission tomography with F-18-deoxyglucose in patients with differentiated thyroid carcinoma, elevated thyroglobulin levels, and negative iodine scans. Langenbecks Arch Surg 383:160–3
8. Alvarez RD, Partridge EE, Khazaeli MB, Plott G, Austin M, Kilgore L, Russell CD, Liu T, Grizzle WE, Schlom J, LoBuglio AF, Meredith RF (1997) Intraperitoneal radioimmunotherapy of ovarian cancer with 177Lu-CC49: a phase I/II study. Gynecol Oncol 65:94–101
9. Alvarez RD, Huh WK, Khazaeli MB, Meredith RF, Partridge EE, Kilgore LC, Grizzle WE, Shen S, Austin JM, Barnes MN, Carey D, Schlom J, LoBuglio AF (2002) A phase I study of combined modality (90)Yttrium-CC49 intraperitoneal radioimmunotherapy for ovarian cancer. Clin Cancer Res 8:2806–11
10. Anthony LB, Woltering EA, Espenan GD, Cronin MD, Maloney TJ, McCarthy KE (2002) Indium-111-pentetreotide prolongs survival in gastroenteropancreatic malignancies. Semin Nucl Med 32:123–32
11. Bander NH, Milowsky MI, Nanus DM, Kostakoglu L, Vallabhajosula S, Goldsmith SJ (2005) Phase I trial of 177lutetium-labeled J591, a monoclonal antibody to prostate-specific membrane antigen, in patients with androgen-independent prostate cancer. J Clin Oncol 23:4591–601
12. Barbaro D, Boni G, Meucci G, Simi U, Lapi P, Orsini P, Pasquini C, Piazza F, Caciagli M, Mariani G (2003) Radioiodine treatment with 30 mCi after recombinant human thyrotropin stimulation in thyroid cancer: effectiveness for postsurgical remnants ablation and possible role of iodine content in L-thyroxine in the outcome of ablation. J Clin Endocrinol Metab 88:4110–5
13. Bartholdi MF, Wu JM, Pu H, Troncoso P, Eden PA, Feldman RI (1998) In situ hybridization for gastrin-releasing peptide receptor (GRP receptor) expression in prostatic carcinoma. Int J Cancer 79:82–90
14. Baselga J (2001) Herceptin alone or in combination with chemotherapy in the treatment of HER2-positive metastatic breast cancer: pivotal trials. Oncology 61 Suppl 2:14–21
15. Behr TM, Gotthardt M, Barth A, Behe M (2001) Imaging tumors with peptide-based radioligands. Q J Nucl Med 45:189–200
16. Behr TM, Jenner N, Behe M, Angerstein C, Gratz S, Raue F, Becker W (1999) Radiolabeled peptides for targeting cholecystokinin-B/gastrin receptor-expressing tumors. J Nucl Med 40:1029–44
17. Behr TM, Jenner N, Radetzky S, Behe M, Gratz S, Yucekent S, Raue F, Becker W (1998) Targeting of cholecystokinin-B/gastrin receptors in vivo: preclinical and initial clinical evaluation

of the diagnostic and therapeutic potential of radiolabelled gastrin. Eur J Nucl Med 25:424–30
18. Behr TM, Liersch T, Greiner-Bechert L, Griesinger F, Behe M, Markus PM, Gratz S, Angerstein C, Brittinger G, Becker H, Goldenberg DM, Becker W (2002) Radioimmunotherapy of small-volume disease of metastatic colorectal cancer. Cancer 94:1373–81
19. Beierwaltes WH (1978) The treatment of thyroid carcinoma with radioactive iodine. Semin Nucl Med 8:79–94
20. Bernal P, Raoul JL, Vidmar G, Sereegotov E, Sundram FX, Kumar A, Jeong JM, Pusuwan P, Divgi C, Zanzonico P, Stare J, Buscombe J, Minh CT, Saw MM, Chen S, Ogbac R, Padhy AK (2007) Intra-arterial rhenium-188 lipiodol in the treatment of inoperable hepatocellular carcinoma: results of an IAEA-sponsored multination study. Int J Radiat Oncol Biol Phys 69:1448–55
21. Bernard BF, Krenning EP, Breeman WA, Rolleman EJ, Bakker WH, Visser TJ, Macke H, de Jong M (1997) D-lysine reduction of indium-111 octreotide and yttrium-90 octreotide renal uptake. J Nucl Med 38:1929–33
22. Bloechl S, Beck R, Seidl C, Morgenstern A, Schwaiger M, Senekowitsch-Schmidtke R (2005) Fractionated locoregional low-dose radioimmunotherapy improves survival in a mouse model of diffuse-type gastric cancer using a 213Bi-conjugated monoclonal antibody. Clin Cancer Res 11:7070s–4s
23. Bodei L, Cremonesi M, Grana C, Rocca P, Bartolomei M, Chinol M, Paganelli G (2004) Receptor radionuclide therapy with 90Y-[DOTA]0-Tyr3-octreotide (90Y-DOTATOC) in neuroendocrine tumours. Eur J Nucl Med Mol Imaging 31:1038–46
24. Bodei L, Cremonesi M, Zoboli S, Grana C, Bartolomei M, Rocca P, Caracciolo M, Macke HR, Chinol M, Paganelli G (2003) Receptor-mediated radionuclide therapy with 90Y-DOTATOC in association with amino acid infusion: a phase I study. Eur J Nucl Med Mol Imaging 30:207–16
25. Bodei L, Handkiewicz-Junak D, Grana C, Mazzetta C, Rocca P, Bartolomei M, Lopera Sierra M, Cremonesi M, Chinol M, Macke HR, Paganelli G (2004) Receptor radionuclide therapy with 90Y-DOTATOC in patients with medullary thyroid carcinomas. Cancer Biother Radiopharm 19:65–71
26. Boerman OC, van Schaijk FG, Oyen WJ, Corstens FH (2003) Pretargeted radioimmunotherapy of cancer: progress step by step. J Nucl Med 44:400–11
27. Bold RJ, Ishizuka J, Yao CZ, Townsend CM, Jr., Thompson JC (1998) Bombesin stimulates in vitro growth of human breast cancer independent of estrogen receptors status. Anticancer Res 18:4051–6
28. Bomanji J, Britton KE, Ur E, Hawkins L, Grossman AB, Besser GM (1993) Treatment of malignant phaeochromocytoma, paraganglioma and carcinoid tumours with 131I-metaiodobenzylguanidine. Nucl Med Commun 14:856–61
29. Boxer GM, Begent RH, Kelly AM, Southall PJ, Blair SB, Theodorou NA, Dawson PM, Ledermann JA (1992) Factors influencing variability of localisation of antibodies to carcinoembryonic antigen (CEA) in patients with colorectal carcinoma–implications for radioimmunotherapy. Br J Cancer 65:825–31
30. Brans B, De Winter F, Defreyne L, Troisi R, Vanlangenhove P, Van Vlierberghe H, Lambert B, Praet M, de Hemptinne B, Dierckx RA (2001) The anti-tumoral activity of neoadjuvant intra-arterial 131I-lipiodol treatment for hepatocellular carcinoma: a pilot study. Cancer Biother Radiopharm 16:333–8
31. Brans B, Van Laere K, Gemmel F, Defreyne L, Vanlangenhove P, Troisi R, Van Vlierberghe H, Colle I, De Hemptinne B, Dierckx RA (2002) Combining iodine-131 Lipiodol therapy with low-dose cisplatin as a radiosensitiser: preliminary results in hepatocellular carcinoma. Eur J Nucl Med Mol Imaging 29:928–32
32. Brouwers AH, Dorr U, Lang O, Boerman OC, Oyen WJ, Steffens MG, Oosterwijk E, Mergenthaler HG, Bihl H, Corstens FH (2002) 131 I-cG250 monoclonal antibody immunoscintigraphy versus [18 F]FDG-PET imaging in patients with metastatic renal cell carcinoma: a comparative study. Nucl Med Commun 23:229–36

33. Buhl T, Mortensen J, Kjaer A (2002) I-123 MIBG imaging and intraoperative localization of metastatic pheochromocytoma: a case report. Clin Nucl Med 27:183–5
34. Burke PA, DeNardo SJ, Miers LA, Kukis DL, DeNardo GL (2002) Combined modality radioimmunotherapy: promise and peril. Cancer 94:1320–31
35. Carney DN, Cuttitta F, Moody TW, Minna JD (1987) Selective stimulation of small cell lung cancer clonal growth by bombesin and gastrin-releasing peptide. Cancer Res 47:821–5
36. Carroll RE, Matkowskyj KA, Chakrabarti S, McDonald TJ, Benya RV (1999) Aberrant expression of gastrin-releasing peptide and its receptor by well-differentiated colon cancers in humans. Am J Physiol 276:G655–65
37. Chatal JF, Campion L, Kraeber-Bodere F, Bardet S, Vuillez JP, Charbonnel B, Rohmer V, Chang CH, Sharkey RM, Goldenberg DM, Barbet J (2006) Survival improvement in patients with medullary thyroid carcinoma who undergo pretargeted anti-carcinoembryonic-antigen radioimmunotherapy: a collaborative study with the French Endocrine Tumor Group. J Clin Oncol 24:1705–11
38. Chen S, Yu L, Jiang C, Zhao Y, Sun D, Li S, Liao G, Chen Y, Fu Q, Tao Q, Ye D, Hu P, Khawli LA, Taylor CR, Epstein AL, Ju DW (2005) Pivotal study of iodine-131-labeled chimeric tumor necrosis treatment radioimmunotherapy in patients with advanced lung cancer. J Clin Oncol 23:1538–47
39. Cheson BD (2006) Radioimmunotherapy of non-Hodgkin's lymphomas. Curr Drug Targets 7:1293–300
40. Chong G, Lee FT, Hopkins W, Tebbutt N, Cebon JS, Mountain AJ, Chappell B, Papenfuss A, Schleyer P, U P, Murphy R, Wirth V, Smyth FE, Potasz N, Poon A, Davis ID, Saunder T, O'Keefe G J, Burgess AW, Hoffman EW, Old LJ, Scott AM (2005) Phase I trial of 131I-huA33 in patients with advanced colorectal carcinoma. Clin Cancer Res 11:4818–26
41. Chrisoulidou A, Kaltsas G, Ilias I, Grossman AB (2007) The diagnosis and management of malignant phaeochromocytoma and paraganglioma. Endocr Relat Cancer 14:569–85
42. Christiansen J, Rajasekaran AK (2004) Biological impediments to monoclonal antibody-based cancer immunotherapy. Mol Cancer Ther 3:1493–501
43. Clarke K, Lee FT, Brechbiel MW, Smyth FE, Old LJ, Scott AM (2000) Therapeutic efficacy of anti-Lewis(y) humanized 3S193 radioimmunotherapy in a breast cancer model: enhanced activity when combined with taxol chemotherapy. Clin Cancer Res 6:3621–8
44. Coakley AJ (1998) Thyroid stunning. Eur J Nucl Med 25:203–4
45. Conti PS, Durski JM, Bacqai F, Grafton ST, Singer PA (1999) Imaging of locally recurrent and metastatic thyroid cancer with positron emission tomography. Thyroid 9:797–804
46. Cooper DS, Doherty GM, Haugen BR, Kloos RT, Lee SL, Mandel SJ, Mazzaferri EL, McIver B, Sherman SI, Tuttle RM (2006) Management guidelines for patients with thyroid nodules and differentiated thyroid cancer. Thyroid 16:109–42
47. Cuttitta F, Carney DN, Mulshine J, Moody TW, Fedorko J, Fischler A, Minna JD (1985) Bombesin-like peptides can function as autocrine growth factors in human small-cell lung cancer. Nature 316:823–6
48. Davis TA, Kaminski MS, Leonard JP, Hsu FJ, Wilkinson M, Zelenetz A, Wahl RL, Kroll S, Coleman M, Goris M, Levy R, Knox SJ (2004) The radioisotope contributes significantly to the activity of radioimmunotherapy. Clin Cancer Res 10:7792–8
49. de Baere T, Taourel P, Tubiana JM, Kuoch V, Ducreux M, Lumbroso J, Roche AJ (1999) Hepatic intraarterial 131I iodized oil for treatment of hepatocellular carcinoma in patients with impeded portal venous flow. Radiology 212:665–8
50. de Jong M, Krenning E (2002) New advances in peptide receptor radionuclide therapy. J Nucl Med 43:617–20
51. de Jong M, Breeman WA, Bernard BF, Bakker WH, Visser TJ, Kooij PP, van Gameren A, Krenning EP (2001) Tumor response after [(90)Y-DOTA(0),Tyr(3)]octreotide radionuclide therapy in a transplantable rat tumor model is dependent on tumor size. J Nucl Med 42:1841–6
52. De Jong M, Valkema R, Jamar F, Kvols LK, Kwekkeboom DJ, Breeman WA, Bakker WH, Smith C, Pauwels S, Krenning EP (2002) Somatostatin receptor-targeted radionuclide therapy of tumors: preclinical and clinical findings. Semin Nucl Med 32:133–40

53. De Kraker J, Hoefnagel CA, Caron H, Valdes Olmos RA, Zsiros J, Heij HA, Voute PA (1995) First line targeted radiotherapy, a new concept in the treatment of advanced stage neuroblastoma. Eur J Cancer 31A:600–2
54. DeNardo GL, Siantar CL, DeNardo SJ (2002) Radiation dosimetry for radionuclide therapy in a nonmyeloablative strategy. Cancer Biother Radiopharm 17:107–18
55. DeNardo GL, Tobin E, Chan K, Bradt BM, DeNardo SJ (2005) Direct antilymphoma effects on human lymphoma cells of monotherapy and combination therapy with CD20 and HLA-DR antibodies and 90Y-labeled HLA-DR antibodies. Clin Cancer Res 11:7075s–9s
56. DeNardo SJ, Kroger LA, Lamborn KR, Miers LA, O'Donnell RT, Kukis DL, Richman CM, DeNardo GL (1997) Importance of temporal relationships in combined modality radioimmunotherapy of breast carcinoma. Cancer 80:2583–90
57. Divgi CR, O'Donoghue JA, Welt S, O'Neel J, Finn R, Motzer RJ, Jungbluth A, Hoffman E, Ritter G, Larson SM, Old LJ (2004) Phase I clinical trial with fractionated radioimmunotherapy using 131I-labeled chimeric G250 in metastatic renal cancer. J Nucl Med 45:1412–21
58. Dohan O, De la Vieja A, Paroder V, Riedel C, Artani M, Reed M, Ginter CS, Carrasco N (2003) The sodium/iodide Symporter (NIS): characterization, regulation, and medical significance. Endocr Rev 24:48–77
59. Dottorini ME, Lomuscio G, Mazzucchelli L, Vignati A, Colombo L (1995) Assessment of female fertility and carcinogenesis after iodine-131 therapy for differentiated thyroid carcinoma. J Nucl Med 36:21–7
60. Dow KH, Ferrell BR, Anello C (1997) Quality-of-life changes in patients with thyroid cancer after withdrawal of thyroid hormone therapy. Thyroid 7:613–9
61. DuBois SG, Messina J, Maris JM, Huberty J, Glidden DV, Veatch J, Charron M, Hawkins R, Matthay KK (2004) Hematologic toxicity of high-dose iodine-131-metaiodobenzylguanidine therapy for advanced neuroblastoma. J Clin Oncol 22:2452–60
62. Eisenhofer G, Bornstein SR, Brouwers FM, Cheung NK, Dahia PL, de Krijger RR, Giordano TJ, Greene LA, Goldstein DS, Lehnert H, Manger WM, Maris JM, Neumann HP, Pacak K, Shulkin BL, Smith DI, Tischler AS, Young WF, Jr. (2004) Malignant pheochromocytoma: current status and initiatives for future progress. Endocr Relat Cancer 11:423–36
63. Ferris HA, Carroll RE, Lorimer DL, Benya RV (1997) Location and characterization of the human GRP receptor expressed by gastrointestinal epithelial cells. Peptides 18:663–72
64. Fitzgerald PA, Goldsby RE, Huberty JP, Price DC, Hawkins RA, Veatch JJ, Dela Cruz F, Jahan TM, Linker CA, Damon L, Matthay KK (2006) Malignant pheochromocytomas and paragangliomas: a phase II study of therapy with high-dose 131I-metaiodobenzylguanidine (131I-MIBG). Ann N Y Acad Sci 1073:465–90
65. Flynn AA, Boxer GM, Begent RH, Pedley RB (2001) Relationship between tumour morphology, antigen and antibody distribution measured by fusion of digital phosphor and photographic images. Cancer Immunol Immunother 50:77–81
66. Forero A, Meredith RF, Khazaeli MB, Shen S, Grizzle WE, Carey D, Busby E, LoBuglio AF, Robert F (2005) Phase I study of 90Y-CC49 monoclonal antibody therapy in patients with advanced non-small cell lung cancer: effect of chelating agents and paclitaxel co-administration. Cancer Biother Radiopharm 20:467–78
67. Froidevaux S, Eberle AN, Christe M, Sumanovski L, Heppeler A, Schmitt JS, Eisenwiener K, Beglinger C, Macke HR (2002) Neuroendocrine tumor targeting: study of novel gallium-labeled somatostatin radiopeptides in a rat pancreatic tumor model. Int J Cancer 98:930–7
68. Goetz C, Riva P, Poepperl G, Gildehaus FJ, Hischa A, Tatsch K, Reulen HJ (2003) Locoregional radioimmunotherapy in selected patients with malignant glioma: experiences, side effects and survival times. J Neurooncol 62:321–8
69. Goldberg SS, DeSantes K, Huberty JP, Price D, Hasegawa BH, Reynolds CP, Seeger RC, Hattner R, Matthay KK (1998) Engraftment after myeloablative doses of 131I-metaiodobenzylguanidine followed by autologous bone marrow transplantation for treatment of refractory neuroblastoma. Med Pediatr Oncol 30:339–46
70. Goldenberg DM, Sharkey RM (2007) Novel radiolabeled antibody conjugates. Oncogene 26:3734–44

71. Goldstein D, Van Hazel G, Pavlakis N, Olver I (2005) Selective internal radiation therapy (SIRT) plus systemic chemotherapy with irinotecan. A phase I dose escalation study. J Clin Oncol 23:(Abstract 3701)
72. Gotthardt M, Dijkgraaf I, Boerman OC, Oyen WJ (2006) Nuclear medicine imaging and therapy of neuroendocrine tumours. Cancer Imaging 6:S178–84
73. Gotthardt M, Boermann OC, Behr TM, Behe MP, Oyen WJ (2004) Development and clinical application of peptide-based radiopharmaceuticals. Curr Pharm Des 10:2951–63
74. Gotthardt M, Battmann A, Beuter D, Bauhofer A, Schipper M, Behe M, et al. (2003) Comparison of In-111-D-Glu-1-Mingastrin, F-18-FDG PET, and CT scanning for detection of metastatic medullary thyroid carcinoma. J Nucl Med 44:169P
75. Gray B, Van Hazel G, Hope M, Burton M, Moroz P, Anderson J, Gebski V (2001) Randomised trial of SIR-Spheres plus chemotherapy vs. chemotherapy alone for treating patients with liver metastases from primary large bowel cancer. Ann Oncol 12:1711–20
76. Grunwald F, Menzel C, Bender H, Palmedo H, Willkomm P, Ruhlmann J, Franckson T, Biersack HJ (1997) Comparison of 18FDG-PET with 131iodine and 99mTc-sestamibi scintigraphy in differentiated thyroid cancer. Thyroid 7:327–35
77. Gugger M, Reubi JC (1999) Gastrin-releasing peptide receptors in non-neoplastic and neoplastic human breast. Am J Pathol 155:2067–76
78. Hajjar G, Sharkey RM, Burton J, Zhang CH, Yeldell D, Matthies A, Alavi A, Losman MJ, Brenner A, Goldenberg DM (2002) Phase I radioimmunotherapy trial with iodine-131–labeled humanized MN-14 anti-carcinoembryonic antigen monoclonal antibody in patients with metastatic gastrointestinal and colorectal cancer. Clin Colorectal Cancer 2:31–42
79. Hajri A, Koenig M, Balboni G, Damge C (1996) Expression and characterization of gastrin-releasing peptide receptor in normal and cancerous pancreas. Pancreas 12:25–35
80. Hall P, Boice JD, Jr., Berg G, Bjelkengren G, Ericsson UB, Hallquist A, Lidberg M, Lundell G, Mattsson A, Tennvall J, et al. (1992) Leukaemia incidence after iodine-131 exposure. Lancet 340:1–4
81. Hanscheid H, Lassmann M, Luster M, Thomas SR, Pacini F, Ceccarelli C, Ladenson PW, Wahl RL, Schlumberger M, Ricard M, Driedger A, Kloos RT, Sherman SI, Haugen BR, Carriere V, Corone C, Reiners C (2006) Iodine biokinetics and dosimetry in radioiodine therapy of thyroid cancer: procedures and results of a prospective international controlled study of ablation after rhTSH or hormone withdrawal. J Nucl Med 47:648–54
82. Haugen BR, Larson LL, Pugazhenthi U, Hays WR, Klopper JP, Kramer CA, Sharma V (2004) Retinoic acid and retinoid X receptors are differentially expressed in thyroid cancer and thyroid carcinoma cell lines and predict response to treatment with retinoids. J Clin Endocrinol Metab 89:272–80
83. Haugen BR, Pacini F, Reiners C, Schlumberger M, Ladenson PW, Sherman SI, Cooper DS, Graham KE, Braverman LE, Skarulis MC, Davies TF, DeGroot LJ, Mazzaferri EL, Daniels GH, Ross DS, Luster M, Samuels MH, Becker DV, Maxon HR, 3rd, Cavalieri RR, Spencer CA, McEllin K, Weintraub BD, Ridgway EC (1999) A comparison of recombinant human thyrotropin and thyroid hormone withdrawal for the detection of thyroid remnant or cancer. J Clin Endocrinol Metab 84:3877–85
84. Heppeler A, Froidevaux S, Eberle AN, Maecke HR (2000) Receptor targeting for tumor localisation and therapy with radiopeptides. Curr Med Chem 7:971–94
85. Herbertson R, Tebbutt N, Gill S, Lee FT, Chapell B, Cavicchiolo T, Skrinos E, Poon A, Saunder T, Scott AM (2007) Targeted chemoradiation for metastatic colorectal cancer: a phase I trial of oral capecitabine combined with 131I-huA33. J Clin Oncol 2007. ASCO Annual Meeting Proceedings 25:183s (Abstract 4078)
86. Hernandez MC, Knox SJ (2004) Radiobiology of radioimmunotherapy: targeting CD20 B-cell antigen in non-Hodgkin's lymphoma. Int J Radiat Oncol Biol Phys 59:1274–87
87. Hessenius C, Bader M, Meinhold H, Bohmig M, Faiss S, Reubi JC, Wiedenmann B (2000) Vasoactive intestinal peptide receptor scintigraphy in patients with pancreatic adenocarcinomas or neuroendocrine tumours. Eur J Nucl Med 27:1684–93
88. Ho S, Lau WY, Leung TW, Johnson PJ (1998) Internal radiation therapy for patients with primary or metastatic hepatic cancer: a review. Cancer 83:1894–907

89. Hoefnagel CA, Voute PA, de Kraker J, Marcuse HR (1987) Radionuclide diagnosis and therapy of neural crest tumors using iodine-131 metaiodobenzylguanidine. J Nucl Med 28:308–14
90. Hoefnagel CA, De Kraker J, Valdes Olmos RA, Voute PA (1994) 131I-MIBG as a first-line treatment in high-risk neuroblastoma patients. Nucl Med Commun 15:712–7
91. Jain RK (1990) Physiological barriers to delivery of monoclonal antibodies and other macromolecules in tumors. Cancer Res 50:814s–9s
92. Jamar F, Barone R, Mathieu I, Walrand S, Labar D, Carlier P, de Camps J, Schran H, Chen T, Smith MC, Bouterfa H, Valkema R, Krenning EP, Kvols LK, Pauwels S (2003) 86Y-DOTA0)-D-Phe1-Tyr3-octreotide (SMT487)–a phase 1 clinical study: pharmacokinetics, biodistribution and renal protective effect of different regimens of amino acid co-infusion. Eur J Nucl Med Mol Imaging 30:510–8
93. Jensen JA, Carroll RE, Benya RV (2001) The case for gastrin-releasing peptide acting as a morphogen when it and its receptor are aberrantly expressed in cancer. Peptides 22:689–99
94. Jungwirth A, Galvan G, Pinski J, Halmos G, Szepeshazi K, Cai RZ, Groot K, Schally AV (1997) Luteinizing hormone-releasing hormone antagonist Cetrorelix (SB-75) and bombesin antagonist RC-3940-II inhibit the growth of androgen-independent PC-3 prostate cancer in nude mice. Prostate 32:164–72
95. Jungwirth A, Pinski J, Galvan G, Halmos G, Szepeshazi K, Cai RZ, Groot K, Vadillo-Buenfil M, Schally AV (1997) Inhibition of growth of androgen-independent DU-145 prostate cancer in vivo by luteinising hormone-releasing hormone antagonist Cetrorelix and bombesin antagonists RC-3940-II and RC-3950-II. Eur J Cancer 33:1141–8
96. Jurcic JG, Caron PC, Scheinberg DA (1995) Monoclonal antibody therapy of leukemia and lymphoma. Adv Pharmacol 33:287–314
97. Jurcic JG, Caron PC, Nikula TK, Papadopoulos EB, Finn RD, Gansow OA, Miller WH, Jr., Geerlings MW, Warrell RP, Jr., Larson SM, et al. (1995) Radiolabeled anti-CD33 monoclonal antibody M195 for myeloid leukemias. Cancer Res 55:5908s–10s
98. Jurcic JG, Larson SM, Sgouros G, McDevitt MR, Finn RD, Divgi CR, Ballangrud AM, Hamacher KA, Ma D, Humm JL, Brechbiel MW, Molinet R, Scheinberg DA (2002) Targeted alpha particle immunotherapy for myeloid leukemia. Blood 100:1233–9
99. Kaminski MS, Zasadny KR, Francis IR, Milik AW, Ross CW, Moon SD, Crawford SM, Burgess JM, Petry NA, Butchko GM, et al. (1993) Radioimmunotherapy of B-cell lymphoma with [131I]anti-B1 (anti-CD20) antibody. N Engl J Med 329:459–65
100. Kaminski MS, Tuck M, Estes J, Kolstad A, Ross CW, Zasadny K, Regan D, Kison P, Fisher S, Kroll S, Wahl RL (2005) 131I-tositumomab therapy as initial treatment for follicular lymphoma. N Engl J Med 352:441–9
101. Kaminski MS, Zasadny KR, Francis IR, Fenner MC, Ross CW, Milik AW, Estes J, Tuck M, Regan D, Fisher S, Glenn SD, Wahl RL (1996) Iodine-131-anti-B1 radioimmunotherapy for B-cell lymphoma. J Clin Oncol 14:1974–81
102. Kaminski MS, Estes J, Zasadny KR, Francis IR, Ross CW, Tuck M, Regan D, Fisher S, Gutierrez J, Kroll S, Stagg R, Tidmarsh G, Wahl RL (2000) Radioimmunotherapy with iodine (131)I tositumomab for relapsed or refractory B-cell non-Hodgkin lymphoma: updated results and long-term follow-up of the University of Michigan experience. Blood 96:1259–66
103. Kaminski MS, Zelenetz AD, Press OW, Saleh M, Leonard J, Fehrenbacher L, Lister TA, Stagg RJ, Tidmarsh GF, Kroll S, Wahl RL, Knox SJ, Vose JM (2001) Pivotal study of iodine I 131 tositumomab for chemotherapy-refractory low-grade or transformed low-grade B-cell non-Hodgkin's lymphomas. J Clin Oncol 19:3918–28
104. Kelly MP, Lee FT, Tahtis K, Smyth FE, Brechbiel MW, Scott AM (2007) Radioimmunotherapy with alpha-particle emitting 213Bi-C-functionalized trans-cyclohexyl-diethylenetriaminepentaacetic acid-humanized 3S193 is enhanced by combination with paclitaxel chemotherapy. Clin Cancer Res 13:5604s–12s
105. Koerber C, Schmutzler C, Rendl J, Koehrle J, Griesser H, Simon D, Reiners C (1999) Increased I-131 uptake in local recurrence and distant metastases after second treatment with retinoic acid. Clin Nucl Med 24:849–51

106. Koong SS, Reynolds JC, Movius EG, Keenan AM, Ain KB, Lakshmanan MC, Robbins J (1999) Lithium as a potential adjuvant to 131I therapy of metastatic, well differentiated thyroid carcinoma. J Clin Endocrinol Metab 84:912–6
107. Kotzerke J, Bunjes D, Scheinberg DA (2005) Radioimmunoconjugates in acute leukemia treatment: the future is radiant. Bone Marrow Transplant 36:1021–6
108. Kraeber-Bodere F, Faivre-Chauvet A, Ferrer L, Vuillez JP, Brard PY, Rousseau C, Resche I, Devillers A, Laffont S, Bardies M, Chang K, Sharkey RM, Goldenberg DM, Chatal JF, Barbet J (2003) Pharmacokinetics and dosimetry studies for optimization of anti-carcinoembryonic antigen x anti-hapten bispecific antibody-mediated pretargeting of Iodine-131-labeled hapten in a phase I radioimmunotherapy trial. Clin Cancer Res 9:3973S–81S
109. Krenning EP, Kwekkeboom DJ, Bakker WH, Breeman WA, Kooij PP, Oei HY, van Hagen M, Postema PT, de Jong M, Reubi JC, et al. (1993) Somatostatin receptor scintigraphy with [111In-DTPA-D-Phe1]- and [123I-Tyr3]-octreotide: the Rotterdam experience with more than 1000 patients. Eur J Nucl Med 20:716–31
110. Kwekkeboom DJ, Bakker WH, Kooij PP, Konijnenberg MW, Srinivasan A, Erion JL, Schmidt MA, Bugaj JL, de Jong M, Krenning EP (2001) [177Lu-DOTAOTyr3]octreotate: comparison with [111In-DTPAo]octreotide in patients. Eur J Nucl Med 28:1319–25
111. Kwekkeboom DJ, Teunissen JJ, Bakker WH, Kooij PP, de Herder WW, Feelders RA, van Eijck CH, Esser JP, Kam BL, Krenning EP (2005) Radiolabeled somatostatin analog [177Lu-DOTA0,Tyr3]octreotate in patients with endocrine gastroenteropancreatic tumors. J Clin Oncol 23:2754–62
112. Kwekkeboom DJ, Bakker WH, Kam BL, Teunissen JJ, Kooij PP, de Herder WW, Feelders RA, van Eijck CH, de Jong M, Srinivasan A, Erion JL, Krenning EP (2003) Treatment of patients with gastro-entero-pancreatic (GEP) tumours with the novel radiolabelled somatostatin analogue [177Lu-DOTA(0),Tyr3]octreotate. Eur J Nucl Med Mol Imaging 30:417–22
113. Kwekkeboom DJ, Mueller-Brand J, Paganelli G, Anthony LB, Pauwels S, Kvols LK, O'Dorisio T M, Valkema R, Bodei L, Chinol M, Maecke HR, Krenning EP (2005) Overview of results of peptide receptor radionuclide therapy with 3 radiolabeled somatostatin analogs. J Nucl Med 46 Suppl 1:62S–6S
114. Ladenson PW, Braverman LE, Mazzaferri EL, Brucker-Davis F, Cooper DS, Garber JR, Wondisford FE, Davies TF, DeGroot LJ, Daniels GH, Ross DS, Weintraub BD (1997) Comparison of administration of recombinant human thyrotropin with withdrawal of thyroid hormone for radioactive iodine scanning in patients with thyroid carcinoma. N Engl J Med 337:888–96
115. Lamberts SW, van der Lely AJ, de Herder WW, Hofland LJ (1996) Octreotide. N Engl J Med 334:246–54
116. Lantry LE, Cappelletti E, Maddalena ME, Fox JS, Feng W, Chen J, Thomas R, Eaton SM, Bogdan NJ, Arunachalam T, Reubi JC, Raju N, Metcalfe EC, Lattuada L, Linder KE, Swenson RE, Tweedle MF, Nunn AD (2006) 177Lu-AMBA: synthesis and characterization of a selective 177Lu-labeled GRP-R agonist for systemic radiotherapy of prostate cancer. J Nucl Med 47:1144–52
117. Lashford LS, Lewis IJ, Fielding SL, Flower MA, Meller S, Kemshead JT, Ackery D (1992) Phase I/II study of iodine 131 metaiodobenzylguanidine in chemoresistant neuroblastoma: a United Kingdom Children's Cancer Study Group investigation. J Clin Oncol 10:1889–96
118. Lau WY, Leung TW, Ho SK, Chan M, Machin D, Lau J, Chan AT, Yeo W, Mok TS, Yu SC, Leung NW, Johnson PJ (1999) Adjuvant intra-arterial iodine-131-labelled lipiodol for resectable hepatocellular carcinoma: a prospective randomised trial. Lancet 353:797–801
119. Leahy MF, Seymour JF, Hicks RJ, Turner JH (2006) Multicenter phase II clinical study of iodine-131-rituximab radioimmunotherapy in relapsed or refractory indolent non-Hodgkin's lymphoma. J Clin Oncol 24:4418–25
120. Leger FA, Izembart M, Dagousset F, Barritault L, Baillet G, Chevalier A, Clerc J (1998) Decreased uptake of therapeutic doses of iodine-131 after 185-MBq iodine-131 diagnostic imaging for thyroid remnants in differentiated thyroid carcinoma. Eur J Nucl Med 25:242–6

121. Leonard JP, Coleman M, Kostakoglu L, Chadburn A, Cesarman E, Furman RR, Schuster MW, Niesvizky R, Muss D, Fiore J, Kroll S, Tidmarsh G, Vallabhajosula S, Goldsmith SJ (2005) Abbreviated chemotherapy with fludarabine followed by tositumomab and iodine I 131 tositumomab for untreated follicular lymphoma. J Clin Oncol 23:5696–704
122. Liebmann J, Cook JA, Teague D, Fisher J, Mitchell JB (1994) Cycloheximide inhibits the cytotoxicity of paclitaxel (Taxol). Anticancer Drugs 5:287–92
123. Liersch T, Meller J, Kulle B, Behr TM, Markus P, Langer C, Ghadimi BM, Wegener WA, Kovacs J, Horak ID, Becker H, Goldenberg DM (2005) Phase II trial of carcinoembryonic antigen radioimmunotherapy with 131I-labetuzumab after salvage resection of colorectal metastases in the liver: five-year safety and efficacy results. J Clin Oncol 23:6763–70
124. Lind P, Kohlfurst S (2006) Respective roles of thyroglobulin, radioiodine imaging, and positron emission tomography in the assessment of thyroid cancer. Semin Nucl Med 36:194–205
125. Loh KC, Fitzgerald PA, Matthay KK, Yeo PP, Price DC (1997) The treatment of malignant pheochromocytoma with iodine-131 metaiodobenzylguanidine (131I-MIBG): a comprehensive review of 116 reported patients. J Endocrinol Invest 20:648–58
126. Luster M, Lippi F, Jarzab B, Perros P, Lassmann M, Reiners C, Pacini F (2005) rhTSH-aided radioiodine ablation and treatment of differentiated thyroid carcinoma: a comprehensive review. Endocr Relat Cancer 12:49–64
127. Maecke HR, Hofmann M, Haberkorn U (2005) (68)Ga-labeled peptides in tumor imaging. J Nucl Med 46 Suppl 1:172S–8S
128. Mahe MA, Fumoleau P, Fabbro M, Guastalla JP, Faurous P, Chauvot P, Chetanoud L, Classe JM, Rouanet P, Chatal JF (1999) A phase II study of intraperitoneal radioimmunotherapy with iodine-131-labeled monoclonal antibody OC-125 in patients with residual ovarian carcinoma. Clin Cancer Res 5:3249s–53s
129. Mandel SJ, Larsen PR, Seely EW, Brent GA (1990) Increased need for thyroxine during pregnancy in women with primary hypothyroidism. N Engl J Med 323:91–6
130. Mandel SJ, Shankar LK, Benard F, Yamamoto A, Alavi A (2001) Superiority of iodine-123 compared with iodine-131 scanning for thyroid remnants in patients with differentiated thyroid cancer. Clin Nucl Med 26:6–9
131. Mantey SA, Weber HC, Sainz E, Akeson M, Ryan RR, Pradhan TK, Searles RP, Spindel ER, Battey JF, Coy DH, Jensen RT (1997) Discovery of a high affinity radioligand for the human orphan receptor, bombesin receptor subtype 3, which demonstrates that it has a unique pharmacology compared with other mammalian bombesin receptors. J Biol Chem 272:26062–71
132. Matthay KK, Panina C, Huberty J, Price D, Glidden DV, Tang HR, Hawkins RA, Veatch J, Hasegawa B (2001) Correlation of tumor and whole-body dosimetry with tumor response and toxicity in refractory neuroblastoma treated with (131)I-MIBG. J Nucl Med 42:1713–21
133. Matthay KK, DeSantes K, Hasegawa B, Huberty J, Hattner RS, Ablin A, Reynolds CP, Seeger RC, Weinberg VK, Price D (1998) Phase I dose escalation of 131I-metaiodobenzylguanidine with autologous bone marrow support in refractory neuroblastoma. J Clin Oncol 16:229–36
134. Matthews DC, Appelbaum FR, Eary JF, Fisher DR, Durack LD, Bush SA, Hui TE, Martin PJ, Mitchell D, Press OW, et al. (1995) Development of a marrow transplant regimen for acute leukemia using targeted hematopoietic irradiation delivered by 131I-labeled anti-CD45 antibody, combined with cyclophosphamide and total body irradiation. Blood 85:1122–31
135. Maxon HR, 3rd, Englaro EE, Thomas SR, Hertzberg VS, Hinnefeld JD, Chen LS, Smith H, Cummings D, Aden MD (1992) Radioiodine-131 therapy for well-differentiated thyroid cancer–a quantitative radiation dosimetric approach: outcome and validation in 85 patients. J Nucl Med 33:1132–6
136. Mazzaferri EL (1999) An overview of the management of papillary and follicular thyroid carcinoma. Thyroid 9:421–7

137. McDevitt MR, Barendswaard E, Ma D, Lai L, Curcio MJ, Sgouros G, Ballangrud AM, Yang WH, Finn RD, Pellegrini V, Geerlings MW, Jr., Lee M, Brechbiel MW, Bander NH, Cordon-Cardo C, Scheinberg DA (2000) An alpha-particle emitting antibody ([213Bi]J591) for radioimmunotherapy of prostate cancer. Cancer Res 60:6095–100
138. Meller S (1997) Targeted radiotherapy for neuroblastoma. Arch Dis Child 77:389–91
139. Meredith RF, Alvarez RD, Partridge EE, Khazaeli MB, Lin CY, Macey DJ, Austin JM, Jr., Kilgore LC, Grizzle WE, Schlom J, LoBuglio AF (2001) Intraperitoneal radioimmunochemotherapy of ovarian cancer: a phase I study. Cancer Biother Radiopharm 16:305–15
140. Miano M, Garaventa A, Pizzitola MR, Piccolo MS, Dallorso S, Villavecchia GP, Bertolazzi C, Cabria M, De Bernardi B (2001) Megatherapy combining I(131) metaiodobenzylguanidine and high-dose chemotherapy with haematopoietic progenitor cell rescue for neuroblastoma. Bone Marrow Transplant 27:571–4
141. Milenic DE, Garmestani K, Brady ED, Albert PS, Ma D, Abdulla A, Brechbiel MW (2005) Alpha-particle radioimmunotherapy of disseminated peritoneal disease using a (212)Pb-labeled radioimmunoconjugate targeting HER2. Cancer Biother Radiopharm 20:557–68
142. Milowsky MI, Nanus DM, Kostakoglu L, Vallabhajosula S, Goldsmith SJ, Bander NH (2004) Phase I trial of yttrium-90-labeled anti-prostate-specific membrane antigen monoclonal antibody J591 for androgen-independent prostate cancer. J Clin Oncol 22:2522–31
143. Miyazaki M, Lamharzi N, Schally AV, Halmos G, Szepeshazi K, Groot K, Cai RZ (1998) Inhibition of growth of MDA-MB-231 human breast cancer xenografts in nude mice by bombesin/gastrin-releasing peptide (GRP) antagonists RC-3940-II and RC-3095. Eur J Cancer 34:710–7
144. Moog F, Linke R, Manthey N, Tiling R, Knesewitsch P, Tatsch K, Hahn K (2000) Influence of thyroid-stimulating hormone levels on uptake of FDG in recurrent and metastatic differentiated thyroid carcinoma. J Nucl Med 41:1989–95
145. Mukherjee JJ, Kaltsas GA, Islam N, Plowman PN, Foley R, Hikmat J, Britton KE, Jenkins PJ, Chew SL, Monson JP, Besser GM, Grossman AB (2001) Treatment of metastatic carcinoid tumours, phaeochromocytoma, paraganglioma and medullary carcinoma of the thyroid with (131)I-meta-iodobenzylguanidine [(131)I-mIBG]. Clin Endocrinol (Oxf) 55:47–60
146. Nelson J, Donnelly M, Walker B, Gray J, Shaw C, Murphy RF (1991) Bombesin stimulates proliferation of human breast cancer cells in culture. Br J Cancer 63:933–6
147. Nock BA, Nikolopoulou A, Galanis A, Cordopatis P, Waser B, Reubi JC, Maina T (2005) Potent bombesin-like peptides for GRP-receptor targeting of tumors with 99mTc: a preclinical study. J Med Chem 48:100–10
148. O'Donoghue JA, Bardies M, Wheldon TE (1995) Relationships between tumor size and curability for uniformly targeted therapy with beta-emitting radionuclides. J Nucl Med 36:1902–9
149. Oberg K (1998) Advances in chemotherapy and biotherapy of endocrine tumors. Curr Opin Oncol 10:58–65
150. Oberg K (2001) Established clinical use of octreotide and lanreotide in oncology. Chemotherapy 47 Suppl 2:40–53
151. Oyen WJ, Bodei L, Giammarile F, Maecke HR, Tennvall J, Luster M, Brans B (2007) Targeted therapy in nuclear medicine–current status and future prospects. Ann Oncol 18:1782–92
152. Oyen WJ (2004) Consolidation therapy with intraperitoneal R1549 (Yttrium-90-labeled HMFG1 murine monoclonal antibody) in epithelial ovarian cancer: a phase III trial (abstract) Cancer Biother Radiopharm 19(4): 508
153. Pacini F, Schlumberger M, Dralle H, Elisei R, Smit JW, Wiersinga W (2006) European consensus for the management of patients with differentiated thyroid carcinoma of the follicular epithelium. Eur J Endocrinol 154:787–803
154. Pacini F, Molinaro E, Castagna MG, Lippi F, Ceccarelli C, Agate L, Elisei R, Pinchera A (2002) Ablation of thyroid residues with 30 mCi (131)I: a comparison in thyroid cancer patients prepared with recombinant human TSH or thyroid hormone withdrawal. J Clin Endocrinol Metab 87:4063–8

155. Pacini F, Molinaro E, Castagna MG, Agate L, Elisei R, Ceccarelli C, Lippi F, Taddei D, Grasso L, Pinchera A (2003) Recombinant human thyrotropin-stimulated serum thyroglobulin combined with neck ultrasonography has the highest sensitivity in monitoring differentiated thyroid carcinoma. J Clin Endocrinol Metab 88:3668–73
156. Pacini F, Ladenson PW, Schlumberger M, Driedger A, Luster M, Kloos RT, Sherman S, Haugen B, Corone C, Molinaro E, Elisei R, Ceccarelli C, Pinchera A, Wahl RL, Leboulleux S, Ricard M, Yoo J, Busaidy NL, Delpassand E, Hanscheid H, Felbinger R, Lassmann M, Reiners C (2006) Radioiodine ablation of thyroid remnants after preparation with recombinant human thyrotropin in differentiated thyroid carcinoma: results of an international, randomized, controlled study. J Clin Endocrinol Metab 91:926–32
157. Palmedo H, Bucerius J, Joe A, Strunk H, Hortling N, Meyka S, Roedel R, Wolff M, Wardelmann E, Biersack HJ, Jaeger U (2006) Integrated PET/CT in differentiated thyroid cancer: diagnostic accuracy and impact on patient management. J Nucl Med 47:616–24
158. Panigone S, Nunn AD (2006) Lutetium-177-labeled gastrin releasing peptide receptor binding analogs: a novel approach to radionuclide therapy. Q J Nucl Med Mol Imaging 50:310–21
159. Patel YC (1999) Somatostatin and its receptor family. Front Neuroendocrinol 20:157–98
160. Postema EJ, Frielink C, Oyen WJ, Raemaekers JM, Goldenberg DM, Corstens FH, Boerman OC (2003) Biodistribution of 131I-, 186Re-, 177Lu-, and 88Y-labeled hLL2 (Epratuzumab) in nude mice with CD22-positive lymphoma. Cancer Biother Radiopharm 18:525–33
161. Press OW, Eary JF, Gooley T, Gopal AK, Liu S, Rajendran JG, Maloney DG, Petersdorf S, Bush SA, Durack LD, Martin PJ, Fisher DR, Wood B, Borrow JW, Porter B, Smith JP, Matthews DC, Appelbaum FR, Bernstein ID (2000) A phase I/II trial of iodine-131-tositumomab (anti-CD20), etoposide, cyclophosphamide, and autologous stem cell transplantation for relapsed B-cell lymphomas. Blood 96:2934–42
162. Preston SR, Woodhouse LF, Jones-Blackett S, Miller GV, Primrose JN (1995) High-affinity binding sites for gastrin-releasing peptide on human colorectal cancer tissue but not uninvolved mucosa. Br J Cancer 71:1087–9
163. Raoul JL, Messner M, Boucher E, Bretagne JF, Campion JP, Boudjema K (2003) Preoperative treatment of hepatocellular carcinoma with intra-arterial injection of 131I-labelled lipiodol. Br J Surg 90:1379–83
164. Raoul JL, Guyader D, Bretagne JF, Heautot JF, Duvauferrier R, Bourguet P, Bekhechi D, Deugnier YM, Gosselin M (1997) Prospective randomized trial of chemoembolization versus intra-arterial injection of 131I-labeled-iodized oil in the treatment of hepatocellular carcinoma. Hepatology 26:1156–61
165. Reardon DA, Akabani G, Coleman RE, Friedman AH, Friedman HS, Herndon JE, 2nd, McLendon RE, Pegram CN, Provenzale JM, Quinn JA, Rich JN, Vredenburgh JJ, Desjardins A, Gururangan S, Badruddoja M, Dowell JM, Wong TZ, Zhao XG, Zalutsky MR, Bigner DD (2006) Salvage radioimmunotherapy with murine iodine-131-labeled antitenascin monoclonal antibody 81C6 for patients with recurrent primary and metastatic malignant brain tumors: phase II study results. J Clin Oncol 24:115–22
166. Reubi JC (2003) Peptide receptors as molecular targets for cancer diagnosis and therapy. Endocr Rev 24:389–427
167. Reubi JC, Waser B (1996) Unexpected high incidence of cholecystokinin-B/gastrin receptors in human medullary thyroid carcinomas. Int J Cancer 67:644–7
168. Reubi JC, Schaer JC, Waser B (1997) Cholecystokinin(CCK)-A and CCK-B/gastrin receptors in human tumors. Cancer Res 57:1377–86
169. Reubi JC, Macke HR, Krenning EP (2005) Candidates for peptide receptor radiotherapy today and in the future. J Nucl Med 46 Suppl 1:67S–75S
170. Reubi JC, Waser B, Schaer JC, Laissue JA (2001) Somatostatin receptor sst1-sst5 expression in normal and neoplastic human tissues using receptor autoradiography with subtype selective ligands. Eur J Nucl Med 28:836–46
171. Reubi JC, Schar JC, Waser B, Wenger S, Heppeler A, Schmitt JS, Macke HR (2000) Affinity profiles for human somatostatin receptor subtypes SST1-SST5 of somatostatin radiotracers selected for scintigraphic and radiotherapeutic use. Eur J Nucl Med 27:273–82

172. Richman CM, Denardo SJ, O'Donnell RT, Yuan A, Shen S, Goldstein DS, Tuscano JM, Wun T, Chew HK, Lara PN, Kukis DL, Natarajan A, Meares CF, Lamborn KR, DeNardo GL (2005) High-dose radioimmunotherapy combined with fixed, low-dose paclitaxel in metastatic prostate and breast cancer by using a MUC-1 monoclonal antibody, m170, linked to indium-111/yttrium-90 via a cathepsin cleavable linker with cyclosporine to prevent human anti-mouse antibody. Clin Cancer Res 11:5920–7
173. Risse JH, Grunwald F, Kersjes W, Strunk H, Caselmann WH, Palmedo H, Bender H, Biersack HJ (2000) Intraarterial HCC therapy with I-131-Lipiodol. Cancer Biother Radiopharm 15:65–70
174. Riva P, Franceschi G, Frattarelli M, Lazzari S, Riva N, Giuliani G, Casi M, Sarti G, Guiducci G, Giorgetti G, Gentile R, Santimaria M, Jermann E, Maeke HR (1999) Loco-regional radioimmunotherapy of high-grade malignant gliomas using specific monoclonal antibodies labeled with 90Y: a phase I study. Clin Cancer Res 5:3275s–80s
175. Robbins RJ, Schlumberger MJ (2005) The evolving role of (131)I for the treatment of differentiated thyroid carcinoma. J Nucl Med 46 Suppl 1:28S–37S
176. Rose B, Matthay KK, Price D, Huberty J, Klencke B, Norton JA, Fitzgerald PA (2003) High-dose 131I-metaiodobenzylguanidine therapy for 12 patients with malignant pheochromocytoma. Cancer 98:239–48
177. Rubino C, de Vathaire F, Dottorini ME, Hall P, Schvartz C, Couette JE, Dondon MG, Abbas MT, Langlois C, Schlumberger M (2003) Second primary malignancies in thyroid cancer patients. Br J Cancer 89:1638–44
178. Safford SD, Coleman RE, Gockerman JP, Moore J, Feldman JM, Leight GS, Jr., Tyler DS, Olson JA, Jr. (2003) Iodine -131 metaiodobenzylguanidine is an effective treatment for malignant pheochromocytoma and paraganglioma. Surgery 134:956–62; discussion 962–3
179. Scemama JL, Zahidi A, Fourmy D, Fagot-Revurat P, Vaysse N, Pradayrol L, Ribet A (1986) Interaction of [125I]-Tyr4-bombesin with specific receptors on normal human pancreatic membranes. Regul Pept 13:125–32
180. Schilder R, Molina A, Bartlett N, Witzig T, Gordon L, Murray J, Spies S, Wang H, Wiseman G, White C (2004) Follow-up results of a phase II study of ibritumomab tiuxetan radioimmunotherapy in patients with relapsed or refractory low-grade, follicular, or transformed B-cell non-Hodgkin's lymphoma and mild thrombocytopenia. Cancer Biother Radiopharm 19:478–81
181. Schlumberger M, De Vathaire F, Ceccarelli C, Delisle MJ, Francese C, Couette JE, Pinchera A, Parmentier C (1996) Exposure to radioactive iodine-131 for scintigraphy or therapy does not preclude pregnancy in thyroid cancer patients. J Nucl Med 37:606–12
182. Schluter B, Bohuslavizki KH, Beyer W, Plotkin M, Buchert R, Clausen M (2001) Impact of FDG PET on patients with differentiated thyroid cancer who present with elevated thyroglobulin and negative 131I scan. J Nucl Med 42:71–6
183. Schmutzler C (2001) Regulation of the sodium/iodide symporter by retinoids–a review. Exp Clin Endocrinol Diabetes 109:41–4
184. Schroeder PR, Haugen BR, Pacini F, Reiners C, Schlumberger M, Sherman SI, Cooper DS, Schuff KG, Braverman LE, Skarulis MC, Davies TF, Mazzaferri EL, Daniels GH, Ross DS, Luster M, Samuels MH, Weintraub BD, Ridgway EC, Ladenson PW (2006) A comparison of short-term changes in health-related quality of life in thyroid carcinoma patients undergoing diagnostic evaluation with recombinant human thyrotropin compared with thyroid hormone withdrawal. J Clin Endocrinol Metab 91:878–84
185. Scopinaro F, De Vincentis G, Varvarigou AD, Laurenti C, Iori F, Remediani S, Chiarini S, Stella S (2003) 99mTc-bombesin detects prostate cancer and invasion of pelvic lymph nodes. Eur J Nucl Med Mol Imaging 30:1378–82
186. Scopinaro F, De Vincentis G, Corazziari E, Massa R, Osti M, Pallotta N, Covotta A, Remediani S, Paolo MD, Monteleone F, Varvarigou A (2004) Detection of colon cancer with 99mTc-labeled bombesin derivative (99mTc-leu13-BN1). Cancer Biother Radiopharm 19:245–52
187. Scott AM, Cebon J (1997) Clinical promise of tumour immunology. Lancet 349 Suppl 2: SII19–22

188. Scott AM, Lee FT, Jones R, Hopkins W, MacGregor D, Cebon JS, Hannah A, Chong G, U P, Papenfuss A, Rigopoulos A, Sturrock S, Murphy R, Wirth V, Murone C, Smyth FE, Knight S, Welt S, Ritter G, Richards E, Nice EC, Burgess AW, Old LJ (2005) A phase I trial of humanized monoclonal antibody A33 in patients with colorectal carcinoma: biodistribution, pharmacokinetics, and quantitative tumor uptake. Clin Cancer Res 11:4810–7
189. Shammas A, Degirmenci B, Mountz JM, McCook BM, Branstetter B, Bencherif B, Joyce JM, Carty SE, Kuffner HA, Avril N (2007) 18F-FDG PET/CT in patients with suspected recurrent or metastatic well-differentiated thyroid cancer. J Nucl Med 48:221–6
190. Sharkey RM, Hajjar G, Yeldell D, Brenner A, Burton J, Rubin A, Goldenberg DM (2005) A phase I trial combining high-dose 90Y-labeled humanized anti-CEA monoclonal antibody with doxorubicin and peripheral blood stem cell rescue in advanced medullary thyroid cancer. J Nucl Med 46:620–33
191. Sharkey RM, Brenner A, Burton J, Hajjar G, Toder SP, Alavi A, Matthies A, Tsai DE, Schuster SJ, Stadtmauer EA, Czuczman MS, Lamonica D, Kraeber-Bodere F, Mahe B, Chatal JF, Rogatko A, Mardirrosian G, Goldenberg DM (2003) Radioimmunotherapy of non-Hodgkin's lymphoma with 90Y-DOTA humanized anti-CD22 IgG (90Y-Epratuzumab): do tumor targeting and dosimetry predict therapeutic response? J Nucl Med 44:2000–18
192. Siegel JA, Yeldell D, Goldenberg DM, Stabin MG, Sparks RB, Sharkey RM, Brenner A, Blumenthal RD (2003) Red marrow radiation dose adjustment using plasma FLT3-L cytokine levels: improved correlations between hematologic toxicity and bone marrow dose for radioimmunotherapy patients. J Nucl Med 44:67–76
193. Silberstein EB (2007) Comparison of outcomes after (123)I versus (131)I pre-ablation imaging before radioiodine ablation in differentiated thyroid carcinoma. J Nucl Med 48:1043–6
194. Singh Jaggi J, Henke E, Seshan SV, Kappel BJ, Chattopadhyay D, May C, McDevitt MR, Nolan D, Mittal V, Benezra R, Scheinberg DA (2007) Selective alpha-particle mediated depletion of tumor vasculature with vascular normalization. PLoS ONE 2:e267
195. Smith CJ, Volkert WA, Hoffman TJ (2005) Radiolabeled peptide conjugates for targeting of the bombesin receptor superfamily subtypes. Nucl Med Biol 32:733–40
196. Smith-Jones PM (2004) Radioimmunotherapy of prostate cancer. Q J Nucl Med Mol Imaging 48:297–304
197. Smith-Jones PM, Vallabhajosula S, Navarro V, Bastidas D, Goldsmith SJ, Bander NH (2003) Radiolabeled monoclonal antibodies specific to the extracellular domain of prostate-specific membrane antigen: preclinical studies in nude mice bearing LNCaP human prostate tumor. J Nucl Med 44:610–7
198. Solcia E, Buffa R, Gini A, Capella C, Rindi G, Polak JM (1988) Bombesin-related peptides in the diffuse neuroendocrine system. Ann N Y Acad Sci 547:83–94
199. Steffens MG, Kranenborg MH, Boerman OC, Zegwaart-Hagemeier NE, Debruyne FM, Corstens FH, Oosterwijk E (1998) Tumor retention of 186Re-MAG3, 111In-DTPA and 125I labeled monoclonal antibody G250 in nude mice with renal cell carcinoma xenografts. Cancer Biother Radiopharm 13:133–9
200. Subramanian S, Goldstein DP, Parlea L, Thabane L, Ezzat S, Ibrahim-Zada I, Straus S, Brierley JD, Tsang RW, Gafni A, Rotstein L, Sawka AM (2007) Second primary malignancy risk in thyroid cancer survivors: a systematic review and meta-analysis. Thyroid 17:1277–88
201. Sunday ME (1988) Tissue-specific expression of the mammalian bombesin gene. Ann N Y Acad Sci 547:95–113
202. Sunday ME, Kaplan LM, Motoyama E, Chin WW, Spindel ER (1988) Gastrin-releasing peptide (mammalian bombesin) gene expression in health and disease. Lab Invest 59:5–24
203. Teunissen JJ, Kwekkeboom DJ, Kooij PP, Bakker WH, Krenning EP (2005) Peptide receptor radionuclide therapy for non-radioiodine-avid differentiated thyroid carcinoma. J Nucl Med 46 Suppl 1:107S–14S
204. Troncone L, Rufini V (1997) 131I-MIBG therapy of neural crest tumours (review). Anticancer Res 17:1823–31
205. Tschmelitsch J, Barendswaard E, Williams C, Jr., Yao TJ, Cohen AM, Old LJ, Welt S (1997) Enhanced antitumor activity of combination radioimmunotherapy (131I-labeled monoclonal antibody A33) with chemotherapy (fluorouracil). Cancer Res 57:2181–6

206. Valkema R, Pauwels S, Kvols LK, Barone R, Jamar F, Bakker WH, Kwekkeboom DJ, Bouterfa H, Krenning EP (2006) Survival and response after peptide receptor radionuclide therapy with [90Y-DOTA0,Tyr3]octreotide in patients with advanced gastroenteropancreatic neuroendocrine tumors. Semin Nucl Med 36:147–56
207. Valkema R, Pauwels SA, Kvols LK, Kwekkeboom DJ, Jamar F, de Jong M, Barone R, Walrand S, Kooij PP, Bakker WH, Lasher J, Krenning EP (2005) Long-term follow-up of renal function after peptide receptor radiation therapy with (90)Y-DOTA(0),Tyr(3)-octreotide and (177)Lu-DOTA(0), Tyr(3)-octreotate. J Nucl Med 46 Suppl 1:83S–91S
208. Valkema R, De Jong M, Bakker WH, Breeman WA, Kooij PP, Lugtenburg PJ, De Jong FH, Christiansen A, Kam BL, De Herder WW, Stridsberg M, Lindemans J, Ensing G, Krenning EP (2002) Phase I study of peptide receptor radionuclide therapy with [In-DTPA]octreotide: the Rotterdam experience. Semin Nucl Med 32:110–22
209. Van de Wiele C, Dumont F, Vanden Broecke R, Oosterlinck W, Cocquyt V, Serreyn R, Peers S, Thornback J, Slegers G, Dierckx RA (2000) Technetium-99m RP527, a GRP analogue for visualisation of GRP receptor-expressing malignancies: a feasibility study. Eur J Nucl Med 27:1694–9
210. Van den Eynde B, Scott AM (1998) Tumor Antigens. Encyclopedia of Immunology. London: Academic press, pp. 2424–31
211. van Hagen PM, Breeman WA, Reubi JC, Postema PT, van den Anker-Lugtenburg PJ, Kwekkeboom DJ, Laissue J, Waser B, Lamberts SW, Visser TJ, Krenning EP (1996) Visualization of the thymus by substance P receptor scintigraphy in man. Eur J Nucl Med 23:1508–13
212. Van Hazel G, Blackwell A, Anderson J, Price D, Moroz P, Bower G, Cardaci G, Gray B (2004) Randomised phase 2 trial of SIR-Spheres plus fluorouracil/leucovorin chemotherapy versus fluorouracil/leucovorin chemotherapy alone in advanced colorectal cancer. J Surg Oncol 88:78–85
213. Van Hazel GA, Price D, Bower G, Sharma RA, Blanshard K, Steward WP (2005) Selective internal radioation therapy (SIRT)for lier metastases with concomitant systemic oxaliplatin, 5-fluorouracil and folinic acid: a phase I/II dose escalation study. J Clin Oncol 23:(Abstract 3657)
214. Van Nostrand D, Wartofsky L (2007) Radioiodine in the treatment of thyroid cancer. Endocrinol Metab Clin North Am 36:807–22, vii–viii
215. Virgolini I, Britton K, Buscombe J, Moncayo R, Paganelli G, Riva P (2002) In- and Y-DOTA-lanreotide: results and implications of the MAURITIUS trial. Semin Nucl Med 32:148–55
216. Virgolini I, Raderer M, Kurtaran A, Angelberger P, Banyai S, Yang Q, Li S, Banyai M, Pidlich J, Niederle B, Scheithauer W, Valent P (1994) Vasoactive intestinal peptide-receptor imaging for the localization of intestinal adenocarcinomas and endocrine tumors. N Engl J Med 331:1116–21
217. von Mehren M, Adams GP, Weiner LM (2003) Monoclonal antibody therapy for cancer. Annu Rev Med 54:343–69
218. Vuillez JP, Kraeber-Bodere F, Moro D, Bardies M, Douillard JY, Gautherot E, Rouvier E, Barbet J, Garban F, Moreau P, Chatal JF (1999) Radioimmunotherapy of small cell lung carcinoma with the two-step method using a bispecific anti-carcinoembryonic antigen/anti-diethylenetriaminepentaacetic acid (DTPA) antibody and iodine-131 Di-DTPA hapten: results of a phase I/II trial. Clin Cancer Res 5:3259s–67s
219. Wahl RL (2003) The clinical importance of dosimetry in radioimmunotherapy with tositumomab and iodine I 131 tositumomab. Semin Oncol 30:31–8
220. Waldherr C, Pless M, Maecke HR, Haldemann A, Mueller-Brand J (2001) The clinical value of [90Y-DOTA]-D-Phe1-Tyr3-octreotide (90Y-DOTATOC) in the treatment of neuroendocrine tumours: a clinical phase II study. Ann Oncol 12:941–5
221. Waldherr C, Pless M, Maecke HR, Schumacher T, Crazzolara A, Nitzsche EU, Haldemann A, Mueller-Brand J (2002) Tumor response and clinical benefit in neuroendocrine tumors after 7.4 GBq (90)Y-DOTATOC. J Nucl Med 43:610–6

222. Waldmann TA, White JD, Carrasquillo JA, Reynolds JC, Paik CH, Gansow OA, Brechbiel MW, Jaffe ES, Fleisher TA, Goldman CK, Top LE, Bamford R, Zaknoen E, Roessler E, Kasten-Sportes C, England R, Litou H, Johnson JA, Jackson-White T, Manns A, Hanchard B, Junghans RP, Nelson DL (1995) Radioimmunotherapy of interleukin-2R alpha-expressing adult T-cell leukemia with Yttrium-90-labeled anti-Tac. Blood 86:4063–75
223. Wiseman GA, White CA, Sparks RB, Erwin WD, Podoloff DA, Lamonica D, Bartlett NL, Parker JA, Dunn WL, Spies SM, Belanger R, Witzig TE, Leigh BR (2001) Biodistribution and dosimetry results from a phase III prospectively randomized controlled trial of Zevalin radioimmunotherapy for low-grade, follicular, or transformed B-cell non-Hodgkin's lymphoma. Crit Rev Oncol Hematol 39:181–94
224. Witzig TE, Flinn IW, Gordon LI, Emmanouilides C, Czuczman MS, Saleh MN, Cripe L, Wiseman G, Olejnik T, Multani PS, White CA (2002) Treatment with ibritumomab tiuxetan radioimmunotherapy in patients with rituximab-refractory follicular non-Hodgkin's lymphoma. J Clin Oncol 20:3262–9
225. Witzig TE, White CA, Wiseman GA, Gordon LI, Emmanouilides C, Raubitschek A, Janakiraman N, Gutheil J, Schilder RJ, Spies S, Silverman DH, Parker E, Grillo-Lopez AJ (1999) Phase I/II trial of IDEC-Y2B8 radioimmunotherapy for treatment of relapsed or refractory CD20(+) B-cell non-Hodgkin's lymphoma. J Clin Oncol 17:3793–803
226. Witzig TE, Gordon LI, Cabanillas F, Czuczman MS, Emmanouilides C, Joyce R, Pohlman BL, Bartlett NL, Wiseman GA, Padre N, Grillo-Lopez AJ, Multani P, White CA (2002) Randomized controlled trial of yttrium-90-labeled ibritumomab tiuxetan radioimmunotherapy versus rituximab immunotherapy for patients with relapsed or refractory low-grade, follicular, or transformed B-cell non-Hodgkin's lymphoma. J Clin Oncol 20:2453–63
227. Wong JY, Shibata S, Williams LE, Kwok CS, Liu A, Chu DZ, Yamauchi DM, Wilczynski S, Ikle DN, Wu AM, Yazaki PJ, Shively JE, Doroshow JH, Raubitschek AA (2003) A Phase I trial of 90Y-anti-carcinoembryonic antigen chimeric T84.66 radioimmunotherapy with 5-fluorouracil in patients with metastatic colorectal cancer. Clin Cancer Res 9:5842–52
228. Yano T, Pinski J, Groot K, Schally AV (1992) Stimulation by bombesin and inhibition by bombesin/gastrin-releasing peptide antagonist RC-3095 of growth of human breast cancer cell lines. Cancer Res 52:4545–7
229. Zalutsky MR, Pozzi OR (2004) Radioimmunotherapy with alpha-particle emitting radionuclides. Q J Nucl Med Mol Imaging 48:289–96
230. Zhang H, Chen J, Waldherr C, Hinni K, Waser B, Reubi JC, Maecke HR (2004) Synthesis and evaluation of bombesin derivatives on the basis of pan-bombesin peptides labeled with indium-111, lutetium-177, and yttrium-90 for targeting bombesin receptor-expressing tumors. Cancer Res 64:6707–15

Chapter 21
Developmental Trends in Targeted Radionuclide Therapy: Biological Aspects

Torgny Stigbrand[1], Jörgen Carlsson[2], and Gregory P. Adams[3]

Summary Targeted radionuclide therapy of hematopoietic malignancies in the clinical setting has been achieved and similar successes with solid tumors and cells disseminated from them are likely within reach. Recombinant technologies have led to the development of a number of new targeting agents and the evaluation of a number of putative new targets is currently in progress. These advances are currently under evaluation in the preclinical setting and are expected to transition into clinical trials before long. Many of these new agents exhibit both improved pharmacological properties and enhanced cellular retention, both of which may lead to substantial improvements over existing compounds. In addition, our knowledge of basic radiobiology and its impact on the different modes of cell death is rapidly expanding, leading to new understanding in the fundamental differences between hematopoietic and epithelial tumor cells. Such knowledge will likely have a significant influence on the development of future treatment modalities. Furthermore, the complex interactions between radiation induced intracellular signaling pathways and the crucial observation that low dose radiation (e.g. less than 15 Gy) is able to significantly affect the growth of disseminated solid tumors cells suggests to us that a new era in targeted radionuclide therapy may soon be here.

Introduction

A paradigm shift is approaching for the targeted radionuclide therapy field. For several decades it has been our goal to increase radionuclide accretion in tumors and disseminated metastases and achieve radiation doses comparable to external therapy while maintaining the tumor specificity that has been the advantage of targeted

[1]Department of Immunology, Clinical Microbiology, University of Umeå, SE-90185, Umeå, Sweden

[2]Unit of Biomedical Radiation Sciences, Department of Oncology, Radiology and Clinical Immunology, Rudbeck Laboratory, Uppsala University, SE-751 85, Uppsala, Sweden

[3]Department of Medical Oncology, Fox Chase Cancer Center, Philadelphia, PA 19111, USA

T. Stigbrand et al. (eds.) *Targeted Radionuclide Tumor Therapy*,

strategies. Quantitative measurements of tumor uptake of radionuclides have dominated reports and parameters such as %ID/g tumor, tumor to non-tumor ratios and dosimetric calculations have been typically used in our attempts to evaluate efficiency of targeting [1–5]. Based upon these parameters we have frequently come up short in our clinical efforts to target solid tumors. However, the optimism surrounding potential future successful treatment of solid tumor cells has been renewed in some members of our field by the widespread evidence that targeted radionuclide therapy is effective in the setting of hematological malignancies (chapter 20 and [6]). Still, it is important to note that the exquisite radiosensitivity of hematopoietic cells has been known and exploited for decades. The ability to successfully transfer targeted radionuclide technology to the treatment of tumor cells originating from solid tumors clearly will not be an easy feat as many of the authors in this book conclude. The therapeutic window, which allows efficient eradication of different populations of lymphoid cells, may be too narrow to allow for similar dramatic and efficient treatment of most common solid tumors (discussed in chapter 16).

On the other hand, reports persist that targeted radionuclide therapy achieving total doses of up to 15 Gy can be associated with responses in the clinic. These doses fall below the range that is considered to be high enough to be associated with clinical efficacy with external beam radiation. Yet they have demonstrated significant growth inhibiting effects on comparatively radioresistant epithelial tumors with dramatic modifications in tumor morphology (e.g. formation of giant cells, vacuoles, changes in connective tissue organization and significant reductions in number of dividing tumor cells). While the clinical breakthrough for targeted radionuclide therapy of solid tumors has though not yet occurred, we are clearly making progress in that direction.

Cell Death

The emergence of the existence of a wide range of cell death mechanisms, including different types of apoptosis, necrosis, senescence, and autophagy will likely have a significant impact on targeted radionuclide therapy. Cell death induction mechanisms that were historically thought of as simply "necrosis causers" in fact vary to a significant extent between different types of cells. This observation will need to be taken into account when the efficacy of targeted treatment is considered. This is extensively discussed in chapter 12.

Hematopoietic cells and corresponding tumors are typically programmed for rapidly induced, rapidly executed, apoptotic deaths occurring within hours or a few days after exposure to very low doses of radiation. In contrast, epithelial cells and various types of carcinoma cells display different death mechanisms and do not directly undergo apoptosis. These cells often develop mitotic catastrophes leading to chaotic disturbances in cell cycle kinetics and cell division mechanisms and finally to delayed apoptosis. This process can take up to one week to occur when low radioactive doses and low dose-rates typical of targeted radionuclide therapy are involved.

These factors have to be carefully considered when new strategies are planned, as they have implications for the choice of radionuclide, the residence time in the tumors of the targeting agent and the kinetics of dose delivery (see chapters 8, 12–15). It is very possible that the treatment window will need to be broader in duration for tumors of epithelial origin than for tumors of hematopoietic origin. A rule of thumb may be that the treatment should cover the period of time required for apoptosis induction (e.g. days for hematological malignancies and a week for solid tumors).

Low Dose-Rate, Radiosensitivity and LET

One of the basic concepts in the expected paradigm shift can be attributed to the growing knowledge of radiobiology (chapters 12–19) and the increasing information regarding signaling pathways within cells that are activated following exposure to low doses and low dose-rate radiation (e.g. chapters 13, 18 and [7]). The significance of these advances cannot be overstated.

Still, there is a need for better characterization of the cellular radiosensitivity of different types of tumor cells to low dose-rate radiation with low LET (e.g. β particle-emitting) radionuclides. Analysis of the growth and clonogenic capacity following irradiation and assays based on analyses of apoptosis, mutations, DNA-expression and protein synthesis could facilitate these efforts.

The ability to apply different quality LET radionuclides to targeted therapy adds an additional optimization parameter that must be addressed (see chapters 9–11). However, the potential to modify radiosensitivity of targeted cells is likely greater for low-LET radiation than for high-LET radiation independent of dose-rate. The use of radiosensitizers for tumor cells and/or radioprotectors for normal cells in combination with low-LET radionuclide therapy needs to be extensively explored.

The Four R:s

The four R:s, which are well known to those working in the field of external radiotherapy [8], stand for:

- *R*epair of sublethal damage (e.g. repair of DNA-damage during or between repeated irradiations).
- *R*eassortment (or redistribution) of cells within the cell cycle due to the radiation (radiation effects on cells in different radiation sensitive phases within the cell cycle giving various patterns of synchronization).
- *R*epopulation or cell-proliferation of the irradiated cells during the therapy session.

– *R*eoxygenation which means that tumor cells, which are radioresistant due to hypoxia, are successively better oxygenated during the therapy session.

These factors are known to modify the effects of external radiotherapy during fractionated radiotherapy and they are probably also factors that impact on the efficacy of low dose-rate irradiation in radionuclide therapy, particularly since this type of low dose-rate treatment occurs over several days. For example, repopulation that occurs during low dose-rate radiation exposure (e.g., cell proliferation generating a larger number of cells which have to be eradicated) can counteract the effects of therapy. However, prolongation of treatment allow also for sparing of normal tissues and reoxygenation of the tumors, as described for external radiotherapy [8].

Thus, the "fractionation related" R-factors mentioned above will also influence normal tissues. It is therefore difficult to foresee the conditions that give the most beneficial tumor/normal tissue effect ratios. More research is clearly needed.

Hyperradiosensitivity

The phenomenon known as hyperradiosensitivity or hypersensitization (chapter 19) implies that a greater biological effect occurs at low doses (<0.5 Gy) of low-LET radiation than would be expected from extrapolations of the effects observed following higher doses (>1 Gy) given at a high dose-rate (about 1–2 Gy/min). However, it is not clear whether this applies to exposure to low dose-rate radiation and whether the cells exposed to low dose-rate are continuously more or less hypersensitive (chapters 16 and 19). A delicate balance between hyperradiosensitivity and "increased radioresistance" occurs with very low dose ranges, described in chapter 19, and required further exploration and exploitation. These phenomena are intimately related to induction of radiation damage sensor and repair systems, as described in chapters 13 and 14.

Bystander Effects

There are many reports of bystander effects following targeted radionuclide therapy in which cells in the vicinity of the irradiated cell are also influenced by the radiation (chapter 17). while the existence of this phenomenon cannot be questioned, the underlying mechanisms are far from fully understood. More research is needed in order to determine the significance of this phenomenon and fully exploit it in future targeted radionuclide therapy.

New Target Structures

In order for an identified tumor-associated gene product to be utilized as a target in radionuclide therapy, it is necessary to verify that it is selectively expressed in relevant amounts and that it is present in both solid tumors and disseminated tumor cells. It is, of course, also necessary to consider the fact that many tumor-associated targets are also expressed to varying degrees in normal cells and tissues. While this does not automatically rule out the use of these gene products as a target for radionuclide therapy, the sensitivity of the targeted normal tissues must be considered. Presumably, the methodological advances in both genomics and proteomics will broaden and accelerate the search for new targets. It is possible that at least half of all disseminated tumors and their corresponding metastases will express cell surface associated structures of potential interest, as a direct or indirect result of the tumor transformation process, [9]. Clearly the choice of a target is a high priority in our field as the present characterizations that have been used to identify the current targets on many tumors are probably of insufficient power to identify the best targets for radionuclide therapy (see chapters 2 and 3).

The need for identification of new targets is especially high for disseminated prostate and colorectal cancer (chapters 2 and 3). While these tumors are two of the most common types of cancer, specific targets that are suitable for radionuclide therapy have yet to be characterized. In the case of prostate cancer it is possible that PSMA (prostate specific membrane antigen) may emerge as a suitable target as it is selectively expressed and unlike PSA, is not extensively shed from the cells. EGFR and HER2 may also prove to be suitable targets in both prostate cancer and colorectal cancer as they are reportedly expressed at reasonable levels in a percentage of both primary tumors and their corresponding metastases (chapter 3), suggesting that a combined approach targeting both receptors at the same time may be effective. This could be achieved with either bifunctional antibodies (chapters 5 and 18) or alternative scaffolds such as affibody molecules (chapter 6). Makers for Cancer stem cells might be targets in the near future (chapter 15).

Changes of Receptor and Antigen Expression

Numerous substances such as cytokines, hormones and other biological response modifiers may up- or down-regulate receptors and cell surface antigens thereby improving their utility as targets. Growth factors and/or kinase inhibiting drugs designed to interfere with signal transduction, e.g. gefitinib, might also modify the cellular uptake of targeted radionuclides and enhance the effects of targeted radionuclide therapy [10, 11]. Another interesting approach that has not yet been examined would be to administer targeting agents according to a fractionation pattern that takes the timing of expression of new receptors or antigens into account. The increasing availability of biologic agents that alter receptor and antigen expression could make such a therapeutic strategy possible.

Influence of Genomic Instability

Genomic instability is most likely a consequence of the multistep carcinogenesis process in which defects in onco-, suppressor-, cell cycle- and apoptosis regulating genes [12] allow the tumor cells to bypass cell cycle checkpoints and successfully divide in the presence of non-repaired DNA damage. Such genomic instability may give rise to unique tumor cell epitopes suitable for targeting. However, it is important to keep in mind that inefficient targeted tumor therapy could subject the tumor to selection pressures leading to antigen escape in which new subclones with little or no expression of the targeted antigen appear. Furthermore, the treatment could itself create additional DNA damage leading to a more extensive selection process.

By choosing appropriate targets for radionuclide therapy it might be possible to minimize the risk of adverse effects due to genomic instability. For example, it is known that the expression of the oncogene product HER2 is surprisingly stable between primary tumors and their corresponding metastases (chapter 3). This suggests that tumor cells overexpressing HER2 are dependent on its expression for growth and possibly for overcoming apoptosis. Thus, downregulation of HER2 would be a growth disadvantage and these cells may be overgrown by cells expressing high levels of HER2. Similar arguments could apply to other tumor-associated receptors such as PDGR, EGFR, IGF1-R and the somatostatin receptor.

Combined Action and Autosensitization

The progress over the last decade in understanding how in basic tumor biology on modified signal transduction relates to growth control and DNA repair has been impressive (see chapter 13 and [12–14]). It is likely that these advances will facilitate for combined or synergistic therapeutic effects such as the combined action or autosensitization described in chapters 13 and 18. For example, radiolabeled EGFR binding agents could deliver radionuclides to the tumor cells while simultaneously triggering signaling events through the receptor that increase the cell's radiosensitivity by inhibiting DNA-repair. While this sounds futuristic it may already be a reality as the EGFR-binding antibody cetuximab (Erbitux) appears to sensitize cells to the effects of radiotherapy [15]. In theory it should be possible to load cetuximab with therapeutic radionuclides that take advantage of this effect. We foresee that additional such additive or synergistic combinations will appear in the near future.

Cellular Binding Affinity, Internalization and Retention

When radionuclide therapy is performed against single disseminated cells, high affinity binding of ligands or antibodies might be optimal. However, in the setting of solid tumor masses it can be preferable to utilize agents with a lower affinity that allow for better tumor penetration (chapter 18).

Intratumoral residence time of the targeted radionuclides is critical for therapeutic success. The longer the radionuclides stay in or near the targeted cell, the higher fraction of the radioactive decays can be utilized for therapy and the higher dose will be delivered per targeting event. Increased retention can be achieved either by a targeting process associated with a high affinity and stable binding or via cellular internalization. In the case of internalization, the radionuclides will come in closer proximity to the critical radiation target, i.e. the nuclear DNA. On the other hand, internalization could be disadvantageous if it leads to quick degradation of the targeting agent followed by elimination of the radionuclide. Intracellular degradation of the targeting agent can be prevented by, e.g. dextranation and other residualizing techniques (chapters 8 and 18). Prolonged intracellular retention of the radioactivity can be achieved by using various residualizing agents for indirect halogen labeling. Cellular excretion can also be limited if the radionuclides are radiometals, e.g. indium or yttrium, due to intracellular adsorbtion of metal containing catabolic products (chapter 8).

Nuclear Localization

Intranuclear localization of radionuclides will possibly decrease the required amounts of targeted α- and β-emitters by one order of magnitude and the doses of Auger emitters by at least three orders of magnitude when therapeutic effects against single disseminated tumor cells are desired. At least three principles can be discussed for tumor specific targeting of the nucleus.

The *first principle* is the use of radionuclide labeled steroids binding to steroid-receptor-rich tumor cells and consequently followed by a transport of the steroid-receptor-complexes to the nuclear DNA. While the mechanism seems clear, it likely has the disadvantage of a too short a residence time in proximity to the DNA. Increased efforts are needed to design steroids associated with prolonged retention of the steroid-receptor-complex by DNA. EGFR could be used in a similar manner as it has been reported, under certain conditions, to be internalized not only into the cytoplasm but all the way into the cell nucleus (chapter 14). while this process is not yet generally accepted it could, if true, allow for the possibility of delivering radionuclides to the cell nucleus via the administration of radiolabeled EGFR binding agents.

The *second principle* is a form of two-step targeting process incorporating separate conjugated cellular and DNA targeting agents. In the first step, a molecular construct enabling peptides or proteins to recognize tumor-associated receptors or antigens would be administered. This molecular construct should then be internalized and degraded to some degree. This leads to the release of the radionuclide containing DNA-binding or nuclear-targeting agent into the cytoplasm (chapter 12).

The *third principle* entails the use of radionuclide-conjugated antisense nucleotides or PNA molecules (protein nucleic acid) that recognize and bind to tumor specific DNA sequences. One major difficulty with this approach is the transport across the cell membrane. A drawback might also be that the antisense or PNA molecules might interact with mRNA to such a degree, that the majority of radionuclides reside in the cytoplasm where they would be less effective.

Clearly additional research is necessary for such principles to be successfully applied to targeted radionuclide therapy.

New Targeting Agents and Their Pharmacokinetics

Our abilities to design and build novel targeting agents are rapidly expanding. Besides exhibiting satisfactory pharmacokinetic properties, an ideal targeting agent should be able to be stably radiolabeled without loss of affinity or tumor specificity. Several different types of targeting agents have been evaluated for radionuclide therapy, e.g. ions, low molecular weight drugs, various forms of peptides, affibody molecules, antibody fragments, intact antibodies and antibody based conjugates and liposomes (chapters 4–7, 20 and [16, 17]). These substances cover a molecular weight range of several orders of magnitude. Thus, radionuclide therapy is not a "monoagent" therapy. Instead, there is potential to consider hundreds of different agents with different molecular weights, lipophilicity and charge. Some of these properties are discussed below.

Limited systemic circulation due to excretion. Molecular weight, lipophilicity and charge of targeting agents are important properties that influence the renal and liver mediated excretion. Small water-soluble peptides, e.g. octreotide (chapter 7), display efficient renal elimination, which is beneficial as it decreases excess circulating radionuclide-labeled compounds. However, if the renal or liver mediated excretion is too rapid it might prevent sufficient quantities of the therapeutic agent from reaching the tumor cells, thereby reducing delivered doses below cytotoxic levels. Thus, the targeting agents must be designed for optimal excretion rate (chapter 8).

High molecular weight and long systemic circulation times. High molecular weight targeting agents may display reduced passage through capillary walls and may hamper the ability to target disseminated tumor cells in normally vascularized tissues. However, high molecular weight provides, in most cases, prolonged circulation which may result in high tumor uptake and improved chances to kill disseminated circulating tumor cells.

Limited penetration in interstitial spaces. The capacity of targeting agents to diffuse within the interstitial space has to be taken into account when treating solid tumors and when single tumor cells have infiltrated normal tissues. This passage can be inhibited or delayed if interactions between the targeting agent and the extracellular matrix or stroma cells take place. Furthermore, it is also possible that an increased interstitial pressure [18] and a net outward flow of liquid in solid tumors inhibit the diffusion and penetration process (chapter 18).

Trapping and degradation of the agents by RES. There are potential advantages in using therapeutic agents designed not to be recognized by the RES, such as low molecular weight substances which are generally not subject to this process.

Additionally, preadministration of non-radioactive antibodies (i.e. "preload") can be used to saturate the RES and thereby modify the distribution of the subsequently administered radiolabeled antibody. The RES uptake of macromolecular agents can also be reduced using pegylation and other preventive molecular modifications.

Immunological responses. Immunogenic epitopes might trigger the patient's immune system to produce antibodies against the targeting agent. The reaction might be intensive and could even induce anaphylactic shock following repeated treatments. The immunoreaction can be minimized if the macromolecular agents mainly contain humanized parts or if they are fully humanized (chapters 4, 5 and 18). Better radiation independent cytotoxic mechanisms (complement fixation, CDC, and antibody-dependent cellular toxicity, ADCC) and also longer half-lives in the circulation might be achieved by appropriate design of the targeting agents.

Efficiency in Clearing Mechanisms

Several approaches, such as extracorporeal adsorption, anti-idiotypic antibody administration and employment of pretargeting techniques, are presently under investigation to decrease the radionuclide uptake in normal tissues.

Extracorporeal elimination. Affinity based extracorporeal elimination of redundant targeting agents in the systemic circulation is one method to decrease the radionuclide uptake in normal tissues. For example, an excess of biotinylated and radionuclide labeled antibodies remaining in the circulation after efficient tumor targeting can be removed if the antibodies are bound to an extracorporeal column with immobilized avidin (chapter 4 and [19]).

Antibodies against targeting agents. One alternative method is to use secondary antibodies with a specificity for the targeting agent in order to generate immuncomplexes, which are taken up and degraded by the RES. A significant amount of the excess targeting agents can be removed from the systemic circulation in this way. A potential approach would be to give radiolabeled antibodies for targeting followed by an anti-idiotype antibody to achieve a RES-mediated clearance. While this has been effective in the experimental setting (chapter 4 and [20]), it has not yet been tested in patients.

Pretargeting. An additional method to reduce the radionuclide uptake in normal tissues is to use pretargeting procedures (chapter 4). One example is to use streptavidin-conjugated primary antibodies with specificity for tumor cells. After allowing sufficient time for the streptavidin-conjugated antibodies to bind to the tumor cells most non-bound antibodies are then cleared from the body. Once the circulating antibody has cleared the circulation, radiolabeled biotin can be injected and the radionuclide will preferentially be retained by a streptavidin-biotin reaction primarily at the surface of tumor cells. This is an example of a two-step method. An example of a corresponding three-step method is to use a suitable injection sequence starting with a biotinylated primary antibody, followed by a streptavidin-based agent that promotes hepatic elimination and finally by radiolabeled biotin.

The advantages and disadvantages of the pretargeting concept are described in chapter 4 and [21]. Bispecific antibodies have also been utilized in two-step targeting approaches [22]. These different "multistep" procedures have recently been very much in focus.

References

1. Goldenberg DM, Sharkey RM (2006) Advances in cancer therapy with radiolabeled monoclonal antibodies. Q J Nucl Med Mol Imaging 50(4):248–64. Review.
2. DeNardo SJ, DeNardo GL (2006) Targeted radionuclide therapy for solid tumors: an overview. Int J Radiat Oncol Biol Phys 66(2 Suppl):S89–95. Review.
3. Wong JY (2006) Systemic targeted radionuclide therapy: potential new areas. Int J Radiat Oncol Biol Phys 66(2 Suppl): S74–82. Review.
4. Oyen WJ, Bodei L, Giammarile F, Maecke HR, Tennvall J, Luster M, Brans B (2007) Targeted therapy in nuclear medicine – current status and future prospects. Ann Oncol 18(11):1782–92. Review.
5. Van Essen M, Krenning EP, De Jong M, Valkema R, Kwekkeboom DJ (2007) Peptide Receptor Radionuclide Therapy with radiolabelled somatostatin analogues in patients with somatostatin receptor positive tumours. Acta Oncol 46(6):723–34. Review.
6. Witzig TE (2006) Radioimmunotherapy for B-cell non-Hodgkin lymphoma. Best Pract Res Clin Haematol 19(4): 655–68. Review.
7. Murray D, McEwan AJ (2007) Radiobiology of systemic radiation therapy. Cancer Biother Radiopharm 22(1):1–23.
8. Hall EJ, Giaccia AJ (2006) Radiobiology for the radiologist. Chapter 22. Lippincott Williams & Wilkins, Philadelphia, PA (ISBN 0-7817-4151-3).
9. Tolmachev V, Carlsson J, Lundqvist H (2004) A limiting factor for the progress of radionuclide based cancer diagnostics and therapy; availability of suitable radionuclides. Acta Oncologica 43(3):264–75.
10. Sundberg AL, Almquist Y, Tolmachev V, Gedda L, Orlova A, Blomquist E, Carlsson J (2003) Combined effect of gefitinib ("Iressa", ZD1839) and targeted radiotherapy with ^{11}At-EGF; Experimental therapy studies in vitro. Eur J Nucl Med 30:1348–1356.
11. Nordberg E, Steffen AC, Persson M, Sundberg AL, Carlsson J, Glimelius B (2005) Cellular uptake of radioiodine delivered by trastuzumab can be modified by the addition of epidermal growth factor. Eur J Nucl Med Mol Imaging 32(7): 771–7.
12. Pecorino L (2005) Molecular biology of cancer. Mechanisms, targets and therapeutics. Oxford University Press, Oxford (ISBN 0-19-926472-4).
13. McGill MA, McGlade CJ (2004) Cellular signaling. In: The basic science of oncology (editors: Tannock IF, Hill RP, Bristow RC and Harrington L). Chapter 8. McGraw-Hill Medical Publishing Division, New York, pp. 142–66 (ISBN-13: 978-0-07-138774-3).
14. Bublil EM, Yarden Y (2007) The EGF receptor family: spearheading a merger of signaling and therapeutics. Curr Opin Cell Biol 19(2):124–34. Review.
15. Bonner JA, Harari PM, Giralt J, et al. (2006) Radiotherapy plus Cetuximab for Squamous-Cell Carcinoma of the Head and Neck. NEJM 354:567–78.
16. Adams GP, Weiner LM (2005) Monoclonal antibody therapy of cancer. Nat Biotechnol 23(9):1147–57. Review.
17. Robinson MK, Shaller C, Garmestani K, Plascjak PS, Hodge KM, Yuan QA, Marks JD, Waldmann TA, Brechbiel MW, Adams GP (2008) Effective treatment of established human breast tumor xenografts in immunodeficient mice with a single dose of the alpha-emitting radioisotope astatine-211 conjugated to anti-HER2/neu diabodies. Clin Cancer Res 14:875–82.

18. Heldin C-H, Rubin K, Pietras K, Östman A (2004) High interstitial fluid pressure - an obstacle in cancer therapy. Nature Rev Cancer 4:806–13.
19. Martensson L, Nilsson R, Ohlsson T, Sjogren HO, Strand SE, Tennvall J (2007) Reduced myelotoxicity with sustained tumor concentration of radioimmunoconjugates in rats after extracorporeal depletion. J Nucl Med 48:269–76.
20. Erlandsson A, Eriksson D, Johansson L, Riklund K, Stigbrand T, Sundstrom BE (2006) In vivo clearing of idiotypic antibodies with antiidiotypic antibodies and their derivatives. Mol Immunol 43:599–606.
21. Goldenberg DM, Sharkey RM, Paganelli G, Barbet J, Chatal JF (2006) Antibody pretargeting advances cancer radioimmunodetection and radioimmunotherapy. J Clin Oncol 24:823–34.
22. Goldenberg DM, Chatal JF, Barbet J, Boerman O, Sharkey RM (2007) Cancer imaging and therapy with bispecific antibody pretargeting. Update Cancer Ther 2:19–31.

Index

MIX
Papier aus verantwortungsvollen Quellen
Paper from responsible sources
FSC® C105338
FSC
www.fsc.org

If you have any concerns about our products,
you can contact us on
ProductSafety@springernature.com

In case Publisher is established outside the EU,
the EU authorized representative is:
Springer Nature Customer Service Center GmbH
Europaplatz 3, 69115 Heidelberg, Germany

Printed by Libri Plureos GmbH
in Hamburg, Germany